# Assisting in
# Long-Term Care

## THIRD EDITION

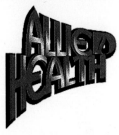

# Assisting in Long-Term Care

## THIRD EDITION

Barbara R. Hegner, MS, RN
*Professor Emeritus*
*Nursing and Life Science*
*Long Beach City College (CA)*

Esther Caldwell, MA, PhD
*Consultant in Vocational Education (CA)*

*Contributing author:*
Joan F. Needham, MSEd, RNC
*Consultant and Educator for*
*Long-Term Care and Gerontology*

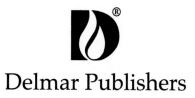

## Delmar Publishers

*an International Thomson Publishing company* I(T)P®

Albany • Bonn • Boston • Cincinnati • Detroit • London • Madrid
Melbourne • Mexico City • New York • Pacific Grove • Paris • San Francisco
Singapore • Tokyo • Toronto • Washington

# NOTICE TO THE READER

Cover Photos: Thomas Stock, Stock Studios, Saratoga Springs, NY

**Delmar Staff**

Publisher: Susan Simpfenderfer
Acquisitions Editor: Dawn Gerrain
Developmental Editor: Marjorie A. Bruce
Project Editor: Coreen Filson
Team Assistant: Sandra Bruce

Art and Design Coordinator: Vincent S. Berger
Production Coordinator: John Mickelbank
Marketing Manager: Katherine Slezak
Marketing Coordinator: Glenna Stanfield
Editorial Assistant: Donna L. Leto

COPYRIGHT © 1998
By Delmar Publishers
a division of International Thomson Publishing Inc.

The ITP logo is a trademark under license.

Printed in the United States of America

For more information, contact:

Delmar Publishers
3 Columbia Circle, Box 15015
Albany, New York 12212-5015

International Thomson Publishing Europe
Berkshire House 168-173
High Holborn
London, WC1V 7AA
England

Thomas Nelson Australia
102 Dodds Street
South Melbourne, 3205
Victoria, Australia

Nelson Canada
1120 Birchmount Road
Scarborough, Ontario
Canada, M1K 5G4

International Thomson Editores
Campos Eliseos 385, Piso 7
Col Polanco
11560 Mexico D F Mexico

International Thomson Publishing GmbH
Konigswinterer Strasse 418
53227 Bonn
Germany

International Thomson Publishing Asia
221 Henderson Road
#05-10 Henderson Building
Singapore 0315

International Thomson Publishing—Japan
Hirakawacho Kyowa Building, 3F
2-2-1 Hirakawacho
Chiyoda-ku, Tokyo 102
Japan

2   3   4   5   6   7   8   9   10   XXX   03   02   01   00   99   98

**Library of Congress Cataloging-in-Publication Data**
Hegner, Barbara R.
    Assisting in long-term care / Barbara R. Hegner, Esther Caldwell ;
contributing author, Joan F. Needham.—3rd ed.
      p.    cm.
    Includes bibliographical references and index.
    ISBN 0-8273-8259-6 (alk. paper)
    1. Long-term care of the sick.   2. Nurses' aides.   I. Caldwell,
Esther.   II. Needham, Joan Fritsch.   III. Title.
    [DNLM:   1. Long-Term Care—methods.   2. Nursing Care—methods.
3. Nurses' Aides.   4. Nursing Homes.    WY 152 H464a 1998]
RT120.L64H44   1998
362.1'6—dc21
DNLM/DLC
for Library of Congress               97-5158
                               CIP

# Table of Contents

About the Authors                                                        xviii

Preface                                                                    xix

Acknowledgments                                                            xxi

About This Book                                                           xxii

## *Section 1*  The Long-Term Care Setting                                   1

**LESSON 1**  **The Long Term Care Facility**                                 3
Community Health Care Facilities                                             4
Types of Long-Term Care Facilities                                           8
Standards and Regulations                                                   10
Facility Surveys                                                            11
Functional Areas in a Long-Term Care Facility                              11

**LESSON 2**  **The Caregivers**                                            19
The Interdisciplinary Team Members                                         20
Administrative Organization                                                26
Quality Assurance Program                                                  28
Staff Development                                                          28

**LESSON 3**  **The Nursing Assistant in Long-Term Care**                  31
Personal Characteristics                                                   32
Attitude                                                                   33
Personal Hygiene                                                           34
Uniforms                                                                   34
Duties and Responsibilities: The Job Description                           35
Staff Relations                                                           37
Assignments                                                               38
Specific Duties                                                           39
Organization of Time                                                      40
Self-Care                                                                 40
Sexual Harassment                                                         41
Continue to Grow                                                          42

## *Section 2*  Communication Skills                                        45

**LESSON 4**  **Communication and Interpersonal Skills**                   47
The Communication Process                                                 48
Communicating with Staff Members                                          49
Oral Communications                                                       49
Written Communications                                                    52

Communicating with Residents                                               54
    **Guidelines for Communicating with Residents**        55
Communicating Through the Use of Touch                                      57
Communicating with Residents Who Have Special Needs                         58

**LESSON 5**   **The Language of Health Care**                 65
The Language of Health Care                                                 66
Word Parts                                                                  66
Expanding Your Vocabulary                                                   67
Common Word Parts                                                           68
Common Abbreviations                                                        71
Understanding the Body                                                      74
Anatomic Terms                                                              75
Organization of the Body                                                    77
Cells                                                                       78
Tissues                                                                     78
Organs                                                                      78
Systems                                                                     78
Membranes                                                                   78
Cavities                                                                    81

**LESSON 6**   **Observation, Documentation, and Reporting**    85
Observation                                                                 86
Reporting                                                                   90
Documentation                                                               90
The Interdisciplinary Health Care Team Process                              92

***Section 3***   **Protecting Residents' Rights and Safety**   97

**LESSON 7**   **Residents' Rights**                           99
Purpose of the Residents' Rights Document                                   100
Residents' Rights                                                           101
Legal Aspects of Health Care                                                116
Ethics and the Health Care Provider                                         117

**LESSON 8**   **Safety**                                      121
Safety in Health Care Facilities                                            122
Employee Safety                                                             122
    **Guidelines for Using Ergonomic Techniques to Reduce
the Risk of Having an Incident**                                            123
Hazards in the Work Environment                                             125
Resident Safety                                                             129
    **Guidelines for the Use of Restraints**             131

Wheelchair Safety                                                       134
Fire Safety                                                            135

**LESSON 9**    **Emergencies**                                              139
Wheelchair Safety
General Measures to Follow for Emergencies                 140
**Guidelines for Responding to an Emergency**       140
Cardiac Arrest                                                        141
Foreign Body Airway Obstruction (Choking)                142
OBRA  OO  PROCEDURE  1  Assisting the Conscious Person with Obstructed
                                    Airway—Heimlich Maneuver              142
OBRA  OO  PROCEDURE  2  Obstructed Airway, Unconscious Person       144
OBRA       PROCEDURE  3  Hemorrhage                             146
Hemorrhage                                                            147
Resident Falls                                                        147
OBRA  OO  PROCEDURE  4  Care of Falling Resident            147
Seizures                                                              148
Burns                                                                 149
Orthopedic Injuries                                                   149
Accidental Poisoning                                                  150
Fainting                                                              150

**LESSON 10**   **Infection**                                               153
Infectious Disease                                                    154
Microbes                                                              154
The Chain of Infection                                                155
Body Flora                                                            156
Natural Body Defenses Against Disease                         156
Immunity                                                              157
Inmmunizations                                                        157
Serious Infections in Health Care Facilities                         157
Bacterial Infections                                                  157
Viral Infections                                                      159
Other Important Infections                                            162
Why the Elderly in Long-Term Care Are at Risk for Infections     162
General Measures to Prevent Infections                        163
Outbreak of Infectious Disease in a Long-Term Care Facility     163

**LESSON 11**   **Infection Control**                                       167
Medical Asepsis                                                       168
Handwashing                                                           170
OBRA  OO  PROCEDURE  5  Handwashing                         170
Protecting Yourself                                                   172
Standard Precautions                                                  173

**Guidelines for Standard Precautions** 173
**Guidelines for Environmental Procedures** 174
Transmission-Based Precautions 176
PROCEDURE  6 Putting on a Mask 179
PROCEDURE  7 Putting on a Gown 180
PROCEDURE  8 Putting on Gloves 181
PROCEDURE  9 Removing Contaminated Gloves 181
PROCEDURE 10 Removing Contaminated Gloves, Mask, and Gown 182
PROCEDURE 11 Caring for Linens in Isolation Unit 185
PROCEDURE 12 Measuring Vital Signs in Isolation Unit 185
PROCEDURE 13 Serving a Meal Tray in Isolation Unit 186
PROCEDURE 14 Specimen Collection from Resident in Isolation Unit 187
PROCEDURE 15 Transferring Nondisposable Equipment Outside
of Isolation Unit 189
PROCEDURE 16 Transporting Resident to and from Isolation Unit 189
Disinfection and Sterilization 190
Sterile Procedures 191
PROCEDURE 17 Opening a Sterile Package 191

*Section 4*   **Characteristics of the Long-Term Care Resident** 195

**LESSON 12**   **The Long-Term Care Resident** 197
Illness and Disability 198
The Process of Normal Aging 200
Stereotypes and Myths 200
The Younger Resident in the Long-Term Care Facility 203
**Guidelines for Caring for Younger Residents** 204

**LESSON 13**   **The Psychosocial Aspects of Aging** 207
Basic Human Needs 208
Cultural Influences 210
Spirituality 210
Religion 212
Sexuality 213
Major Challenges to Adjustments 215
Using Defense (Coping) Mechanisms 217
Meeting Residents' Psychosocial Needs 217
Stress Reactions 218
Reactive Behaviors 218

**LESSON 14**   **The Physical Effects of Aging** 223
The Process of Normal Aging 224
Theories of Aging 224

About Aging 224
Changes Caused by Aging 224

## Section 5  Meeting the Residents' Basic Needs 231

**LESSON 15  Care of the Residents' Environment** 233
Resident Environment 234
Personal Space 234
Resident Unit 235
Extended Resident Environment 235
Critical Procedure Actions 237
    **Guidelines for Ensuring a Safe and Comfortable Environment** 238
Bedmaking 241
    **Guidelines for Handling Linens and Making the Bed** 241
OBRA  PROCEDURE 18  Unoccupied Bed: Changing Linens 242
OBRA  PROCEDURE 19  Occupied Bed: Changing Linens 247

**LESSON 16  Caring for the Residents' Personal Hygiene** 251
Epidermis 252
Dermis 252
Skin Functions 253
Skin Changes Caused by Aging 253
Skin Lesions 254
    **Guidelines for Preventing Skin Breakdown** 257
Backrub 261
Bathing Residents 261
OBRA  PROCEDURE 20  Backrub 261
OBRA  PROCEDURE 21  Bed Bath 264
OBRA  PROCEDURE 22  Tub Bath or Shower 267
OBRA  PROCEDURE 23  Partial Bath 268
OBRA  PROCEDURE 24  Female Perineal Care 270
OBRA  PROCEDURE 25  Male Perineal Care 271
Daily Hair Care 273
OBRA  PROCEDURE 26  Daily Hair Care 274
Facial Hair 274
OBRA  PROCEDURE 27  Shaving Male Resident 275
Hand and Fingernail Care 276
OBRA  PROCEDURE 28  Hand and Fingernail Care 276
Foot and Toenail Care 277
OBRA  PROCEDURE 29  Foot and Toenail Care 278
Oral Hygiene 278
OBRA  PROCEDURE 30  Assisting Resident to Brush Teeth 280

| OBRA | | PROCEDURE 31 Cleaning and Flossing Resident's Teeth | 281 |
| OBRA | 👓 | PROCEDURE 32 Caring for Dentures | 282 |
| OBRA | 👓 | PROCEDURE 33 Assisting with Special Oral Hygiene | 283 |
| | | Dressing Resident | 284 |
| OBRA | 👓 | PROCEDURE 34 Dressing and Undressing Resident | 284 |

**LESSON 17   Meeting the Residents' Nutritional Needs**   289

The Digestive System   290
The Digestive Process   291
Aging Changes   293
Nutrients   293
Food Groups   294
Nutritional Status   297
Diets   297
Personal Dietary Practices   299
Intake and Output (I&O)   299

| OBRA | 👓 | PROCEDURE 35 Measuring and Recording Fluid Intake | 302 |

Ensuring Proper Nutrition   303
Nursing Assistant Responsibilities   304

| OBRA | 👓 | PROCEDURE 36 Assisting the Resident Who Can Feed Self | 306 |
| OBRA | 👓 | PROCEDURE 37 Feeding the Dependent Resident | 308 |

Nourishments and Supplements   309
Providing Water   310
Alternate Methods of Feeding   311
Disorders of the Digestive System   312

**LESSON 18   Meeting the Residents' Elimination Needs**   319

Introduction   321
The Continent Resident   321
Equipment to Assist Elimination   321

| OBRA | 👓 | PROCEDURE 38 Giving and Receiving the Bedpan | 323 |
| OBRA | 👓 | PROCEDURE 39 Giving and Receiving the Urinal | 325 |
| OBRA | 👓 | PROCEDURE 40 Assisting with the Use of the Bedside Commode | 326 |
| OBRA | 👓 | PROCEDURE 41 Assisting Resident to Use the Bathroom | 326 |

Elimination from the Lower Digestive Tract   327
The Resident with Constipation   328
Bowel Aids   328

| | | PROCEDURE 42 Checking for Fecal Impaction | 329 |
| | 👓 | PROCEDURE 43 Giving an Oil-Retention Enema | 330 |
| | 👓 | PROCEDURE 44 Giving a Soapsuds Enema | 331 |
| | 👓 | PROCEDURE 45 Giving a Commercially Prepared Enema | 334 |
| | | PROCEDURE 46 Inserting a Rectal Suppository | 336 |

Rectal Tube and Flatus Bag   337

PROCEDURE 47 Inserting a Rectal Tube and Flatus Bag 338
Ostomies 338
PROCEDURE 48 Giving Routine Stoma Care (Colostomy) 340
Fecal Incontinence 342
Collecting a Stool Specimen 343
PROCEDURE 49 Collecting a Stool Specimen 343
Urinary System 344
Changes in the Urinary System Caused by Aging 346
Urine Elimination 347
Urinary Retention and Incontinence 347
Internal Urinary Catheter Drainage 347
PROCEDURE 50 Routine Drainage Check 348
PROCEDURE 51 Giving Indwelling Catheter Care 349
PROCEDURE 52 Disconnecting the Catheter 351
Intake and Output (I&O) 352
PROCEDURE 53 Measuring and Recording Fluid Output 353
PROCEDURE 54 Emptying a Urinary Drainage Unit 355
Leg Bag Drainage 356
PROCEDURE 55 Emptying a Leg Bag 357
PROCEDURE 56 Connecting Catheter to Leg Bag 357
PROCEDURE 57 Collecting a Routine Urine Specimen 358
PROCEDURE 58 Collecting a Clean-Catch Urine Specimen 360
External Urinary Drainage (Male) 361
PROCEDURE 59 Applying a Condom for Urinary Drainage 362
Common Conditions 363

*Section 6* **Special Nursing Assistant Activities** 367

**LESSON 19** **Measuring and Recording Residents' Data** 369
Measuring Vital Signs 370
Temperature 371
PROCEDURE 60 Measuring an Oral Temperature (Glass Thermometer) 373
PROCEDURE 61 Measuring a Rectal Temperature (Glass Thermometer) 375
PROCEDURE 62 Measuring an Axillary Temperature (Glass Thermometer) 376
PROCEDURE 63 Measuring an Oral Temperature (Electronic Thermometer) 377
PROCEDURE 64 Measuring a Rectal Temperature (Electronic Thermometer) 378
PROCEDURE 65 Measuring an Axillary Temperature (Electronic Thermometer) 379

OBRA ⊙⊙   PROCEDURE 66 Measuring a Tympanic Temperature   380
Pulse and Respiration   381
OBRA ⊙⊙   PROCEDURE 67 Counting the Radial Pulse Rate   382
⊙⊙   PROCEDURE 68 Counting the Apical-Radial Pulse Rate   383
Blood Pressure   385
OBRA ⊙⊙   PROCEDURE 69 Counting Respirations   385
**Guidelines for Preparing to Measure Blood Pressure**   387
OBRA ⊙⊙   PROCEDURE 70 Taking Blood Pressure   389
Weighing and Measuring the Resident   391
OBRA ⊙⊙   PROCEDURE 71 Weighing and Measuring the Resident Using an
Upright Scale   393
OBRA ⊙⊙   PROCEDURE 72 Measuring Weight with an Electronic Wheelchair
Scale   394
OBRA ⊙⊙   PROCEDURE 73 Weighing the Resident in a Chair Scale   395
OBRA ⊙⊙   PROCEDURE 74 Measuring and Weighing the Resident in Bed   396
Recording Vital Signs   396

**LESSON 20**   **Admission, Transfer, and Discharge**   401
Admitting the Resident   402
⊙⊙   PROCEDURE 75 Admitting the Resident   405
Transferring the Resident   407
Discharging the Resident   409
⊙⊙   PROCEDURE 76 Transferring the Resident   410
⊙⊙   PROCEDURE 77 Discharging the Resident   411

**LESSON 21**   **Warm and Cold Applications**   417
Safety   418
Commercial Preparations   418
Use of Warm Applications   419
⊙⊙   PROCEDURE 78 Applying an Aquamatic K-Pad®   420
Use of Cold Applications   421
⊙⊙   PROCEDURE 79 Applying a Disposable Cold Pack   421
⊙⊙   PROCEDURE 80 Applying an Ice Bag   422
PROCEDURE 81 Assisting with the Application of a Hypothermia
Blanket   423

*Section 7*   **Introduction to Restorative Care**   427

**LESSON 22**   **Restorative Care of the Resident**   429
Restorative Care and the Interdisciplinary Health Care Team   431
Purposes of Restorative Care   432
Preventing Complications from Inactivity   433
Activities of Daily Living   436

Setting Up Restorative Programs    437
    **Guidelines for Nursing Assistant Responsibilities
    in General Restorative Program**    443
The Restorative Environment    444
Progressive Mobilization    445
Range of Motion    445
    **Guidelines for Passive Range of Motion Exercises**    445
`OBRA` 👓 PROCEDURE 82 Passive Range of Motion Exercises    448
Self Range of Motion Exercises    456
Active Range of Motion Exercises    456
Positioning the Resident    457
    **Guidelines for Positioning**    457
Turning the Dependent Resident with a Turning Sheet    461
`OBRA` 👓 PROCEDURE 83 Moving the Resident Toward the Head of the Bed    462
`OBRA` PROCEDURE 84 Moving the Resident Toward the Foot of the Bed    463
`OBRA` 👓 PROCEDURE 85 Moving the Resident Toward the Side of the Bed    463
`OBRA` 👓 PROCEDURE 86 Turning the Resident to the Side    464
`OBRA` PROCEDURE 87 Log Rolling the Resident Onto the Side    465
Positioning the Dependent Resident    467
`OBRA` 👓 PROCEDURE 88 Supine Position    467
`OBRA` 👓 PROCEDURE 89 Semisupine or Tilt Position    468
`OBRA` 👓 PROCEDURE 90 Lateral (Side-Lying) Position    468
`OBRA` PROCEDURE 91 Lateral Position on the Affected Side    469
`OBRA` 👓 PROCEDURE 92 Semiprone Position    470
`OBRA` 👓 PROCEDURE 93 Fowler's Position    470
`OBRA` PROCEDURE 94 Chair Positioning    472
`OBRA` 👓 PROCEDURE 95 Repositioning a Resident in a Wheelchair    473
`OBRA` 👓 PROCEDURE 96 Wheelchair Activities to Relieve Pressure    474
Independent Bed Movement    476
`OBRA` PROCEDURE 97 Assisting with Independent Bed Movement    476
Continuing with Progressive Mobilization    477
Bowel and Bladder Programs    477
    **Guidelines for Bowel and Bladder Programs**    478

**LESSON 23**    **Restoring Residents' Mobility**    483
Transfers    484
    **Guidelines for Transfers**    485
`OBRA` 👓 PROCEDURE 98 Using a Transfer Belt (Gait Belt)    485
`OBRA` 👓 PROCEDURE 99 Bringing the Resident to a Sitting Position at the
    Edge of the Bed    487
`OBRA` 👓 PROCEDURE 100 Assisted Standing Transfer    489
`OBRA` 👓 PROCEDURE 101 Transferring the Resident from Chair to Bed    490
`OBRA` 👓 PROCEDURE 102 Assisted Standing Transfer/Two Assistants    491

| OBRA ▣ | PROCEDURE 103 Wheelchair to Toilet Transfer | 492 |
| OBRA ▣ | PROCEDURE 104 Toilet to Wheelchair Transfer | 493 |
| OBRA | PROCEDURE 105 Transferring to Tub Chair or Shower Chair | 494 |
| OBRA | PROCEDURE 106 Transferring a Nonstanding Resident from Wheelchair to Bed | 495 |
| | Using Mechanical Lifts | 496 |
| OBRA ▣ | PROCEDURE 107 Transferring Resident with a Mechanical Lift | 496 |
| | Sliding Board Transfer | 499 |
| | **Guidelines for Sliding Board Transfers** | 499 |
| | PROCEDURE 108 Sliding Board Transfer | 499 |
| | Ambulation | 500 |
| | **Guidelines for Ambulation** | 504 |
| OBRA ▣ | PROCEDURE 109 Ambulating a Resident | 504 |
| OBRA ▣ | PROCEDURE 110 Assisting Resident to Ambulate with Cane or Walker | 505 |
| | Using a Wheelchair | 506 |
| | Special Maneuvers with a Wheelchair | 507 |
| | Positioning the Dependent Resident in the Wheelchair | 511 |
| | Wheelchair Activity | 513 |

### *Section 8*  Residents with Specific Disorders   517

| **LESSON 24** | **Caring for Residents with Cardiovascular System Disorders** | 519 |
| | Introduction | 520 |
| | The Heart | 521 |
| | Blood Vessels | 522 |
| | Lymph | 523 |
| | The Blood | 526 |
| | Disorders of the Blood | 526 |
| | Disorders of the Blood Vessels and Circulation | 526 |
| | **Guidelines for Caring for Residents with Peripheral Vascular Disease** | 529 |
| | Heart Disease | 531 |
| ▣ | PROCEDURE 111 Applying Elasticized Stockings | 533 |

| **LESSON 25** | **Caring for Residents with Respiratory System Disorders** | 539 |
| | Introduction | 540 |
| | The Respiratory Organs | 540 |
| | Voice Production | 541 |
| | Changes in the Respiratory System Caused by Aging | 542 |
| | Introduction to Pathology | 542 |
| ▣ | PROCEDURE 112 Collecting a Sputum Specimen | 544 |
| | Chronic Obstructive Pulmonary Disease | 545 |

Treatment and Care of Residents with COPD 545
PROCEDURE 113 Refilling the Humidifier Bottle 548

**LESSON 26  Caring for Residents with Endocrine System Disorders** 551
Introduction 552
Endocrine Glands 553
Aging Changes 554
Electrolyte Balance 555
Glucose Metabolism 555
Diabetes Mellitus 556

**LESSON 27  Caring for Residents with Reproductive System Disorders** 563
Introduction 564
The Male Reproductive System 564
The Female Reproductive System 566
Menstrual Cycle 568
Menopause 568
Changes in the Reproductive System as a Result of Aging 568
Related Conditions 569
PROCEDURE 114 Breast Self-Examination 569
Sexually Transmitted Diseases 571

**LESSON 28  Caring for Residents with Musculoskeletal System Disorders** 577
The Musculoskeletal System 578
Changes in the Musculoskeletal System Caused by Aging 581
Conditions Affecting the Musculoskeletal System 581

**LESSON 29  Caring for Residents with Nervous System Disorders** 591
Components of the Nervous System 593
Central Nervous System 594
Autonomic Nervous System 596
Sense Organs 596
Changes in the Nervous System Caused by Aging 598
Causes of Severe Vision Impairment 598
OBRA  PROCEDURE 115 Care of Eyeglasses 599
**Guidelines for Assisting Visually Impaired Residents** 600
Hearing Loss 600
OBRA  PROCEDURE 116 Applying and Removing In-The-Ear
or Behind-The-Ear Hearing Aids 602
Nervous System Disorders 602
**Guidelines for Caring for Residents with Parkinson's Disease** 604
**Guidelines for Caring for Residents Who Have Had a Stroke** 606
**Guidelines for Caring for Residents with Multiple Sclerosis** 608

Guidelines for Caring for Residents
with Huntington's Disease | 609
Guidelines for Caring for Residents Who Have
Amyotrophic Lateral Sclerosis | 610
Guidelines for Caring for Residents Who Have
Myasthenia Gravis | 610

**Section 9   Residents with Special Needs   615**

**LESSON 30   Alzheimer's Disease and Related Disorders
(Caring for the Cognitively Impaired Resident)** | 617
Definition of Alzheimer's Disease | 618
Stages and Symptoms of Alzheimer's Disease | 620
Caring for Residents with Dementia | 622
Guidelines for Caring for Residents with Alzheimer's Disease | 623
Guidelines for Activities of Daily Living | 626
Special Problems | 628
Special Management Techniques | 629

**LESSON 31   Caring for Residents with Developmental Disabilities** | 633
Characteristics of a Developmental Disability | 634
Mental Retardation | 635
Other Forms of Developmental Disabilities | 637
Caring for Residents with Developmental Disabilities | 639

**LESSON 32   Caring for the Dying Resident** | 643
Introduction | 644
The Dying Process | 644
Signs of Approaching Death | 648
Postmortem Care | 648
PROCEDURE 117 Giving Postmortem Care | 650

**LESSON 33   Caring for the Person in Subacute Care** | 653
Description of Subacute Care | 654
Special Procedures Provided in the Subacute Care Unit | 655
Pulse Oximetry | 655
Intravenous Therapy | 656
Pain Management Procedures | 657
Guidelines for Caring for Residents with Intravenous Lines | 658
PROCEDURE 118 Changing a Gown on a Resident with a Peripheral
Intravenous Line in Place | 658
Caring for Residents with Tracheostomies | 660

Caring for the Resident Receiving Dialysis Treatments ............................................... 661
Oncology Treatments ............................................... 662

*Section 10*  **Employment** ............................................... **665**

**LESSON 34**  **Surviving a Survey** ............................................... 667
Purpose of a Survey ............................................... 667
Survey Preparation by Surveyors and Staff ............................................... 668
Survey Process ............................................... 669
Responsibilities of the Nursing Assistants During Survey ............................................... 671
Survey Completion ............................................... 672

**LESSON 35**  **Seeking Employment** ............................................... 675
Congratulations Are in Order ............................................... 675
Step I—Self-Appraisal ............................................... 676
Step II—Possibility Search ............................................... 676
Step III—The Résumé ............................................... 677
Step IV—References ............................................... 678
Step V—Taking the Step ............................................... 678
Step VI—The Interview (Putting Your Best Foot Forward) ............................................... 678
Keeping the Job ............................................... 679
Growing ............................................... 680
Resigning ............................................... 681

Glossary ............................................... 685
Index ............................................... 705

# About the Authors

## BARBARA R. HEGNER

Barbara Robinson Hegner, RN, MSN, is a graduate of a three-year diploma nursing program where direct and total care was the focus. She earned a BSN at Boston College and an MS in nursing from Boston University, with a minor in biologic sciences. She is Professor Emeritus of Nursing and Life Sciences at Long Beach City College, Long Beach (CA).

Throughout her professional career, she has had a deep interest in both hospital-based and long-term care nursing. She continues to update her nursing knowledge and skills and has kept performance levels current with nursing practice. She is an active participant in clinical symposia.

It has long been Ms. Hegner's belief that to ensure the rights and well-being of residents in long-term care requires the care of competent, caring nursing assistants under the supervision of professional nurses. The nursing assistants who provide this care should be thoroughly trained and consistently encouraged, evaluated, and given the opportunity for continued learning. Providing the tools to prepare these health care providers in the most effective and efficient way is the goal of *Assisting in Long-Term Care*, third edition. She is the author of the following texts, also from Delmar Publishers: *Geriatrics, A Study of Maturity*, fifth edition, and *Nursing Assistant, A Nursing Process Approach*, seventh edition revised.

## JOAN F. NEEDHAM

Joan Fritsch Needham, MSEd, RNC, is a contributing author to the third edition of *Assisting in Long-Term Care*. She also graduated from a three-year diploma nursing program. She received her BS from the College of Saint Francis and her MS from Northern Illinois University. She is certified by the American Nurses Association in Gerontological Nursing. Ms. Needham was Director of Education at a long-term care facility where she was responsible for staff development, curriculum development and instruction for basic and advanced nursing assistant training, and development and instruction in continuing education courses for licensed nurses. In addition, she is a part-time instructor at a community college for nursing assistant and nursing continuing education courses.

She contributed to *Nursing Assistant, A Nursing Process Approach*, sixth and seventh editions, is the coauthor of the *Pocket Reference for the Long-Term Care Nursing Assistant* (Delmar), and is the author of *Gerontological Nursing—A Restorative Approach* (Delmar) and *Plans of Care for Specialty Practice, Gerontological Nursing* (Delmar).

# Preface

## Introduction

Long-term care facilities provide services to an ever-changing population that includes:

- The elderly
- People who have had an acute illness and still require nursing care during recuperation and restoration before returning home
- People of various ages who need assistance and supervision because of developmental disabilities or mental incapacity
- Those who have experienced severe trauma and have been transferred from an acute care facility for continued care and rehabilitation
- People who have a chronic illness that interferes with their ability to live independently

These residents need well-trained and highly motivated people to provide care. Nursing assistants provide the majority of direct personal care and are in a unique position to enhance the quality of life for residents.

The goal of *Assisting in Long-Term Care* is to serve as a critical resource in the education and training of nursing assistants as essential care providers. The text stresses core concepts and provides clearly written explanations of principles. Examples, illustrations, guidelines, and procedures serve to reinforce the principles and help learners gain a firm understanding of topics and develop competence in essential skills. The text also helps learners appreciate their value to the interdisciplinary health care team that is the basis of care in the long-term care facility.

## Elements of the Text

The text is designed to enhance the learning process. Among the elements provided are the table of contents with the procedures identified for OBRA content or a video component, Clinical Focus in each unit, objectives, vocabulary lists with phonetic pronunciations, highlighted vocabulary terms in the text content, guidelines, procedures, photos and line drawings, cultural awareness notes, lesson synthesis, and lesson reviews. Refer to the section "About This Book" following the acknowledgments for an explanation of each of these features and how they contribute to enhanced learning.

## Changes for the Third Edition

The third edition of *Assisting in Long-Term Care* was significantly revised to achieve a better organization of content, more consistency between lessons, less repetition of content, an improved reading level, and updated content. Some of the changes made include:

- Elimination of repetitive content between lessons so that each lesson covers its topic (topics) thoroughly to facilitate class planning
- Reorganized Lesson 5, "Language of Health Care," to present an introduction to medical terminology and basic anatomy (body organization). Specific body system anatomy is covered in the lessons in Section 8
- New Lesson 6, "Observation, Reporting, and Documentation," with the introduction of the Minimum Data Set (MDS)
- Reorganized Lesson 7, "Residents' Rights," to highlight these rights and show how the nursing assistant can help to guarantee the rights for residents
- New content on ergonomics in Lesson 8, "Safety," and expanded content relating to prevention of employee injuries; in addition, safety for nursing assistants and residents is emphasized throughout the text
- Expanded Lesson 10, "Infections," with additional content on TB, HIV, HBV, MRSA, and VRE
- Expanded Lesson 11, "Infection Control," with a discussion of Standard Precautions and transmission-based precautions and more detailed guidelines on the use of personal protective equipment (PPE); the principles of infection control are applied and emphasized throughout the text

- Content on pressure ulcers was updated to reflect guidelines from the Agency for Health Care Policy and Research (AHCPR)
- Expanded Lesson 17, "Meeting the Residents' Nutritional Needs"
- New procedures added to Lesson 19, "Measuring and Recording Resident Data": measuring temperature using tympanic thermometer, weighing resident on a wheelchair scale, weighing residents in bed and measuring residents in bed
- New and expanded Lesson 20, "Admission, Transfer, and Discharge"
- Expanded Lesson 22, "Introduction to Restorative Care," with new content on orthoses
- Expanded Lesson 30, "Alzheimer's Disease and Related Disorders"
- New Lesson 33, "Caring for the Person in Subacute Care," with current information on the responsibilities of nursing assistants working in subacute care units
- New Lesson 34, "Surviving a Survey," to introduce nursing assistants to the process of a facility survey by representatives from licensing agencies
- Expanded Lesson 35, "Seeking Employment," with new content on drug testing, health care worker background checks, cross training, and career laddering

## SUPPLEMENTS

The supplements package consists of an Instructor's Guide, Student Workbook, Instructor's Resource Kit, and Computerized Test Bank. Also available is the third edition of Delmar's Nursing Assistant Video Series.

- The Instructor's Guide consists of teaching strategies, teaching and learning resources, supplementary learning aids, answers to end of lesson reviews, answers to workbook exercises, procedure evaluation forms, and transparency masters.
- The Student Workbook consists of information on the learning process, tips on studying effectively, student activities, exercises, student performance record form, procedure evaluation forms, and medical terminology flash cards.
- The Instructor's Resource Kit contains teaching methods and strategies, resource materials (including internet addresses), lesson plans, clinical situations, classroom activities, procedure guidelines, curriculum guides, and quizzes and final examination with answer keys.
- Computerized Test Bank with additional questions organized by lesson. Question types include multiple choice, true and false, completion, brief answer, and matching. Instructors have the capability of generating a multitude of combinations of questions for testing purposes.

Join us on the web: www.DelmarAlliedHealth.com for the latest information on health care assisting and related topics.

# Acknowledgments

The authors and staff of Delmar Publishers Allied Health Team wish to thank the Saratoga Hospital Nursing Home (Saratoga Springs, NY) for permitting the facility to be used as a photo shoot site. The photographer and editorial personnel were given full access to the staff, residents, and physical space of the facility. Our deepest appreciation is extended to Susan M. Manti, Director of Nursing, and her staff.

For a period of five days the photo crew worked closely with staff members in setting up each shot. The intense schedule could not have been met without the enthusiastic support and technical assistance provided by the staff. At all times during this period, the primary concern was to maintain the privacy, safety, and well-being of the residents, both those who participated in the photo shoot and those who were bystanders. The photo crew left the facility much enriched by their experiences with the residents who were so very enthusiastic and giving. We were impressed by the professionalism and dedication of the staff, especially the nursing assistants who served as models while performing their daily tasks.

Special thanks are due to Thomas Stock of Stock Studios (Saratoga Springs, NY) for bringing to the photo shoot his technical knowledge, good humor, and creative eye.

## Reviewers

The revision was aided by a dedicated group of instructors who reviewed content at different stages of the revision process. For their valuable suggestions and corrections, we thank:

Barbara Acello
Innovations in Health Care, Denton, TX

Paula Baker
Angelina College, Lufkin, TX

Myrna Bartel
Manhattan Area Technical Center,
Manhattan, KS

Susan Brooks
Community College of Southern Nevada, Las Vegas, NV

Helen Lee
Chula Vista Adult School, Chula Vista, CA

Karen Neighbors
Trinity Valley Community College, Athens, TX

Mary Pasqual
Central County Occupational Center,
San Jose, CA

Carol DeLong Pyles, EdD
Miami-Dade Community College, Miami, FL

Joan Rose
Board of Cooperative Educational Services,
Poughkeepsie, NY

Cathy Schley
Joliet Junior College
Joliet, IL

J. Elaine Seiden
Blue Ridge Community College, Flat Rock, NC

Mary Therriault
Our Lady of Mercy Life Center, Albany, NY

Karla Uhde
Indiana Vocational Technical College,
Evansville, IN

# About this **Book**

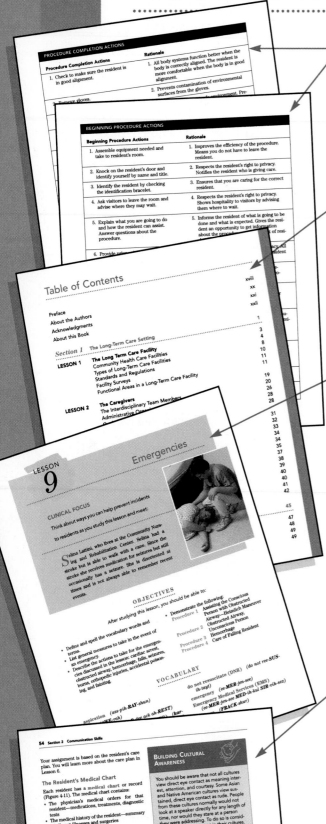

## Inside Cover Content

The listings of beginning and ending procedure actions give the essential steps to be performed before beginning any direct resident care procedure. These steps assure the rights of the resident and the safety of the resident and you, the nursing assistant. The ending procedure actions are performed at the end of each procedure to ensure that the resident is comfortable and safe, the resident's environment is clean, all equipment used is cleaned or discarded according to facility policy, and the proper documentation is completed.

## Table of Contents

The table of contents lists, for each lesson, the lesson title, major topic headings, general guidelines for specific areas of care or topics of importance to the nursing assistant, and resident care procedures. Each procedure is identified as appropriate for:

 Essential OBRA procedures that students must master for certification.

 Procedures for which there is a corresponding segment on *Delmar's Nursing Assisting Video Series, 3rd edition*

## Lesson Opening Page

The **Clinical Focus** presents a common resident care situation and asks you to think about ways to address the situation as the lesson content is studied.

The **Objectives** help you know what is expected of you as you read the text. Your success in achieving each objective is measured by your completion of the unit end reviews.

The **Vocabulary** list alerts you to new terms presented in the lesson. When each term is first presented in the text, it is highlighted in boldface and color. (The color of the term in the vocabulary list matches the color of the term in the text.) Each term is defined at this point. Read the definition and note the context of the term until you feel comfortable using the term.

The vocabulary list also contains the **phonetic pronunciation** for each new term. This is a system in which common sounds are used consistently to indicate the pronunciation. The part of the word that receives the primary emphasis is shown in **boldface** and **CAPITAL LETTERS**. The part or parts that receive the secondary emphasis is in boldface lower case letters.

## Building Cultural Awareness

These brief examples are designed to help you become aware of the differences between people from different groups. They help you recognize that people react differently to health and sickness and that their reactions are determined largely by the culture of which they are a part. The text suggests that if you observe, listen and learn and accept people as they are, you will provide a high level of caring service.

## Procedures

The text contains 118 clinical procedures that provide step-by-step directions for a specific aspect of care. Each procedure reminds you to perform the beginning procedure actions (and you can refer to the inside of the front cover if you need to refresh your memory of these actions). A list of equipment and supplies needed for the procedure follows. Any notes or cautions about performing the precaution are given. The steps take you carefully through the procedure, emphasizing at all times the need to work safely and to protect the resident's dignity. At the end, you are reminded of the procedure completion actions (refer to the inside back cover to refresh your memory of these actions).

Three icons may be used with the procedures:

 **OBRA** to indicate an essential procedure required for certification

 **gloves** to indicate the need to observe Standard Precautions and wear personal protective equipment

 **video** to indicate that there is a companion video segment for the procedure in *Delmar's Nursing Assistant Video Series, 3rd edition*

## Photographs and Line Drawings

Many new photographs and line drawings were created for this new edition. Many of these are used to illustrate the procedures to help you visualize critical actions. Drawings of human physiology help you to locate body components and understand body organization. Simple callouts identify the components.

## Guidelines

The table of contents identifies the guidelines included in each lesson. These guidelines highlight important points that you need to remember for specific situations or types of care. They are presented in an easy to use format that you can refer to repeatedly until you know the actions you must take when confronted with the situation.

## Lesson Synthesis: Putting it all Together

At the end of each lesson, you are asked to return to the situation presented in the **Clinical Situation** at the beginning of the lesson. Based upon what you have learned from the lesson, you are to answer a series of questions related to the resident or nursing assistant discussed. This exercise helps you to integrate what you have learned and apply it to a common clinical situation.

## Review

A variety of review questions tests your understanding of the lesson content. For additional activities and exercises to reinforce your learning, refer to the Student Workbook. Your instructor has the answers to the Lesson Reviews and the Workbook Activities (exercises) in the accompanying Instructor's Guide. Your instructor may give you additional questions and tests from the Instructor's Resource Kit or the Computerized Test Bank accompanying this text.

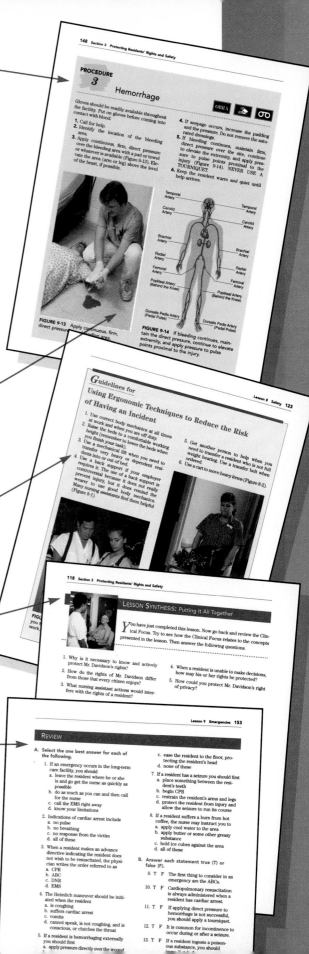

# The Long-Term Care Setting

## LESSONS

*1*  The Long-Term Care Facility

*2*  The Caregivers

*3*  The Nursing Assistant
    in Long-Term Care

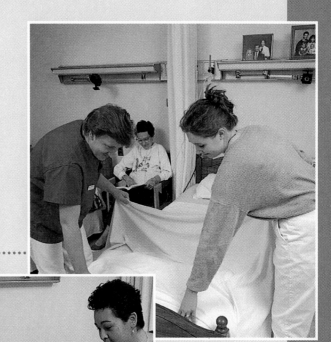

# The Long-Term Care Facility

**CLINICAL FOCUS**

Think how people in need of health care can move from one agency to another when health care needs change as you study this lesson and meet:

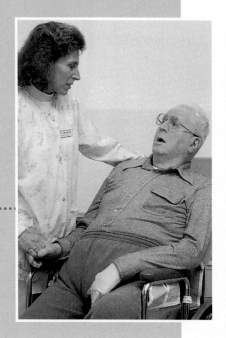

*R*udolph McCarver. Mr. McCarver is recovering from a stroke. He is 79 years old. Although he no longer needs the services of an acute care hospital, he will still require weeks of rehabilitation in long-term care before he can return to his home.

## OBJECTIVES

*After studying this lesson, you should be able to:*

- Define and spell vocabulary words and terms.
- Name community facilities offering health care services.
- Explain the differences in services offered by health care facilities.

- List names applied to types of long-term care facilities.
- Describe state and federal licensing standards and regulations.
- Describe the functional areas and equipment related to a long-term care facility.

## VOCABULARY

**care plan**   (*KAIR plan*)
**client**   (*KLIGH-ent*)
**communal**   (*kum-MYOU-nul*)
**confidential**   (*kon-fih-DEN-shul*)
**day room**   (*day room*)
**emesis basin**   (*EM-eh-sis BAY-sin*)
**geriatric**   (*jer-ee-AT-rick*)
**Kardex**   (*KAR-dex*)

**long-term care facility**   (*lawng turm kair fah-SILL-ih-tee*)
**nurses' station**   (*nur-ses STAY-shun*)
**patient**   (*PAY-shent*)
**policy book**   (*POL-ah-see book*)
**procedure book**   (*proh-SEE-jur book*)
**rehabilitation**   (*ree-hah-BILL-ih-tay-shun*)
**resident**   (*REZ-ih-dent*)

# VOCABULARY

resident unit  (**REZ**-ih-dent **YOU**-nit)
restoration  (reh-stor-**AY**-shun)
skilled nursing facility  (skilled nursing
  fah-**SILL**-ih-tee)

subacute care  (**sub**-ah-**KYOUT** kair)
terminal  (**TER**-mih-nul)

Nursing assistants make valuable contributions in providing health care. Nursing assistants are trained to care for people who are ill or need help in caring for themselves. The care given is always under the guidance and supervision of licensed health care providers such as nurses or physicians.

## COMMUNITY HEALTH CARE FACILITIES

The health needs of the nation are met in various community settings (Figure 1-1). Although trained nursing assistants may work in each type of agency or facility, they find their greatest opportunity for employment in agencies or facilities that provide:

- Health and personal care for people in their homes
- Hospice care for the terminally ill
- Care for the developmentally disabled
- Health services in acute care hospitals
- Extended (long-term) care
- Subacute care services

Each care setting provides basic care in addition to special services to meet individual needs. Figure 1-2 compares some of the characteristics of three care settings where nursing assistants are employed.

Home health care, hospices, and homes for the developmentally disabled offer similar services:

- They are conducted in a homelike setting.
- They stress supportive psychosocial services.
- They provide for physical needs.
- They assist clients to maintain and achieve the maximum level of personal control and functioning.

**FIGURE 1-1**  Different types of health care facilities are needed to meet the nation's health needs.

- Acute care hospitals
- Facilities for the mentally ill
- Physician's offices
- Clinics of various kinds
- Hospices for the terminally ill
- Facilities for the developmentally disabled
- Facilities for long-term care
- Rehabilitation facilities
- Community nursing centers
- Subacute care facilities
- Residential care facilities for the elderly
- Day care facilities
- Group homes

### Home Health Care

Home health services provide for the health and daily living activity needs of people who are ill or have disabilities when family members cannot provide the necessary care in the home.

The care needed is assessed and planned by the nurse along with other health care specialists. The nursing assistant, who works for the home health care agency, carries out the care in the person's home. The person who receives the care is called a **client**. The home care nursing assistant is supervised by professionals but usually works alone with clients. The client is assisted in performing activities of daily living (ADL) and needed personal and basic nursing care is given. The nursing assistant reports directly to the supervising nurse and is involved in the planning, implementation, and documentation of care.

## Hospice Care

Hospice care is provided in a special area of a hospital, in a nursing home, in the client's own home, or in a special hospice facility (Figure 1-3). The nursing assistant helps meet the physical and psychosocial needs of the person who has a limited life span, usually less than 6 months. Clients are encouraged to be as independent as possible for as long as possible. The nursing assistant working in hospice care uses skills to provide physical care but needs well-developed interpersonal skills to effectively help clients and their families during this difficult period.

## Care for the Developmentally Disabled

Services for the developmentally disabled are designed to assist in the care and training of persons whose mental and physical limitations affect self-care (Figure 1-4).

**FIGURE 1-2**  Comparison of the health care provided in three different settings: acute care, long-term care, and home care

| Facility | Care Recipient | Length of Stay | Characteristics/Service | Nursing Assistant Participation |
|---|---|---|---|---|
| **Acute care** | Patient | Few days to weeks | Cure oriented; frequent physician visits; high-level skilled nursing; high-technology equipment; multiple support services; multiple support departments; multiple personnel; may be specialized according to patient needs; care of acutely ill persons; limited term. | Employed by the hospital; may or may not require certificate; cares for a few patients at one time; gives basic care under direct supervision; assists professionals in more complex care; carries out special techniques under supervision and for which they have been specially trained; contributes to nursing care plan through observing and reporting. |
| **Long-term care** | Resident | Weeks, months, years | Subacute care; restoration, maintenance oriented; assistance with activities of daily living; rehabilitative techniques; less sophisticated equipment; stress on social and psychological needs; fewer physician visits; professional nursing supervision; long-term care of chronically ill, infirmed, and developmentally disabled. | Requires certification; encourages self-care when possible; provides complete personal care for those who are unable to help themselves; participates in rehabilitative efforts; contributes to nursing care plan through observing and reporting. |

*(continues)*

| | | | | |
|---|---|---|---|---|
| **Facility** | **Care Recipient** | **Length of Stay** | **Characteristics/ Service** | **Nursing Assistant Participation** |
| **Home care** | Client | Continuous, may have periodic hospital stays | Restoration, maintenance oriented; help in activities of daily living; special nursing care procedures; in some cases may provide for minimal household tasks. | Employed by the agency; may or may not require certification; time spent with a client may range from 1 hour to a full 8-hour shift; may visit several clients in one day for 1–3 hours each; must interact with family members to provide required services to client and offers emotional support to family; carries out basic care under indirect supervision; promotes self-care and rehabilitation; carries out special nursing skills after demonstrating competence; contributes to the nursing care plan by observing, reporting, and documenting; keeps records related to reimbursements. |

FIGURE 1-2 *(continued)*

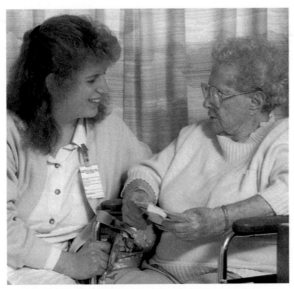

**FIGURE 1-3** Hospice care assists people with a limited life span.

Many developmentally disabled clients live in a long-term care facility. Some clients live at home but spend time daily in the facility for care and training, such as in ADL. The nursing assistant working with this group of clients also needs basic nursing and interpersonal skills.

## Acute Care Hospitals

People receiving care in an acute care hospital are called **patients**. These people are usually seriously ill or injured, or they have some special health need. They require a high level of skilled professional care. Nursing assistants provide basic care and are supervised as they perform special technical skills that they have been taught. Patients stay in hospitals for a limited time and may then be transferred to long-term care facilities or home as their conditions improve.

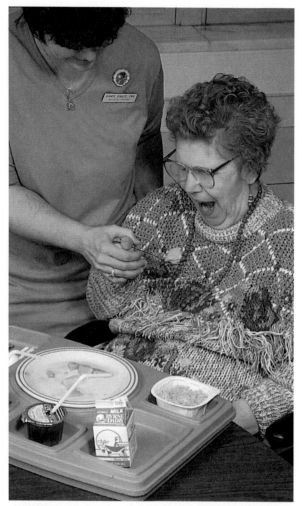

**FIGURE 1-4** Developmentally disabled people are limited in their ability to care for themselves.

Because the patients in an acute care facility need closer attention and more care, the nursing assistant is assigned to care for a specific number of people at a time and is always under the direct supervision of a professional health provider. The nursing assistant working in an acute care facility needs basic nursing skills and interpersonal relationship skills and may be trained by the facility in special technical skills.

## Physicians' Offices/Clinics

People visit physicians' offices for acute short-term care and referrals. Nursing assistants may assist the professional staff by receiving patients and performing basic procedures such as measuring temperature, pulse, respiration, and blood pressure. Nursing assistants may be asked to measure and weigh patients and record and report the information. Selected nursing assistants are trained to do other special procedures under the direct supervision of the physician or nurse.

## Facilities for the Mentally Ill

Patients are admitted to facilities for mental illness to receive care and therapy. Some patients may stay for a short time, whereas others are admitted for long periods of time. The trend today is to move patients out of institutions as soon as possible and into community-based outpatient programs. Nursing assistants employed by the facility perform basic care skills and make a major contribution to the nursing care plan through careful observation and reporting of the patients' behavior and response to care.

## Rehabilitation Clinics

Patients visit rehabilitation clinics as outpatients. The focus is on evaluating, maintaining, and restoring the patient's mobility and independence in carrying out ADL. Generally, the patients make many visits over a period of weeks to months. Nursing assistants work with nurses and therapists in positioning patients, caring for equipment, and providing emotional support and encouragement. For example, a person who is recovering from a fractured leg received in an automobile accident may live at home but receive rehabilitation therapy as an outpatient.

## Community Nursing Centers

These outpatient centers offer short-term care and staff see clients on a regular basis. Nurses in the centers provide health teaching and monitor chronic conditions such as diabetes and high blood pressure (hypertension). They also offer weight control counseling. Nursing assistants provide basic skills such as measuring and weighing clients and taking vital signs. They may also help with examinations and care for equipment and records.

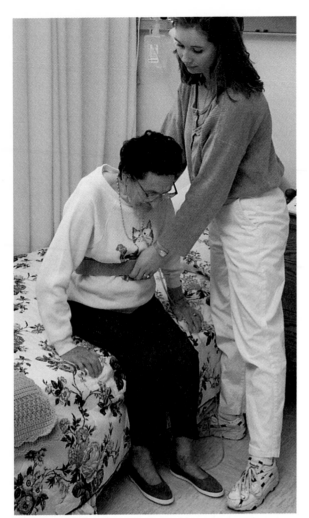

**FIGURE 1-5** The nursing assistant helps the resident get out of bed.

## Long-Term Care Facilities

The person cared for in a **long-term care facility** is called a **resident**. The facility becomes this person's home for an extended period. This period may be for weeks or months as the resident is restored to health. In some cases the facility may become the resident's permanent home.

People are discharged from an acute care facility because they no longer need the specialized care provided there. However, they may still require skilled care and not be ready to return home. Often they are admitted to the **subacute care** unit in a long-term care facility. Here, they receive short-term nursing care until they are ready to go home.

The different types of long-term care facilities employ many nursing assistants who play a vital role in the success of the care given (Figure 1-5). Nursing assistants who work in long-term care must be certified. This text is designed to help students become successful certified nursing assistants.

## TYPES OF LONG-TERM CARE FACILITIES

Several different names are applied to long-term care (LTC) facilities. Some of the names you will hear include:

- Nursing facility (NF)
- Skilled nursing facility (SNF)
- Rest home
- Assisted living facility

People who need long-term care are those who:

- Need to regain the ability to care for themselves (restoration or rehabilitation)
- Cannot, because of illness or disability, care for themselves, and have no one else to provide such care
- Are elderly and frail and need continuous skilled nursing care (**geriatric** care)

All long-term care facilities provide housing, protection, and assistance as needed to meet individual needs (Figure 1-6). Most also provide some skilled nursing care. Placement in a specific long-term care facility is determined by the level

| **FIGURE 1-6** Health care facility functions |
| --- |
| All Care Facilities Provide: |
| • Physical care |
| • Emotional care |
| • Help with activities of daily living (ADL) |
| • Restorative care |
| • Safety and security |
| • Opportunities for social interaction |

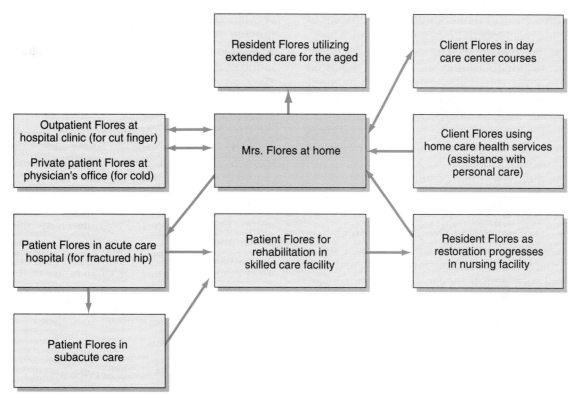

FIGURE 1-7 boxes:

- Resident Flores utilizing extended care for the aged
- Client Flores in day care center courses
- Outpatient Flores at hospital clinic (for cut finger)
- Private patient Flores at physician's office (for cold)
- Mrs. Flores at home
- Client Flores using home care health services (assistance with personal care)
- Patient Flores in acute care hospital (for fractured hip)
- Patient Flores for rehabilitation in skilled care facility
- Resident Flores as restoration progresses in nursing facility
- Patient Flores in subacute care

**FIGURE 1-7**   People move from one health care service to another as their needs change.

of care and type of services needed (Figure 1-7). Much of the service is supported by governmental funds such as Medicare and Medicaid.

## The Skilled Nursing Facility

The **skilled nursing facility** (SNF) offers professional nursing care to chronically ill or disabled persons and those who are recovering but do not require the high-cost services of an acute hospital setting. Many of these people are elderly; some are in the **terminal** (last) stage of life. They have many needs and require the services of many skilled professionals. Highly trained team members provide this specialized care. Physicians, professional nurses, and pharmacy services are readily available. Other support personnel and specialists are available as required.

Skilled nursing facilities are able to provide many but not all of the services offered in the acute hospital setting. The care is aimed at maintenance and **restoration (rehabilitation)** (Figure 1-8) rather than acute care. Maintenance is aimed at preventing further loss and limitations.

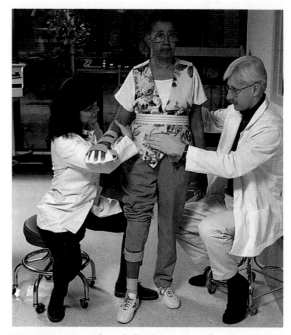

**FIGURE 1-8**   The skilled nursing facility (SNF) provides technical nursing care and emphasizes rehabilitation.

Restoration or rehabilitation is the process of assisting residents to do as much as they can, as well as they can, for as long as they can for themselves. Residents of any age who are admitted primarily for rehabilitation usually stay about 3 months before they are discharged. The cost of care in such an SNF is higher than in some other types of extended care because more services are available. As soon as appropriate, residents are transferred, usually to a less expensive care setting such as a nursing facility.

## The Nursing Facility

In the nursing facility (NF), the rehabilitation effort is continued, but at a less intensive level, requiring fewer specialists. Supervision and care are still provided, however, on a 24-hour basis. When a person in an NF has made as much progress toward self-care as possible, that person is again transferred. It might be to his or her own home or, if further help is necessary, to a still less intensive care facility such as an assisted living facility.

## Assisted Living Facility

Residents in this type of facility can provide most of their own care. Services include meals, assistance with medications, and housekeeping. These facilities are often associated with skilled care facilities, subacute units, or acute care hospitals. This allows the resident to move easily from one level of care to another as health needs change.

# STANDARDS AND REGULATIONS ·····

All facilities must adhere to standards that are set by official public agencies. These standards govern the:

- Qualifications of the caregivers
- Care that is given
- Safety of the facility
- Sanitary conditions

## Nursing Assistant Certification Under the Omnibus Budget Reconciliation Act

Nursing assistants must be certified by the state before they can work in long-term care. State regulations for the training and certification of nursing assistants are guided by the Federal legislation known as the Omnibus Budget Reconciliation Act (OBRA) of 1987. Since October 1, 1990, all persons working as nursing assistants must complete a competency evaluation program or approved course.

The National Council of State Boards of Nursing, Inc. developed the Nurse Aide Competency Evaluation Program (NACEP) to meet the requirements of OBRA. NACEP is a guide for individual training programs to certify and register nursing assistants. NACEP specifies the minimum skills required. Programs may exceed these minimums.

Nursing assistants who wish to be certified must complete a minimum of 75 hours of theory and practice. Some states require a minimum of 80 to 120 program hours in written or oral and clinical skills in several areas, including:

- Basic nursing skills
- Basic restorative services
- Mental health and social service needs
- Personal care skills
- Residents' rights
- Safety and emergency care
- Standard precautions and transmission-based precautions

Nursing assistants who are not certified have three opportunities to meet the requirements for certification. In most states a new training and competency evaluation program must be completed by nursing assistants who previously finished such a program but have not performed nursing-related services for pay for a continuous 24-month period. Certified nursing assistants must complete at least 12 hours of continuing education per year. In some states, the continuing education requirement is 24 hours per year.

The OBRA regulations are important because they:

- Give nursing assistants recognition through certification and listing on the state registry
- Help define the scope of nursing assistant practice
- Ensure better uniformity of care by nursing assistants
- Promote educational standards for nursing assistants

Be sure you are familiar with any specific state regulations or legislation that relate to your job as a nursing assistant.

## FACILITY SURVEYS

Representatives of various agencies visit each facility to check that the standards that apply to the facility are being met. The standards help ensure both the quality of care and the safety of the residents.

Survey teams visit the facility for several days to study the facility operation, the residents, the care they receive, and the caregivers. The team arrives unannounced. During the survey, each team member:

- Reviews the quality of care provided to the residents
- Examines the quality of life for the residents
- Determines areas of deficient care
- Checks the physical well-being of the residents
- Observes care given and questions policy, procedures, and equipment used by nursing assistants
- Evaluates how well care plans are being followed

During a survey period there is always a higher level of tension and anxiety among the caregivers. You can give your best level of care all the time if you remember the following:

- Be calm and confident.
- Know the residents you care for.
- Know and follow the care plan for each resident in your care.
- Cooperate with the surveyors.
- Keep all work areas clean and tidy.
- Perform each procedure as outlined in the facility procedures manual.
- Know the policies that affect you in your facility.
- Know how to operate all equipment properly.
- Respect the residents' rights.
- Report for duty where and when assigned even though the survey is being conducted. Continue with your normally assigned duties as the surveyors visit the unit in which you are working.
- Attend in-service education programs and cooperate in presurvey audits conducted by

the quality assurance committee of the facility. You will be given specific directions by your supervisor.

The findings of the survey are important. They are discussed with the facility administration, including the nursing supervisor. If deficiencies are found, the facility is usually given 10 days to prepare a plan to correct them. Up to 60 days are allowed for the facility to correct deficiencies.

Serious defects can result in:

- Fines up to $10,000 per day until all deficiencies are corrected
- Loss of certification
- Loss of licensure to operate as a long-term care facility and loss of your job

Nursing assistants and how they provide care are important to the success of the survey. Additional information about a survey is given in Lesson 34.

## FUNCTIONAL AREAS IN A LONG-TERM CARE FACILITY

Facilities vary to some degree in physical layout but certain elements are common to all.

### The Resident Room

The resident's room is called the **resident unit**. An adjustable bed, bedside stand, overbed table, chair, and a storage area (closet) are provided for each person (Figure 1-9).

Resident rooms may be designed for occupancy by a single individual, but usually accommodate two persons. In some instances several residents share a single room.

Many facilities encourage residents who will be making the facility their home to bring personal articles as space permits. A familiar chest of drawers, a lamp, or bedside table may replace some of the facility's equipment to add a sense of familiarity and security for the resident. Personal mementos such as pictures or religious articles are important to residents and are kept at the bedside or displayed.

**The Bed.** The bed is usually adjustable for height. It can be raised during care (eliminating

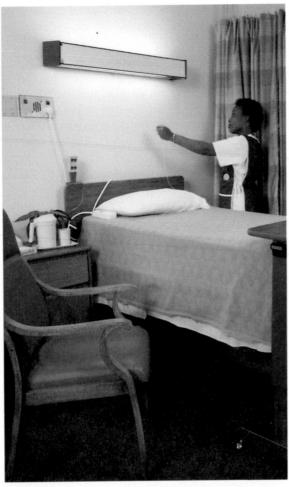

**FIGURE 1-9**  Standard furniture provided in a resident unit

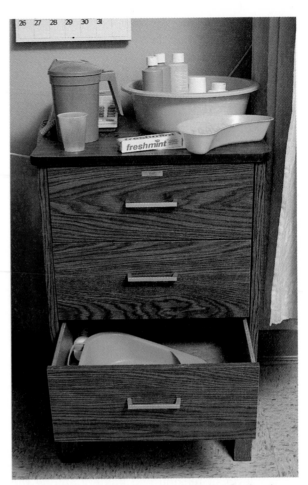

**FIGURE 1-10**  The top two areas of a bedside stand—whether drawers or shelves—contain clean equipment.

bending for the caregiver) and lowered so that residents can get into or out of bed safely. The head and bottom of the bed can also be raised or lowered for resident comfort.

Each bed is equipped with side rails. Side rails should be securely in place if they are ordered for a specific resident. Not all residents need the side rails up. When giving personal care with the bed elevated, only the side rail nearest the caregiver should be lowered.

Some beds are electric; others are adjusted by hand with a crank. The assistant should be thoroughly familiar with the bed controls before attempting to operate them.

**Personal Equipment.**  The bedside stand in each unit is equipped with articles for the resi-

dent's personal care and use. Many of the articles are purchased by the resident or the resident's family. These articles should not be shared with other residents.

The equipment included in each unit is kept in two areas of the bedside stand. The top shelf and two drawers (Figure 1-10) are "clean areas" and hold the following:

- Resident's personal toilet articles
- Wash basin
- Kidney-shaped emesis (vomit) basin
- Soap/dish

The **emesis basin** is usually used when performing personal care procedures such as brushing the teeth.

The drawer holds personal toilet articles such as:

- Toothbrush
- Toothpaste
- Denture cup
- Comb
- Lotion
- Makeup

The bottom drawer is a "dirty area" and holds the:

- Bedpan or bedpan and urinal
- Toilet tissue

**Call Lights.**   Each unit has a signaling device, such as a call light (Figure 1-11). Call lights may be attached to the wall or may be part of a more complex panel attached to the side rail. The panel may also control a radio, television, or telephone. Call lights are also located in the bathroom and shower area. When a resident needs help and uses the call bell, a light at the nurses' station comes on, showing the room number of the resident who called (Figure 1-12).

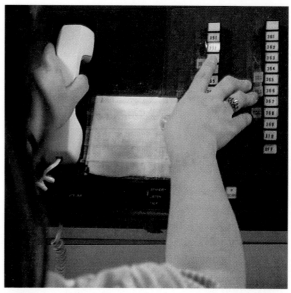

**FIGURE 1-12**   When the resident pushes the button, a light shows at the communications center at the nurses' station and over the door of the resident's room to indicate which resident is calling for assistance.

The call light should always be within reach of the resident.

An overbed table, which is adjustable in height, may be placed over the bed, providing a place to serve meals or hold equipment during care. Each unit has a closet for storing the resident's personal articles.

## Dining Room/Day Room

Residents who are able are encouraged to eat in a **communal** (group) setting, so each facility has a common dining room.

Dining rooms can sometimes function as **day rooms** where residents can meet for activities and socialization at times other than meals. Many facilities have separate day rooms and dining rooms.

Because talking, watching television, and playing cards are enjoyable activities for those whose physical abilities may be limited, a television set, playing cards, and other quiet games are available. Group exercises, singing, and parties that celebrate a special occasion such as a resident's birthday or a holiday are also usually held in the day room or dining room.

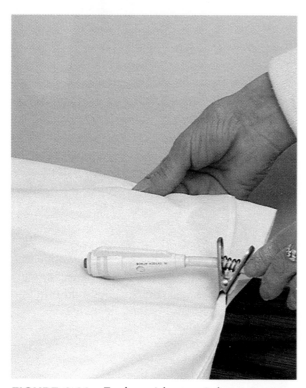

**FIGURE 1-11**   Each resident unit has a means for signaling for assistance.

## Nurses' Station

Every facility has an area where records of care are kept. This area is called the **nurses' station**. Part of the nurses' station is set aside for the control and dispensing of medications; unauthorized persons are not permitted in this area. Authorized persons include the physician, the pharmacist, the registered nurse, and the licensed vocational/practical nurse (LVN or LPN). This part of the nurses' station is kept locked when unattended.

Medications are delivered to residents by the medication nurse using a medicine cart. Residents are not permitted near an unattended medication cart because a confused resident might be hurt by accidentally sampling medications. Medication carts must always be locked when unattended.

Reports of residents' needs and care are usually given within the nurses' station. This is **confidential** (private, personal) information and should not be discussed within hearing of the residents or guests. This information should never be discussed outside the facility. Nursing assistants use this area to report and record their observations and the care given. Directions and assignments are received at the nurses' station.

**Records.** Seven important types of records are found in the nurses' station. They are the:

1. Procedure book
2. Policy book
3. Resident's chart
4. Kardex or resident profile
5. Assignment sheet
6. Care plans
7. Fire and safety manual

The **procedure book** explains how care is to be given. The **policy book** (Figure 1-13) outlines the rules for the facility and explains what will be done for the residents. The resident's chart contains a record of the care given and the progress reported, as well as information about the resident. The resident profile or **Kardex** contains information about the specific daily care to be given to a particular resident. The information on the Kardex reflects a plan called the interdisciplinary **care plan** that has been developed for each resident. The assignment sheet

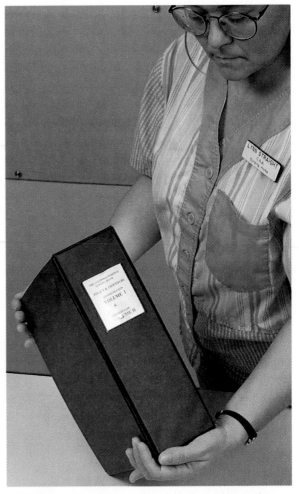

**FIGURE 1-13** The policy book outlines the rules of the facility.

lists the specific assignments and duties for the staff for the shift. The fire and safety manual outlines procedures to follow if a fire or accident occurs in the facility.

## Computers

Computers are used in health care facilities to:

- Maintain records such as care plans, nursing assessments, physicians' orders, and required reports to state and federal agencies
- Inventory supplies
- Record medications and treatments
- Schedule appointments
- Set work schedules

If your facility uses computers to process information, you may be asked to use one. You

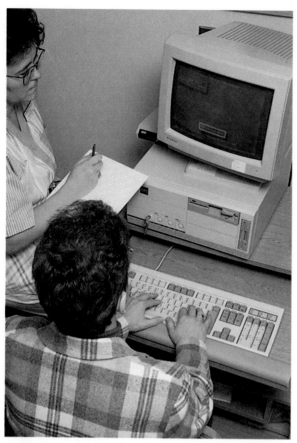

**FIGURE 1-14** Computers provide immediate access to resident information.

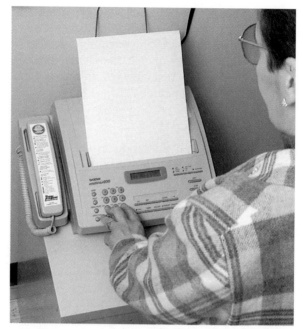

**FIGURE 1-15** Fax machines make it possible to transmit information rapidly from one place to another.

will be trained to use the computer and then be supervised until you can operate it properly.

Computers have a central processing unit, a drive, a display screen, and a keyboard. The keyboard is like the keyboard of a typewriter. The information typed appears on the screen. Information can be stored in the drive of the computer or on disks. A disk has a menu that lists the files of information on the disk. Once information is entered and named, the file name can be selected on the menu and opened. The information can then be reviewed and revised as needed.

Computers provide ready access to essential information that can be used to make medical and nursing decisions (Figure 1-14).

### Fax Machines

Fax machines (Figure 1-15), allow you to send information from printed sheets over telephone lines to other locations. These locations may be within the same building, the same city, across the United States, or in another country. The sending and receiving of information by fax machines can be accomplished in a few minutes. To operate the fax machine, you dial a telephone number that prepares a machine at the other end to receive and print the message.

### Areas for Specific Rehabilitation

Rehabilitation is a main goal of all nursing activity. To make it easier to work with residents, facilities have special areas devoted to the rehabilitation process.

- In the physical therapy department, physical therapists and physical therapy aides focus on exercises to strengthen the muscles of residents. Residents are also taught to use prostheses (artificial limbs), canes, walkers, or crutches to increase their mobility and independence.
- In the occupational therapy department, occupational therapists and occupational therapy aides focus on improving the flexibility of the smaller muscles of the residents' hands and

arms. This is especially helpful when a resident has arthritis and for rehabilitation after a stroke.

- In the speech therapy department, residents are evaluated for speech problems. Speech therapists assist residents to improve their ability to communicate.

## Kitchen

Meals are prepared and food is stored in the kitchen. Meals are then delivered to residents in the day room, dining room or, when necessary, in their rooms.

Both regular and special diets are prepared for residents in this area and then delivered in special carts.

## Laundry

Some facilities have laundries that wash and dry residents' personal clothes. Basic linens needed in resident care may be commercially laundered and delivered to the facility and soiled laundry and clothing may be picked up for cleaning. Some facilities may handle all laundry needs on the premises.

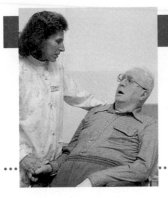

## LESSON SYNTHESIS: Putting It All Together

You have just completed this lesson. Now go back and review the Clinical Focus at the beginning of the lesson. Try to see how the Clinical Focus relates to the concepts presented in the lesson. Then answer the following questions.

1. Why would Mr. McCarver not remain in the acute care facility until he had entirely recovered?

2. What services would be provided for Mr. McCarver in the long-term care facility?

3. How does the organization of the long-term care facility and the equipment provided for each resident contribute to the comfort, safety, and well-being of the resident?

## REVIEW

**A. Match each term with the proper definition.**

   a. geriatric care     c. resident
   b. long-term care    d. restoration
      facility        e. terminal

  1. _____ rehabilitation

  2. _____ last or final

  3. _____ care concerned with the medical problems and nursing care of the elderly

  4. _____ person cared for in long-term care

  5. _____ skilled care facility

**B. List five community health agencies that provide health care.**

  6. _____

  7. _____

  8. _____

  9. _____

  10. _____

## C. Select the one best answer for each of the following.

11. Mr. Jackson has cancer and is expected to live not more than 3 months. He probably would be cared for in
    a. an acute care hospital
    b. a hospice program
    c. a long-term care facility
    d. an outpatient clinic

12. A person being cared for in a long-term care facility is usually called the
    a. patient
    b. resident
    c. client
    d. recipient

13. The care in a skilled care facility is aimed at
    a. acute short-term care
    b. terminal care
    c. restoration
    d. providing a homelike atmosphere

14. Which articles are kept in the "dirty" area of the bedside table?
    a. denture cup
    b. comb
    c. toothbrush and toothpaste
    d. bedpan, urinal

15. When giving personal care with the side rails in use
    a. side rails can be down
    b. side rail nearest the caregiver is down and the far side rail is up
    c. far side rail is down and side rail nearest the caregiver is up
    d. both side rails must be up

16. The resident's room is called the
    a. resident's space
    b. resident's bedroom
    c. resident's area
    d. resident's unit

17. The nurses' station is the area where
    a. personal care is given
    b. food is stored
    c. residents' records and charts are kept
    d. residents' clothes are laundered

18. Which of the following contains confidential resident records?
    a. resident's chart
    b. Kardex
    c. care plans
    d. all of the above

## D. Indicate where each of the following areas is found by selecting from the list (items a.–d.). (More than one answer may apply.)

a. nurses' station     c. resident unit
b. dining room         d. day room

19. _____ bedside stand

20. _____ medication storage

21. _____ meal service area

22. _____ emesis basin

23. _____ bed

24. _____ group activities area

25. _____ television

26. _____ reports

27. _____ resident's health record

28. _____ Kardex

## E. Clinical Experience

Amelia Walters, 85, has lived in the same community all of her life. She has lived alone since her husband died 3 years ago. Her only living relative, a daughter, lives some distance away. The daughter has little contact with her mother.

Mrs. Walters had frequent upper respiratory infections and received care from her neighborhood physician.

During wet weather, Mrs. Walters fell and broke her right ankle and both wrists. Mrs. Walters is unable to perform personal care. She requires full-time care. Healing is slow and her generally frail health makes it impossible for her to live independently. Despite care, her condition declines.

Tests ordered by her physician reveal advanced cancer of the colon, a terminal condition. Mrs. Walters insists that she wants to go home and remain there as long as possible. Answer the following questions relating to Mrs. Walters. Select your answers from the list provided.

a. hospice care
b. acute care hospital
c. skilled nursing facility
d. physician's office
e. home care

29. _____ Mrs. Walters received care here for her upper respiratory infections.

30. _____ Care was given here when Mrs. Walters fell, breaking an ankle and both wrists.

31. _____ Mrs. Walters received restorative care here as her ankle and wrists healed.

32. _____ What help may make it possible for Mrs. Walters to go home once more?

33. _____ What kind of care is available to Mrs. Walters during the final stage of her life?

# 2

# The Caregivers

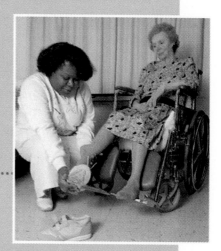

## CLINICAL FOCUS

Think about how staff members contribute their

special knowledge and expertise to the resident's

well-being as you study this lesson and meet:

**M**s. Esther Patterson, who is 74 years old and complains every time her shoes are put on her feet and she is assisted to walk. You are asked to help the podiatrist who is visiting her. Consider how this care will help Ms. Patterson become more active.

## OBJECTIVES

*After studying this lesson, you should be able to:*

- Define and spell vocabulary words and terms.
- Describe the purpose of the interdisciplinary team.

- Name three or more members of the interdisciplinary team.
- List the members of the nursing staff.
- State the purpose of the organizational chart.

## VOCABULARY

**activities of daily living (ADL)**  *(ack-**TIV**-ih-tees of **DAY**-lee **LIV**-ing)*

**adaptive device**  *(ah-**DAP**-tiv dih-**VICE**)*

**administrator**  *(ad-**MIN**-iss-tray-tor)*

**ambulation**  *(am-byou-**LAY**-shun)*

**assessment**  *(ah-**SESS**-ment)*

**assistive device**  *(ah-**SIS**-tiv dih-**VICE**)*

**audiologist**  *(**awe**-dee-**OL**-oh-jist)*

**care plan conference**  *(kair plan **KON**-fer-ens)*

**consultant**  *(kon-**SUL**-tant)*

**dental hygienist**  *(**DEN**-tal high-**JEE**-nist)*

**dentist**  *(**DEN**-tist)*

**diagnosis**  *(die-ag-**NOH**-sis)*

**dietitian**  *(die-eh-**TISH**-un)*

**environmental services**  *(en-**vire**-un-**MEN**-tal **SIR**-vuh-sez)*

**interdisciplinary health care team**  *(in-ter-**DISS**-sih-plin-air-ee health kair team)*

# VOCABULARY

licensed practical nurse   *(**LICE**-enst **PRACK**-tih-kul nurs)*

mobility   *(moh-**BILL**-ih-tee)*

nursing assistant   *(**NUR**-sing ah-**SIS**-tant)*

occupational therapist   *(ock-you-**PAY**-shun-al **THER**-ah-pist)*

ophthalmologist   *(**off**-thal-**MOL**-oh-jist)*

optometrist   *(op-**TOM**-eh-trist)*

orthotic device   *(or-**THAW**-tick dih-**VICE**)*

physical therapist   *(**FIZ**-ih-kul **THER**-ah-pist)*

podiatrist   *(poh-**DYE**-ah-trist)*

quality assurance program   *(**KWAL**-ih-tee **AH**-shur-ans **PROH**-gram)*

registered nurse   *(**REJ**-is-terd nurs)*

rehabilitation aide   *(ree-hah-**BILL**-ah-**tay**-shun ayd)*

social worker   *(**SO**-shul **WERE**-ker)*

speech-language pathologist   *(speech **LAN**-gwehj pah-**THOL**-oh-jist)*

support services   *(sup-**PORT SIR**-vuh-sez)*

therapeutic diet   *(**ther**-ah-**PEW**-tick **DIE**-et)*

therapeutic recreational specialist   *(**ther**-ah-**PEW**-tick **reck**-ree-**AY**-shun-al **SPEH**-shul-ist)*

total care   *(**TOH**-tal kair)*

## THE INTERDISCIPLINARY TEAM MEMBERS

Many workers help care for the resident. These caregivers represent many professions or "disciplines," and each has a specific function. As a group they are called the **interdisciplinary health care team** (Figure 2-1). Each member of the interdisciplinary health care team helps plan the care of the residents. This process is completed at the resident's **care plan conference**. You will learn more about this in Lesson 6. The

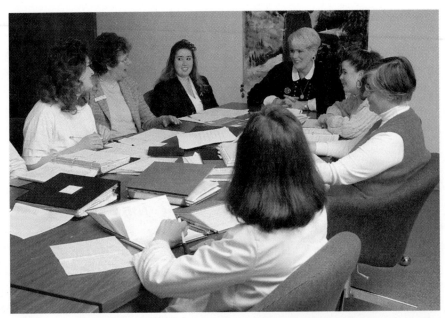

**FIGURE 2-1**   The interdisciplinary health care team is responsible for the care of the resident.

team members who attend the care plan conference include the:

- Resident
- Resident's family (if resident gives permission)
- Members of the nursing staff
- Members of the rehabilitation staff
- Social worker
- Activities director
- Dietitian or dietary supervisor

By using the interdisciplinary team approach, the residents receive **total care**. This considers the emotional, spiritual, physical, and social needs of each person. The resident and the resident's family are also considered members of the team. Most of the direct care is given by the nursing staff. Figure 2-2 defines the jobs of people who are commonly part of the interdisciplinary health care team.

## The Nursing Staff

The nursing staff in a long-term care facility includes **registered nurses** (RNs), **licensed practical nurses** (LPNs), and **nursing assistants**. (In some states LPNs are called licensed vocational nurses or LVNs.)

The *director of nursing* must be a registered nurse. This person has had, besides nursing school, some additional training in administration. The director of nurses is at the head of the nursing staff and is responsible for all nurses, nursing assistants, and residents in the facility. If the facility is very large, there may also be an assistant director of nursing and supervisors, as well as other nurses in charge of education, infection control programs, and quality assurance. These programs ensure that all residents receive appropriate care.

An *assistant director of nursing* works with the director. *Supervisors* are in charge of the entire building during a specific shift. *Charge nurses* are responsible for a nursing unit. There may be one or several nursing units within a facility. *Staff nurses* are in charge of a specific number of residents. They pass medications, perform treatments, and supervise the residents' direct care (Figure 2-3). There may be a *rehabilitation nurse* who coordinates activities between the therapists and the nurses. The nursing assistants are responsible for carrying out most of the personal resident care (Figure 2-4).

The use of advance practice nurses is becoming more frequent. An advance practice nurse has completed additional educational programs leading to a master's degree or doctoral degree. The course of study qualifies them to work as nurse practitioners or clinical nurse specialists.

The *unit secretary* is responsible for the clerical tasks of the nursing staff. These duties include answering the telephone, writing out daily reports, filing, entering reports into the medical records, making out assignment sheets, and ordering supplies.

## Social Services

The social services department provides for many of the nonmedical needs of the residents (Figure 2-5). The department works closely with the nursing staff. In many facilities they are responsible for the admission of new residents. **Social workers** plan the discharge for residents going home. This may involve coordination of community services for the resident, such as making arrangements for homemaking services or for the services of a home health agency. The social workers may arrange for appointments with dentists, podiatrists, audiologists, or mental health consultants. They may organize religious services and other programs with local religious groups or leaders.

## The Physician

Each resident has a physician who makes the medical **diagnosis** and writes medical orders for the resident. In addition to writing new orders, the physician evaluates the health and well-being of the residents. The physician may also participate in care plan conferences.

## The Dietitian

A **dietitian** plans and supervises the preparation of resident meals and therapeutic diets (Figure 2-6). The dietitian performs a nutritional **assessment** for each resident. Monitoring residents' weights is another duty of the dietitian. Special meals and supplements are provided for residents requiring **therapeutic diets** (special diets designed to meet a resident's specific needs). Therapeutic diets are ordered by the physician. (Lesson 17 has more details on therapeutic diets.)

**FIGURE 2-2** Who's who on the interdisciplinary health care team

Each of these disciplines requires a specified course of study (usually a minimum of a college degree and clinical training). Most require either licensing by a state agency or certification from a professional association. Requirements for some disciplines may vary from state to state.

| | |
|---|---|
| **Activities director:** | Requirements vary. Plans and implements activities for residents to meet the goals on the plan of care. |
| **Administrator:** | Licensed and meets state requirements to provide general administration and supervision of a long-term care facility. |
| **Audiologist:** | Certified in audiology and qualified to test hearing and prescribe hearing aids. |
| **Chaplain:** | Provides services to meet the spiritual needs of the residents. |
| **Dental hygienist:** | Licensed by the state and provides dental services under the supervision of a dentist. |
| **Dentist:** | Licensed by the state to provide services for the prevention and treatment of diseases and disorders of the teeth and oral cavity. |
| **Dietitian:** | Licensed by the state and responsible for the provision of all nutritional assessments and food services for residents. |
| **Licensed practical nurse (LPN or LVN):** | Licensed by the state and provides direct resident care under the supervision of a registered nurse. Sometimes called licensed vocational nurse. |
| **Medical record practitioner:** | Certified or licensed to review and audit all medical records. |
| **Nursing assistant:** | Has completed at least 75 hours of a state-approved course and is certified to provide direct resident care under the supervision of a licensed or registered nurse. |
| **Occupational therapist:** | Licensed to provide rehabilitative services to evaluate and treat persons with physical injury or illness, psychosocial problems, or developmental disabilities. Occupational therapy assistants and aides have completed specified courses of study and work under the supervision of an occupational therapist. |
| **Optometrist:** | Licensed by the state to examine eyes and prescribe glasses. |
| **Orthotist:** | Licensed by the state and designs and fits braces and splints for the extremities. |
| **Pharmacist:** | Licensed by the state and fills prescriptions for medications as ordered by the physician. Resource to nurses and physicians for updates on new medications and for maintaining safe drug therapy for residents. |
| **Physical therapist:** | Licensed by the state to provide rehabilitative services to evaluate and treat persons with neuromuscular and musculoskeletal problems due to disease, injury, or developmental disability. Physical therapy assistants and aides have completed specified courses of study and work under the supervision of a physical therapist. *(continues)* |

## FIGURE 2-2   *(continued)*

| | |
|---|---|
| **Physician:** | Licensed by the state to diagnose and treat disease and to prescribe medications. The many specialty areas within medicine require additional education. |
| **Podiatrist:** | Licensed by the state to treat diseases and disorders of the feet. |
| **Prosthetist:** | Licensed by the state to design and fit artificial limbs for persons who have had amputations. |
| **Registered nurse (RN):** | Licensed by the state to make assessments, plan, implement, and evaluate nursing care. Supervises other nursing staff and may coordinate the interdisciplinary health care team. The many specialty areas within nursing require additional education. |
| **Rehabilitation aide:** | A certified nursing assistant with additional training to perform procedures under the direction of the licensed physical therapist and licensed occupational therapist. |
| **Resident:** | The most important member of the interdisciplinary team and has input into the planning and implementation of care. The family may participate with the resident or in place of the resident if the resident is unable to do so. |
| **Respiratory therapist:** | Licensed by the state to evaluate and treat diseases and problems associated with breathing and the respiratory tract. |
| **Social worker:** | Licensed by the state to assess and provide services for the nonmedical, psychosocial needs of the residents. |
| **Speech-language pathologist:** | Licensed by the state to evaluate and provide services for residents with problems in hearing, language, speech production, and swallowing. |
| **Therapeutic recreational specialist:** | Certified to evaluate and provide recreational services to treat mental and physical disorders. |
| **Unit secretary:** | Certified nursing assistant with additional training, responsible for clerical duties of nursing staff; may also be a person with no previous health care experience who is trained as a unit secretary for a specific period of time. |

In addition to these members of the interdisciplinary health care team, many other employees in the long-term care facility provide services that benefit the quality of life for the residents.

- Environmental services staff maintain a clean, comfortable, and homelike environment. These services may include housekeeping, laundry, and building and grounds maintenance.
- The business office handles the personal funds of the residents as well as the financial affairs of the facility.
- Assistants in all departments provide services to residents as part of the interdisciplinary team.
- Volunteers may provide direct services to residents and may raise funds to provide equipment for resident care.

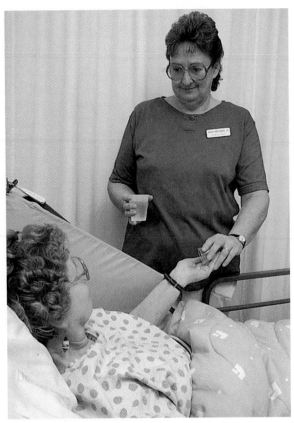

**FIGURE 2-3** Staff nurses pass medications and perform treatments.

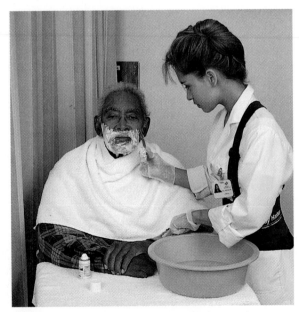

**FIGURE 2-4** Nursing assistants provide most of the resident's personal care.

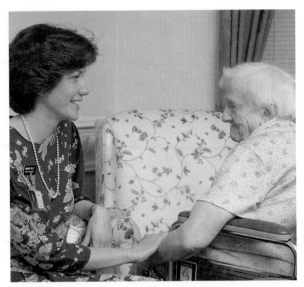

**FIGURE 2-5** The social services department is responsible for the admission of new residents.

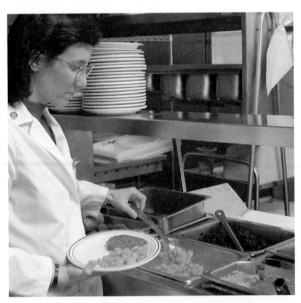

**FIGURE 2-6** The dietitian supervises the nutritional services of the facility.

## Special Therapists

In large facilities many different types of therapists are in the facility every day. In smaller facilities, the therapists may be **consultants**. Consultants come to the facility regularly to evaluate the residents' conditions and recommend treatment.

The **physical therapist** works to improve the **mobility** (ability to move) of the resident (Figure 2-7). After an initial evaluation, a plan is developed to restore and maintain optimum body functioning. This may include teaching the resident how to use an **assistive device**. Canes and walkers are examples of assistive devices. Many times the nursing assistant helps to carry out the program prescribed by the therapist. For example, range of motion exercises are part of daily care. These are ordered by the physician but they are done by the nursing assistant or in the rehabilitation department.

The **occupational therapist** helps residents learn new ways of doing basic self-care (**activities of daily living** or **ADL**). For example, the therapist may teach the resident to dress or eat with the use of **adaptive devices**. An adaptive device is a piece of equipment designed to assist a resident to carry out ADL. The occupational therapist may evaluate and fit an **orthotic device** (splint) for a resident's hand. Orthotic devices are appliances used to protect and support a body part. Such a device can hold a paralyzed hand in position to prevent contractures (permanent deformities) from forming (Figure 2-8).

There may be other members of the rehabilitation team. Physical therapy assistants and occupational therapy assistants must complete 2 years of an approved educational program. They work under the direct supervision of the therapists. Some states allow occupational and physical **rehabilitation aides** to perform some of the less complex, routine procedures. They also work under the direction and supervision of the therapists. The rehabilitation aides are nursing assistants who have taken additional courses to prepare them for this job.

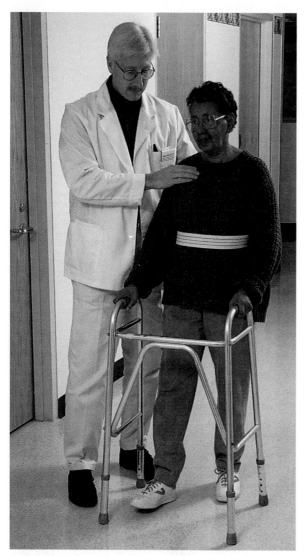

**FIGURE 2-7**   The physical therapist works to improve the resident's mobility.

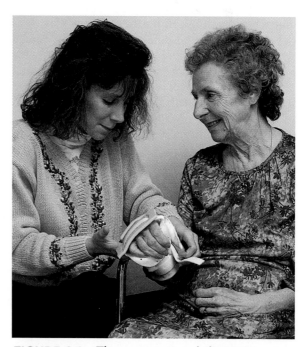

**FIGURE 2-8**   The occupational therapist applies an orthotic device to support the resident's weak right hand and wrist.

The occupational therapist or **therapeutic recreational specialist** may direct recreational, educational, spiritual, artistic, or social activities for the resident. Activities aides also work with the resident in doing the activities.

The **speech-language pathologist** (speech therapist) works with residents who have speech and language problems. The speech-language pathologist may help a resident regain the ability to talk. If a resident is unable to do this, the resident will be taught other means of communication. Speech-language pathologists also work with residents who have trouble swallowing. They are qualified to do swallowing evaluations and to suggest techniques for feeding residents.

### Consultants

Some of the services provided by the facility are not needed on a daily basis. Not all residents need all of the services. Consultants are hired to perform these services.

The **audiologist** tests and evaluates hearing. For residents with impaired hearing, the audiologist may prescribe a hearing aid.

**Dentists** or **dental hygienists** examine and clean teeth. They also evaluate the resident's dental health. Maintaining good nutrition is difficult when teeth are in poor condition. The dentist will recommend dentures or denture repair when needed. Choking is always a concern with improperly fitting dentures.

The **podiatrist** is another special caregiver who visits periodically. Many older persons have foot and toenail problems that make **ambulation** (walking) difficult. The podiatrist examines and may treat foot problems, such as bunions, hammer toes, calluses, and corns. This increases the resident's comfort and mobility because these conditions are very painful.

An **ophthalmologist** examines the resident's eyes and prescribes glasses. The ophthalmologist may also perform surgery to correct or improve vision problems. The **optometrist** is licensed by the state to examine eyes and prescribe glasses.

### Support Services

Many other workers provide **support services** These workers:
- Maintain the building and grounds
- Perform housekeeping duties (Figure 2-9)

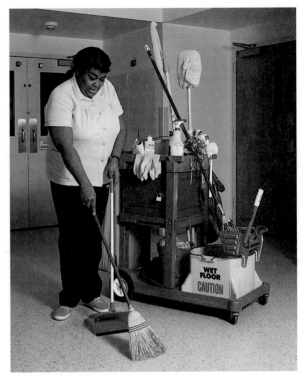

**FIGURE 2-9** Housekeeping staff maintain a clean and comfortable environment.

- Do the laundry
- Work in the kitchen
- Handle administrative duties
- Manage the financial affairs of the facility

Buildings and grounds, housekeeping, and laundry departments are sometimes called **environmental services**

## ADMINISTRATIVE ORGANIZATION ···

Each facility has an organizational chart that shows the line of authority or command. Each department is represented on the chart. All employees are recognized within these departments. The organizational chart is also used as a guide for communication so all employees know to whom they should report.

The **administrator** of the long-term care facility provides leadership for all departments and employees. The administrator may be called the Chief Executive Officer (CEO) or President. This person is responsible for the financial aspects of the facility. The requirements for administrator vary from state to state.

The facility is managed and directed by a Board of Directors that delegates authority for day-to-day operation to the administrator and department heads. You should become familiar with the lines of authority in your facility. Each facility also has a physician who serves as medical director.

An example of a line of authority is that from the Board of Directors to the administrator. The administrator is assisted by designated heads of various departments (Figure 2-10). The authority for care is passed from the physician to the director of nursing, nursing supervisor, charge nurse, and on to the nursing assistant. Your immediate supervisor is the instructor, charge nurse, or staff nurse designated for this role. The supervising nurse will give you your assignment and you will report your observations and the completion of the assigned tasks to this person. The supervising nurse is your primary line of communication and authority. It is important that you know and follow the proper chain of command.

Any questions about your assignment should be directed to your supervising nurse for clarification. *Never attempt to carry out an assignment for which you have not been trained or an assignment you do not fully understand.* Inform the supervisor and ask for help. Never feel embarrassed. It is better to ask for help than to injure a resident.

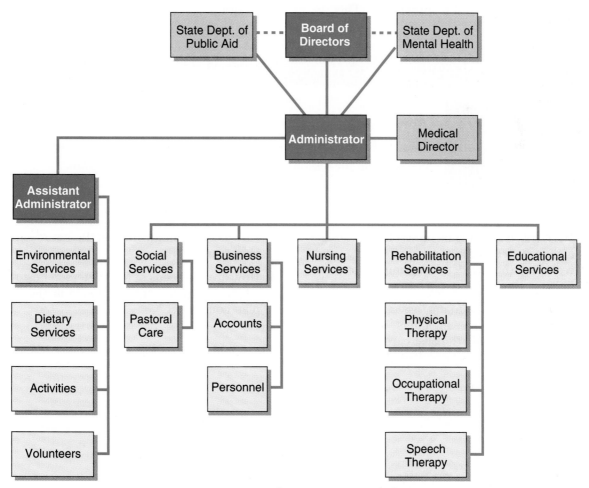

**FIGURE 2-10**  The organizational chart

## QUALITY ASSURANCE PROGRAM ···

Every employee of the long-term care facility is involved in the **quality assurance program**. This program provides a method of ensuring that all residents are receiving appropriate and adequate care. All facilities have a quality assurance coordinator. This person is responsible for organizing the projects carried out by the quality assurance team. The team is made up of employees from every department. Nursing assistants are frequently appointed to assist the team. You will learn more about quality assurance in Lesson 34.

## STAFF DEVELOPMENT ···············

All staff members are expected to participate in continuing education programs. This is called staff development. Some of the programs will be attended by all members of the interdisciplinary team. Other programs may be presented specifically for nursing assistants. OBRA requires that all nursing assistants participate in 12 hours of continuing education each year. Some states may require more than 12 hours. At these programs, you will learn about:

- New facility policies
- New procedures involving resident care
- Use of new equipment
- Caring for residents with unusual diagnoses or problems
- Issues in health care
- Topics related to residents' rights, safety, and infection control

The more you learn, the better you can care for the residents and the more you will enjoy your work.

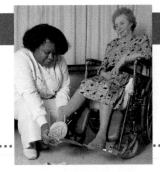

## LESSON SYNTHESIS: Putting It All Together

You have just completed this lesson. Now go back and review the Clinical Focus. Try to see how the Clinical Focus relates to the concepts presented in the lesson. Then answer the following questions.

1. What role does each member of the interdisciplinary team play in maintaining and restoring the resident's optimum level of independent functioning?

2. How does the nursing assistant interact with other team members to provide Ms. Patterson with the best care?

3. How do consultants fit into the interdisciplinary team?

4. How are the needs of Ms. Patterson best met when care plans are developed at the care plan conference?

## REVIEW

**A. Select the one best answer for each of the following.**

1. The many professions responsible for the care of the resident in the long-term care facility are members of the
   a. medical staff
   b. interdisciplinary health care team
   c. employee council
   d. residents' council

2. Employees who attend the resident's care plan conference include
   a. the resident
   b. activities director
   c. members of the nursing staff
   d. all of these

3. The person who is responsible for helping residents learn new ways of doing the activities of daily living is the
   a. occupational therapist
   b. physician
   c. pharmacist
   d. physical therapist

4. An adaptive device is a
   a. piece of equipment designed to assist a resident with activities of daily living
   b. cane or walker
   c. hearing aid
   d. set of dentures

5. A splint is a device that
   a. helps the resident walk
   b. prevents deformities
   c. helps the resident breathe
   d. restrains the resident

6. The social worker may be responsible for
   a. admission and discharge of residents
   b. giving medications
   c. giving physical therapy
   d. supervising nursing assistants

7. Most of the direct care of residents is given by the
   a. director of nursing
   b. nursing assistants

   c. administrator
   d. dietitian

8. The purpose of the organizational chart is to
   a. indicate the lines of authority
   b. provide a guide for communication
   c. indicate the chain of command
   d. all of these

9. The housekeeping, laundry, and maintenance departments may be referred to as
   a. rehabilitation services
   b. food services
   c. environmental services
   d. nursing services

10. The Omnibus Budget Reconciliation Act (OBRA) requires that all nursing assistants participate in
    a. 12 hours of in-service education each year
    b. annual college courses
    c. providing social services
    d. food preparation

11. The purpose of the quality assurance program is to
    a. ensure that all residents are receiving appropriate and adequate care
    b. ensure that employees receive pay raises every year
    c. provide service for the physicians
    d. all of these

**B. Match the team members (items a.–j.) with their responsibilities.**

a. physician
b. dietitian
c. physical therapist
d. respiratory therapist
e. administrator
f. audiologist
g. dentist
h. podiatrist
i. ophthalmologist
j. housekeeper

12. _____ cares for residents with mobility problems

13. _____ provides leadership to staff

14. _____ performs housekeeping duties

15. _____ examines and cleans teeth

16. _____ provides eye examinations and prescriptions

17. _____ defines the medical diagnosis and writes orders

18. _____ treats diseases associated with breathing

19. _____ cares for foot problems

20. _____ plans and supervises preparation of meals

21. _____ tests and evaluates residents' hearing

# The Nursing Assistant in Long-Term Care

## CLINICAL FOCUS

Think about the characteristics that are needed to

be a successful nursing assistant as you study this

lesson and meet:

*R*ay Rodriquez, who is 20 years old. He did not finish high school because he needed to earn money to help at home. Ever since he was a little boy he has known responsibility and the need to be prompt and dependable. While growing up, he helped his mother care for an elderly grandmother and younger brothers and sisters. He learned to be patient as he helped his grandmother eat. Ray comes from a very close and loving family and is putting his skills to positive use.

## OBJECTIVES

*After studying this lesson, you should be able to:*

- Define and spell vocabulary words and terms.
- List five personal characteristics needed to be a successful nursing assistant in long-term care.
- Describe how to dress properly for work.
- Define the job description.
- List 10 duties that the nursing assistant performs.

- List five ways to use time efficiently.
- Explain how interpersonal relations influence the effectiveness of resident care.
- State the responsibilities the nursing assistant has for personal and clinical growth.

## VOCABULARY

accuracy   (*ACK*-your-ah-see)

assignments   (ah-*SIGHN*-ments)

attitude   (*AT*-ih-tood)

burnout   (*BURN*-out)

dependability   (dee-*pen*-dah-*BILL*-ih-tee)

empathy   (*EM*-pah-thee)

harmony   (*HAR*-mun-ee)

job description   (job dih-*SKRIP*-shun)

maturity   (mah-*CHUR*-rih-tee)

procedure   (proh-*SEE*-jur)

sensitivity   (*sen*-sih-*TIV*-ih-tee)

## PERSONAL CHARACTERISTICS ·········

Nursing assistants working in long-term care are very special people. They feel pride in themselves when they fulfill their role with enthusiasm and dedication. They will be successful if they:

- Possess maturity and sensitivity
- Are dependable and accurate
- Can be satisfied with small gains
- Bring a positive attitude to their job
- Carry out **assignments** (work to be completed during the shift) as they have been taught in a safe manner

Not everyone can be a successful, satisfied long-term care nursing assistant. Nursing assistants care for many people who cannot care for themselves. Some of them may be confused; others need a great deal of patience and assistance in carrying out even the most intimate parts of their own personal hygiene.

### Sensitivity and Maturity

Because the residents have so many needs, the nursing assistant must have the **sensitivity** to recognize the needs that are expressed and those that are not expressed. The need for dry, clean linen is obvious if the bed is wet. The need for a close human relationship may be less obvious. It is just as important to be aware of and to meet residents' emotional needs as their physical needs (Figure 3-1).

The sensitive, mature care provider quickly recognizes both the physical and emotional needs of residents and willingly reaches out. **Maturity** means that you can control your emotions. Angry responses have no place in the facility. You must relate to residents and coworkers with courtesy, kindness, and respect. The mature individual can accept and learn from constructive evaluation and criticism. Maturity and sensitivity are also required to make the observations (assessments) that are part of a nursing assistant's job. Maturity is not a matter of age; it is one of attitude.

In the acute care hospital, patients who have been very ill or who have had extensive surgery can make rapid, dramatic gains as their health improves. They look forward to returning home. The resident in a long-term care facility makes small strides at best—for example,

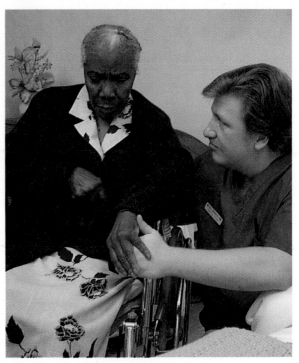

**FIGURE 3-1** The nursing assistant must be sensitive to the resident's needs.

relearning to hold a spoon or walking a corridor with the help of a cane. The facility becomes their home, and often the staff becomes their only family and friends. The enthusiasm and patience that the nursing assistant brings to work can spread like sunshine throughout the unit. A smile or the therapeutic use of touch in the recognition of a resident's successful efforts can brighten the day for those in your care.

### Dependability and Accuracy

**Dependability** and **accuracy** are also essential qualities of the nursing assistant. You demonstrate these qualities when you:

- Arrive for duty on time (Figure 3-2)
- Come prepared to do your job
- Carry out your assignment correctly

### Empathy

The ability to put yourself in another person's position is called **empathy**. Being able to see a situation from another person's viewpoint helps you become more sensitive to that person.

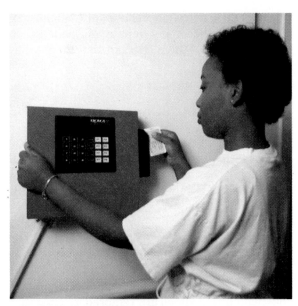

**FIGURE 3-2**   Reporting for duty on time demonstrates dependability.

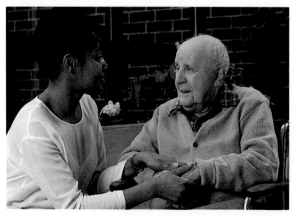

**FIGURE 3-3**   The nursing assistant brings a positive attitude to her job.

Your attitude is reflected in the way you relate to your coworkers as well. Each time you willingly help another worker, you show your shared concern for each other and for the welfare of the residents (Figure 3-4).

Just for a moment, pretend you are one of the residents. What qualities do you want in the nursing assistants who care for you? Imagine what it must be like to:

- Have to sit for hours in a geri-chair
- Have thoughts you cannot express in words
- Need to go to the toilet and have to wait for help
- Need help to take a bath
- Not be able to feed yourself
- Have a tube in your bladder to drain urine
- Be separated from family and friends
- Be demeaned by wearing a protective brief for incontinence

As you do this, you will begin to understand the situation of the residents, and your empathy for those in your care will grow.

# ATTITUDE

The most important characteristic that you bring to your job is your **attitude** (Figure 3-3). The other characteristics described here are an outer reflection of your inner feelings, of your attitude about yourself and others.

Residents have the right to be cared for in a calm, unhurried atmosphere. Your attitude and behavior are critical in providing such an environment.

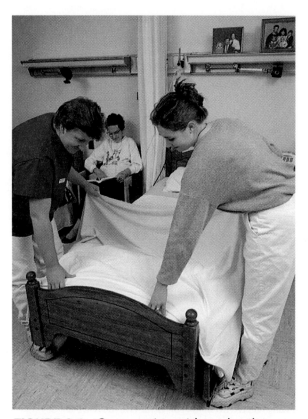

**FIGURE 3-4**   Cooperating with each other demonstrates your concern for maintaining a calm environment for the resident.

## PERSONAL HYGIENE

The work of a long-term care nursing assistant is physically demanding. Because you will be in close contact with the residents, your personal hygiene and grooming must be the very best (Figure 3-5). Good grooming starts with a daily bath or shower and the use of a deodorant to control body odor. Careful attention to the cleanliness of teeth and nails is also important; teeth should be cleaned at least twice each day and fingernails kept trimmed and smooth. Hair should be neatly arranged and controlled. Hair should not fall over the face or shoulders. It should be pulled up or back neatly. Beards and mustaches should be neatly trimmed. Makeup should be moderate.

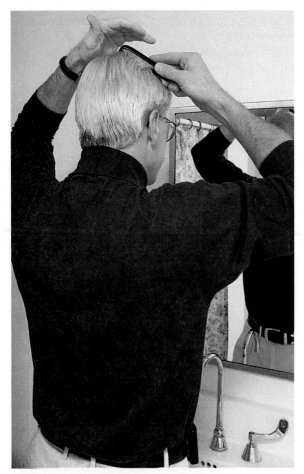

**FIGURE 3-5** Good grooming starts with a daily bath or shower and the use of a deodorant and includes the brushing of teeth and a neat hair style.

Strongly scented aftershave lotions and perfumes can bother many people and cause allergic reactions in others. Do not use them while you are on duty.

## UNIFORMS

The uniform of nursing assistants in long-term care facilities is often a matter of preference. If your facility has a dress code and specifies how nursing assistants should dress, you must follow that code (Figure 3-6).

The uniform includes shoes and stockings or socks. Shoes are usually white and should be cleaned daily, and white shoelaces should be laundered frequently. Because nursing assistants spend many hours on their feet, good, comfortable, well-fitting shoes are required.

Wear your uniform only while on duty. When you arrive home, remove your uniform, fold it inside out so that the dirtiest part is on the inside, and put it in the laundry. When doing the laundry, use bleach if possible to kill the bacteria that may be present on the uniform.

Wear a fresh, clean uniform each day that you report to work. Make sure that the uniform is presentable with no broken zippers, missing buttons, hanging hems, or tears.

Do not smoke while in uniform. Clothing absorbs the odor of tobacco, which is offensive to many people. If you do smoke, storing clean uniforms in plastic garment bags at home will help reduce the exposure to the smoke.

### Accessories

Bracelets, rings, earrings, and necklaces are not to be worn (although most facilities do permit the wearing of a wedding ring and small stud earrings). Jewelry tends to harbor germs, may scratch or injure a resident, and can easily be lost.

A watch with a second hand and an identification badge are part of your official uniform. You will need the watch to do certain procedures. The identification badge lets other staff members know who you are and helps residents remember your name. It should always be worn when you are in uniform.

You should keep a pen and a small notepad in your uniform pocket to jot down your observations of the residents and their responses to care.

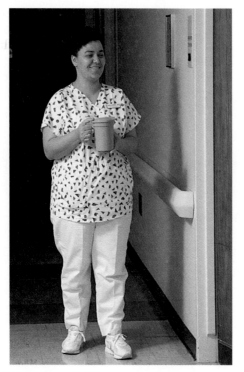 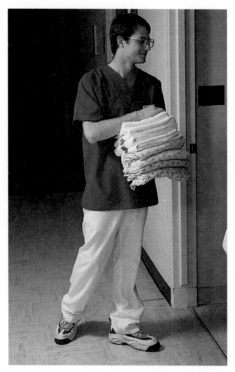

**FIGURE 3-6**   Well-groomed nursing assistants wear a fresh, clean uniform each day.

## Pride in Appearance

Always remember that your appearance declares your pride in yourself and your work. Remember that you are a representative of your facility to residents and visitors. You are ready to work if you:

- Demonstrate personal cleanliness
- Use an antiperspirant or deodorant
- Wear an appropriate, clean uniform
- Wear clean shoes and stockings or socks, including clean shoelaces
- Arrange your hair so that it is neat and controlled
- Neatly trim your beard and mustache (if you are a man)
- Trim fingernails smoothly; do not use colored polish
- Do not use strong perfumes or aftershave lotion
- Wear a watch with a second hand
- Carry a pen and notepad in your uniform pocket
- Properly pin identification badge on your uniform
- Do not smoke while in uniform

## DUTIES AND RESPONSIBILITIES: THE JOB DESCRIPTION ·················

The duties and responsibilities of nursing assistants in long-term care are stated in the policy book as a **job description**. During the pre-employment interview, you should review the job description to be sure you can perform the work required before you accept employment. As you learned in Lesson 1, each facility has:

- A policy book that describes the role and responsibilities of each staff member
- A procedure book that describes how each task should be performed

Find each of these books in your unit and become familiar with them. Both books are usually found in the nurses' station.

Basic **procedures** may be varied in some ways to meet individual needs. You must know any differences in basic procedures preferred in your facility. Differences in procedure may be explained during the orientation period after you are hired. You can also check the procedure book for exact details of how procedures are to be performed.

Be willing to learn new techniques and different ways to perform tasks, taking instruction from your charge nurse or staff development coordinator. If you are asked to perform a procedure that you have not learned but is within the scope of practice for nursing assistants, ask

for a demonstration. You will be supervised until both you and your supervisor are confident in your ability to do the procedure correctly and safely.

The job description is the basis for specific assignments (Figure 3-7).

---

**FIGURE 3-7**   Typical nursing assistant duties. Specific duties will vary depending on state regulations and facility policy.

**Some of the duties performed by nursing assistants include activities that:**

1. Protect the rights of residents
   a. Treat resident with respect.
   b. Protect resident's privacy and maintain confidentiality.
   c. Keep call bells within resident's reach and answer promptly.
   d. Give resident choices whenever possible.
   e. Assist in recreational and spiritual activities of the resident's choice.

2. Help the unit function smoothly
   a. Report for duty on time and ready to work.
   b. Cooperate with other team members.
   c. Communicate effectively with residents, their families, and other members of the interdisciplinary health care team.
   d. Follow facility policies.
   e. Know and carry out assignments.

3. Protect the safety of residents
   a. Keep units clean and clutter free.
   b. Know how to operate equipment properly.
   c. Use standard precautions for routine care.
   d. Follow the principles of medical asepsis, including transmission-based isolation precautions when appropriate.
   e. Make beds properly.
   f. Report potential hazards as soon as noted.
   g. Useing bed side rails and restraints properly.
   h. Know and practice the fire safety plan of the facility.
   i. Know and practice the disaster plan of the facility.
   j. Know and practice emergency procedures for obstructed airway (Heimlich maneuver) and cardiopulmonary resuscitation.
   k. Follow oxygen precautions carefully.

4. Help residents by observing and collecting data
   a. Measure and record vital signs (temperature, pulse, respirations, and blood pressure).
   b. Measure weight and height.
   c. Measure intake and output.
   d. Collect specimens.
   e. Document and report observations of resident's condition.

*(continues)*

| **FIGURE 3-7** *(continued)* |
| --- |
| 5. Help residents meet personal hygiene needs<br>   a. Bathe residents.<br>   b. Give oral hygiene.<br>   c. Provide denture care.<br>   d. Provide nail and hair care.<br>   e. Assist residents to dress and undress.<br>   f. Shave residents.<br>   g. Apply support hose. |
| 6. Help residents meet nutritional needs<br>   a. Check food trays.<br>   b. Serve food trays.<br>   c. Assist residents who can help themselves.<br>   d. Feed dependent residents.<br>   e. Provide fresh water, nourishments, and supplements. |
| 7. Help residents meet elimination needs<br>   a. Assist with bedpans, urinals, and commodes.<br>   b. Empty urine collection bags.<br>   c. Give enemas.<br>   d. Assist with colostomy care. |
| 8. Help residents with restoration and mobility<br>   a. Turn and position residents in bed, wheelchair, or geri-chair to prevent complications of immobility.<br>   b. Assist in transfer activities.<br>   c. Carry out range of motion exercises.<br>   d. Help with ambulation.<br>   e. Assist with restorative activities.<br>   f. Encourage independence. |
| 9. Help in carrying out special procedures (as defined by the facility)<br>   a. Admitting, transfer, and discharge.<br>   b. Warm and cold applications.<br>   c. Providing catheter care.<br>   d. Providing ostomy care. |

## Staff Relations

All members of the interdisciplinary health care team are expected to be friendly and to cooperate with each other. This kind of relationship promotes a sense of **harmony**, which is important to create a calm atmosphere. Older residents are adversely affected by any discord among staff members. While you are in the facility, you must be supportive of and pleasant to everyone.

If a staff member or resident complains to you about another nursing assistant, tactfully refuse to comment. Never criticize your coworkers to the residents. Suggest that the matter be referred to the charge nurse.

Listen to residents and offer to help with legitimate problems according to facility policy. Always remember that the effectiveness of care is affected by interpersonal relationships. Good relationships improve care; poor ones can harm the quality of care.

## ASSIGNMENTS

The charge nurse makes out assignments based on the needs of the residents and availability of staff (Figure 3-8). At times your care load will be lighter than usual and at times much heavier. Remember that the staff works as a team. Develop a positive attitude and be ready to help when someone needs it.

Your assignment must be carried out with the resident's personal wishes in mind. Talk with the resident about the care plan so that the resident is involved in making decisions about how and when the plan can best be carried out.

Although you will be responsible for the care of specific residents, do not ignore a resident who needs help but is not part of your assignment. Never allow any resident to be uncomfortable or in danger. For exam-

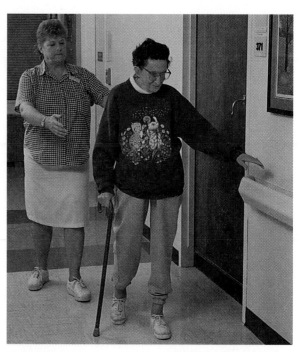

**FIGURE 3-9**   A nursing assistant saw that a resident needed help and moved quickly to assist.

ple, a resident who needs assistance to walk becomes impatient waiting in the day room for her assistant to help her return to her room. She stands up and starts unsteadily down the hall. You see potential danger and without hesitation assist her to her room even though she is not part of your specific assignment (Figure 3-9).

### Unfinished Assignments

Be sure to report any difficulty you have in performing a procedure or finishing an assignment. Tell the charge nurse of any tasks that are not completed at the time indicated. This can be very important. For example, you are assigned to give an enema before 10 o'clock in the morning. You have been very busy with a new admission and will not be able to do this procedure on time. Tell the charge nurse right away so the resident can receive the necessary care. Always tell the nurse if you believe there is any part of your assignment that you might not be able to complete. Plan ahead so that someone else may be assigned to take care of it and will have time to do the task.

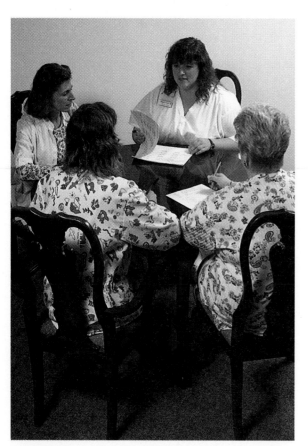

**FIGURE 3-8**   The supervising nurse gives an assignment to each nursing assistant.

## SPECIFIC DUTIES

The duties of a nursing assistant can be divided into four groups of activities:

1. Assisting in the activities of daily living (ADL)
2. Carrying out special procedures
3. Performing support services
4. Documentation (keeping records)

### Activities of Daily Living

Much of the nursing assistant's duties are centered on helping residents carry out the ADL that meet their physical, emotional, spiritual and social needs. The major physical needs of the resident include:

- Being clean
- Receiving proper exercise and positioning
- Receiving proper nourishment (Figure 3-10)
- Being able to eliminate wastes

Remember that each time residents participate in their own care or are able to contribute to making decisions, the residents feel they have some control over their own lives, which fosters independence.

### Special Procedures

Special procedures are required to care for residents with special needs. Special procedures include:

- Catheter care
- Ostomy care
- Measuring urine
- Giving enemas
- Collecting specimens

### Support Services

The third group of tasks does not necessarily involve resident contact. These tasks support the nursing care and include:

- Supplying drinking water
- Placing and removing meal trays (Figure 3-11)
- Making beds
- Caring for equipment
- Carrying messages

Each activity makes the nursing care better and more effective. For example, elderly per-

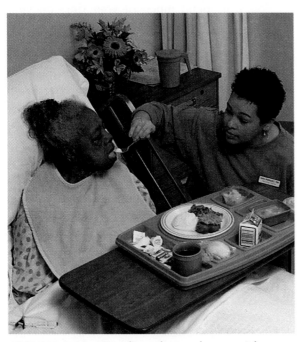

**FIGURE 3-10** Feeding dependent residents is a required nursing assistant duty that provides an essential ADL.

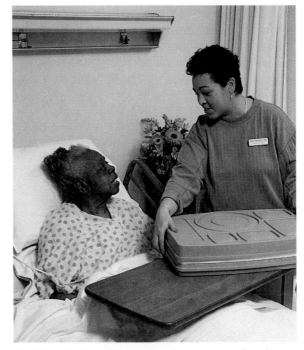

**FIGURE 3-11** Placing and removing food trays is a nursing assistant function.

sons often do not drink enough fluids, and part of your assignment is to encourage them to drink more liquids. Offer them liquids each time you enter the room.

### Documentation

The fourth group of nursing assistant tasks involves documentation of observations. These tasks are described in Lesson 6.

## ORGANIZATION OF TIME

Nursing assistants have many tasks to carry out during their on-duty time. The better organized you are, the more easily you will complete your tasks. You can become more organized by:

- Reporting for duty on time
- Listening to report
- Planning your work
- Working while on duty
- Trying to improve your performance

### Report for Duty at the Correct Time

Your job is your first responsibility. People are depending on you. If you are ill, you must call the facility as soon as you know that you will be unable to work so that someone can cover your responsibilities. If you have personal responsibilities that might affect your availability, you should discuss these with your employer when you are hired. Be sure that you and your employer agree as to how these responsibilities are to relate to your on-duty time.

Know who you should call if you cannot report for duty. Keep the telephone number and name beside your home telephone and in your wallet.

### Listen to the Report/Review Your Assignment

Note any changes in the care plans and any special orders that are to be followed. Make special note of orders that must be carried out at a specific time. Do not assume that because a resident has been at the facility for a long time, orders remain the same.

### Plan Your Work

Take a few moments to rearrange your plans if something unexpected develops during your shift. Refer to your plan frequently so that you can reorganize if necessary. *Remember that you are employed and paid to work for a whole shift.* Do not waste time chatting with coworkers. Be on time returning from breaks and lunch and do not leave early without permission. At the end of your shift review your assignment. Think of ways you might have used your time and energy more efficiently. Learn to organize activities and tasks in order of importance.

## SELF-CARE

Caregivers may get so involved in caring for others that they do not pay enough attention to their own well-being. You must take care of your own mental and physical health if you are to have the energy and enthusiasm to work successfully. When people are tired or stressed, they may find it hard to be cooperative, patient, and pleasant. Mistakes are more likely to be made. For your own sake and that of the residents in your care, you need to be at your best.

You will spend much of your time on your feet—walking corridors, pushing wheelchairs, handling equipment, and moving, supporting, and lifting residents—and carrying out detailed procedures. In addition you will be offering emotional support in a variety of situations. All of these activities require physical and emotional energy. To stay fit you will need:

- Sufficient rest
- Good nutrition
- Balanced recreation

There are some additional actions that you can take to promote your own well-being:

- Have regular physical examinations, including immunizations.
- Limit alcohol intake; do not drink alcohol while on duty or before reporting for duty.
- Limit or stop smoking.
- Always use proper body mechanics.
- Wear a support belt.
- Get help and use mechanical lifts when residents are heavy.
- Practice safe sex.

## Career Health

Nursing assistants also need to care for their careers. A nursing assistant who feels insecure in skills and knowledge cannot perform at a high level. You can increase your confidence when you:

- Follow procedures as they are taught
- Do only those activities that are within your job description
- Attend staff development programs
- Seek other opportunities to increase your nursing care knowledge and skills

## Emotional Health

You give so much of yourself to those in your care that you face the risk of burnout.

**Burnout** is mental and emotional—and sometimes physical—fatigue. People who work with the sick or infirm often experience burnout because of the emotional and physical demands of providing care. You can reduce the stress that leads to burnout by balancing your work with rest and recreation.

You can also learn stress-reducing techniques. Food and cigarettes are used by some people to reduce stress, but these can cause other serious health problems. To reduce stress try the following:

- Exercise at least three to five times a week, doing something you enjoy.
- Sit for a few moments with your feet up.
- Shut your eyes and take deep breaths.
- With your eyes shut, picture a special place you like, and be there in your mind.
- Take a warm relaxing bath.
- Listen to some quiet music.
- Carry out a specific relaxation exercise.
- Make yourself a cup of herbal tea and sip it slowly.
- Find a hobby that you really enjoy.
- Take a few minutes to talk with a friend (Figure 3-12).
- Meditate on your higher power or value belief system.

## SEXUAL HARASSMENT ···················

People cannot perform at their best when they are subjected to insensitive remarks or inappro-

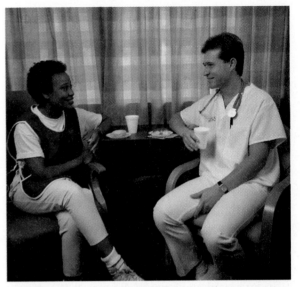

**FIGURE 3-12**  A quiet moment relaxing with a friend is a good way to reduce stress.

priate behavior by coworkers or supervisors. The anxiety these situations produce is increased by the fear of losing their jobs if they take action against the person responsible.

Sexual harassment may be expressed by actions, words, or implied threats. These behaviors create an environment that is hostile and nonproductive. Examples of sexual harassment include:

- The administrator makes sexual advances when you deliver reports to the office.
- A coworker rubs your neck as you document your completed tasks in the nurses' station.
- A coworker repeatedly tells off-color jokes in your presence even though you have asked him not to do so.
- A coworker makes remarks related to the size of your breasts, buttocks, or genitalia.
- Sexually explicit cartoons are posted on the staff bulletin board.
- A coworker reads and shows pornographic magazines during lunch.
- A supervisor tells you that your performance evaluation will be better if you are more "friendly."
- A charge nurse tells you that your assignments will be reduced if you agree to a date.

It is important to understand that you have the right to work in an environment that is free of sexual harassment. However, handling these situations requires sensitivity and tact. First, be sure that the situation is truly sexual harassment. Then:

- Tell the offender that you are displeased with the action.
- Document the incident so the details stay fresh in your mind.
- Report the situation to your supervisor.
- If the offender is your supervisor, follow the chain of command upward.

## CONTINUE TO GROW

Your training program prepares you to perform as a beginning level nursing assistant. You have a responsibility to continue your education and personal growth (Figure 3-13). If you are willing to do so, you may learn much from team leaders, charge nurses, and other nursing assistants.

The procedure and policy books kept at the nursing station are ready references when you have questions about a new procedure or how to handle a new situation. Become familiar with each of these sources and with the medical dictionary on your unit. Use the dictionary to look up and learn the correct spelling of medical words. Learn at least two new words each week and practice using them. Remember, always ask for help when in doubt. Always be ready to learn.

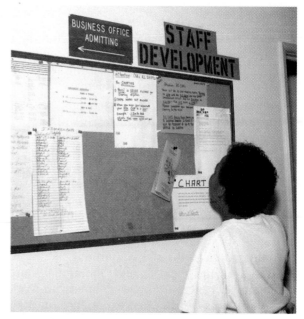

**FIGURE 3-13** Once employed, take advantage of staff development programs to advance your education.

Many facilities have professional magazines for staff use. Take advantage of this opportunity to increase your knowledge.

Care planning conferences can be an excellent way to expand your knowledge. Listen carefully. Remember, learning is a lifelong challenge.

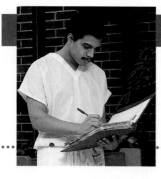

## LESSON SYNTHESIS: Putting It All Together

You have just completed this lesson. Now go back and review the Clinical Focus. Try to see how the Clinical Focus relates to the concepts presented in the lesson. Then answer the following questions.

1. How does Ray's attitude and maturity affect the level of care the residents receive?

2. How does the pride Ray has in himself show in his own appearance and work?

3. What important contributions do nursing assistants make to the well-being of residents through the activities they perform?

4. What responsibility does a nursing assistant have to maintain personal mental and physical health?

## REVIEW

**A. Match each term (items a.–e.) with the proper definition.**

a. accuracy      d. empathy
b. attitude      e. harmony
c. burnout

1. _____ friendly, cooperative atmosphere

2. _____ ability to put yourself in another person's position

3. _____ total emotional and mental fatigue

4. _____ outer reflection of inner feelings

5. _____ performing correctly

**B. Select the one best answer for each of the following.**

6. Recognizing needs that are expressed and those that are not expressed shows that the nursing assistant is
   a. dependable
   b. mature
   c. sensitive
   d. accurate

7. Maturity is related to
   a. age
   b. attitude
   c. accuracy
   d. none of these

8. The nursing assistant should bathe
   a. daily
   b. once a week
   c. twice each week
   d. every other day

9. Which of the following is a proper part of your uniform?
   a. earrings
   b. bracelets
   c. identification badge
   d. necklace

10. The nursing assistant is ready for work when
    a. fingernails are polished bright red
    b. strong aftershave lotion is applied
    c. wearing a watch with a second hand
    d. wearing bracelets

11. The activities and responsibilities of nursing assistants are
    a. stated in the procedure manual
    b. called a job description
    c. located in the nurses' manual
    d. the same all over the country

12. Nursing assistant assignments are based on
    a. the needs of the assistant
    b. the needs of the residents
    c. the wishes of visitors
    d. the wishes of social workers

13. The nursing assistant's uniform is
    a. worn on shopping trips
    b. worn for 3 days without washing it
    c. folded so the dirtiest side is on the outside when it is put into the laundry
    d. worn only on duty

14. The nursing assistant notices that a resident who is not assigned to him is walking unsteadily down the hall. He should
    a. ignore the situation
    b. assist the resident as needed
    c. notify the supervisor
    d. inform the assigned nursing assistant of the situation.

15. The nursing assistant has not had the time to carry out the exercises that had been ordered for the resident. It is now time to go off duty. She should
    a. tell another assistant to do the exercises
    b. go off duty because it is not really important that the exercises be done
    c. tell the supervisor right away
    d. plan to do double the amount of exercises the next day

**C. For each of the following duties, indicate if it is a duty of the nursing assistant by answering yes (Y) or no (N).**

16. Y  N   giving bed baths

17. Y  N   measuring temperatures

18. Y  N   serving trays

19. Y  N   starting intravenous fluids

20. Y  N   making beds

21. Y  N   applying sterile dressings

22. Y  N   calling physicians for orders

23. Y  N   weighing residents

24. Y  N   carrying messages

**D. Clinical Experiences**

Read each case history and answer the questions.

25. Mary was assigned to make the bed of a resident who was able to get out of bed. The supervisor was not satisfied with the way the bed was made and told Mary she would have to remake the bed. Mary was very angry. After the supervisor left, she complained to the resident.
    a. Did Mary show maturity in her reaction?
    b. How should Mary have reacted?

26. Mrs. Randolph is a very slow eater. She had a stroke and lost the use of her left side. She is naturally left-handed. Star, the nursing assistant, can feed Mrs. Randolph faster than she can feed herself, but Star lets Mrs. Randolph feed herself.
    a. Do you think Star has a special reason for letting Mrs. Randolph feed herself?
    b. What do you think her purpose is?

27. John did not complete his assignment on time and his supervisor told him he must plan more carefully. John said nothing but slammed the door on the way out of the office.
    a. Do you think John responded in a mature way?
    b. How can you tell?
    c. Is maturity a matter of age or attitude?

28. Even though they can feed themselves slowly, Carrie feeds her residents to save time.
    a. Is her method of feeding best?
    b. Is it more or less satisfying to the resident to be fed?
    c. What benefit is there in allowing residents to feed themselves?

29. Eric always comes to work on time, has a pleasant attitude, and finishes his assignment correctly.
    a. What important characteristic does Eric show by arriving on time?
    b. What characteristic does he show by being sure his assignments are correctly done?

30. Lois is very patient with the residents in her care because she says she would find it so hard to need help to go to the bathroom or to have to sit all day.
    a. By her actions Lois is showing what important characteristic?

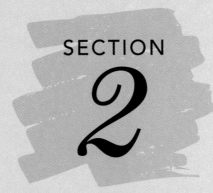

# Communication Skills

## LESSONS

*4*  Communication and
Interpersonal Skills

*5*  The Language of Health Care

*6*  Observation, Documentation,
and Reporting

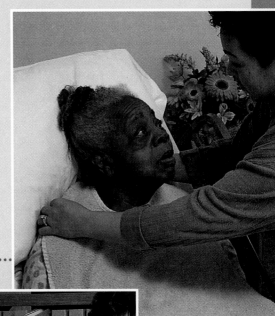

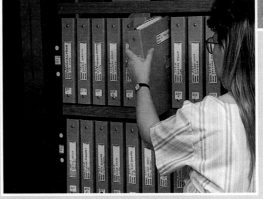

# 4

# Communication and Interpersonal Skills

## CLINICAL FOCUS

Think about how successful messages are sent

and received and how people communicate with

one another as you study this lesson and meet:

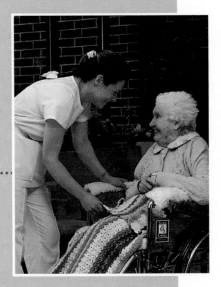

*D*oris Greene, age 83, who broke her hip and had no one to care for her at home. She has been a resident in long-term care for 4 years. She has no immediate family and her only sister lives 3,000 miles away. The staff and residents have become her family and friends.

## OBJECTIVES

*After studying this lesson, you should be able to:*

- Define and spell vocabulary words and terms.
- State two ways in which people communicate.
- Describe situations when nursing assistants must communicate with other staff members.

- Identify barriers to effective communications with residents.
- List general guidelines for communicating with residents.
- Describe ways in which a nursing assistant can improve communications with residents who have impaired hearing, impaired vision, aphasia, or disorientation.

## VOCABULARY

**aphasia**  *(ah-**FAY**-zee-ah)*
**articulation**  *(are-**tick**-you-**LAY**-shun)*
**assignment**  *(ah-**SIGHN**-ment)*
**body language**  *(**BAH**-dee **LAN**-gwihj)*
**Braille**  *(brayl)*
**care plan**  *(kair plan)*

**communication**  *(kom-**myou**-nih-**KAY**-shun)*
**disorientation**  *(dis-**oh**-ree-en-**TAY**-shun)*
**medical chart**  *(**MED**-ih-kul chart)*
**memo**  *(**MEM**-oh)*
**nonverbal communication**  *(**NON**-ver-bal kom-**myou**-nih-**KAY**-shun)*

# VOCABULARY

......................

shift report *(shift ree-***PORT***)*
symbol *(***SIM***-bull)*

verbal communication *(***VER***-bal kom-***myou***-nih-***KAY***-shun)*

..............................................................

## THE COMMUNICATION PROCESS....

Communication involves the exchange of information (Figure 4-1). For successful **communication**, you must have a:

* Sender
* Message
* Receiver

As a nursing assistant, you can assist in this process by using effective methods of communication with residents and coworkers. Some of the residents you care for will have barriers to effective communication. These may be caused by difficulties in hearing, seeing, or understanding what is being communicated. You can improve the quality of life for residents by communicating appropriately with each one (Figure 4-2). When residents speak a different language, you may need an interpreter to communicate effectively.

The two ways to communicate are:

* Verbally—using spoken language
* Nonverbally—using **body language** and **symbols**

## Verbal Communication

**Verbal communication** includes more than the words you speak. How you say the words also sends a message to the listener. When communicating verbally with others, be aware of:

* The tone of your voice
* Loudness (volume) of your voice
* Articulation
* Words or phrases with double meanings or cultural meanings
* Swearing or the use of slang

The tone of voice you use and its volume can convey a message of happiness, anger, sadness, or caring. Keep the volume of your voice at a moderate level. A harsh, loud voice is disturbing to others.

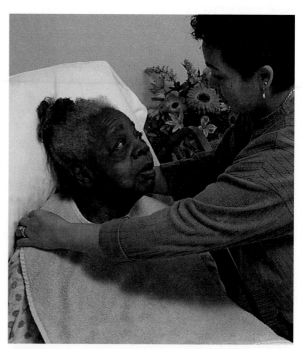

**FIGURE 4-2** The nursing assistant is listening to the resident relay the message.

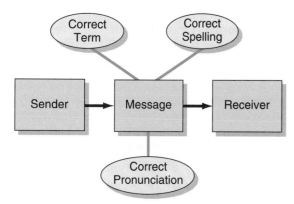

**FIGURE 4-1** The message can only be interpreted correctly if the words are chosen carefully and pronounced and spelled correctly.

**Articulation** is the clarity with which you pronounce words. If you do not articulate (speak clearly), others will not be able to understand you.

You will be caring for residents from many cultures and ethnic groups. Remember that certain words in your culture may have an entirely different meaning to someone else. Swearing is never permissible in a health care facility and slang is not to be used.

### Nonverbal Communication

Your **nonverbal communication** or body language can sometimes say more than words. Be aware of the message that is being sent through your:

- Body posture/position
- Body movements
- Facial expressions
- Activity level
- Overall appearance

Your body movements send messages that can give the receiver either a negative or positive reaction about you. Your appearance gives others their first impression about you. This impression is usually lasting; it is important that it be positive. As you work in the facility, be aware that your body language is sending messages to those around you (Figure 4-3). Remember that

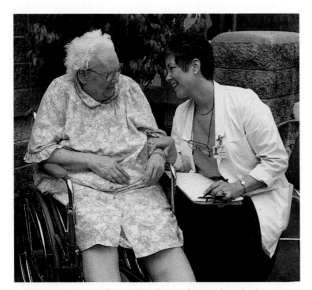

**FIGURE 4-3** The social worker's body language shows caring and interest in the resident's message.

residents may be looking at you when you are not aware of their attention.

## COMMUNICATING WITH STAFF MEMBERS

In Lesson 2 you learned that the organizational chart is a guide for communication. The organizational chart tells you the lines of authority. All facilities have an organizational chart that illustrates how each department relates to other departments. Some of the larger departments such as nursing have their own chart that indicates the line of authority within the nursing department (Figure 4-4). You will need to develop methods of communication with other staff members in nursing and with members of other departments.

## ORAL COMMUNICATIONS

When you first come on duty, you will listen to **shift report** (Figure 4-5). The nurse who worked the previous shift will report to staff coming on duty. This report will include:

- Changes in residents' conditions
- Information about new residents
- Names of residents who were discharged or died
- Any incidents that occurred to residents
- Physicians' new orders
- Special events for the residents that will occur during your shift

Listen carefully to the report because it will help you plan your **assignment** (Figure 4-6). Your assignment includes:

- Which residents you will care for during your shift
- The procedures you will need to do for these residents

Your supervising nurse will then give you additional information about your assignment based on the shift report. This information may include orders to complete procedures for specific residents:

- Take temperature, pulse, and respirations on designated residents

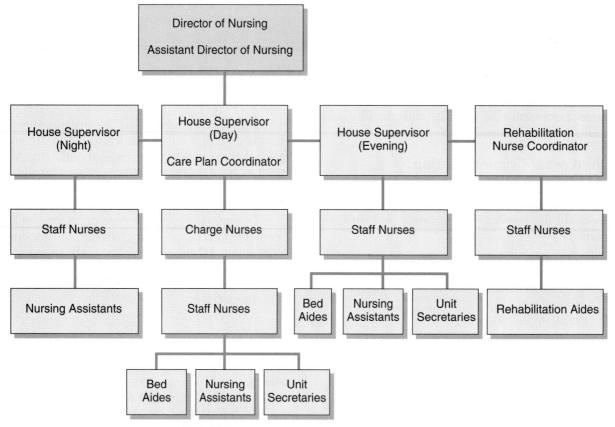

**FIGURE 4-4** Nursing organizational chart

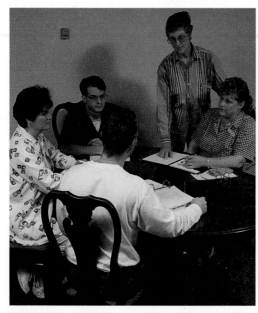

**FIGURE 4-5** A shift report is given at the beginning of every shift.

- Obtain weights on designated residents
- Allow a resident to remain in bed because of a change in condition
- Make observations on a resident who has had a change of condition

During your shift you will give oral reports to the nurse about procedures you have completed and observations you have made. At the end of the shift you will summarize your assignment to the nurse so that the information can be included in the shift report to the employees coming on duty when you leave. When leaving the nursing unit for any reason during your shift, always report to the nurse.

## Answering the Telephone

Many telephone calls come into a long-term care facility. Families call to ask about the condition of a loved one. Physicians call to leave new medical orders. The laboratory may call to give

| Rm. | Resident | Bath | Pos. Sched. | PROM | V.S. | WT. | B+B | ADL Prog. | Transfer | Safety |
|-----|----------|------|-------------|------|------|-----|-----|-----------|----------|--------|
| 101ᴬ | J. Damski | X | X | X | | | X | X | 2+TB | X |
| 101ᴮ | G. Jones | | X | X | X | X | | | Mech Lift | |
| 102ᴬ | C. Hernandez | X | | | | X | | | Indep. | |
| 102ᴮ | R. Lattini | X | X | X | | | X | | 2+ TB | X |
| 103 | N. Goldberg | X | | | X | X | X | | SBA | |
| 104ᴬ | M. Welch | | X | X | | | | | Mech Lift | |
| 104ᴮ | L. Ordoni | | X | X | | | X | X | 1+TB | X |
| 105 | B. Brinzoski | X | | | X | | X | | Indep. | |
| 106ᴬ | A. Feinstein | X | | | | X | | X | 1+TB | |
| 106ᴮ | D. Farmell | | X | X | X | | X | X | 2+TB | |
| 107 | T. Green | X | X | X | | X | X | | 2+TB | |
| 108ᴬ | H. Johnson | X | X | X | X | | | X | 2+TB | |
| 108ᴮ | B. Miller | | X | X | | X | | | 1+TB | X |

*Title row:* **CNA ASSIGNMENT SHEET**  **DATE** 4-18-XX

**FIGURE 4-6**  The assignment sheet gives directions for the duties to be completed.

results of diagnostic tests. Remember that nursing assistants are not allowed to take physician's orders or results of diagnostic tests or to give information to families. You must call the nurse to do this. If you answer the telephone:

- Identify the nursing unit: "third floor, north," for example.
- Identify yourself and your position: "Mary Smith, nursing assistant, how may I help you?"
- Ask the caller's name and ask the caller to wait while you locate the person called.
- If the person is unavailable, take a message (Figure 4-7) and write down the following information:
  - Date and time of call
  - Caller's name and telephone number
  - Message left by caller
  - Whether the person is to return the call or whether the caller will telephone again later
  - Your signature

Some facilities have more complex telephone systems. You will be taught how to transfer calls or to voice page. Most facilities do not allow employees to make or receive personal telephone calls while they are on duty.

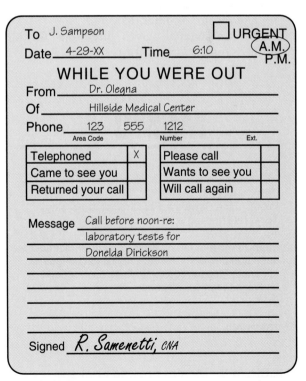

**FIGURE 4-7**  Telephone messages must be accurate and clear.

## WRITTEN COMMUNICATIONS··········

Many situations rely on written communications. The ability to accurately write or read the communication is essential to the care of the resident.

### Memos

A **memo** (Figure 4-8) is a brief communication that informs or reminds employees of:

• Changes in policies or procedures
• Upcoming meetings or staff development classes
• Admission of new residents
• Promotions of staff members

Be sure you know where memos are posted so that you will be aware of the facility activities.

### Manuals

All facilities have several manuals that provide information about policies and procedures (Figure 4-9). These may include:

• Employee personnel handbook—describes all the personnel policies and benefits
• Disaster manual—gives directions for actions to take for fire or other disasters
• Procedure manual—gives directions for all procedures performed for residents

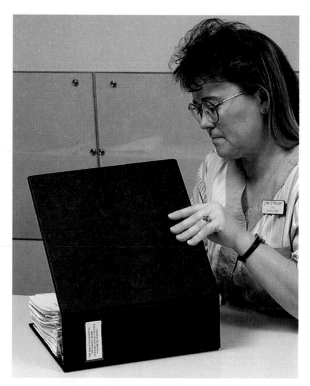

**FIGURE 4-9** The procedure manual provides information on all nursing procedures performed in the facility.

• Quality assurance manual—describes all quality control policies and procedures
• Nursing policy manual—describes rules and regulations pertaining to the care of the residents
• Dietary manual—explains therapeutic diets

You are not expected to memorize all the information contained in the manuals but you should know where they are kept on the nursing unit and be able to look up information when it is needed.

### The Resident Care Plan

Each resident has a **care plan** that has been developed by the interdisciplinary health care team (Figure 4-10). The care plan:

• Lists the resident's medical diagnoses
• Identifies the resident's problems
• Gives directions for resolving the resident's problems
• Lists the expected outcomes for resolving the problems

# MEMO

**Date:** April 21, 19XX
**From:** Jane Sowalski, RN Director of Nursing
**To:** All nursing staff

Please note that the Nursing Procedure Manual has been updated and revised. The list of changes is attached. Please read the indicated procedures and sign the attached page.

Thank you.

**FIGURE 4-8** Memos provide brief and important information.

| MARYSVILLE CARE CENTER | CARE PLAN | 02/06/1997 |
|---|---|---|
| | | FORM # 280L |

| PROBLEM | SHORT TERM GOAL | APPROACH |
|---|---|---|
| (1) Potential for impaired skin integrity<br>  a) Related to altered circulation in legs<br>  b) Related to flexion contracture of neck<br><br>    ONSET    TARGET    RESOLVE<br>    02/06/97  05/07/97   / / | (1) Will remain ulcer free (legs) through 5/7/97<br><br>    BEGIN    TARGET    RESOLVE<br>    02/06/97  05/07/97   / /<br><br>(2) Skin intact lower neck through 5/7/97<br><br>    BEGIN    TARGET    RESOLVE<br>    02/06/97  05/07/97   / / | (1) R.N. check legs q a.m.<br>    DISC: NSG<br><br>(2) Elevate legs when up in w/c.<br>    DISC: NA<br><br>(3) Wash and dry area b.i.d.<br>    DISC: NA<br><br>(4) Apply 4 x 4 to separate skin surfaces.<br>    DISC: NSG  NA<br><br>(5) Use Mycalog cream for increased redness prn.<br>    DISC: NSG |
| (2) Alteration in comfort<br>  a) Related to impaired circulation<br>  b) Related to joint pain<br><br>    ONSET    TARGET    RESOLVE<br>    02/06/97  05/07/97   / / | (1) 2 nocs/week without leg cramps by 5/7/97<br><br>    BEGIN    TARGET    RESOLVE<br>    02/06/97  05/07/97   / /<br><br>(2) States relief of pain with heat packs through 5/7/97.<br><br>    BEGIN    TARGET    RESOLVE<br>    02/06/97  05/07/97   / / | (1) Administer Procardia as ordered and assess effectiveness.<br>    DISC: NSG<br><br><br>(1) Heat packs to neck, shoulder, knees 5x/wk.<br>    DISC: RA |

| PHYSICIAN / ALT. PHYSICIAN | PHONE NO. | ALLERGIES / NOTES | | | | |
|---|---|---|---|---|---|---|
| WASHINGTON, JAMES M.D.<br>KEELEY, JANICE M.D. | (555) 555-8888 | PENICILLIN, ASPIRIN | | | | |

| RESIDENT | STATION / ROOM / BED | ADMISSION NUMBER / DATE | | SEX | DATE OF BIRTH | CARE PLAN DATE | PAGE # |
|---|---|---|---|---|---|---|---|
| | | | | | (73) | | |
| JAMES, FIONA | NORTH-122-B | 33652 | 10/18/1995 | F | 02/28/1923 | 02/06/1997 | 1 |

**FIGURE 4-10**  The care plan gives information for the resident's care.

Your assignment is based on the resident's care plan. You will learn more about the care plan in Lesson 6.

### The Resident's Medical Chart

Each resident has a **medical chart** or record (Figure 4-11). The medical chart contains:

- The physician's medical orders for that resident—medications, treatments, diagnostic tests
- The medical history of the resident—summary of all past illnesses and surgeries
- Results of physical examinations
- Results of all diagnostic tests—blood tests and x-rays

- Progress notes from the physician and from all disciplines involved in the resident's care—brief, periodic descriptions of the resident's condition and response to treatment
- Assessments from all disciplines—identifies the resident's problems
- Nursing notes—information that describes the resident's condition, nursing care given, and the resident's response to the care

The information entered into the chart is called documentation. The chart is a legal document. It may be used to:

- Determine payments by insurance companies
- Determine settlement of law suits

This means that all entries must be made in black ink and are considered permanent.

## COMMUNICATING WITH RESIDENTS

The ability to communicate with the resident is a skill that will develop with experience. It is not

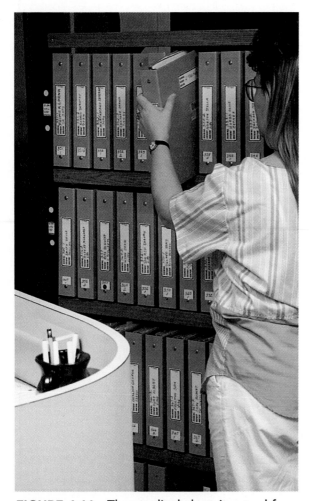

**FIGURE 4-11** The medical chart is a tool for communication.

### BUILDING CULTURAL AWARENESS

You should be aware that not all cultures view direct eye contact as meaning interest, attention, and courtesy. Some Asian and Native American cultures view sustained, direct eye contact as rude. People from these cultures normally would not look at a speaker directly for any length of time, nor would they stare at a person they were addressing. To do so is considered a sign of disrespect in their cultures. Do not make assumptions about the behavior of the residents in your care. If they are not of your culture, find out as much as you can about their culture. Refer to the resident assessment and care plan for information that is resident specific. This may be done if people from specific cultures are residents in the facility.

always the words you choose that are important, but the way in which they are said. Your tone of voice, facial expression, and even the way you touch a resident, all communicate a sense of honest caring, or lack of caring, to the resident. Looking directly at the resident as you speak and addressing the person respectfully by name are also indications of caring.

Listening actively is a special skill requiring more than just being physically present. When you listen actively, all of your attention is focused on the speaker. You maintain eye contact and do not interrupt while the other person is speaking. You ask questions that encourage the speaker to continue and respond to specific questions being asked. To communicate effectively:

- Face the resident.
- Speak slowly.
- Maintain eye contact.
- Listen carefully.
- Be patient and take your time.
- Use touch appropriately.
- Be aware of your body language.
- Do not sit or stand too close to the resident.
- Avoid finishing their sentences for them.

# *G*uidelines for
# Communicating with Residents

Remember these guidelines when you are communicating with residents.

## Sending a Message

First, be aware of the message you are sending to the resident:

1. Use nonthreatening words or gestures.
   - Be calm. Avoid rapid, jerky movements.
   - Speak clearly and courteously.
   - Use a pleasant tone of voice.
   - Use the name of the resident's choice. Some residents may wish to be called by Mr., Mrs., or Miss with the last name. Others will ask you to use their first names. Avoid using names like "dear" or "honey."
2. Use appropriate body language.
   - This includes your general appearance. Think about the first impression that you make. Do your uniform and grooming show pride in yourself and your work?
   - Your posture and movements will tell the residents whether or not you are enthusiastic about your work.

3. Show interest and concern when the resident is talking.
   - Use eye contact that is natural.
   - Try to communicate at eye level. Many residents are in wheelchairs so you may need to squat down or sit to do this.
   - Remain at a comfortable distance from the resident. For most people, this is about 2 feet away. If a resident is disoriented, this may be too close (Figure 4-12).

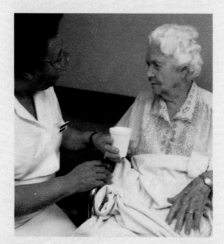

**FIGURE 4-12** Remain a comfortable distance from the resident.

*(continues)*

# *G*uidelines *(continued)*

4. Be considerate when you are working with residents.
   - Do not talk as if the resident is not present. Include the resident in the conversation.
   - Do not discuss personal activities with other staff members in the presence of the residents (Figure 4-13).
   - Do not interrupt when the resident is speaking.
   - Ask for clarification if you do not understand the resident.

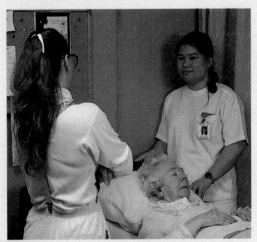

**FIGURE 4-13** It is inappropriate to discuss personal activities with other staff in the presence of residents.

5. Give the resident only factual information, not your personal feelings, opinions, or beliefs. Your responsibility as a nursing assistant is to listen in a nonjudgmental manner. Remember:
   - Do not give orders or advice to residents.
   - Do not use threats or warnings to get residents to do what you want them to do.
   - Do not criticize or make fun of residents' beliefs or ideas.
6. Information concerning the resident's condition, medications, and treatments should be given only by the nurse.

## Receiving a Message

Be sensitive to the message you are receiving from the resident.

1. Be alert to the resident's needs to communicate with you. Allow time for the resident to talk and respond.
2. Observe the resident's body language. This is especially important if a resident is unable to communicate verbally.
   - Does the resident's posture indicate the presence of pain?
   - Do the resident's gestures and movements indicate that the resident may be anxious or frightened? (Figure 4-14)

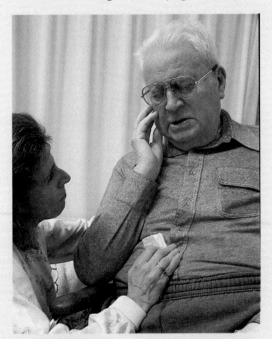

**FIGURE 4-14** The resident's body language indicates fear and anxiety.

3. Consider whether the resident can see and hear you. A resident may have difficulty paying attention if there are many distractions in the environment. This includes other people, televisions, and radios.

*(continues)*

---

### *G*uidelines *(continued)*

4. Report problems to the nurse if you are concerned with the resident's statements. Do not argue or try to talk a resident out of a belief.

5. Ask for clarification if you are unsure of what the resident is saying.
6. Reflect the feelings and thoughts of the resident by rewording the resident's statements into questions.

---

## COMMUNICATING THROUGH THE USE OF TOUCH

All human beings have a need to touch and be touched by others. Infants go through a "bonding" process when they are held close to another human being. This human contact is essential to the growth and development of infants and children. The need for touching is never outgrown. However, as people age, there are fewer opportunities for touching. Many older people no longer have a spouse. As one gets older, the circle of friends and relatives becomes smaller.

Nursing assistants can learn to use touch appropriately with the residents. First, you must know the residents. The way people touch each other may mean different things to different people. This is because everyone comes from a different background. Cultural meanings may be attached to touching. Be aware of these factors:

1. You will touch residents frequently while you are giving care. Be gentle and patient.
2. Touching others is not just physical contact. We touch others with our eye contact, facial expressions, and body language.
3. Some residents may have been physically abused in their past. They may associate all forms of physical contact with abuse. It may be difficult for them to accept nonthreatening forms of touch.
4. Some individuals view touching only as a preliminary to sexual intercourse. You will need to avoid touching these individuals in a way that can be misinterpreted.
5. Touching can be patronizing. An example of this is patting a resident on the head.

6. Holding a resident's hand can demonstrate a sense of caring (Figure 4-15).
7. For some residents, a hug may be suitable (Figure 4-16).

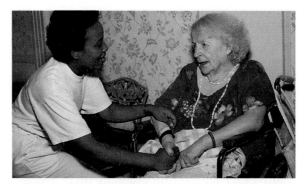

**FIGURE 4-15** Holding a resident's hand can show a sense of caring.

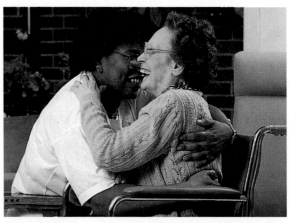

**FIGURE 4-16** Some residents may appreciate a hug.

8. Disoriented residents may be startled if you touch them unexpectedly. They may react aggressively. Be sure they are aware of your approach.
9. Touching residents appropriately can increase their self-esteem. It gives the message that you accept and care about them.

## COMMUNICATING WITH RESIDENTS WHO HAVE SPECIAL NEEDS

Some residents may have difficulty communicating with you. This may be caused by:

- Hearing impairment
- Vision impairment
- Aphasia
- Disorientation

Always check the care plan before attempting to communicate with a resident who has special communication needs. Specific approaches may be established for all staff members to use with the resident. Lack of consistency in the use of these approaches is confusing and frustrating to the resident.

### Communicating with Hearing Impaired Residents

Many older adults lose some of their hearing. Some of them may wear hearing aids. Even those who do may still have problems understanding others when they speak.

1. Get the resident's attention first.
   - Make sure the resident sees you.
   - Touch the resident lightly to indicate you wish to speak.
2. If the resident uses a hearing aid, be sure the resident is wearing it and that the hearing aid is on.
3. If the resident has a "good" ear, stand or sit on that side when you are talking.
4. Do not chew gum, eat, or cover your mouth while you are talking.
5. The light should be behind the resident, so your face can be clearly seen.
6. Face the resident; many hearing impaired people can read lips or interpret your facial expressions.

7. Reduce outside distractions. Turn off the television and move the resident to a quieter place.
8. Speak quietly and calmly.
9. Keep your voice pitch low.
10. Speak slowly, distinctly, and naturally.
11. Start conversation with a key word or phrase to identify the topic for the resident.
12. Form words carefully, use familiar words, and keep sentences short.
13. Rephrase words as needed.
14. Shouting, exaggerating words, or speaking very slowly only make it harder for the resident to understand you.
15. Use facial expressions, gestures, and body language to help express your meanings.
16. Some hearing impaired residents use sign language. Signing depends on hand and finger movements and facial expressions. It is a skill that requires learning and practice. There are different forms of sign language just as there are different spoken languages. Recognizing some basic signs may be helpful (Figure 4-17).
17. Residents who have been hearing impaired for several years may have speech that is difficult to understand.
18. Some hearing impaired people are embarrassed to tell you when they do not understand you. Watch the resident's facial expressions. You may be able to tell whether or not your message was understood.
19. People who cannot hear may appear confused when they are not.

### Communicating with Visually Impaired Residents

As people age, vision changes usually occur. These can generally be corrected with glasses. However, some older people have eye diseases that may seriously impair their vision. Even though they are not completely blind, they may be unable to see clearly.

Having a visual impairment does not necessarily mean the resident will have problems with communication. However, some actions you can take will make the resident feel more at ease.

1. When approaching a visually impaired resident, address the person by name and then touch him or her lightly on the hand or arm to avoid startling.

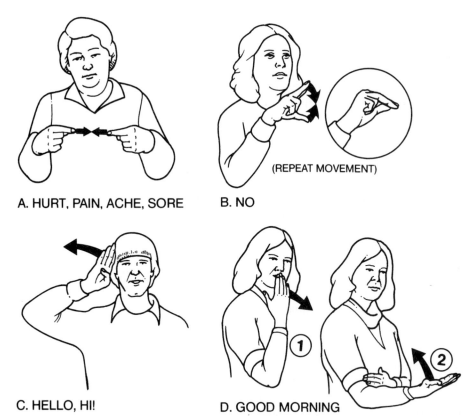

A. HURT, PAIN, ACHE, SORE          B. NO

(REPEAT MOVEMENT)

C. HELLO, HI!          D. GOOD MORNING

**FIGURE 4-17**   Signing: A. Palms facing chest, index fingers extended toward, but not touching one another. Thrust them toward one another several times: hurt, pain, ache, sore. B. Extend index and middle fingers, bringing them down to meet the thumb in two quick movements: no. C. Start with the index finger of the right hand at the right temple, palm forward and fingers pointing up. Bring the hand outward to the right: hello, hi. D. Start with the fingertips of the right open hand toward face. Touch lips and bring hand down, bending elbow. Touch inner elbow with left open hand as the right hand is brought upward: good morning.

2. After you speak to the resident, identify yourself and explain why you are there. "Hello, Mr. Smith. My name is Mary Jones and I would like to check your blood pressure."
3. Be specific when giving directions: "I am putting your mail on the right side of your bedside stand."
4. When giving directions for locating an area in the building, tell the resident how many doors to pass and when the resident should turn right or left.
5. When you leave the resident, make sure you announce your departure, "I am leaving your room now. May I get you anything else?"
6. Offer to read mail to visually impaired residents (Figure 4-18).

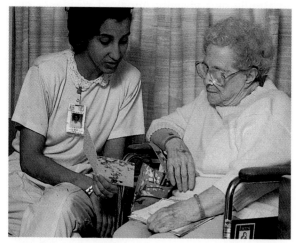

**FIGURE 4-18**   Offer to read mail to visually impaired residents.

7. Help the resident use a telephone by counting the numbers on the dial or otherwise guiding the resident verbally to make calls.
8. Tactfully inform a visually impaired person if clothing is soiled, unmatched, or in need of repair.
9. Encourage the resident to listen to the radio or television to keep up with news and current events.
10. Make sure the resident is aware of talking book machines. Inform social services or activities departments if the resident wishes to use these.
11. Describe the environment and objects around the resident. This helps avoid disorientation.
12. Describe the food served to the resident. Use an example of a clock. "Your meat is at 12:00, the peas are at 3:00, and the potato is at 9:00."

**Using Braille.**  Some residents with impaired vision may know how to read **Braille**. This is a system in which each letter of the alphabet and numbers 0 through 9 are translated into a unique pattern of raised dots. Rather than reading the printed letters with their eyes, those who know Braille "read" with their fingers as they touch the raised dots and spell out words. Many books and other printed materials are produced in Braille. In addition, most elevator controls are marked in Braille. Braille telephones are also available. Room numbers in facilities may also be marked in Braille and visually impaired residents may have their names marked in Braille outside their rooms.

## Communicating with Residents with Aphasia

**Aphasia** is a condition that results from damage to the area of the brain that controls speech. This can happen after a stroke or a severe brain injury. Some residents with aphasia:

- Have trouble expressing themselves, but may be able to understand some of the words you say
- Express themselves better than they can understand others

Aphasia can be frustrating to the resident and the caregivers. To communicate more effectively with residents with aphasia, follow these suggestions:

1. Face the resident and make eye contact before speaking.
2. Say the resident's name and include a social greeting ("Good morning, Mrs. Jones.") before asking questions or giving instructions.
3. Speak slowly and clearly. Use short, complete sentences.
4. Pause between sentences to allow the resident time to understand and interpret what you said.
5. Check the resident's comprehension before you proceed. Ask a question based on information you just gave the resident.
6. Use nonverbal cues to reinforce spoken communication. Gestures, facial expressions, or pictures are helpful.
7. Ask questions that require only short responses or answers that can be made nonverbally.
8. Repeat what the resident just said to help her keep focused on the conversation.
9. Find out if the speech therapist has devised methods of nonverbal communication such as communication boards or picture books.
10. Do not avoid talking to persons with aphasia. Do not shout to try and make them understand.
11. If you sense frustration, let the resident know that you are aware of the frustration. Suggest that you talk about something else for a while and then try again.

## Communicating with Disoriented Residents

Some residents in long-term care facilities are disoriented. **Disorientation** means the resident is not aware of time and place. This may be permanent, as a result of a mental impairment such as Alzheimer's disease. Sometimes disorientation is temporary. This is common in new residents until they get used to their new surroundings. Residents who have an acute illness such as an infection may also be temporarily disoriented. You can improve communication with disoriented residents when you:

1. Begin conversation by identifying yourself and calling the resident by name. Do not ask the resident if he remembers you or knows who you are. This puts the resident "on the spot" and may embarrass him.
2. Talk to the resident at eye level and maintain eye contact.
3. Maintain a pleasant facial expression while you are talking and listening.
4. Place a hand on the resident's arm or hand unless this causes agitation.
5. Make sure the resident can hear you.
6. Use a lower tone of voice.
7. Provide a calm and quiet environment.
8. Use short, common words and short, simple sentences.
9. Give the resident time to respond.
10. Ask only one simple question at a time. If you must repeat it, say it exactly the same way.
11. Ask the resident to do only one task at a time.
12. Residents with dementia will eventually be unable to understand any verbal communication.
    - Use pictures; point, touch, or hand things to the resident.
- Demonstrate the action when you want the resident to complete a task. For example, put the washcloth in your hand and make face washing movements. Then instruct the resident to do the same. If this does not work, use a hand-over-hand technique.
13. Understand the word substitutes used by the resident. If these are consistent, find out what they mean. Use them yourself to see if the resident understands you better.
14. Avoid abstract, common expressions that may be misunderstood. For example, "You can hop into bed now," means just that to the resident. The resident may indeed try to "hop" into bed.
15. Repeat the resident's last words to help stay on track during conversation.
16. Do not try to force the resident to understand. Avoid lengthy explanations and excessive verbal communication. This tends to agitate people who are disoriented.
17. Use nonverbal praise freely and always respect the resident's feelings.

The way in which you communicate with residents can make a difference in their lives. Be caring, considerate, and sensitive to their feelings and needs.

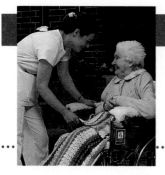

## LESSON SYNTHESIS: Putting It All Together

You have just completed this lesson. Now go back and review the Clinical Focus. Try to see how the Clinical Focus relates to the concepts presented in the lesson. Then answer the following questions.

1. How can Doris Greene meet her physical, emotional, and social needs if communications with the staff are ineffective?

2. How can the nursing assistant improve the flow of communication or make it more difficult?

3. What special situations may make communications especially difficult with this resident?

4. What can the nursing assistant do to improve communications in the situations listed for question 3?

5. Why is it especially important for communications to be open with Doris Greene?

## REVIEW

**A. Select the one best answer for each of the following.**

1. Successful communication requires a
   a. sender
   b. message
   c. receiver
   d. all of these

2. Verbal communication includes
   a. talking and listening
   b. facial expressions
   c. writing reports
   d. using a fax machine

3. Verbal communication is influenced by
   a. tone of voice
   b. choice of words used
   c. articulation
   d. all of these

4. Examples of nonverbal communication include
   a. gestures and body language
   b. answering the telephone
   c. listening to shift report
   d. conversing with residents

5. A nursing assistant may give or take which information over the telephone?
   a. report of a resident's condition
   b. physician's orders
   c. results of laboratory tests
   d. name of person leaving the message

6. The shift report is given by the
   a. administrator
   b. physician
   c. the nurse who worked the previous shift
   d. director of nursing

7. The purpose of the shift report is to
   a. give information about all the residents on the nursing unit
   b. discuss the social activities of the staff
   c. tell the nursing assistants when they are scheduled for days off
   d. rest before starting work

8. You must report to the nurse when you
   a. take a break or go to lunch
   b. leave the nursing unit for any reason
   c. have finished your shift
   d. all of these

9. One purpose of a memo is to inform staff of
   a. meetings or educational programs
   b. residents' conditions
   c. physicians' new orders for specific residents
   d. weather conditions

10. Examples of manuals that are found on nursing units include
    a. procedure manual
    b. disaster manual
    c. quality assurance manual
    d. all of these

11. The resident's care plan provides information for
    a. the nursing assistant assignments
    b. employee benefits
    c. the procedure for fire drills
    d. all of these

12. The resident's medical record or chart is
    a. used only by the physician
    b. used by all members of the interdisciplinary health care team
    c. a temporary record
    d. a report of the nursing assistant's competencies

13. You may receive messages from the resident's
    a. body language
    b. verbal statements
    c. facial expressions
    d. all of these

14. If a resident is disoriented it means the resident is
    a. mentally ill
    b. unaware of the environment and the time
    c. unable to communicate with you
    d. unable to hear

15. Aphasia means the resident
    a. has an infection of the respiratory tract
    b. is hearing impaired
    c. is disoriented
    d. is unable to speak or to understand the spoken language of others

16. When working with hearing impaired residents you should
    a. speak in a calm, quiet manner
    b. talk louder
    c. avoid speaking if possible
    d. speak very slowly

17. When working with residents with aphasia, it is best to
    a. use only hand gestures to communicate
    b. speak louder
    c. avoid communication if at all possible
    d. face the resident and make eye contact before speaking

18. Residents who are visually impaired should
    a. stay in their rooms to avoid getting lost in the facility
    b. have identification on their clothing so everyone realizes they are visually impaired
    c. learn to use sign language
    d. be given directions for locating various areas in the building

19. When working with disoriented residents you should
    a. ask the resident if he remembers you or knows who you are
    b. try to make the resident understand you
    c. avoid distractions of noise and activity when communicating with them
    d. get as close as possible to the resident when talking or giving care

20. Touching the resident can be a successful method of communication if you
    a. are gentle and caring
    b. use appropriate gestures, facial expressions, and eye contact
    c. hold a resident's hand
    d. all of these

**B.  Fill in the blanks by selecting the correct word or phrase from the list provided.**

| | |
|---|---|
| aphasia | medical chart |
| body language | memo |
| Braille | nonverbal communication |
| care plan | shift report |
| disorientation | verbal communication |

21. Persons who cannot express themselves verbally or understand verbal communications have _____.

22. Loss of recognition of time, place, location, or person is called _____.

23. The exchange of information given by the nurse going off duty to those coming on duty is called the _____.

24. The _____ is a legal document.

25. A brief, written message that provides information is a _____.

26. _____ is an example of nonverbal communication.

27. The record that contains a description of the resident's problems, the goals for resolving the problems, and the approaches used is the _____.

28. Sign language is an example of _____.

29. Talking orally is _____.

30. _____ is used by persons who are visually impaired.

# LESSON 5

## The Language of Health Care

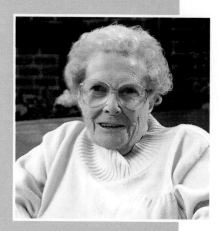

### CLINICAL FOCUS

Think about how your knowledge of the

language of health care and the human body

can improve your understanding of the

conditions of the residents in your care as you

study this lesson and meet:

*G*eorgina England, who is 74 years old, and has just been admitted to your facility because she can no longer care for herself. Her Hx reveals long-term arthritis, cardialgia, and recurrent cystitis. Her current admission Dx is ASHD, arthritis, and UTI. Part of her care plan includes: ass't c̄ ADL, Amb & Ass't c̄ cath care, I & O, VS q4h.

## OBJECTIVES

*After studying this lesson, you should be able to:*

- Define and spell vocabulary words and terms.
- Recognize the meanings of common suffixes and prefixes.
- Use combining forms to develop new words.
- Write terms and abbreviations commonly used in health care communications and documentation.

- Explain the organization of the body into cells, tissues, organs, and systems.
- Locate body parts and organs, using the proper anatomic terms.
- List body systems and their functions.

## VOCABULARY

**abbreviation**   *(ah-**BREE**-vee-**ay**-shun)*

**abdominal**   *(ab-**DOM**-ih-nal)*

**anatomic position**   *(**an**-ah-**TOM**-ick poh-**ZISH**-un)*

**anatomy**   *(ah-**NAT**-oh-mee)*

**anterior**   *(an-**TEER**-ee-or)*

**cardiac muscle**   *(**KAR**-dee-ack **MUS**-ell)*

**cavity**   *(**KAV**-ih-tee)*

# VOCABULARY

cell  *(sell)*

combining forms  *(kom-**BUY**-ning forms)*

connective tissue  *(kuh-**NECK**-tiv **TISH**-you)*

connective tissue cell  *(kuh-**NECK**-tiv **TISH**-you sell)*

cutaneous membrane  *(kyou-**TAY**-nee us **MEM**-brain)*

distal  *(**DIS**-tal)*

dorsal  *(**DOR**-sal)*

epithelial cell  *(**ep**-ih-**THEE**-lee-al sell)*

epithelial tissue  *(**ep**-ih-**THEE**-lee-al **TISH**-you)*

gerontology  *(**jer**-on-**TOL**-oh-jee)*

inferior  *(in-**FEER**-ee-or)*

kidneys  *(**KID**-nees)*

lateral  *(**LAT**-er-al)*

medial  *(**MEE**-dee-al)*

membrane  *(**MEM**-brain)*

meninges  *(meh-**NIN**-jeez)*

mucous membrane  *(**MYOU**-kus **MEM**-brain)*

mucus  *(**MYOU**-kus)*

muscle cell  *(**MUS**-ell sell)*

muscle tissue  *(**MUS**-ell **TISH**-you)*

nerve cell  *(nurv sell)*

nervous tissue  *(**NUR**-vus **TISH**-you)*

organ  *(**OR**-gan)*

pancreas  *(**PAN**-kree-as)*

pathology  *(pah-**THOL**-oh-jee)*

pericardium  *(**pair**-ih-**KAR**-dee-um)*

peritoneum  *(**pair**-ih-toh-**NEE**-um)*

physiology  *(**fiz**-ee-**OL**-oh-jee)*

pleura  *(**PLOOR**-ah)*

posterior  *(pos-**TEER**-ee-or)*

prefix  *(**PREE**-fix)*

proximal  *(**PROX**-ih-mal)*

quadrant  *(**KWAHD**-rant)*

serous membrane  *(**SEE**-rus **MEM**-brain)*

skeletal muscle  *(**SKEL**-eh-tal **MUS**-ell)*

skin  *(skin)*

smooth muscle  *(smooth **MUS**-ell)*

suffix  *(**SUF**-fix)*

superior  *(soo-**PEE**-ree-or)*

synovial membrane  *(sih-**NOH**-vee-al **MEM**-brain)*

system  *(**SIS**-tum)*

tissue  *(**TISH**-you)*

umbilicus  *(um-**BILL**-ih-kus)*

ventral  *(**VEN**-tral)*

word root  *(werd root)*

## THE LANGUAGE OF HEALTH CARE

You have learned that people communicate information to one another in different ways. It is important that the sender and receiver understand the same message.

Two ways to help keep the message clear in written and oral communications are:

- Choosing the correct word or term to express the message
- Spelling or pronouncing the word properly

Health care has its own language and sometimes a single letter or two can change the entire meaning.

For example:

- *Ilium* is part of the pelvic bone.
- *Ileum* is part of the intestinal tract.
- *Perineum* is an area of the body between the vagina and anus.
- *Peritoneum* is a membrane that lines one of the body cavities.

You can see how important it is to use the correct scientific terms and to spell them accurately.

## WORD PARTS

The language of health care is formed by building on common word parts (Figure 5-1).

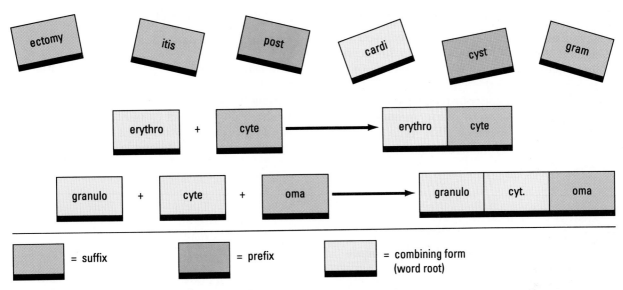

**FIGURE 5-1**   New words can be formed by putting different combining forms together.

These parts include:

- **Word roots**—usually refer to the part of the body described or the condition being treated.
- **Combining forms**—combinations of root words and other forms. Sometimes vowels are added at the end of the root to make it easier to connect other word parts.
- **Prefixes**—word parts found at the beginning of a word to change or add to its meaning.
- **Suffixes**—word parts found at the end of a word to change or add to its meaning.
- **Abbreviations**—shortened forms of words (often just letters).

For example, the word form *cyte* means cell. It is a common combining form because the human body is made up of many different kinds of cells. *Cyte* is seen in different positions in many words and the letter *C* may refer to cell in abbreviations.

Look at the following examples carefully:

- *Cyto*logy—(prefix) study of the cell
- Erythro*cyte*—(suffix) red blood cell
- Granulo*cyt*oma—(root word) a tumor made up of cells called granulocytes
- WB*C*—(abbreviation) white blood cell

## EXPANDING YOUR VOCABULARY...

During your career you will continue to add to your understanding and ability to use scientific terms. Here are some ways to help yourself.

- Use the facility medical dictionary to check new words.
- Look up new words; note spelling, meaning, and pronunciation.
- Get a medical dictionary and keep it available at home.
- Keep a notebook of new words (Figure 5-2), writing down:
  - Definitions
  - Spelling
  - Pronunciation
- Practice writing new words until you spell them correctly without checking your notebook or the dictionary.

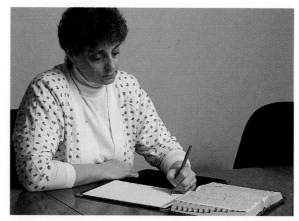

**FIGURE 5-2**   Keep a notebook of new terms to expand your vocabulary.

- Try to use each new term correctly three times in the next month. If you succeed, you can claim it as your own. You might do this in your conversation, in your documentation, or by simply explaining the word to a coworker.
- Be willing to accept your teacher's or supervisor's suggestions as to proper pronunciation and usage. Remember, this is a learning process and everyone needs a guide.

## COMMON WORD PARTS

### Combining Forms

The basic combining forms listed in the following tables will serve as a foundation for your learning. Your teacher may make selections from this list. Study each set carefully and do the exercises in the text and workbook and you will have started on a path of lifelong learning.

## Combining Forms

| Combining Form | Meaning | Example | Meaning |
|---|---|---|---|
| abdomin (o) | abdomen | abdominal | portion of body between the thorax and the pelvis |
| arthr (o) | joint | arthritis | inflammation of a joint |
| bronch (i)(o) | bronchus | bronchiectasis | abnormal enlargement of passageways that carry air into and out of the lungs |
| cardi (o) | heart | cardialgia | pain in the region of the heart |
| cephal (o) | head | cephalic | pertaining to the head |
| cerebr (o) | brain | cerebro-vascular accident | another name for a stroke |
| chol (e) | bile | cholecystitis | inflammation of the gallbladder |
| col (o) | colon, large intestine | colectomy | excision of the colon |
| crani (o) | skull | craniotomy | opening of the skull |
| cyst (o) | bladder, cyst | cystitis | inflammation of the bladder |
| cyt (o) | cell | cytology | study of cells |
| dent (i) (o) | tooth | dentist | person licensed to practice dentistry |
| dermat (o) | skin | dermatitis | inflammation of the skin |
| enter (o) | small intestine | enteritis | inflammation of the intestines |
| gastr (o) | stomach | gastritis | inflammation of the lining of the stomach |
| glyc (o) | sugar | glycemia | sugar in the blood *(continues)* |

## Combining Forms *(continued)*

| Combining Form | Meaning | Example | Meaning |
|---|---|---|---|
| hem (o), hemat (o) | blood | hematuria | discharge of blood in urine |
| hepat (o) | liver | hepatitis | inflammation of the liver |
| hydr (o) | water | dehydration | not having adequate water |
| hyster (o) | uterus | hysterectomy | surgical removal of the uterus |
| laryng (o) | larynx | laryngectomy | partial or total removal of the larynx by surgery |
| mast (o) | breast | mastitis | inflammation of the breast |
| men (o) | menstruation | menstrual | pertaining to menstruation |
| my (o) | muscle | myalgia | muscular pain |
| nephr (o) | kidney | nephrolithiasis | presence of renal calculi |
| neur (o) | nerve | neuropathy | any disease of the nervous system |
| oste (o) | bone | periosteum | specialized connective tissue covering all bones of the body |
| ot (o) | ear | otitis media | inflammation of the middle ear |
| pharyng (o) | throat, pharynx | pharyngitis | inflammation of the pharynx |
| pneum (o) | lung, air, gas | pneumonectomy | resection of lung tissue |
| proct (o) | rectum | proctoscopy | rectal exam with a proctoscope |
| psych (o) | mind | psychology | study of human behavior |
| pulm (o) | lung | pulmonary | pertaining to the lungs |
| py (o) | pus | pyogenic | producing pus |
| rect (o) | rectum | rectocele | hernial protrusion of part of the rectum into the vagina |
| thorac (o) | chest | thoracotomy | opening of the chest |
| thromb (o) | clot | thrombosis | formation of blood clots inside a blood vessel |
| trache (i) (o) | trachea | tracheotomy | incision of the trachea |
| ur (o) | urine | urinalysis | analysis of the urine   *(continues)* |

## Combining Forms *(continued)*

| Combining Form | Meaning | Example | Meaning |
|---|---|---|---|
| urin (o) | urinary tract | urinopathy | disease in any part of the urinary system |

## Common Prefixes

| Prefix | Meaning | Example | Meaning |
|---|---|---|---|
| a- | without | asepsis | without infection |
| ante- | before | antemortem | before death |
| anti- | against, counteracting | antidote | substance that counteracts the effects of a poison |
| brady- | slow | bradycardia | slow heart rate |
| dys- | pain or difficulty | dysuria | painful urination |
| hyper- | above, excessive | hypertension | high blood pressure |
| hypo- | low, deficient | hypotension | low blood pressure |
| poly- | many | polyuria | excessive urine |
| post- | after | postoperative | after surgery |
| pre- | before | premenstrual | before the menses |
| tachy- | fast | tachycardia | pulse rate above normal |

## Common Suffixes

| Suffix | Meaning | Example | Meaning |
|---|---|---|---|
| -ectomy | excision of | mastectomy | excision of a breast |
| -emia | blood | anemia | lacking sufficient quality or quantity of blood |
| -gram | record | electro-cardiogram | record produced by electrocardiography |
| -itis | inflammation of | bronchitis | inflammation of the bronchi |
| -logy | study of | hematology | study of blood                        *(continues)* |

## Common Suffixes (continued)

| Suffix | Meaning | Example | Meaning |
|--------|---------|---------|---------|
| -oma | tumor | fibroma | a tumor containing fibrous tissue |
| -otomy | incision | tracheotomy | incision of the trachea |
| -plegia | paralysis | hemiplegia | paralysis of one side of the body |
| -pnea | breathing, respiration | apnea | temporary cessation of breathing |
| -scope | examination instrument | otoscope | instrument for inspecting the ear |
| -scopy | examination using a scope | proctoscopy | rectal exam with a proctoscope |

## COMMON ABBREVIATIONS

Lists of abbreviations and their meanings follow. They have been grouped according to most common usage for easier learning.

Specific abbreviations may have different meanings in different parts of the country and in different facilities. For example, drg in one facility may mean *drainage*, yet in another facility it is used to mean *dressing*. Both facilities may use IDDM to mean *insulin-dependent diabetes mellitus*. Lists of facility approved terms and abbreviations are usually found in the policy or procedure manual.

### Body Parts

| | |
|---|---|
| **abd** abdomen | **GU** genitourinary |
| **AU** auditory | **lt (L)** left |
| **AX** axillary | **os** mouth |
| **bld** blood | **sh** shoulder |
| **GI** gastrointestinal | **vag** vagina, vaginal |

### Diagnoses

**AIDS** acquired immune deficiency syndrome

**AKA** above knee amputation

*(continues)*

### Diagnoses (continued)

**ASHD** arteriosclerotic heart disease

**BKA** below knee amputation

**CA** cancer

**CAD** coronary artery disease

**CHD** coronary heart disease

**CHF** congestive heart failure

**COPD** chronic obstructive pulmonary disease

**CVA** cerebrovascular accident; stroke

**DJD** degenerative joint disease

**FUO** fever of unknown origin

*(continues)*

## Diagnoses *(continued)*

**Fx** fracture

**HBV** hepatitis B virus (infection)

**HIV** human immune deficiency virus (infection)

**IDDM** insulin-dependent diabetes mellitus

**KS** Kaposi's sarcoma

**MI** myocardial infarction; refers to the death of heart tissues due to loss of blood supply (heart attack)

**MRSA** methicillin-resistant *Staphylococcus aureus*

**MS** multiple sclerosis

**NIDDM** non–insulin-dependent diabetes mellitus

**NSU** nonspecific urethritis

**PID** pelvic inflammatory disease

**PVD** peripheral vascular disease

**RF** renal failure

**SDAT** senile dementia of Alzheimer's type

**STD** sexually transmitted disease

**TIA** transient ischemic attack

**URI** upper respiratory infection

**UTI** urinary tract infection

## Patient Orders and Charting

**ā** before

**ADL** activities of daily living

**ad lib.** as desired

**adm** admission

*(continues)*

## Patient Orders and Charting *(continued)*

**ADT** admission, discharge, transfer

**amb** ambulate, ambulatory

**ASAP** as soon as possible

**as tol** as tolerated

**B.M., bm** bowel movement

**BP** blood pressure

**B.R.** bed rest, bathroom

**BRP** bathroom privileges

**BSC** bedside commode

**c̄** with

**cath** catheterize/catheter

**CBB** complete bed bath

**CBR** complete bed rest

**ck** check

**cl liq** clear liquid

**c/o** complains of

**CP** care plan

**DAT** diet as tolerated

**DC, D/C** discontinue

**disch** discharge

**DNR** do not resuscitate

**DR** doctor

**drg** dressing, drainage

**DSD** dry, sterile dressing

**Dx** diagnosis

**E** enema

**GT** gastrostomy tube

*(continues)*

## Patient Orders and Charting
*(continued)*

**HOB** head of bed

**HOH** hard of hearing

**ht** height

**Hx** history

**I & O** intake and output

**irrig** irrigation

**isol** isolation

**IV** intravenous

**lg** large

**liq** liquid

**MDS** minimum data set

**N/C** no complaints

**neg** negative

**NGT** nasogastric tube

**NPO** nothing by mouth

**N & V** nausea and vomiting

**NVD** nausea, vomiting, diarrhea

**O** oral

**O₂** oxygen

**OOB** out of bed

**p̄** after

**per** by

**p.o. (per os)** by mouth

**PPE** personal protective equipment

**p.r.n.** whenever necessary

**pt** patient; pint (500 mL)

**Px** prognosis (prog)

*(continues)*

## Patient Orders and Charting
*(continued)*

**q.s.** sufficient quantity

**qt** quiet

**R** rectal

**rehab** rehabilitation

**resp** respiration

**rt (R)** right, routine

**Rx** treatment

**s̄** without

**sm** small

**spec** specimen

**SSE** soap suds enema

**stat** at once, immediately

**Sx** symptoms

**TIAN** toilet in advance of need

**TPN** total parenteral nutrition

**TPR** temperature, pulse, respiration

**TWE** tap water enema

**Tx** traction

**TY** tympanic

**ung.** ointment (oint)

**VS** vital signs

**w/c** wheelchair

**wt** weight

## Tests

**AFB** acid-fast bacillus

**CBC** complete blood count  *(continues)*

## Tests (continued)

**FBS** fasting blood sugar

**UA** urinalysis

## Places or Departments

**CS** central supply

**Lab** laboratory

**MRD** medical record department

**OT** occupational therapy

**PT** physical therapy

## Time Abbreviations

**a.c.** before meals

**AM** morning

**b.i.d.** twice a day

**h** hour

**h.s.** hour of sleep (bedtime)

**noc, noct** night

**p.c.** after meals

**PM** evening or afternoon

**qd** every day

**qh** every hour

**q2h** every 2 hours

**q.i.d.** four times a day

**qm (qAM)** every morning

**qn** every night

**qod** every other day

**t.i.d.** three times a day

**WA** while awake

## Roman Numerals

| | |
|---|---|
| **I** 1 | **VI** 6 |
| **II** 2 | **VII** 7 |
| **III** 3 | **VIII** 8 |
| **IV** 4 | **IX** 9 |
| **V** 5 | **X** 10 |

## Measurements and Volume

**cc** cubic centimeter

**mL** milliliter

**L** liter

## Weight/Height

**kg** kilogram

**lb** pounds

**in** inches

## Temperature

**F** Fahrenheit

**C** Celsius

**°** degree

## UNDERSTANDING THE BODY

The reasons for the type of care given to residents are based on an understanding of how the body is made, how it functions normally, and the changes caused by age and disease.

These reasons, or principles, are derived from four sciences:

- **Anatomy:** the study of structure
- **Physiology:** the study of function
- **Gerontology:** the study of aging
- **Pathology:** the study of disease

## ANATOMIC TERMS

Special terms are used to describe the location and relationship of body parts and organs. Knowing these terms will help you to study and learn more easily. You will also be able to communicate more accurately as you report and record your observations.

### The Anatomic Position

Health care providers must use the same frame of reference when describing the resident's body, the position of the resident, and actions to be taken. For example, everyone who works with the resident must understand and describe precisely where the back of the resident's left wrist is and which is the resident's right hand.

It is helpful to view the resident as if he or she were standing in the **anatomic position.** This means the resident:

- Is standing
- Is facing the observer
- Has hands at the sides
- Has palms forward (Figure 5-3)

This means that the heels will always be toward the back, even if the resident is resting on the abdomen or lying on the side. The breasts will always be described as facing front even if she is sitting in a wheelchair or walking away from you. Notice also that the resident's left hand will be on the same side as your right hand. It is the same as looking at a mirror image.

### Descriptive Terms

Imaginary lines drawn through the body (Figure 5-4) can provide us with other reference terms.

- A line drawn down the center of the body from head to foot divides the body into equal right and left sides. Note that the body has the same parts on either side. For example, there is an

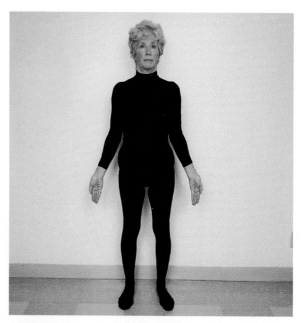

**FIGURE 5-3** In the anatomic position, the person is standing, facing forward, with palms forward.

arm, a leg, an eye, and half of a nose on each side of the line.

- Parts close to this line are **medial** to the line.
- Parts farther away from the line are **lateral** to the line.
- For example, in the anatomic position, the thumbs are more lateral to the line and the little fingers are more medial to the line.

Another line drawn parallel to the floor divides the body into upper and lower parts. This line can be drawn at any level on the body as long as it is parallel to the floor.

- Parts located above this line are **superior** to the line.
- Parts located below this line are **inferior** to the line.
- For example, if the line is drawn between the knees and ankles, the knees are superior to the ankles and the ankles are inferior to the knees.

A third line can be drawn to divide the body into front and back.

- Parts in front of this line are **anterior** or **ventral** to the line.
- Parts in back of this line are **posterior** or **dorsal** to the line.

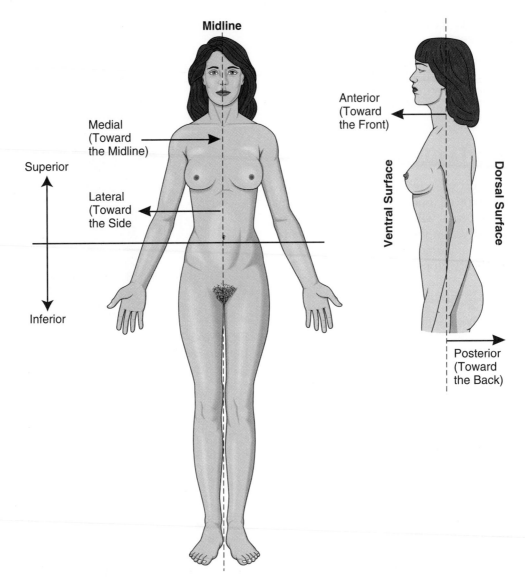

**FIGURE 5-4** Imaginary lines can be used to section the body to make it easier to locate parts.

## Points of Attachment

The arms and legs are called the extremities of the body. The arms are attached to the body at the shoulders. The legs are attached to the body at the hips. Two terms are used to describe the relationship between the parts of the extremities and their points of attachment to the body.

- **Proximal**—means closest to the point of attachment
- **Distal**—means farthest away from the point of attachment

Because the upper arm is closest to the shoulder, where it is attached, this part is described as proximal when compared to the fingers, which are farthest away. The fingers are distal or farthest away from the point of attachment of the upper extremity. Figure 5-5 presents a summary of terms.

## Abdominal Quadrants

If a resident places his or her hand on the anterior **abdominal** wall, complaining of pain, you

**FIGURE 5-5** Summary of terms relating to the anatomic position and the location of parts

- **Anterior** or **ventral** refers to the front.

- **Posterior** or **dorsal** refers to the back.

- **Lateral** refers to the side (away from the midline).

- **Medial** refers to the center of the body (midline).

- **Proximal** means closest to the point of attachment.

- **Distal** refers to the point farthest away from the point of attachment.

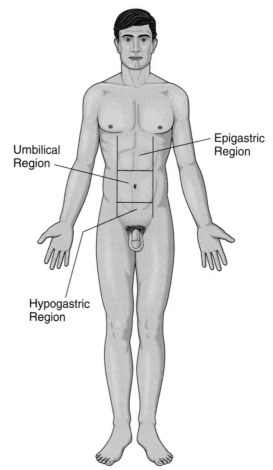

FIGURE 5-7 The abdomen can also be described as having three medial regions.

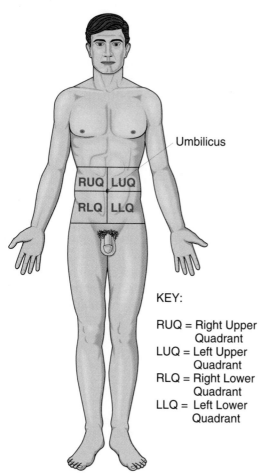

KEY:

RUQ = Right Upper
Quadrant
LUQ = Left Upper
Quadrant
RLQ = Right Lower
Quadrant
LLQ = Left Lower
Quadrant

**FIGURE 5-6** The abdominal quadrants

must be able to describe the area in proper terms. For reference, the anterior wall of the abdomen is divided into four parts or **quadrants** (Figure 5-6). The center of the area is the **umbilicus**. The abdomen can also be described as having regions (Figure 5-7).

## ORGANIZATION OF THE BODY

All parts of the body are interdependent. The basic unit of the body is the **cell**. Groups of similar cells are organized into **tissues**. Different tissues form **organs**. The organs are organized into **systems** that perform the body functions.

# CELLS

Each cell performs the same basic functions that the total body performs, but on a smaller scale. These functions are breathing (respiration), reproduction, nutrition, and excretion (eliminating wastes). Some cells perform different kinds of work necessary for the body as a whole to function. Some of the various specialized types of cells are:

- Epithelial cells
- Nerve cells
- Muscle cells
- Connective tissue cells

**Epithelial cells**, which are very close together, form protective coverings and sometimes produce body fluids.

**Nerve cells** carry electrical messages to and from the different parts of the body, coordinating activities and making us aware of changes in the environment.

**Muscle cells** are special in their ability to shorten or lengthen, changing their shape and the position of parts to which they are attached. They also surround body openings, such as the mouth, to control the size of these openings.

**Connective tissue cells** are present throughout the body in many different types. They support and connect body parts.

# TISSUES

Groups of similar cells are organized into tissues. The basic tissue types are:

- Epithelial tissue
- Connective tissue
- Nervous tissue
- Muscle tissue

**Epithelial tissue** is specialized in its ability to absorb, secrete (produce) fluids, excrete (eliminate) waste products, and protect.

**Nervous tissue** forms the brain and spinal cord and the nerves throughout the body. This tissue is also found in the special sense organs such as the eyes, ears, and tastebuds. The activities of the rest of the body are directed and coordinated through the nervous tissues.

Three kinds of **muscle tissue** are found in the body:

- **Skeletal muscle** is attached to bones for movement.
- **Cardiac muscle** forms the heart wall.
- **Smooth muscle** (visceral) forms the walls of body organs such as the stomach and intestines.

**Connective tissue** forms blood, bone, and fibrous and elastic tissues to hold the skin on the body, attach muscles to bones, and support delicate cells throughout the body. Generally, connective tissues support and form connections for other tissue types.

# ORGANS

Each organ is made up of more than one kind of tissue and performs special functions that contribute to the function of the body systems. Some organs, like the **kidneys**, are found in pairs. Some single organs contribute to more than one system. For example, the **pancreas** contributes secretions to both the endocrine and digestive systems.

# SYSTEMS

The body has 10 major body systems. Figure 5-8 lists the organs that contribute to the function of each system. Notice that some organs are included with more than one system. For example, the ovaries contribute to the endocrine system by producing female hormones and to the reproductive system by producing the female egg.

# MEMBRANES

**Membranes** are sheets of epithelial tissues supported by connective tissues. Membranes:

- Cover the body
- Line body cavities
- Produce some body fluids

**FIGURE 5-8**  Systems of the body

| System | Function | Organs |
|---|---|---|
| Cardiovascular | Transports materials around the body; carries oxygen and nutrients to the cells and carries waste products away; part of the immune system that provides protective cells and chemicals to fight current infections and protect against future infections | Heart, arteries, capillaries, veins, spleen, lymph nodes, lymphatic vessels, blood, lymph |
| Endocrine | Produces hormones that regulate body processes | Pituitary gland, thyroid gland, parathyroid glands, thymus gland, adrenal glands, testes, ovaries, pineal body, islets of Langerhans in pancreas |
| Gastrointestinal (Digestive) | Digests, transports food, absorbs nutrients, and eliminates wastes | Mouth, esophagus, pharynx, stomach, small intestine, large intestine, salivary glands, teeth, tongue, liver, gallbladder, pancreas |
| Integumentary | Protects the body from injury and against infection, regulates body temperature, eliminates some wastes | Skin, hair, nails, sweat and oil glands |
| Skeletal | Supports and protects body parts, produces blood cells, acts as levers in movement | Bones, joints |
| Muscular | Protects organs by forming body walls, forms walls of some organs, assists in movement by changing position of bones at joints | *Smooth* muscles—form walls of organs<br>*Skeletal* muscles—attached to bones<br>*Cardiac* muscles—form wall of heart |
| Nervous | Coordinates body functions | Brain, spinal cord, spinal nerves, cranial nerves, special sense organs such as eyes and ears |
| Reproductive | Reproduces the species, fulfills sexual needs, develops sexual identity | *Male:* Testes, epididymis, urethra, seminal vesicles, ejaculatory duct, prostate gland, bulbourethral glands, penis, spermatic cord<br>*Female:* Breasts, ovaries, oviducts, uterus, vagina, Bartholin glands, vulva |
| Respiratory | Brings in oxygen and eliminates carbon dioxide | Sinuses, nose, pharynx, larynx, trachea, bronchi, lungs |
| Urinary | Manages fluids and electrolytes of body, eliminates liquid wastes | Kidneys, ureters, urinary bladder, urethra |

**FIGURE 5-9** Body cavities and the organs contained within each cavity

| | Cavity | Organs | |
|---|---|---|---|
| **Dorsal Cavity** | Cranial | Brain, pineal body, pituitary gland | |
| | Spinal | Nerves, spinal cord | |
| **Ventral Cavity** | Thoracic | Lungs, heart, great blood vessels, thymus gland | |
| | Abdominal Peritoneal | Stomach, small intestine, most of large intestine, liver, gallbladder, pancreas, spleen | |
| | Pelvic | *Male* Seminal vesicles, prostate gland, ejaculatory ducts, urinary bladder, urethra, rectum | *Female* Uterus, oviducts, ovaries, urinary bladder, urethra, rectum |
| | Retroperitoneal Space | Kidneys, adrenal glands, ureters | |

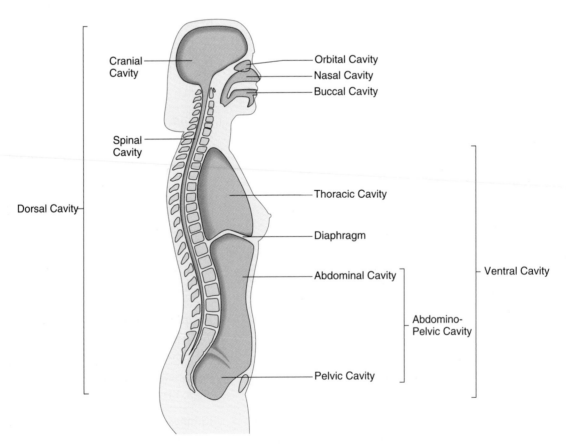

**FIGURE 5-10** Lateral view of body cavities

Important membranes include:

- **Mucous membranes**
  - Produce a fluid called **mucus**
  - Line body cavities that open to the outside

Because the respiratory, digestive, and genitourinary systems all open to the outside they are lined with mucous membranes. The eyelids are also lined with a mucous membrane; a mucous membrane covers the eyeballs.

- **Synovial membranes**
  - Produce synovial fluid
  - Line joint cavities

The synovial fluid is a clear fluid resembling the white of an egg. It reduces the friction between the bones of active joints and the tendons.

- **Serous membranes**
  - Produce serous fluid
  - Cover the organs and line the closed cavities of the body

Serous fluid reduces friction as the organs work and move. Important serous membranes are the:

- **Pericardium**—surrounds the heart
- **Pleura**—surrounds the lungs and lines the thoracic cavity

- **Meninges**—cover the brain and spinal cord and line the dorsal cavity
- **Peritoneum**—covers the digestive organs and lines the abdominal cavity
- **Cutaneous membrane (skin)**
  - Protects the body
  - Covers the entire body
  - Helps to control body temperature
  - Eliminates wastes through sweat glands
  - Produces vitamin D when exposed to sunlight

Special epithelial cells in this membrane, called glands, secrete perspiration and oils.

## CAVITIES

The body seems like a solid structure, but **cavities** (spaces) within it contain the organs. Figure 5-9 lists the two main cavities, the dorsal cavity and the ventral cavity. Each of these cavities is lined by and divided into other cavities by serous membranes. These other cavities are also listed in Figure 5-9, as are the organs contained in each.

Figure 5-10 is a simple drawing of the location of these cavities.

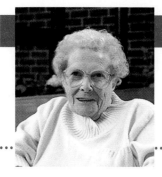

## LESSON SYNTHESIS: Putting It All Together

*Y*ou have just completed this lesson. Now go back and review the Clinical Focus. Try to see how the Clinical Focus relates to the concepts presented in the lesson. Then answer the following questions.

1. What health problems has Mrs. England had prior to her present problem?

2. What health problems have made admission to the long-term facility necessary?

3. Which activities would you be performing as part of Mrs. England's care?

4. What value to you, as a nursing assistant, is knowing the language of health care?

## REVIEW

**A. Complete the definition by crossing out the incorrect term in each sentence.**

1. The word part found at the end of a word to change or add to its meaning is the (prefix) (suffix).

2. A word that means the study of aging is (gerontology) (pathology).

3. The term that means the front of the body is (ventral) (dorsal).

4. The term meaning closest to the point of attachment is (distal) (proximal).

5. Cells that are specialized to produce body fluids like mucus are called (nerve cells) (epithelial cells).

**B. Based on the prefixes in each of the words, match the correct meaning (items a.–e.) with the word.**

a. excessive urine
b. high blood pressure
c. painful urination
d. rapid pulse
e. slow pulse

6. _____ bradycardia

7. _____ hypertension

8. _____ dysuria

9. _____ tachycardia

10. _____ polyuria

**C. Based on the suffixes in each of the words, match the correct meaning (item a.–e.) with the word.**

11. _____ electrocardiogram

12. _____ mastectomy

13. _____ hematology

14. _____ bronchitis

15. _____ anemia

a. excision of a breast
b. record produced by electrocardiography
c. inflammation of the bronchi
d. study of blood

e. insufficient quantity or quality of blood

**D. Match the tissue with its function.**

*Tissue*
a. connective       c. muscle
b. epithelial       d. nervous

*Function*

16. _____ coordinates body activities

17. _____ attached to bones for movement

18. _____ forms the walls of the stomach and intestines

19. _____ connects and supports body parts

20. _____ specialized in its ability to excrete waste products

21. _____ found in the eyes, ears, and tastebuds

22. _____ specialized in its ability to absorb

23. _____ forms the heart wall

24. _____ forms blood and bone

25. _____ forms nerves

**E. Match the organ to the system of which it is a part.**

*System*
a. cardiovascular    d. digestive
b. respiratory       e. reproductive
c. endocrine         f. urinary

*Organ*

26. _____ kidney

27. _____ uterus

28. _____ small intestines

29. _____ heart

30. _____ lungs

31. _____ urinary bladder

32. _____ mouth

33. _____ thyroid gland

34. _____ veins

35. _____ gallbladder

**F. Using your knowledge of combining forms, prefixes, and suffixes, write a medical word that means each of the following. Then check to see if you can find it in the glossary at the back of the book.**

36. without infection

_____

37. instrument for inspecting the ear

_____

38. study of the cells

_____

39. tumor containing fibrous tissue

_____

40. after surgery

_____

**G. Name the areas indicated in the diagram. Select from the list provided.**

left lower quadrant       right lower quadrant
left upper quadrant       right upper quadrant

41. _____

42. _____

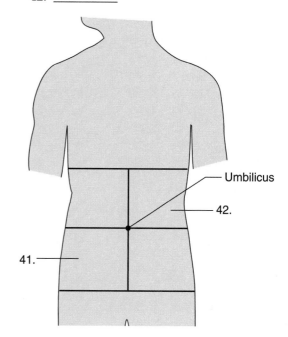

Umbilicus

42.

41.

## LESSON 6

# Observation, Documentation, and Reporting

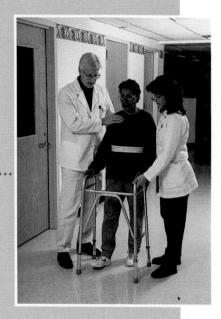

## CLINICAL FOCUS

Think about using your vision, hearing, sense of smell, and your sense of touch to learn about the residents as you study this lesson and meet:

Mrs. Sara Bass, who was admitted to the facility from the local hospital after having surgery for a fractured hip. She is going to rehabilitation every day in the hope that she will be able to return to her home. The hospital reported that she was disoriented after surgery.

## OBJECTIVES

*After studying this lesson, you should be able to:*

- Define and spell vocabulary words and terms.
- Describe one observation to make for each body system.
- Explain the difference between an objective observation and a subjective observation.
- Explain the difference between signs and symptoms.

- List the information to include when reporting off duty.
- List the guidelines for documentation.
- Name the four components of the interdisciplinary health care team process.
- Describe the responsibilities of the nursing assistant for each component of the interdisciplinary health care team process.

## VOCABULARY

**approach**  *(ah-**PROHCH**)*
**assessment**  *(ah-**SESS**-ment)*
**care plan conference**  *(kair plan **KON**-fer-ens)*
**document**  *(**DOCK**-you-ment)*
**evaluation**  *(ee-**val**-you-**AY**-shun)*

**goal**  *(gohl)*
**implementation**  *(**im**-plih-men-**TAY**-shun)*
**intervention**  *(**in**-ter-**VEN**-shun)*
**Minimum Data Set (MDS 2.0)**  *(**MIN**-ih-mum **DAY**-tah set)*

# VOCABULARY

nurse's notes   *(NUR-sez nohts)*

nursing diagnosis   *(NURS-ing die-ag-NOH-sis)*

objective observation   *(ob-JECK-tiv ob-sir-VAY-shun)*

observation   *(ob-sir-VAY-shun)*

resident care plan   *(REZ-ih-dent kair plan)*

sign   *(sighn)*

symptom   *(SIMP-tum)*

subjective observation   *(sub-JECK-tiv ob-sir-VAY-shun)*

## OBSERVATION

One of the most important skills you will develop is the ability to make accurate observations. An **observation** is something you notice about the resident. Some observations must be reported immediately. Other observations may be reported later to the nurse. You must carry a pen and paper with you at all times. You can then make notes of your observations. If you try to rely on your memory, you may forget some vital information when you give your report. You make observations by using your senses:

- You use your eyes to see observations:
    - Blood in the urine
    - Bruises or breaks in the skin
    - The resident crying
    - A change in the way the resident walks
- Your ears to hear observations:
    - Wheezing when the resident breathes
    - Pulse or blood pressure with a stethoscope
    - Comments from the resident such as "I am very tired today"
- Your nose to smell observations:
    - Body odor
    - Stool or urine when the resident is incontinent
- Your hands and fingers to use your sense of touch:
    - A lump under the resident's skin
    - Radial pulse
    - Warmth or coolness of the resident's skin

### Sign and Symptoms

The things you notice are called signs and symptoms. A **sign** is objective evidence of disease. These are facts that can be seen or measured by the observer (Figure 6-1). Examples of signs are:

- Rashes, bruises, pressure ulcers
- Elevated temperature
- Vomiting
- Rapid heartbeat

When you observe a sign, you are making an **objective observation**

**Symptoms** are subjective evidence of disease. These are facts that need to be relayed from the resident to the observer; that is, the resident tells you either verbally or through body language (Figure 6-2). Examples of symptoms are:

- The resident tells you he has nausea
- Anxiety—may be noted by the resident's behavior such as pacing or the resident may tell you she is nervous
- Pain—may be noted by the resident's position or he may tell you he has pain

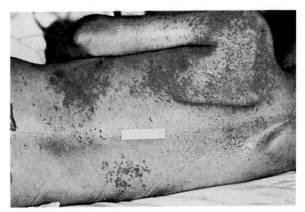

**FIGURE 6-1** A rash is an example of a sign—it is an objective observation.

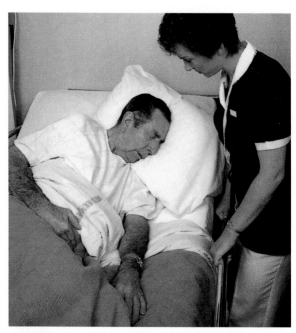

**FIGURE 6-2**   The resident's body language and facial expression are examples of subjective observations.

When a resident reports a symptom to you, you are making a **subjective observation**.

Observations provide evidence of:

- A change in the resident's physical condition. Example: A resident with diabetes may be having an insulin reaction.
- A new condition that is developing. Example: A pressure ulcer may be noted (Figure 6-3).
- A change in the resident's mental condition. Example: A resident who has shown no signs of disorientation is now wandering about stating he does not know where he is.
- A change in the resident's emotional condition. Example: A resident is crying and states she "does not want to continue living."
- The effectiveness of a medication or treatment. Example: A resident may be taking an antibiotic for a urinary tract infection. If the signs and symptoms of the infection are not going away, then the medication may not be effective and the physician will need to change the order.
- A change in the resident's ability to function. Example: The resident may not be able to walk as far or may not be able to complete an activity of daily living independently.

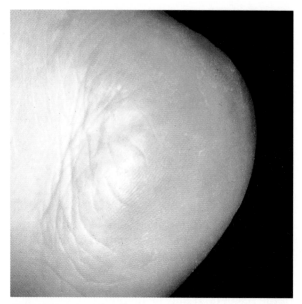

**FIGURE 6-3**   The first sign of a pressure ulcer should be reported immediately.

Remember that observations:

- Must be accurate and timely
- Are reported to the nurse immediately
- Are documented in the resident's record either by you or the nurse

## Making Initial Observations

To make accurate observations you must first know what is expected or normal for an individual. For this reason, baseline information is collected when the resident is admitted to the facility. If you help admit a resident, make observations while you are completing your assignment. It is especially important to note any signs of injury or skin breakdown. Think of the body systems as an organized way of making observations. This information will provide you with a basis for making future comparisons. For example, one resident may have a blood pressure of 110/68 on admission. If you take the resident's blood pressure later and it is 140/88 you should report this to the nurse because this is not the usual blood pressure for this person.

## Body System Observations

Try to establish a routine way of making observations. Keep in mind the age and known illness

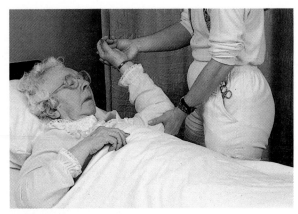

**FIGURE 6-4** Noting the resident's ability to move the joints is an observation of the musculoskeletal system.

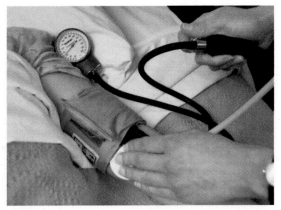

**FIGURE 6-5** Taking blood pressure provides important information about the circulatory system.

of the resident. It may be helpful to think of each body system and note the following:

- Integumentary system (skin, nails)
  - Color: flushed, pale, jaundiced (yellow color), or cyanotic (bluish gray color); nails pale, pink, or cyanotic
  - Temperature: warm, hot, cool
  - Moisture: dry, moist, perspiring
  - Abnormalities: rashes, bruises, scars, pressure ulcers, areas of redness, skin tears
- Musculoskeletal system (muscles, bones, joints)
  - Posture: stooped, curled up in bed, straight
  - Mobility: ability to move in bed, to get out of bed, to stand, and to walk
  - Range of motion: ability to move all joints (Figure 6-4)
- Circulatory system (heart, blood vessels, blood)
  - Pulse: strength, regularity, rate
  - Skin: color, temperature, moisture (see integumentary system)
  - Nails: (see integumentary system)
  - Blood pressure: within normal limits or high (hypertension) or low (hypotension) (Figure 6-5)
- Respiratory system (nose, throat, trachea, bronchi, lungs)
  - Respirations/breathing: rate, regularity, depth, difficulty breathing, shortness of breath on exertion or while still, wheezing or crackling heard
  - Cough: frequency; dry, loose, or productive; color, amount, and consistency of sputum (if any)

- Nervous system (brain, spinal cord, nerves)
  - Mental status: orientation to time, place, person; ability to make verbal or nonverbal responses
- Senses (eyes, ears, nose, sense of touch)
  - Eyes: reddened, drainage, pupils equal in size
  - Ears: drainage
  - Nose: drainage, bleeding
  - Sense of touch: ability to feel pressure and pain
- Urinary system (kidneys, ureters, bladder, urethra)
  - Urination: frequency, amount, color, clarity, presence of blood or sediment (Figure 6-6), ability to hold urine, incontinence, pain on urination (dysuria)
- Digestive system (mouth, teeth, throat, esophagus, stomach, large and small intestines, gallbladder, liver, pancreas)
  - Appetite: amount of fluids and food consumed, tolerance to foods, belching or burping
  - Eating: difficulty chewing or swallowing, nausea or vomiting or both
  - Bowel elimination: frequency, amount, consistency, color of stools, diarrhea, constipation, incontinence, flatus, difficulty passing stool
- Endocrine system (glands)
  - Signs and symptoms of diabetes: blood sugar imbalance
- Reproductive system (male and female internal and external sex organs)

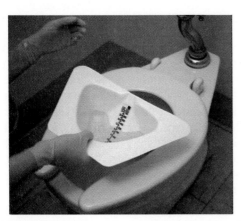

**FIGURE 6-6**  Before discarding urine check the amount, color, clarity, and the presence of blood or sediment.

- Female
  - Breasts: condition of nipples, presence of lumps, discolorations, scars, bleeding, or discharge
  - Menstrual periods: frequency, amount and character of bleeding, cramping
  - Vaginal drainage: amount, odor, character
- Male
  - Testes: lumps
  - Penis: amount, odor, character of drainage

## Observations of Pain and Behavior

You also need to note facts related to the resident's pain and behavior.

- Pain: location, type (sharp, burning, dull, aching), constant or intermittent or related to specific activities
- Behavior: actions, conduct, functioning

It is important that you be very objective in reporting observations of pain and behavior. Never try to judge whether a resident really has pain or how severe it is. Some individuals are expressive about pain and others try not to show their discomfort. Never compare residents. One person may seem to have more pain than another person with the same diagnosis. It is not appropriate to think that they should both respond in the same way.

When you report to your supervisor about the resident's behavior, do not use "labels" based on your judgment of the resident. Describe only what you see and hear. Refer to Figure 6-7 for examples of how certain behaviors should be reported.

You will make additional observations that are related to the resident's medical diagnoses. For example, if a resident has a kidney condition, you will look for edema (swelling) of the face, hands, and ankles. You will also monitor the person's fluid intake and output. You will

**FIGURE 6-7**  When reporting observations of residents' behavior, you will report only what you see and hear (second column). The words in the first column are judgments, opinions, or assumptions.

| Resident's Actions | What You Will Report |
| --- | --- |
| agitating other residents | 0300 Out of bed, talking to roommates, attempting to get them out of bed |
| confused | 0210 States over and over that he "wants to go to Maywood to see his mother." |
| disoriented | 0100 States "I want to go to church today because it is Sunday." |
| combative | 2130 Hit nursing assistant 2x on upper arm with fist when nursing assistant attempted to change incontinent pad. |
| uncooperative | 1300 Refused to get up from chair when nursing assistant tried to take to bathroom. |
| verbally abusive | 1420 Called resident in next bed a "stupid, ignorant idiot." |
| physically abusive | 1000 Scratched nursing assistant on face when bed was being changed. |

learn more about observations related to medical diagnoses as you study these conditions.

In some situations you may be expected to report "normal" observations. This information tells the nurse and physician whether the resident's condition is improving. For example, if a resident has a respiratory tract infection and the signs and symptoms have decreased, it is important to report that "no coughing or respiratory distress is noted."

# REPORTING

When you make observations, you must report your findings to the nurse. Be specific when you describe your observations. If you are relaying a subjective observation (something the resident has told you), repeat it exactly the way the resident told it to you. Here are examples:

- "Mr. Jones in 249 says it hurts every time he urinates."
- "Mrs. Bernetti says her heart is racing and feels like it's skipping beats."
- "Mrs. Goldberg was wandering around in the hall and said she did not know where she was."

When you report off duty at the end of your shift, report to the nurse:

- The condition of each of the residents you cared for
- The care you gave each resident
- Observations you made while giving care

# DOCUMENTATION

In some facilities you may be expected to document your observations on the resident's medical chart. A document is a legal record. The resident's care, response to treatment, and progress are documented (charted) in the resident's chart. To **document** means to write out your findings. Nursing assistants may document on flow sheets in the chart or on the **nurse's notes** (sometimes called nurse's progress notes, Figure 6-8). The charting must:

- Address the problems listed in the resident's care plan
- Describe the interventions listed in the care plan and note whether or not the interventions are effective
- Indicate the progress the resident is making toward meeting the goals on the care plan

## Charting Guidelines

A resident's medical record (chart) is a legal document and may be used in court as legal evidence. Everything *must* be correct and legible. All charting and records must be in clear, simple, and accurate language. Entries must be printed or written carefully so that the meaning is not misunderstood. If you follow the established rules of charting, you will avoid problems (Figure 6-9).

Each chart relates only to one resident so it is unnecessary to use the term *resident* or to use the resident's name. Phrases rather than sen-

| NURSE'S PROGRESS NOTES | | |
|---|---|---|
| DATE AND TIME | NURSING CARE NOTES | SIGNATURE |
| 3-16-XX | 2200 Found lying on floor beside bed. Responds verbally. States was "trying to get to the bathroom." Nurse notified immediately_____ | *C. Simmons CNA* |
| | 2205 ROM satisfactory. Denies having pain. No injuries noted. Assisted back to bed. Call light within reach. Instructed to use call light when having to go to B.R. Pulse 86, strong and regular. B/P 136/84. Oriented to time, place, person. Incontinent after fall. Pajamas chgd._____ | |
| | 2300 Sleeping s̄ distress_____ | *B. Selici RN* |
| 3-17-XX | 2400-0200 Sleeping soundly. Respirations regular. Pulse 78 strong and regular._____ | |
| | 0230 Awake. c/o "arthritis pain" in both hips. Acetaminophen tabs ii given with water. Assisted to bathroom. Voided large amt. clear urine._____ | |
| | 0230-0630 Slept soundly. Pulse 72 strong and regular. B/P 128/80. T 98⁶(0). Denies pain anywhere. No other c/o distress._____ | *P. Hernandez RN* |
| 3-17-XX | ~~2400 Up to B.R. c̄ assistance~~_____Error ES | *E. Seldes LPN* |

**FIGURE 6-8** Nursing assistants may document on the nurse's notes in the resident's chart.

tences should be used and there should *never* be erasures or empty spaces on the record. All entries are made in black or blue ink because it is a permanent record; no erasable ink or correction fluid is allowed. If you make an error, draw one line through the error, write "error" above it, and sign your initials.

If you use medical terms in your charting, make sure you are using the correct words and that spelling is correct. Use a medical dictionary if you are not sure. Abbreviations are allowed but they must be on the approved list of your facility. Do not make up your own abbreviations. You must chart only for yourself and only when the procedure or assignment has been completed.

The time of entry must be noted when the entry is made. Most health care facilities use international (24-hour) time (Figure 6-10) to

| **FIGURE 6-9**　Guidelines for accurate charting |
|---|
| • Check for: Right resident<br>　　　　　　 Right chart<br>　　　　　　 Right room |
| • Fill out new headings completely. |
| • Use correct color of ink. |
| • Date and time each entry. |
| • Make entries in proper time sequence. |
| • Make entries brief, objective, and accurate. |
| • Spell each word correctly. |
| • Print or write clearly. |
| • Leave no blank spaces or lines between entries. |
| • Do not use the term *resident*. |
| • Do not use ditto marks. |
| • Sign each entry with first initial, last name, and job title. |
| • Make corrections by drawing one line through entry; then print the word "error" and your initials above. |

**FIGURE 6-10**　24-Hour clock

| Standard Clock | International Time (24-Hour Clock) |
|---|---|
| 12:00 midnight | 2400 or 0000 |
| 1:00 AM | 0100 "oh one hundred" |
| 2:00 AM | 0200 "oh two hundred" |
| 3:00 AM | 0300 |
| 4:00 AM | 0400 |
| 5:00 AM | 0500 |
| 6:00 AM | 0600 |
| 7:00 AM | 0700 |
| 8:00 AM | 0800 |
| 9:00 AM | 0900 |
| 10:00 AM | 1000 "ten hundred" |
| 11:00 AM | 1100 "eleven hundred" |
| 12:00 noon | 1200 |
| 1:00 PM | 1300 |
| 2:00 PM | 1400 |
| 3:00 PM | 1500 |
| 4:00 PM | 1600 |
| 5:00 PM | 1700 |
| 6:00 PM | 1800 |
| 7:00 PM | 1900 |
| 8:00 PM | 2000 |
| 9:00 PM | 2100 "twenty-one hundred" |
| 10:00 PM | 2200 |
| 11:00 PM | 2300 |

avoid confusion between AM and PM. With international time, the 24 hours of each day are identified by the numbers 0100 (1:00 AM) through 2400 (12:00 AM, midnight). The last two digits indicate the minutes of each hour, from 01 to 59. Thus, 0101 is 1 minute after 1:00 AM; 1210 is ten minutes after 12 PM (noon); 1658 is 4:58 PM and so on.

## THE INTERDISCIPLINARY HEALTH CARE TEAM PROCESS

The interdisciplinary health care team provides the right care for the residents. The members of the team are responsible for completing activities that will result in a care plan for each resident. To do this, the team members must have a foundation of knowledge on which to base their recommendations (Figure 6-11). The team members and other staff are accountable for implementing the care. Nursing assistants help in each step of this process.

### Step 1: Assessment

**Assessment** means to make an evaluation of the resident's mental, physical, and emotional status. This evaluation is completed by gathering information about the resident's past and present problems. The information is called data. Each discipline completes an assessment when the resident is admitted and annually. This assessment is called the **Minimum Data Set (MDS 2.0)** and is required by law. A less complex assessment is repeated every 3 months. If the resident's condition changes, the assessment is again completed. In addition to the MDS 2.0, the resident may be evaluated for specific risk factors. Examples include:

- Pressure ulcer risk assessment. If data indicate the resident is at risk for developing pressure ulcers, a preventive program is initiated.
- Safety assessment. If the resident is at risk for falling or getting lost, a program to prevent incidents is initiated.
- Mental status examination. This is done to determine the resident's orientation to time and place and mental capabilities.

Data for the MDS 2.0 and the other assessments are collected by the nurse and other members of the team from many sources:

- Interviewing the resident, the family, and nursing staff on all shifts
- Reading the results of the physician's history and physical examination and progress notes
- Reading the results of all diagnostic tests
- Performing a physical assessment (Figure 6-12)
- Performing a functional assessment

When the data are collected, nursing diagnoses are established.

The **nursing diagnosis** is a statement of a problem and its probable cause. Although these are called nursing diagnoses, each member of the interdisciplinary team uses the same system for making problem statements. Here are some examples:

- Impaired physical mobility related to pain and stiffness due to osteoarthritis
- Altered thought processes related to deficits in attention, concentration, and memory resulting from stroke
- Altered family processes related to long-term illness of the resident and the role changes experienced by family members

**Nursing Assistant Responsibility: Assessment.** The nursing assistant's responsibility for Step 1: Assessment is to:

- Make accurate and thorough observations.
- Report and document observations factually.

### Step 2: Planning

After the assessments are completed and the nursing diagnoses have been developed, the care plan is written. The **resident care plan** is the "blueprint" for giving care. Members of the interdisciplinary team attend the **care plan conference**. The resident is invited to attend. Family members are also invited to participate if the resident agrees. At the care plan conference the team:

- Establishes goals for the resident. A **goal** is an outcome; it states what the team (including the resident) plans for the resident to accomplish or be able to do. The goals are developed by determining the resident's potential. For example, if one of the nursing diagnoses is impaired mobility, the team would set goals to maintain or improve mobility. In some situations goals may come from more than one discipline. A mobility problem may involve goals

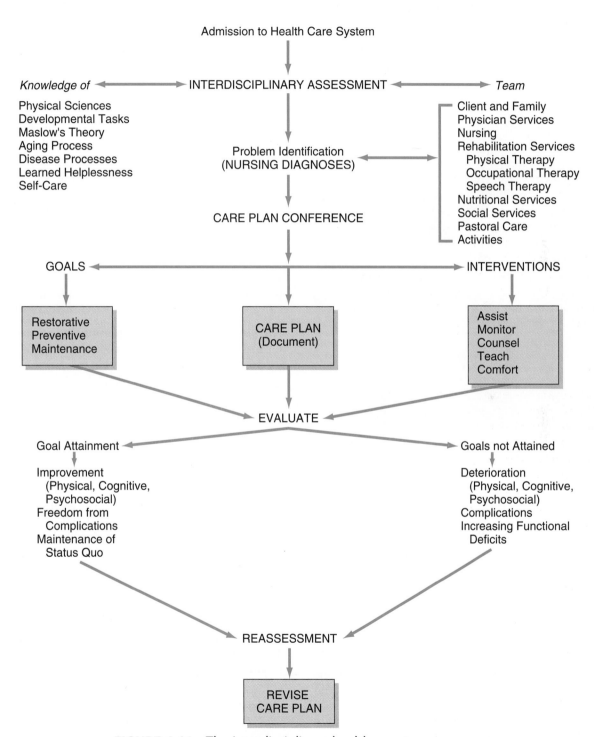

**FIGURE 6-11**  The interdisciplinary health care team process

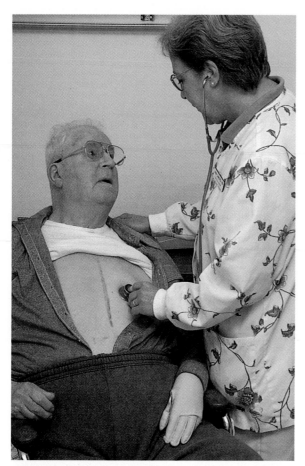

**FIGURE 6-12** The registered nurse collects information by doing a physical assessment of the resident.

from both the physical therapist and the nursing staff. The goals must be realistic and measurable. A nursing goal for impaired mobility might be: resident will walk 100 feet with a walker and one assistant two times a day by a certain date. Goals may be restorative (improvement), preventive (prevent complications such as pressure ulcers or infection), or maintenance (the resident's current state will not change).

• Determines the approaches or interventions to use to help the resident meet the goals. The **approach** or **intervention** states exactly which members of the team are responsible for the approach—what they will do, how they will do it, and when. The approach for the impaired mobility goal might be: place transfer belt on resident, assist to standing posi-

tion, place walker in front of resident, and instruct resident to use three-point gait to walk; to be done by nurse or nursing assistant after breakfast and before supper.

**Nursing Assistant Responsibility: Planning.** The nursing assistant responsibility for Step 2: Planning is to:

• Give suggestions to the nurse if you think a specific approach may be successful. Example: Mrs. Donetti becomes agitated when you try to give her a shower. You tell the nurse you think Mrs. Donetti might prefer a tub bath instead.

• Attend care plan conference if you have the opportunity to do so.

## Step 3: Implementation

**Implementation** is putting the care plan into practice. Members of the interdisciplinary team carry out the approaches listed on the care plan.

**Nursing Assistant Responsibility: Implementation.** The nursing assistant responsibility for Step 3: Implementation is to:

• Read the residents' care plans.
• Carry out the approaches assigned to nursing assistants consistently and correctly.

## Step 4: Evaluation

The purpose of **evaluation** is to determine whether or not the resident is meeting the goals as set forth in the care plan. If the goals are not met, the problems are not resolved. The resident's condition may be deteriorating; there may be complications or decreasing functional abilities. The team needs to determine why the resident is unable to meet the goals. Then different goals will be written or different approaches will be used.

**Nursing Assistant Responsibility: Evaluation.** The nursing assistant responsibility for Step 4: Evaluation is to:

• Report to the nurse when you are unable to carry out an approach as stated in the care plan.
• Relay to the nurse any ideas you have about why there is a problem.
• Report to the nurse the resident's progress toward meeting the care plan goals.

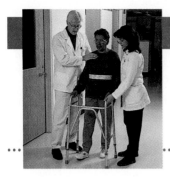

## LESSON SYNTHESIS: Putting It All Together

*Y*ou have just completed this lesson. Now go back and review the Clinical Focus. Try to see how the Clinical Focus relates to the concepts presented in the lesson. Then answer the following questions.

1. Which systems would be most important in making observations for Mrs. Bass?

2. Which members of the interdisciplinary health care team would attend Mrs. Bass's care plan conference?

3. Which senses would you use to determine whether or not Mrs. Bass was disoriented?

4. What information could you gain by observing her facial expressions and body language?

## REVIEW

**A. Select the one best answer for each of the following.**

1. Which of the following examples is a subjective observation?
   a. Mrs. Pochoski tells you she feels sick to her stomach.
   b. You take Mr. Johnson's temperature and it is 99.6°.
   c. Miss Dominick has a reddened area around her tailbone.
   d. Mr. Flores has a blood pressure of 126/84.

2. Which of the following examples is an objective observation?
   a. You feel a lump when you are giving Mrs. Smith her bath.
   b. Mrs. Smith tells you she has a lump in her breast.
   c. Mr. Johnson tells you he thinks he has a fever.
   d. Miss Dominick says she has pain in her tailbone.

3. When you make observations they must be
   a. accurate and timely
   b. reported to the nurse immediately
   c. documented in the resident's record by you or the nurse
   d. all of these

4. Initial observations or baseline information is collected when the resident
   a. is discharged from the facility
   b. is admitted to the facility
   c. has a care plan conference
   d. has a change in condition

5. When observing the integumentary system you would note the
   a. resident's ability to move his arms and legs
   b. resident's blood pressure
   c. color of the resident's skin
   d. resident's ability to respond

6. When you observe the resident's breathing, you are observing the resident's
   a. circulatory system
   b. digestive system
   c. respiratory system
   d. reproductive system

**B. Answer each statement true (T) or false (F).**

7. T  F  Charting is done in pencil in case you make a mistake and need to erase.

8. T  F  Each statement in the chart begins with the word resident.

9. T   F   The resident and the resident's family (if the resident agrees) are invited to attend the care plan conference.

10. T   F   The nursing diagnosis is the physician's statement of the resident's problem.

11. T   F   Goals must be realistic and measurable.

**C.   Fill in the blanks by selecting the correct word or phrase from the list.**

| | |
|---|---|
| approach | intervention |
| assessment | nurse's notes |
| baseline | objective |
| goal | planning |
| implementation | subjective |

12. A sign is a/an _____ observation.

13. A symptom is a/an _____ observation.

14. Making initial observations provides _____ information.

15. The MDS 2.0 is used to make a/an _____ of the resident.

16. The second step of the interdisciplinary health care team process is _____.

17. Carrying out the instructions on the resident's care plan is called _____.

18. Nursing assistants may be expected to document on the _____ in the resident's medical record.

19. A statement of what the interdisciplinary team hopes the resident will be able to accomplish is called a _____.

20. The actions taken by members of the interdisciplinary team to help the resident is called a/an _____ or a/an _____.

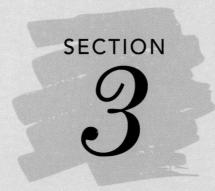

SECTION

3

Protecting Residents'
Rights and Safety

LESSONS

7 Residents' Rights

8 Safety

9 Emergencies

10 Infection

11 Infection Control

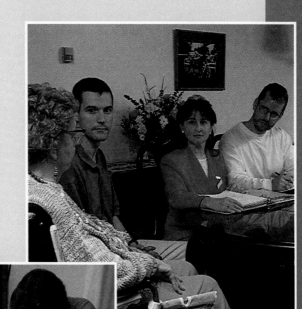

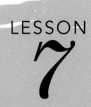
# Residents' Rights

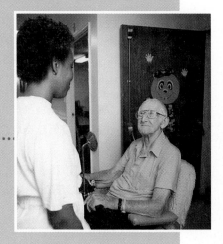

## CLINICAL FOCUS

Think about the basic rights guaranteed to each

resident as you study this lesson and meet:

*S*tanley Davidson. Mr. Davidson has no close relatives and has chosen you to be a confidant. He has shared many personal facts that he would not want anyone else to know.

## OBJECTIVES

*After studying this lesson, you should be able to:*

- Define and spell vocabulary words and terms.
- Describe the purpose of the Residents' Rights document.
- List four situations when the nursing assistant should provide privacy for the resident.
- Explain the nursing assistant's responsibilities for meeting (accommodating) the resident's needs.

- State the differences between physical abuse, sexual abuse, mental abuse, and verbal abuse.
- Give two examples of neglect.
- List five situations when the resident can make choices.
- Describe the term involuntary seclusion.
- Describe four ways the nursing assistant can help residents meet their psychosocial needs.

## VOCABULARY

**advance directives**  *(ad-VANS dih-RECK-tivs)*

**advocate**  *(AD-voh-kit)*

**artificial nutrition**  *(are-tih-FISH-al new-TRIH-shun)*

**assault**  *(ass-SALT)*

**battery**  *(BAT-er-ee)*

**cardiac arrest**  *(KAR-dee-ack ah-REST)*

**cardiopulmonary resuscitation (CPR)**  *(kar-dee-oh-PUL-moh-nair-ee ree-sus-ih-TAY-shun)*

**chemical restraint**  *(KEM-ih-kal ree-STRAYNT)*

**corporal punishment**  *(KOR-poh-ral PUN-ish-ment)*

**defamation of character**  *(def-eh-MAY-shun of KAIR-ack-ter)*

**ethics**  *(ETH-icks)*

**false imprisonment**  *(falls im-PRIHS-on-ment)*

**grievance**  *(GREE-vans)*

# VOCABULARY

hospice  (*HAHS*-*piss*)

hot-line number  (*hot-line NUM*-*ber*)

incontinent  (*in-KON*-*tin-ent*)

informed consent  (*in-FORMD kon-SENT*)

invasion of privacy  (*in-VAY*-*shun of PRY-vah-see*)

involuntary seclusion  (*in-VOL*-*un-ter-ee sih-KLUE*-*zhun*)

legal guardian  (*LEE*-*gul GAR*-*dee-un*)

libel  (*LIE*-*bul*)

Living Will  (*LIV*-*ing will*)

mental abuse  (*MEN*-*tal ah-BYOUSE*)

neglect  (*neh-GLECKT*)

no-code (DNR) (do not resuscitate)  (*no-kohd*)

ombudsman  (*OM*-*buds-man*)

physical abuse  (*FIZ*-*ah-kul ah-BYOUSE*)

physical restraint  (*FIZ*-*ah-kul ree-STRAYNT*)

Power of Attorney for Health Care  (*POW-er of ah-TUR*-*nee for helth kair*)

prostheses  (*pros-THEE*-*sees*)

reprisal  (*ree-PRY*-*zul*)

Self-Determination Act  (*self dee-ter-mih-NAY*-*shun akt*)

sexual abuse  (*SEX*-*you-al ah-BYOUSE*)

sexuality  (*sex*-*you-AL*-*ih-tee*)

slander  (*SLAN*-*der*)

terminal condition  (*TER*-*mih-nal kon-DIH*-*shun*)

theft  (*theft*)

verbal abuse  (*VER*-*bal ah-BYOUSE*)

## PURPOSE OF THE RESIDENTS' RIGHTS DOCUMENT

The Residents' Rights document was legislated by federal and state governments. It is the same as any other law. This document ensures that residents in long-term care facilities are allowed the same rights as any citizen of this country. When these rights are respected by the caregivers, the residents have a higher quality of life.

The resident and family or a court appointed representative of the resident (**legal guardian**) must be given a copy of this document before admission to the facility. Any questions they have should be discussed with the staff member who is coordinating the admission (Figure 7-1).

The resident has the right to an environment that:

- Promotes quality of life
- Promotes dignity and respect for each resident's individuality
- Is safe, clean, comfortable, and homelike
- Helps the resident maintain the highest practical physical, mental, and psychological well-being

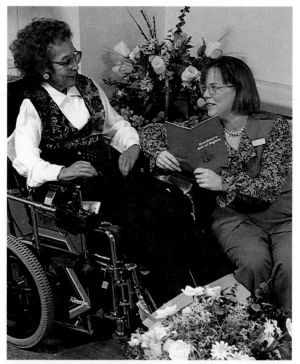

**FIGURE 7-1**  The resident must receive a full explanation of the residents' rights before admission to the facility.

As a nursing assistant, you can assist residents to exercise their rights by:

- Being courteous
- Showing respect at all times
- Being considerate
- Giving residents the opportunity to make decisions about matters that relate to their care

## RESIDENTS' RIGHTS

### The Right to Free Choice

The resident has the right to make choices regarding medical treatment, including:

- The right to choose an attending physician. If the attending physician refuses to obey certain federal regulations regarding the resident's care, the facility may replace the physician after notifying the resident.

- The right to full advance information about changes in care or treatment that affect the resident. This includes the right to refuse treatment. Treatment refers to procedures ordered by the physician. The resident must be consistent and persistent in refusing treatment. State laws must be followed. For example, if a resident cannot take in food and fluids, the resident may refuse to have a feeding tube inserted (**artificial nutrition**). In this case, the specific laws of that state would be obeyed. Whenever a resident refuses treatment, the nurse or physician must explain the possible consequences of the refusal.

- The right to be part of the assessment and care planning process. This means the resident must be told of the evaluations made by the members of the care team. The resident and the family (if the resident agrees) are invited to the care plan conference so they may help with the planning process (Figure 7-2).

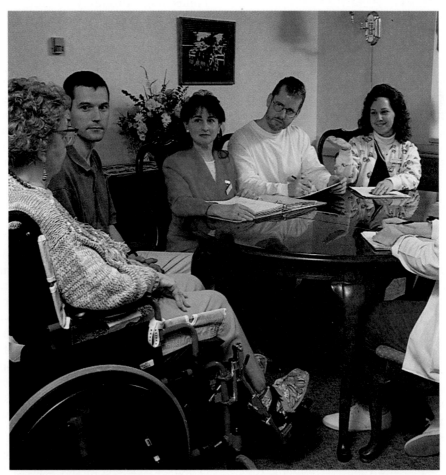

**FIGURE 7-2**  The resident and family are invited to participate in the care planning conference.

- The resident may self-administer medications if the assessment demonstrates that this is possible and the resident wishes to do so. The nurse is responsible for overseeing this process.
- The right to consent to participate in experimental research. Research that personally affects the resident cannot be done without the resident's consent.

## The Right to Freedom from Abuse and Restraints

The term abuse refers to mistreatment of a person. Residents may be abused by staff members, family members, other residents, or visitors. The different forms of abuse are physical abuse, sexual abuse, verbal abuse, and mental abuse. Improperly used or applied restraints is another form of abuse.

**Physical abuse** is:

- Hitting, slapping, pinching, or kicking
- Any physical contact that intentionally causes pain or discomfort
- **Corporal punishment**—inflicting pain on residents to force them to follow orders

**Sexual abuse** is:

- Using physical means or verbal threats to force a resident to perform any sexual act, including fondling, kissing, or sexual intercourse
- Tormenting or teasing a resident with sexual gestures or words

**Verbal abuse** is:

- Talking to the resident in a sarcastic or rough manner
- Using crude slang or swearing
- Using gestures that are considered demeaning or obscene

**Mental abuse** is:

- Making verbal threats to hurt or punish a resident, that is, telling a resident you will put him in a restraint if he does not obey you
- Humiliating a resident, that is, embarrassing a resident who wets her pants
- Separating a resident from other residents against the resident's will (**involuntary seclusion**), unless it is part of a therapeutic plan and is documented. Involuntary seclusion may be used if a resident's actions endanger or offend other residents, such as cursing or being physically aggressive.

Physical and psychosocial neglect may be considered forms of abuse. **Neglect** is the failure to provide safe care. Some examples are:

- Not meeting the resident's physical need for food, fluids, rest, activity, oxygen, cleanliness, shelter, and elimination. This is physical neglect.
- Actions by staff that make the resident agitated or depressed. This is psychosocial neglect.

No resident deserves to be abused or live in fear. Preventing all forms of abuse is everyone's responsibility. If staff members, family members, volunteers, or visitors appear to be abusive or on the verge of becoming so, report this immediately to your supervisor. If you witness abuse and do not report it, you are also guilty. Family members are also under a great deal of stress and may need counseling. Promptly report any bruises or wounds that you observe or any statements of the resident that may possibly be a result of abuse.

Caring for residents requires patience and tolerance. If you feel yourself becoming tense or short-tempered, take action to calm yourself. Take a short break and some deep breaths. If you notice coworkers who appear "uptight," help them to regain their composure. Staff members need to care for each other as well as the residents. Working together with a true team spirit can help prevent abuse.

There are two forms of restraints:

- Chemical restraints
- Physical restraints

**Chemical Restraints.** At times medications to alter behavior are needed. These situations must be carefully evaluated by the interdisciplinary team, resident, and family. **Chemical restraints** are medications that affect the resident's behavior so that mental powers such as thinking are changed. Residents receiving such medications are monitored for unusual reactions. The ordering and dispensing of medications is not the responsibility of the nursing assistant. The nursing assistant should report a resident's unusual behavior or a change in behavior.

**Physical Restraints.** A **physical restraint** (Figure 7-3) is any device that:

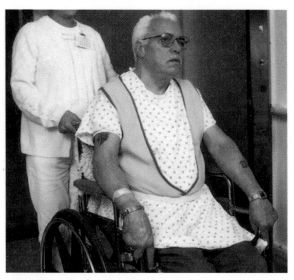

**FIGURE 7-3** A physical restraint is a device that inhibits the resident's movements.

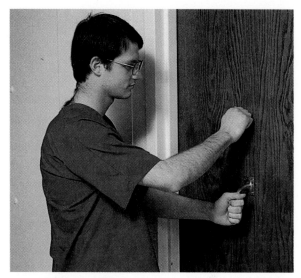

**FIGURE 7-4** Always knock before you enter a resident's room.

- A resident cannot easily remove
- Restricts a resident's movement
- Does not allow resident normal access to body

Physical restraints are discussed in Lesson 8.

### The Right to Privacy

The right to privacy includes:

- Privacy during medical treatment and nursing care
- Receiving and sending unopened mail
- Privacy during telephone calls
- Privacy when visitors are present

Here are some suggestions for ensuring the resident's right to privacy:

- Always knock before entering a resident's room whether the door is closed or open (Figure 7-4). Wait for a response before entering.
- Close the door, the window curtain, and pull the privacy curtains when you are working with residents in their rooms (Figure 7-5).
- Keep residents covered as much as possible when you perform procedures.
- No other people should be present when you are helping the resident go to the bathroom, to dress, or to complete personal care procedures. The exceptions include times when more than one staff person is required to complete a procedure, for example, to position a dependent person.

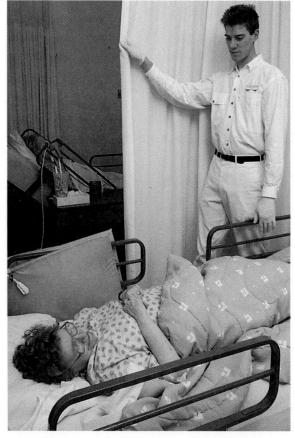

**FIGURE 7-5** Pull the privacy curtain when you are working with residents in their rooms.

• Close the doors to tub rooms, showers, and bathrooms when these areas are in use.

## The Right to Confidentiality of Personal and Clinical Records

This means that information about the resident is available only to those who need the information to provide care. This includes information on the resident's chart and care plan. It also includes any information about the resident's personal life and relationship with the family. The caregivers who receive this information must keep the information confidential.

To protect this right:

• Avoid talking about residents or families during breaks or when you are off duty. When you have to discuss a resident with a coworker, do so in private. Family members, other residents, and visitors should not be able to overhear your conversation.
• Shift reports and other conferences should be held in areas of privacy.
• If a resident or family member wishes to see the medical records, relay the request to the nurse.
• Avoid talking about residents to other residents in the facility.

## The Right to Accommodation of Needs

This includes the right to make choices about life that are important to the resident. This includes activities, schedules, and health care that are consistent with the resident's interests and care plan.

This right means the resident may make choices about:

• Nutrition and eating
• Times for getting up and going to bed
• Clothing, use of makeup, hair style
• Bath or shower and when to take it
• Use of free time
• Visitors

## Accommodation of Needs

The resident has the right to expect the assistance of the staff in meeting both physical needs and psychosocial needs.

**Physical Needs.** As a nursing assistant, you help residents meet their physical needs when you:

• Assist residents to maintain personal hygiene and cleanliness.
    • Give baths or showers.
    • Clean and trim fingernails and toenails.
    • Shave daily.
    • Give shampoos and allow residents to wear the hair style of their choice.
    • Give regular and thorough oral hygiene.
    • Allow residents to choose their own clothing (Figure 7-6).

Provide clothing that is:

• Clean
• In good repair and fits properly

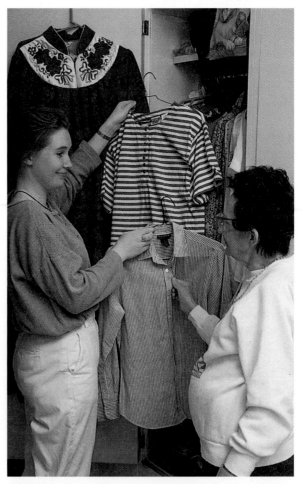

**FIGURE 7-6** Allow residents to choose their own clothing.

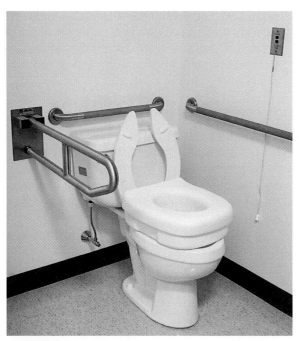

**FIGURE 7-7**   Raised toilet seats and grab bars assist residents to be more independent.

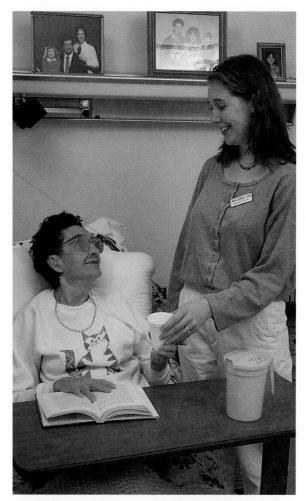

**FIGURE 7-8**   Residents should always have access to fresh drinking water.

- Appropriate for the season and the weather
- Appropriate for the resident's age and sex

- Assist residents with toileting needs as necessary.
  - Take residents to the bathroom as needed or at regularly scheduled times. The bathroom is designed to meet the physical needs of the residents, with grab bars and elevated toilet seats (Figure 7-7).
  - Attend to **incontinent** residents (those unable to control bladder or bowel) immediately.
- Assist residents to remain adequately nourished.
  - Consider the residents' food choices as much as possible.
  - Give residents the assistance necessary to eat independently.
  - Feed residents who cannot feed themselves in a dignified manner.
  - Never force residents to eat.
  - Provide access to fresh drinking water throughout the day (Figure 7-8).
  - Give dependent residents drinks of fresh water regularly.

- Assist residents with the use of devices to meet their needs.
  - Make sure they have their eyeglasses and that the glasses are clean and in good repair.
  - Assist residents with insertion of hearing aids and report improperly functioning hearing aids to the proper person.
  - Assist with the use of canes and walkers.
  - Help residents with **prostheses** (artificial body parts) or other devices.

**Psychosocial Needs.**   Residents have the right to expect the staff to help them meet their psychosocial needs as much as possible. This may require the attention of various members of the interdisciplinary team. The staff needs to remember:

- The medical condition of a resident when providing these rights
- That the rights of all residents are equal
- That no resident has the right to infringe on the right or safety of other residents

The team works together to:

- Allow residents to:
    - Spend their free time as they wish
    - Move about the facility (if their medical condition permits) as long as they respect the privacy of other residents and staff members
    - Participate, if desired, in structured activities offered by the facility (Figure 7-9)
    - Visit other residents in the facility
- Allow married couples who both reside in the facility to share a room, if they both so desire and if it is medically appropriate.
- Respect the **sexuality** and sexual needs of the resident. Sexuality is one aspect of human psychosocial needs. Whether married to each other or not, residents have the right to express their needs and to experience satisfaction as long as this is mutually agreeable. Residents must be mentally and physically able to agree to the relationship.

## Environmental Needs

The resident has the right to expect that the environment is adapted to meet the needs of individuals with disabilities. This means:

- The residents must be able to safely move about and function within the facility. This requires:
    - Handrails attached to corridor walls (Figure 7-10)
    - Elevators for resident use
    - Ramps that allow for wheelchair access into and out of the facility

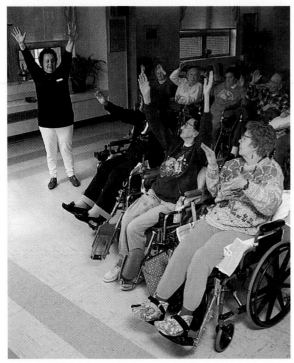

**FIGURE 7-9** Facilities must offer an activity program to all residents.

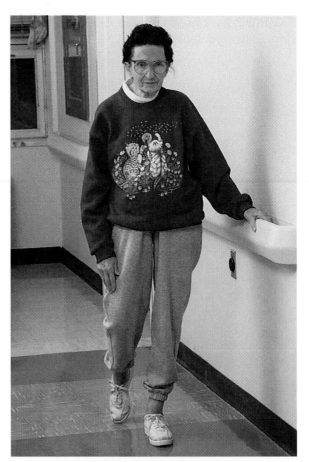

**FIGURE 7-10** Handrails attached to the wall allow residents more independence.

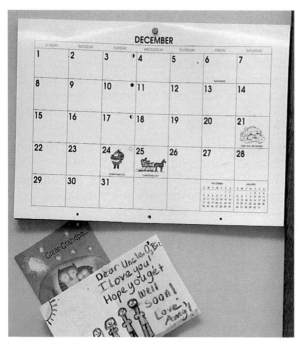

**FIGURE 7-11** Calendars with large numbers help residents remain oriented.

- Permanent grab bars in bathrooms and elevated toilet seats
- Signal lights in the residents' rooms and in the bathrooms and showers
- Safety measures for residents who wander
- Clocks and calendars with large numerals located throughout the building to help residents remain oriented (Figure 7-11)
- The facility environment is expected to be homelike and to allow social interaction, including:
  - Furniture arrangements in public areas that allow for visiting (Figure 7-12)
  - The use of color, plants, and artwork to create a cheerful environment

## Advance Directives

Residents also have the right to make **advance directives**. In 1990, the federal government passed a law called the **Self-Determination Act**. This law states that all competent adults have the right to:

- Accept or refuse any medical treatment, including life-sustaining treatments

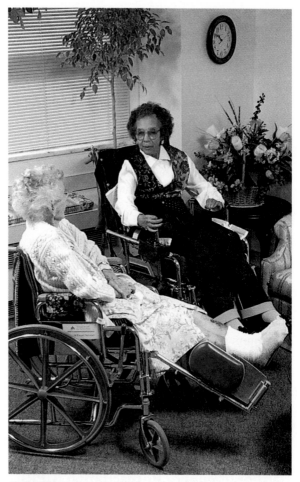

**FIGURE 7-12** Facilities should have comfortable visiting areas.

- Be adequately informed about:
  - Their medical condition
  - Treatment alternatives
  - Likely risks of each treatment alternative
  - Benefits of each alternative
  - Possible consequences of each alternative

The law applies to competent adults entering hospitals, nursing homes, home health care, or **hospice** (an agency that provides care for terminally ill persons). The law requires that residents:

- Be informed of what kinds of advance directives are available to ensure that their wishes are carried out when they are no longer able to make or communicate their decisions

- Be informed that it is the right of every competent adult to choose whether or not he or she wants to execute an advance directive

There are two types of advance directives:
- **Living Will** (Figure 7-13)
- **Power of Attorney for Health Care** (Figure 7-14)

A Living Will:
- Allows individuals to describe their wishes about discontinuing procedures that delay death if they have a **terminal condition**. This means that death is expected soon and the person's condition is incurable and irreversible.
- Is legal in most states
- Must be witnessed by two people who will not benefit from the resident's death. (In most facilities, the nursing assistant should not be a witness for the signing of legal forms.)

Durable Power of Attorney for Health Care:
- Permits a person (called the principal) to delegate to another person (called the agent) the power to make any health care decision that the principal is unable to make

Even though these advance directives have been completed, the resident must still make decisions regarding other support measures.

## Cardiopulmonary Resuscitation (CPR)

- The resident must inform the physician whether **cardiopulmonary resuscitation** is to be administered if **cardiac arrest** occurs. In most states, the law requires that all persons be resuscitated unless they have previously made their wishes known.
- The physician must write the order on the resident's chart if a resident or the person with Power of Attorney for Health Care determines that CPR should not be administered. This is called **no-code** or **DNR (do not resuscitate)**.

When there is a DNR order, resuscitation is not performed when the resident stops breathing. The resident is allowed to die with peace and dignity. All personnel should be aware when a DNR order is written. It is often difficult to carry out a DNR order when you have come to know and love the resident. Try to remember that life needs to be meaningful and that quality of life is limited for a person on life support systems.

If a resident has chosen to be resuscitated in the event that cardiac arrest occurs, then every effort is made to keep the resident alive. A "code" is called and CPR is initiated. An ambulance is called to transport the resident to the hospital for additional life support measures.

## Hospitalization

- Some technical procedures cannot be performed in the long-term care facility.
- When residents become acutely ill, hospitalization may be necessary if lifesaving measures are to be taken.
- Residents may choose not to go to the hospital, but to remain in the facility for supportive care only.

## Feeding Restrictions

- Residents who are terminally ill frequently do not wish to eat or drink.
- The physician may suggest inserting a feeding tube into the stomach.
- In most states this procedure will not be done if the resident has made his wishes clear in the advance directives.

## Medication and Treatment Restrictions

The resident has the right to refuse:
- Life-sustaining medications such as chemotherapy or antibiotics
- Blood transfusions
- Surgery
- Being placed on a ventilator
- Any medical treatment

Residents always have the right to change their mind. For example, if the advance directives state that a feeding tube is not to be inserted, the resident may change this directive if the time comes.

## The Right to Voice Grievances

This means the resident may voice **grievances** (complaints) to the facility without fear of retaliation (**reprisal**) or discrimination. The facility must take prompt action to resolve the grievances (Figure 7-15).

The resident may have a grievance about:
- The way in which care is given
- Treatment or care that is not given

# FLORIDA LIVING WILL

| INSTRUCTIONS | |
|---|---|

**PRINT THE DATE**

Declaration made this _____ day of _____, 19_____.

**PRINT YOUR NAME**

I, _____, willfully and voluntarily make known my desire that my dying not be artificially prolonged under the circumstances set forth below, and I do hereby declare:

If at any time I have a terminal condition and if my attending or treating physician and another consulting physician have determined that there is no medical probability of my recovery from such condition, I direct that life-prolonging procedures be withheld or withdrawn when the application of such procedures would serve only to prolong artificially the process of dying, and that I be permitted to die naturally with only the administration of medication or the performance of any medical procedure deemed necessary to provide me with comfort care or to alleviate pain.

It is my intention that this declaration be honored by my family and physician as the final expression of my legal right to refuse medical or surgical treatment and to accept the consequences for such refusal.

In the event that I have been determined to be unable to provide express and informed consent regarding the withholding, withdrawal, or continuation of life-prolonging procedures, I wish to designate, as my surrogate to carry out the provisions of this declaration:

**PRINT THE NAME, HOME ADDRESS AND TELEPHONE NUMBER OF YOUR SURROGATE**

Name: _____

Address: _____

_____ Zip Code: _____

Phone: _____

© 1995
CHOICE IN DYING, INC.

*(continues)*

**FIGURE 7-13** A Living Will allows individuals to describe their choices if they become terminally ill. (Reprinted by permission of Choice In Dying 200 Varick Street, New York, NY 10014 212/366-5540)

| | |
|---|---|
| | **FLORIDA LIVING WILL — PAGE 2 OF 2** |

I wish to designate the following person as my alternate surrogate, to carry out the provisions of this declaration should my surrogate be unwilling or unable to act on my behalf:

**PRINT NAME, HOME ADDRESS AND TELEPHONE NUMBER OF YOUR ALTERNATE SURROGATE**

Name: _____

Address: _____

_____ Zip Code: _____

Phone: _____

**ADD PERSONAL INSTRUCTIONS (IF ANY)**

Additional instructions (optional):

I understand the full impo[...] [...]is declaration, and I am emotionally and mentally competent to make t[...] declaration.

**SIGN THE DOCUMENT**

Signed: _____

**WITNESSING PROCEDURE**

Witness 1:

Signed: _____

Address: _____

**TWO WITNESSES MUST SIGN AND PRINT THEIR ADDRESSES**

Witness 2:

Signed: _____

Address: _____

| |
|---|
| *Courtesy of Choice In Dying*          9/95 |
| 200 Varick Street, New York, NY 10014 1-800-989-WILL |

**FIGURE 7-13** *(continued)*

## INSTRUCTIONS

# FLORIDA DESIGNATION OF HEALTH CARE SURROGATE

**PRINT YOUR NAME**

Name: _____

(Last)                    (First)                    (Middle Initial)

In the event that I have been determined to be incapacitated to provide informed consent for medical treatment and surgical and diagnostic procedures, I wish to designate as my surrogate for health care decisions:

**PRINT THE NAME, HOME ADDRESS AND TELEPHONE NUMBER OF YOUR SURROGATE**

Name: _____

Address: _____

_____ Zip Code: _____

Phone: _____

If my surrogate is unwilling or unable to perform his duties, I wish to designate as my alternate surrogate:

**PRINT THE NAME, HOME ADDRESS AND TELEPHONE NUMBER OF YOUR ALTERNATE SURROGATE**

Name: _____

Address: _____

_____ Zip Code: _____

Phone: _____

I fully understand that this designation will permit my designee to make health care decisions and to provide, withhold, or withdraw consent on my behalf; to apply for public benefits to defray the cost of health care; and to authorize my admission to or transfer from a health care facility.

*(continues)*

© 1995
CHOICE IN DYING, INC.

**FIGURE 7-14** The Power of Attorney for Health Care is a document that delegates another person to make decisions for the resident. (Reprinted by permission of Choice In Dying 200 Varick Street, New York, NY 10014 212/366-5540)

| FLORIDA DESIGNATION OF HEALTH CARE SURROGATE — PAGE 2 OF 2 |
|---|

**ADD PERSONAL INSTRUCTIONS (IF ANY)**

Additional instructions (optional):

I further affirm that this designation is not being made as a condition of treatment or admission to a health care facility. I will notify and send a copy of this document to the following persons other than my surrogate, so they may know who my surrogate is:

**PRINT THE NAMES AND ADDRESSES OF THOSE WHO YOU WANT TO KEEP COPIES OF THIS DOCUMENT**

Name: _____

Address: _____

Name: _____

Address: _____

**SIGN AND DATE THE DOCUMENT**

Signed: _____

Date: _____

**WITNESSING PROCEDURE**

**TWO WITNESSES MUST SIGN AND PRINT THEIR ADDRESSES**

Witness 1:

    Signed: _____

    Address: _____

Witness 2:

    Signed: _____

    Address: _____

© 1995
CHOICE IN DYING, INC.

| *Courtesy of* **Choice In Dying**        9/95<br>200 Varick Street, New York, NY 10014 1-800-989-WILL |
|---|

**FIGURE 7-14** *(continued)*

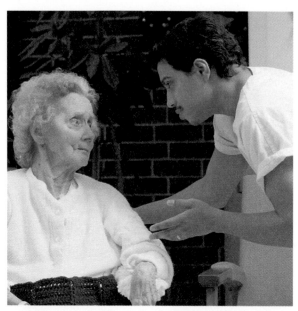

**FIGURE 7-15** Residents have the right to voice grievances.

As a nursing assistant you can help avoid problems by following these guidelines.

1. Relay concerns of the resident to the nurse in charge.
2. Carry out all instructions you may be given for solving the problem.
3. Never withhold care or attention from a resident because of grievances or complaints voiced by the resident.
4. Avoid discussing grievances with other staff members unless there is a valid need for such discussion. You may, for example, discuss a grievance at a care plan conference as a way of trying to solve the problem.

## The Right to Organize and Participate in Family and Resident Groups

This means:
- The facility must provide space for meetings.
- A staff member from the facility will attend if invited.
- The staff will address written recommendations from the meetings that concern decisions affecting the residents' care and life in the facility.

Most long-term care facilities have resident councils. These councils meet regularly and all residents are invited to participate in the meetings. The councils give the residents a method for communication with each other and with staff in a constructive and organized manner.

To assist in providing these residents' rights, you can:

1. Cooperate in assisting residents to attend council meetings.
   - Help residents to get dressed to attend the meeting.
   - Arrange the residents' care so it does not interfere with their attendance at the meetings.
   - Toilet residents if necessary before they go to the meeting.
   - Help transport residents to the meeting if necessary.
2. Cooperate in carrying out recommendations of the council that are implemented by the facility administration.

## The Right to Participate in Social, Religious, and Community Activities

**Social Activities.**   Someone from the activities staff meets with each resident shortly after admission to the facility. Residents are given an opportunity to express their choices for activities. Activities must include:

1. Empowerment activities
   - Activities that increase self-respect by providing opportunities for self-expression such as doing artwork or creative crafts
   - Activities that require personal responsibility and choices. Voting is an example of this type of activity. Residents have the right to vote in all local, state, and federal elections. Residents are given the opportunity to vote by absentee ballot or they are taken to the polls.
2. Maintenance activities
   - Maintenance activities promote physical, mental, social, and emotional health.
   - Maintenance activities include physical exercise, current events discussion groups, picnics, and musical or dramatic presentations.
3. Supportive activities
   - Supportive activities provide stimulation to residents with severe mental or physi-

cal disabilities who cannot participate in other types of programs.

As a nursing assistant, follow these guidelines for supporting the residents' participation in activities.

1. Cooperate with the activities staff schedule of events. Schedule resident care so it does not interfere with the residents' attendance.
2. Be aware of the activities that are scheduled. Give residents information if they ask about the nature and time of the activities being offered.

Residents also have the right to refuse to participate in any of these activities. They can develop their own individual activities, for example, reading or doing needlework or crossword puzzles.

**Religious Activities.** Worship and religious activities are an important aspect of living in a long-term care facility. Freedom of worship must be allowed for each resident.

1. Respect the residents' religious beliefs and practices.
2. Assist residents to attend church services and other religious activities within the facility.
3. Treat religious articles such as Bibles, crucifixes, and rosaries with respect (Figure 7-16).
4. Provide privacy for residents' visits with the clergy (such as priest, pastor, or rabbi).
5. Allow residents privacy for prayer and meditation.
6. Remember that the resident also has the right to not have religious beliefs or practices.

**Community Activities.** Involvement with the community can be important for the residents' interest and enthusiasm. Many long-term care facilities have large vans or buses with wheelchair access that enable residents to attend community events. These activities might include entertainment, educational, religious, or recreational programs. Groups from the community visit the long-term care facility to provide these events for residents who cannot leave the facility.

## The Right to Examine Survey Results and Correction Plans

Surveys of all facilities are completed on a regular basis by regulatory agencies. The surveyors

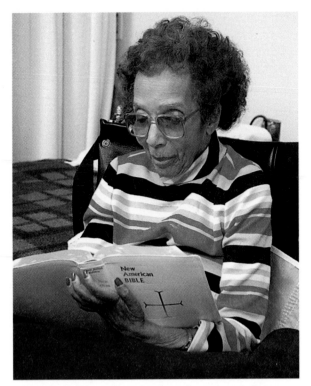

**FIGURE 7-16** The resident has the right to keep religious items in the room.

write up their findings from the survey. If any problems are found, the facility must write a plan of correction that states how the problems will be solved. The resident (or family, if resident wishes) may inspect these records during normal business hours or by special appointment.

## The Right to Manage Personal Funds

This means:

- The resident may request the facility to manage the funds. The resident must give written authorization.
- If the account exceeds $50, it must earn interest, which is given to the resident.

## The Right to Information About Eligibility for Medicare/ Medicaid Benefits

This means:

- The resident has the right to receive these benefits if the resident is eligible for the benefits, and the facility participates in the programs.

## The Right to File Complaints About Abuse, Neglect, or Misappropriation of Property

This means:

- If the resident believes there has been abuse, neglect, or property stolen, the resident can file a complaint with the state agency that inspects the facility.

## The Right to Information About Advocacy Groups

This means:

- Each state has an **ombudsman** program. An ombudsman may visit facilities to question residents about the care they are receiving. This person is trained by a state agency to perform this responsibility.
- Each facility also has agencies in the area that serve as **advocates** (spokespersons) for the residents to ensure that they receive appropriate care.
- The telephone numbers of these groups must be available to residents. Each facility must also post a **hot-line number** that can be used to register complaints about a facility or caregiver (Figure 7-17).

## The Right to Immediate and Unlimited Access to Immediate Family or Relatives

This also includes:

- The long-term care ombudsman
- Government agency representatives
- The attending physician

The resident may also withdraw consent to visit with any of these people.

## The Right to Share a Room with Spouse

If spouses are residents in the facility, they may share a room. This may not be possible if there are medical reasons to keep one of the couple in a special unit.

## The Right to Perform or Not Perform Work for the Facility

The resident may perform work at the facility if it is medically appropriate for the resident to do so. In addition:

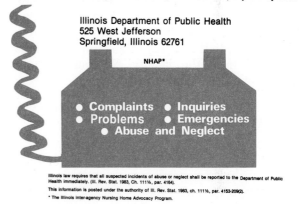

# NURSING HOME

## HOTLINE

### CALL TOLL FREE 24 HOURS

# 1-800-252-4343

If you have a complaint concerning this long-term care facility, you may discuss it with the administrator or a person designated by the administrator to discuss complaints. If this does not resolve your complaint, you have the right to contact the Illinois Department of Public Health's Nursing Home Hotline, 1-800-252-4343, or you may write

Illinois Department of Public Health
525 West Jefferson
Springfield, Illinois 62761

NHAP*

- **Complaints**  • **Inquiries**
- **Problems**  • **Emergencies**
- **Abuse and Neglect**

Illinois law requires that all suspected incidents of abuse or neglect shall be reported to the Department of Public Health immediately. (Ill. Rev. Stat. 1983, Ch. 111½, par. 4164).

This information is posted under the authority of Ill. Rev. Stat. 1983, ch. 111½, par. 4153-209(2).

* The Illinois inter-agency Nursing Home Advocacy Program.

**FIGURE 7-17**  Each resident must have access to the hot-line number. (Courtesy of Illinois Department of Public Health)

- The resident must formally agree to any work arrangement.
- If the work is for pay, the resident earns the prevailing rate for the services.

## The Right to Remain in the Facility

The resident can remain in the facility unless one or more of the following items applies:

- Resident no longer needs the care.
- Resident's welfare requires transfer.
- Facility no longer meets the resident's needs.
- Health or safety of others in the facility is endangered.
- Resident fails to pay for services.
- Facility ceases to operate.

- In these cases, 30 days notice must be given except where health is improved, there is an emergency, or there is danger to the health or safety of individuals in the facility.

## The Right to Use Personal Possessions

This means:

- Personal clothing and jewelry (Figure 7-18)
- Personal furnishings when these can be used in accordance with health and safety regulations

The residents' right to retain and use personal possessions ensures that the residents' environment is homelike. Using personal possessions gives residents some control over their lives. The facility is responsible for taking reasonable measures to safeguard residents' belongings. Each resident's record contains a personal possession list. It must be noted on this list any time an item is brought into the facility or any time an item is removed from the facility. Nursing assistant responsibilities include the following:

1. Encourage residents to display pictures and family photos in their rooms.

2. Assist residents to arrange their personal items if they need help.
3. Report any lost items immediately and take measures to find the items.
4. Do not rearrange furniture in a resident's room without the person's permission, unless there is a valid health or safety reason.
5. Do not go through dresser drawers, closets, lockers, or purses without the resident's permission.
6. Be careful what you throw out when tidying the room.

## The Right to Notification of Change in Condition

This means the facility will notify the resident's attending physician, legal representative, and family member of:

- An accident involving the resident
- A significant change in the resident's condition
- A need to alter treatment significantly
- A decision for transfer or discharge

The members of the interdisciplinary team work together to provide the residents with the rights expressed in this document.

## LEGAL ASPECTS OF HEALTH CARE

The Residents' Rights document has a legal foundation. Contained within the document are several rights which, if violated, could result in legal action against the facility or care provider. This action may be a fine or imprisonment for the offender. Each employee is responsible for personal actions. The OBRA legislation requires that a facility report any case of abuse and the names of the persons involved. Each state has a designated agency that investigates such reports.

### Assault and Battery

Assault and battery are examples of actions that violate the residents' rights and are criminal offenses. Any type of abuse of a resident may be a form of assault or battery. **Assault** is a threat or an attempt to harm another person. Threatening to restrain a resident if he does not stay in bed is an example of assault. **Battery** is touching another

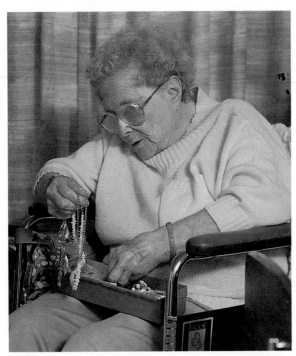

**FIGURE 7-18** Residents can wear their own clothing and jewelry.

person without that person's consent. Grabbing a resident to give him a bath when he does not want one is battery. To protect the caregivers, legal permission is required from the resident, family, or legal guardian for certain procedures. This permission must be obtained with the **informed consent** of the resident. This means the resident fully understands the procedure. This formal consent is not required for routine personal care and procedures. However, you must explain what you are going to do to the resident before you do it. If the resident objects, discuss the situation with the nurse.

### False Imprisonment

The unauthorized use of restraints can be considered **false imprisonment** (detaining an individual without a reason and against that individual's will).

### Invasion of Privacy

Violating a resident's right to privacy and confidentiality of personal and medical records is an example of **invasion of privacy**.

### Defamation of Character

If a person spreads false information about a resident, then that person may be guilty of **defamation of character**. If the false information is verbal or spoken, it is called **slander**. If it is written, it is called **libel**.

### Neglect

Neglect may also be considered a criminal offense. Neglect was discussed earlier in this lesson.

### Theft

The resident has the right to use personal possessions. To take anyone's personal possessions is **theft**.

You will avoid problems as a health care provider if you:

- Always do the very best job possible.
- Treat the resident with respect.
- Remember the rights of the resident.
- Do only those tasks that you are legally qualified to perform.

## ETHICS AND THE HEALTH CARE PROVIDER

The term **ethics** refers to conduct or behavior. Every profession has a code of ethics for its members. For example:

- Health care providers do not accept tips. If a resident offers to give you money for services you perform, thank the resident and explain that you are not allowed to accept the money.
- Health care providers are expected to be mature, responsible adults. This means accepting assignments willingly and helping others as needed.
- Health care providers do not discuss their personal problems at work. If you have problems that may affect your work, discuss them only with your supervisor.
- Avoid horseplay, joking around, and loud laughter when you are working on the resident unit. Humor is necessary but should be appropriate and tasteful; never make fun of a resident.
- Avoid gossip and "griping." A negative attitude from one person can be depressing to everyone else.

A code of ethics is based on respect for all people and for your employer. Your employer also deserves your loyalty. You will find your work enjoyable and rewarding if you follow an ethical code of behavior.

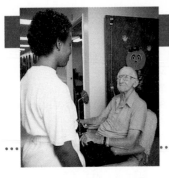

## LESSON SYNTHESIS: Putting It All Together

*Y*ou have just completed this lesson. Now go back and review the Clinical Focus. Try to see how the Clinical Focus relates to the concepts presented in the lesson. Then answer the following questions.

1. Why is it necessary to know and actively protect Mr. Davidson's rights?

2. How do the rights of Mr. Davidson differ from those that every citizen enjoys?

3. What nursing assistant actions would interfere with the rights of a resident?

4. When a resident is unable to make decisions, how may his or her rights be protected?

5. How could you protect Mr. Davidson's right of privacy?

## REVIEW

**A. Select the one best answer for each of the following.**

1. The purpose of the Residents' Rights document is to
   a. promote dignity and respect for residents
   b. provide a safe, clean, and comfortable environment
   c. help the resident maintain the highest level of well-being
   d. all of these

2. The right to free choice means the resident can choose
   a. which room he will stay in
   b. his attending physician
   c. which nursing assistants will provide his care
   d. all of these

3. An example of mental abuse is
   a. not taking the resident to the bathroom when she needs to go
   b. swearing at the resident
   c. slapping the resident when she refuses to eat
   d. fondling the resident's breasts

4. Corporal punishment means
   a. isolating the resident without providing care
   b. using chemical restraints
   c. using painful treatment for correction of behavior
   d. using physical restraints

5. Involuntary seclusion is
   a. helping the resident to his room and closing the door when the resident wants to lie down
   b. isolating the resident when it is not part of a therapeutic plan
   c. placing a resident with a communicable disease in isolation
   d. giving the resident medication to put him to sleep

6. A chemical restraint is
   a. a medication that influences behavior
   b. any device that limits the resident's mobility
   c. an alcoholic beverage
   d. all of these

7. The resident has the right to privacy when
   a. going to the bathroom
   b. receiving nursing care or medical treatment
   c. talking on the telephone
   d. all of these

8. The right to confidentiality means
   a. the resident cannot see her chart or medical record
   b. that only the physician can read the chart
   c. information about the resident is available only to those who need it to provide care
   d. that nursing assistants cannot read the chart

9. Accommodation of needs means that the staff must
   a. provide the resident with fresh fruit at every meal
   b. escort the resident to the church of his or her choice
   c. give every resident a private room with bath
   d. assist the resident to maintain personal hygiene and cleanliness

10. Residents are not allowed to
    a. move about the facility
    b. visit other residents
    c. enter other residents' rooms without permission of that resident
    d. have visitors in their rooms

11. If a husband and wife are both admitted to the facility, they are
    a. not allowed to have sexual activity
    b. allowed to share the same room if their medical conditions permit
    c. expected to help take care of each other
    d. all of these

12. Providing an environment to meet the needs of the residents means that
    a. the resident can choose the color of his room and drapes
    b. there are permanent grab bars in the bathrooms
    c. there must be wall-to-wall carpeting throughout the facility
    d. the residents' personal furnishings are not allowed

13. A Living Will provides instructions for
    a. who will inherit the resident's money
    b. how the resident will pay her bill
    c. carrying out the resident's wishes if she has a terminal illness
    d. the resident's funeral in the event of her death

14. A person who has Power of Attorney for Health Care
    a. must be a lawyer
    b. makes decisions for the resident even if he is able to do so himself
    c. can make health care decisions if the resident is unable to do so
    d. can decide how the resident's money is spent

15. A grievance is a
    a. complaint
    b. sad feeling
    c. lawsuit
    d. all of these

16. An ombudsman
    a. is the person who has Power of Attorney for Health Care
    b. visits facilities to make sure residents are receiving adequate care
    c. is the administrator
    d. has an office in the facility

17. The hot-line number is used
    a. by a resident or family member to call a state agency to register a complaint about the facility
    b. to call the fire department in the event of fire
    c. to order meals to be sent in to the resident
    d. by staff members to register complaints about their supervisors

18. Assault is the legal term for
    a. touching another person without consent
    b. a threat or an attempt to harm another person

c. placing a restraint on a resident
d. invasion of privacy

19. The term slander means
    a. spreading false information about a resident verbally
    b. writing false information about a resident
    c. mental abuse
    d. false imprisonment

20. Which situation would be considered unethical?
    a. accepting a tip from a resident
    b. accepting a homemade cookie from the resident's daughter
    c. calling in sick when you have an elevated temperature and the flu
    d. asking another nursing assistant to help you get a heavy resident out of bed

B. **Match the resident right (items a.–e.) with the nursing assistant actions that protect that right.**

a. freedom from abuse
b. providing privacy
c. ensuring confidentiality
d. accommodating individual needs
e. participation in religious activities

21. _____ encouraging the resident to feed himself

22. _____ frequently visiting a disoriented resident

23. _____ informing the nurse that the resident wishes a visit from a clergyperson

24. _____ knocking before entering a room

25. _____ refusing to discuss one resident's condition with another

26. _____ assisting the resident to the telephone

27. _____ gently handling the resident when turning him

28. _____ leaving all written notes regarding residents in the facility

29. _____ drawing the curtains during a bedbath

30. _____ encouraging residents to choose their own clothing

C. **Fill in the blanks by selecting the correct word or phrase from the list.**

chemical restraints     physical restraint
empowerment             supportive care
maintenance

31. Medications that affect the resident's behavior and alter thinking are called _____.

32. A device that restricts a resident's movement and does not allow normal access to the body is called a _____.

33. An activity that promotes self-respect by providing opportunities for self-expression is a(an) _____ activity.

34. _____ activities promote physical, mental, social, and emotional health.

35. Providing comfort measures to a person who is dying is called giving _____.

# Safety

## CLINICAL FOCUS

Think about the role the nursing

assistant can play in ensuring a

safe environment for each

resident as you study this lesson

and meet:

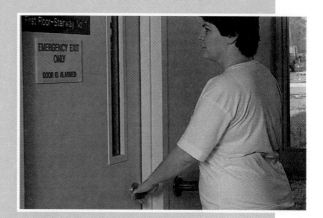

*D*ebra, a nursing assistant who works at the Great Neck Nursing Center. Each month, Debra and members of the staff carry out a fire drill. This practice means that they will all be prepared to act promptly in case of a real emergency.

## OBJECTIVES

*After studying this lesson, you should be able to:*

- Define and spell vocabulary words and terms.
- List the ergonomics techniques you can use to prevent incidents on the job.
- Demonstrate the correct use of body mechanics.
- Describe the types of information contained in the Material Safety Data Sheets (MSDS).
- Use equipment safely.
- Describe three safety rules when oxygen is in use.
- Identify residents who are at risk for having incidents.

- List three alternatives to the use of physical restraints.
- Describe the guidelines for the use of restraints.
- Demonstrate the correct application of restraints.
- Describe three measures for preventing resident incidents: accidental poisoning, thermal injuries, skin injuries, falls, and choking.
- List four measures to follow for safe wheelchair use.
- Describe three procedures to follow in the event of fire.

# VOCABULARY

**aspiration**   *(ass-pih-RAY-shun)*

**body mechanics**   *(BAH-dee mih-KAN-icks)*

**ergonomics**   *(er-goh-NOM-icks)*

**incident**   *(IN-sih-dent)*

**lacerations**   *(las-er-AY-shuns)*

**Material Safety Data Sheets (MSDS)**   *(mah-TEER-ee-al SAYF-tee DAY-tah sheets)*

**Occupational Safety and Health Administration (OSHA)**   *(ock-you-PAY-shun-al SAYF-tee and helth ad-min-iss-TRAY-shun)*

**physical restraint**   *(FIZ-ih-kul ree-STRAYNT)*

## SAFETY IN HEALTH CARE FACILITIES

A major concern in health care facilities is the prevention of injuries to residents, employees, volunteers, and visitors. An **incident** (accident) is any unexpected situation that can cause a resident, employee, or any other person harm. Prevention of incidents depends on:

• Employees knowing their jobs and all policies and procedures related to safety
• Maintaining a safe environment
• Knowing the residents and using safety measures to decrease their risk of injury

When an incident occurs, it must be reported immediately. Report to your supervisor and follow the policy of your facility.

## EMPLOYEE SAFETY

Health care workers are required to perform many physical tasks. You must learn how to use your body correctly while you are completing your assignments. This is called using good **body mechanics**. This means you are using your muscles correctly when you lift or move residents or heavy objects. If you always apply the rules of body mechanics, you will avoid injury to yourself and to the residents.

### Ergonomics

The word **ergonomics** means adapting the environment and using techniques and equipment to prevent injury to the body. If certain risk factors are present, it is likely that an ergonomic (work-related) problem will occur. These risk factors include:

1. Performance of the same motion or motion pattern every few seconds for more than 2 to 4 hours at a time
2. Being in a fixed or awkward posture for more than 2 to 4 hours
3. Using forceful hand movements for more than 2 to 4 hours at a time
4. Doing heavy lifting, unassisted for more than 1 to 2 hours

### Body Mechanics

The use of proper body mechanics at all times can prevent fatigue and body injury. Good body mechanics means to:

1. Maintain good standing posture.
   • Stand with your feet flat on the floor.
   • Separate your feet about 12 inches (shoulder width apart).
   • Bend your knees slightly.
   • Keep your back straight.
   • Tighten your abdominal muscles.
2. Use the weight of your body to help to push or pull an object.
3. Use the strongest muscles to do the job.
   • It is easier to bring the resident or object toward you than to lift the resident or object away from you.
   • Use stronger muscles (leg muscles) rather than weaker muscles (back muscles) when lifting, pushing, or pulling.

# *G*uidelines for

## Using Ergonomic Techniques to Reduce the Risk of Having an Incident

1. Use correct body mechanics at all times at work and when you are off duty.
2. Raise the beds to a comfortable working height (remember to lower the beds when you finish your task).
3. Use a mechanical lift when you need to transfer very heavy or dependent residents into or out of bed.
4. Use a back support if your employer requires it. The use of a back support is controversial because it does not really prevent injury, but it does remind the wearer to use good body mechanics. Many nursing assistants find them helpful (Figure 8-1).
5. Get another person to help when you need to transfer a resident who is not full weight bearing. Use a transfer belt when ordered.
6. Use a cart to move heavy items (Figure 8-2).

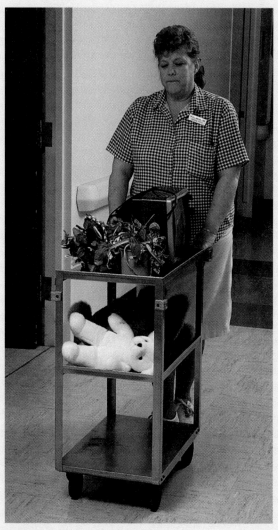

**FIGURE 8-2** Use a cart to move heavy items.

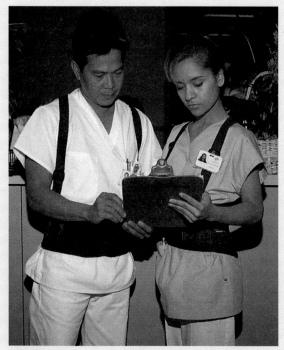

**FIGURE 8-1** Your employer may require you to wear a back support while you work.

4. Avoid twisting your body and overreaching as you work.
5. Avoid bending for long periods of time.
6. Use the method that has been ordered to move a resident. For example, if the care plan states that two people are needed to transfer a resident from bed to chair, always get another person to help you.
7. Follow the eight commandments of lifting to greatly decrease the risk of injuring yourself:

   - Plan your lift and test the load (Figure 8-3A).
   - Ask for help (Figure 8-3B).
   - Get a firm footing (Figure 8-3C).
   - Bend your knees (Figure 8-3D).
   - Tighten your stomach muscles (Figure 8-3E).
   - Lift with your legs (Figure 8-3F).
   - Keep the load close (Figure 8-3G).
   - Keep your back straight (Figure 8-3H).

8. Ask your physician or a physical therapist for specific exercises for the back that can help prevent injuries.
9. Warm up before working to help prevent strains. Perform the exercises shown in Figures 8-4A–J before each work shift. Remember that you can avoid many problems if you also:

   - Exercise every day. Get outside if possible and take several deep breaths.
   - Eat a nourishing, well-balanced diet.
   - Get adequate sleep.
   - Avoid alcohol, tobacco, and drug use and too much caffeine.
   - Wear comfortable shoes with good support and nonskid soles.

10. Remember that most back injuries can be prevented if you follow the rules for good body mechanics and if you complete all lifting procedures correctly.

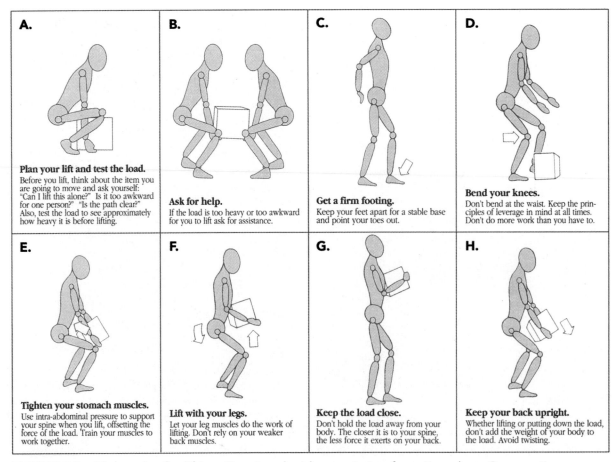

**A.**

**Plan your lift and test the load.**
Before you lift, think about the item you are going to move and ask yourself: "Can I lift this alone?" "Is it too awkward for one person?" "Is the path clear?" Also, test the load to see approximately how heavy it is before lifting.

**B.**

**Ask for help.**
If the load is too heavy or too awkward for you to lift ask for assistance.

**C.**

**Get a firm footing.**
Keep your feet apart for a stable base and point your toes out.

**D.**

**Bend your knees.**
Don't bend at the waist. Keep the principles of leverage in mind at all times. Don't do more work than you have to.

**E.**

**Tighten your stomach muscles.**
Use intra-abdominal pressure to support your spine when you lift, offsetting the force of the load. Train your muscles to work together.

**F.**

**Lift with your legs.**
Let your leg muscles do the work of lifting. Don't rely on your weaker back muscles.

**G.**

**Keep the load close.**
Don't hold the load away from your body. The closer it is to your spine, the less force it exerts on your back.

**H.**

**Keep your back upright.**
Whether lifting or putting down the load, don't add the weight of your body to the load. Avoid twisting.

**FIGURE 8-3**  Eight rules for lifting (Reprinted with permission from Ergodyne Corporation, St. Paul, MN)

**FIGURE 8-4** Warm-up exercises (Reprinted with permission from Ergodyne Corporation, St. Paul, MN)

The student should check with a physician before beginning any exercise program.

**A.**

**Neck Flexion and Extension:**
SLOWLY tip your head forward and touch your chin to your chest. Then SLOWLY tip your head back as far as possible. Repeat five times.

**B.**

**Neck Rotation:**
Keep your chin tucked down and look over your right shoulder as far as possible, then look over your left shoulder as far as possible. Repeat five times in each direction.

**C.**

**Shoulder Flexion:**
Clasp your hands together and inhale as you raise your arms over your head as far as possible with palms pointing up. Exhale as you bring your hands down behind your back. Repeat five times.

**D.**

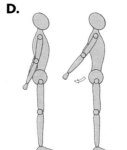

**Shoulder Extension:**
Stand erect. Clasp hands behind your back and push them out as far as possible. Hold for a count of three. Repeat five times.

**E.**

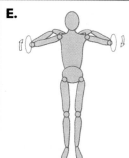

**Shoulder Circles:**
Place your hands on top of your shoulders and make circles as big as possible with your elbow. Circle five times forward and then five times backward.

**F.**

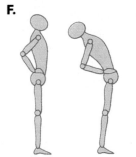

**Back Extension:**
Standing, put your hands on your hips and lean back, slowly arching your back. Repeat five times.

**G.**

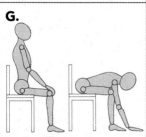

**Low Back Flexion:**
Sit in a chair with your knees shoulder width apart. Tip your chin to your chest and place your arms between your knees. SLOWLY lean forward and touch the floor. Repeat five times.

IF CHAIRS ARE ABSENT: Stand with feet shoulder width apart. Move into a squat position with your arms between your knees and your feet flat on the floor. Hold the position for a count of ten.

**H.**

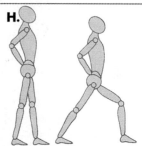

**Heel Cord Stretching:**
Place one foot forward and one foot in back, keep your back heel on the floor and back foot pointing forward. SLOWLY lean forward until you feel stretching in your calf muscles. Hold this position for five counts, then repeat with the opposite leg.

**I.**

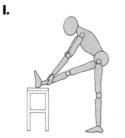

**Hamstring Stretching:**
Place your heel on a stool or chair and pull your toes toward your head. Keep your chin up and your back straight as you SLOWLY lean forward until you feel a stretch in the hamstring and calf muscles. Hold this position for ten counts, then repeat with opposite leg.

**J.**

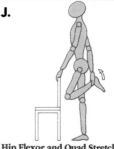

**Hip Flexor and Quad Stretching:**
While standing, hold on to the back of a chair, grab your right ankle with your left hand and pull your heel towards your right buttock. Do do not bend forward and do not arch your back. Hold this position for ten counts, then repeat with the opposite leg.

# HAZARDS IN THE WORK ENVIRONMENT

## Chemical Hazards

All health care facilities have hazards that may injure employees. Many of these items are chemicals that you may have in your own home (for example, chlorine bleach). A nursing unit may contain cleaning supplies, disinfectants, and other hazardous products. Injuries can be prevented if you know what the hazards are and how to protect yourself and others. The **Occupational Safety and Health Administration (OSHA)** is a part of the federal government under the Department of Labor. OSHA requires that all manufacturers of these items supply **Material Safety Data Sheets** or **MSDS** (Figure 8-5) with all hazardous products they sell. The MSDS provide hazard information that explains:

- What precautions to take in the presence of a hazard, for example, wearing personal protective equipment
- Instructions for safe use of the potentially dangerous substance
- How to clean up and dispose of the hazardous product
- First aid measures to use if exposure occurs

OSHA has established other rules for a safe environment. Employers are required to inform employees of:

- The location of the MSDS
- The hazards in the work environment and where they are in the building
- The location of information related to the hazards
- How to read and understand chemical labels and hazard signs
- What type of personal protective equipment should be worn if working with these hazards and where the personal protective equipment is stored
- How to manage spills and where cleaning equipment is stored

All hazardous products must be kept in the original container with the original label intact and legible. Long-term care facilities must keep all chemicals in locked cabinets.

## Equipment Safety

Learn to use equipment correctly. Report equipment that is broken or needs repair. Your facility may have a system of tagging equipment that needs repair. The tag will have the words "DO NOT OPERATE." NEVER attempt to use equipment that has been tagged. Your facility designates who is responsible for removing the tag. The equipment is returned to service only after it has been repaired and tested.

1. Beds
   - The wheels of the bed should always be locked, unless you need to move the bed.
   - Raise the bed to a comfortable working height when giving resident care.
   - Put the bed in the lowest horizontal position when you are finished giving care.
   - Make sure gatch handles on manually operated beds do not stick out.
   - Raise side rails if ordered, and check for security.
   - Do not attach restraints, supports, drainage bags, or tubing to side rails.
   - Ensure that all therapeutic, support, and protective devices are attached securely and properly to the bed. These devices include bed cradles, side rail pads, restraints, wandering alerts, special mattresses, and pads.

2. Signal cords (call lights)
   - Check call lights to make sure they are in working order.
   - Residents must always have access to caregivers. If a resident is physically or mentally unable to use a signal cord, the resident must be monitored frequently. The call light must still be within reach.
   - Answer call lights promptly.

3. Other equipment
   - Use equipment only if you know how to use it correctly.
   - Report needed repairs promptly.
     Lost screws
     Frayed straps or cords
     Loose wheels
     Broken control knobs
     Latches that do not hook
     Side rails that do not fasten correctly

4. Avoid injury from "sharps." These are needles, blades, disposable razors, or instruments that can puncture your skin.
   - Dispose of needles and blades in puncture-resistant, leakproof containers that are labeled or color coded. (This is described further in Lesson 11).
   - Never handle broken bits of glass with your bare hands. Before cleaning up broken glass, put on disposable gloves or utility gloves. Then hold several thicknesses of moist paper towels to pick up the pieces of glass (Figure 8-6). Discard the glass according to facility policy. Glassware that may be contaminated should be cleaned up with a brush and dust pan, tongs, or forceps.

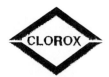

**The Clorox Company**
7200 Johnson Drive
Pleasanton, California  94588
Tel. (510) 847-6100

# Material Safety
# Data Sheet

| **I  Product:** | REGULAR CLOROX BLEACH |
|---|---|
| **Description:** | CLEAR, LIGHT YELLOW LIQUID WITH CHLORINE ODOR |

| **Other Designations** | **Manufacturer** | **Emergency Telephone No.** |
|---|---|---|
| Sodium hypochlorite solution<br>Liquid chlorine bleach<br>Clorox Liquid Bleach | The Clorox Company<br>1221 Broadway<br>Oakland, CA  94612 | Notify your Supervisor<br>Rocky Mountain Poison Center<br>(800) 446-1014<br>For Transportation Emergencies Chemtrec<br>(800) 424-9300 |

## II  Health Hazard Data

*Causes substantial but temporary eye injury. May irritate skin. May cause nausea and vomiting if ingested. Exposure to vapor or mist may irritate nose, throat and lungs. The following medical conditions may be aggravated by exposure to high concentrations of vapor or mist; heart conditions or chronic respiratory problems such as asthma, chronic bronchitis or obstructive lung disease. Under normal consumer use conditions the likelihood of any adverse health effects are low.

FIRST AID:  EYE CONTACT: Immediately flush eyes with plenty of water. If irritation persists, see a doctor. SKIN CONTACT:  Remove contaminated clothing. Wash area with water. INGESTION:  Drink a glassful of water and call a physician. INHALATION:  If breathing problems develop remove to fresh air.

## III  Hazardous Ingredients

| Ingredients | Concentration | Worker Exposure Limit |
|---|---|---|
| Sodium hypochlorite<br>CAS # 7681-52-9 | 5.25% | not established |

None of the ingredients in this product are on the IARC, NTP or OSHA carcinogen list. Occasional clinical reports suggest a low potential for sensitization upon exaggerated exposure to sodium hypochlorite if skin damage (e.g. irritation) occurs during exposure. Routine clinical tests conducted on intact skin with Clorox Liquid Bleach found no sensitization in the test subjects.

## IV  Special Protection and Precautions

Hygienic Practices:  Wear safety glasses. With repeated or prolonged use, wear gloves.

Engineering Controls:  Use general ventilation to minimize exposure to vapor or mist.

Work Practices:  Avoid eye and skin contact and inhalation of vapor or mist.

Keep out of the reach of children.

## V  Transportation and Regulatory Data

U.S. DOT Hazard Class:          Not restricted

U.S. DOT Proper Shipping Name:   Hypochlorite solution with not more than 7% available chlorine.   Not Restricted per 49CFR172.101(c)(12)(iv).

Section 313 (Title III Superfund Amendment and Reauthorization Act):
As a consumer product, this product is exempt from supplier notification requirements under Section 313 Title III of the Superfund Amendment and Reauthorization Act of 1986 (reference 40 CFR Part 372).

## VI  Spill or Leak Procedures

Small Spills (<5 gallons)
1) Absorb, containerize, and landfill in accordance with local regulations.
(2) Wash down residual to sanitary sewer.*
Large Spills (>5 gallons)
1) Absorb, containerize, and landfill in accordance with local regulations; wash down residual to sanitary sewer.* - OR - (2) Pump material to waste drum(s) and dispose in accordance with local regulations; wash down residual to sanitary sewer.*

* Contact the sanitary treatment facility in advance to assure ability to process washed-down material.

## VII  Reactivity Data

Stable under normal use and storage conditions. Strong oxidizing agent. Reacts with other household chemicals such as toilet bowl cleaners, rust removers, vinegar, acids or ammonia containing products to produce hazardous gases, such as chlorine and other chlorinated species. Prolonged contact with metal may cause pitting or discoloration.

## VIII  Fire and Explosion Data

Not flammable or explosive. In a fire, cool containers to prevent rupture and release of sodium chlorate.

## IX  Physical Data

Boiling point . . . . . . . . . . . . . . . . . . . . . . . 212°F/100°C decomposes)
Specific Gravity (H₂O=1) . . . . . . . . . . . . . . . . . . . . . . . . . . . . . . . . 1.085
Solubility in Water . . . . . . . . . . . . . . . . . . . . . . . . . . . . . . . . . complete
pH . . . . . . . . . . . . . . . . . . . . . . . . . . . . . . . . . . . . . . . . . . . . . . 11.4

DATE PREPARED   11/92

**FIGURE 8-5**  Example of a Material Safety Data Sheet (MSDS) (Courtesy of The Clorox Company, Pleasanton, CA)

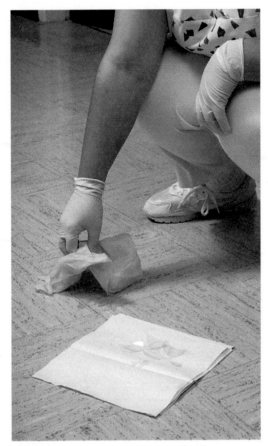

**FIGURE 8-6** Small pieces of glass may be picked up carefully with several thicknesses of damp paper towels. (The nursing assistant must wear gloves.)

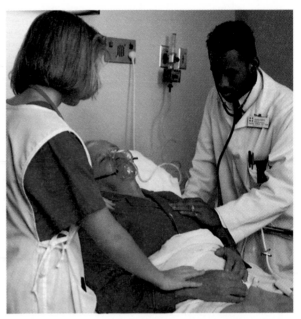

**FIGURE 8-7** Oxygen is piped into the resident's room and attached to a gauge and humidifying jar.

## Oxygen Safety

All health care facilities have oxygen in the building. It is usually piped in through the walls (Figure 8-7). Small, portable tanks of oxygen (Figure 8-8) are also kept on hand. Oxygen is flammable in the presence of a spark or open flame. For safety when a resident is using oxygen, remember:

- Do not allow smoking.
- Do not use woolen blankets.
- Do not allow an open flame such as matches, lighters, or candles.
- Disconnect oxygen before using electrical equipment.
- Do not adjust the liter flow.
- Be sure oxygen source (if a tank) is secure.
- Post oxygen safety signs.

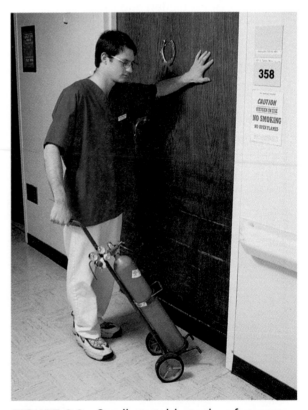

**FIGURE 8-8** Small portable tanks of oxygen are kept on hand.

# RESIDENT SAFETY ·····················

You can contribute to resident safety by performing procedures as taught and correctly following orders. Review the care plans for the residents in your care as soon as you receive your assignments after the shift report. This will allow you to see any changes in the orders for the residents. For example, on your previous shift, a resident was up and about with minimal supervision; now the resident is anxious and disoriented because of a slight stroke during the night.

All staff members in long-term care facilities are responsible for monitoring residents as they move about the building.

## Risk Factors for Incidents

Residents in long-term care facilities are at risk for incidents. There are several reasons why residents may have incidents:

- The changes in vision and hearing that most older people experience cause a loss of "warning systems." They are unaware of dangerous situations.
- Problems with mobility result from arthritic changes. These changes cause the joints to be less flexible.
- Residents may tire more easily. This increases the risk of an incident.
- Inner ear changes can cause a loss of balance and coordination.
- Frequency of urination often leads to fear of incontinence. This can result in unsafe toileting habits.
- Disorientation can cause residents to have poor judgment and an inability to recognize unsafe conditions.
- Some elderly persons experience dizziness when they stand up too quickly. This can cause them to fall.
- Certain medications can affect mental status, balance, and coordination.
- Residents may use assistive mobility devices (canes, walkers) unsafely.

## Restraints

A **physical restraint** is defined as any device or equipment that:

- A resident cannot easily remove
- Restricts a resident's movement

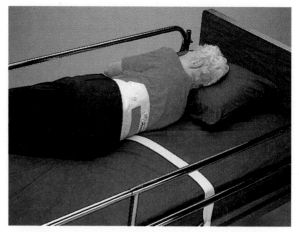

**FIGURE 8-9**   Any device that restricts movement is considered a restraint.

- Does not allow normal access to one's body

Restraints include wrist or arm and ankle or leg restraints, vests, jackets, hand mitts, geriatric and cardiac chairs, and wheelchair safety belts and bars. Side rails may be considered restraints.

The term *safety device* is often used when referring to a physical restraint. However, if a device meets the definition given above, it is still a physical restraint (Figure 8-9). Postural supports used to maintain a resident's position are not considered restraints unless they fit the description for a restraint.

Alternatives to restraints should be tried before restraints are applied. Restraints are used only as a last resort in situations where the resident may harm himself or others. Nursing assistants can take a number of actions to help reduce the resident's need for restraints:

1. Care for residents' personal needs promptly.
   - Take residents to the bathroom regularly.
   - Meet their needs if they are hungry or thirsty.
   - Report signs and symptoms of pain or illness promptly.
   - Follow all instructions for assisting residents with exercise.
   - Be sure that residents have their eyeglasses and hearing aids if they need them.
   - Answer call signals promptly.
   - Check residents often to see if they need anything.

2. Know which residents are at risk for falling. Monitor these residents during your shift. All staff members should help with monitoring.
3. Check with the nurse to see if a resident can be instructed on safe mobility skills.
4. Observe residents who walk and transfer independently. Sometimes falls occur because they use incorrect and unsafe methods. Report these situations and learn how to teach residents the correct way.
5. Report immediately any physical or mental changes that can increase the resident's risk for an incident, such as:
   • Disorientation (the resident does not know time, place, or self)
   • A resident's complaints of dizziness
   • A resident's problems with balance and coordination
6. Maintain a calm, quiet, consistent environment. Too much noise and too many distractions can agitate residents.
7. Help maintain a homelike environment. Small, cozy seating areas located throughout the building give residents the opportunity to sit down if they become tired.
8. Provide comfortable chairs for residents. Position residents for comfort and to prevent slumping to the side and sliding. Use supportive devices and pillows as necessary.
9. Work with the activities personnel to provide residents with activities that prevent boredom (Figure 8-10).
10. Make sure residents have access to signal lights at all times.
11. Use side rails only if necessary.
12. Wandering residents should be allowed to wander. Security devices are available that alert staff to residents who try to wander into unsafe areas (Figure 8-11).

The inappropriate use of restraints or safety devices can lead to physical and psychosocial complications. Restraints reduce physical mobility. This can lead to contractures, pressure ulcers, and other complications that result from inactivity. Restraints can cause disorientation, depression, hostility, and agitation in residents.

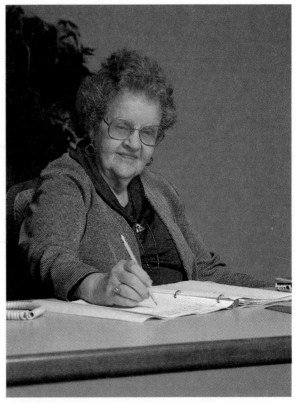

**FIGURE 8-10** Providing appropriate activities can reduce the need for restraints.

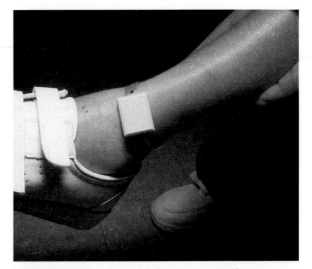

**FIGURE 8-11** A special sensor may be attached to the leg of the wandering, disoriented resident. Some manufacturers recommend that the sensor be worn on the wrist.

# *G*uidelines for

## The Use of Restraints

Restraints may be needed in life-threatening situations. They are never used for staff convenience or as a substitute for good nursing care. The need for a restraint or safety device must be continually evaluated. If physical restraints are necessary, follow these guidelines.

1. The reasons for the restraint and all actions taken to avoid restraints must be carefully documented.

    * The resident, resident's family, or legal guardian must give written consent to the use of the restraint.
    * The charge nurse is responsible for the documentation and obtaining approval.

2. The physician must write an order for the restraint. The order must include:

    * The reason for the restraint or safety device

* The type of device
* The length of time it can be used
* Where it can be used (chair, bed, or both)

3. The least restrictive device is always tried first. The restraint or safety device should be clean and in good repair.

4. Always apply restraints or safety devices according to the manufacturer's directions.

    * Make sure the restraint or safety device is the right size for the resident.
    * Apply restraints over clothing; never apply them next to the resident's skin.
    * Use only the type of restraint or safety device that is ordered (Figures 8-12 through 8-15).

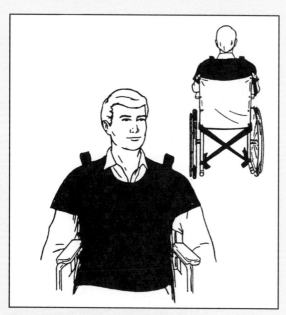

**FIGURE 8-12** Example of a jacket restraint (Courtesy of The J. T. Posey Co., Inc., Arcadia, CA)

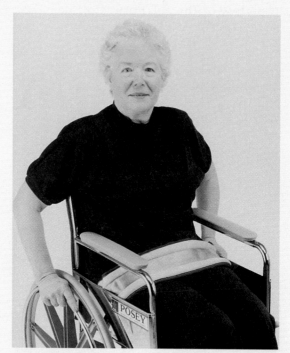

**FIGURE 8-13** A soft belt may be used when the resident is in a wheelchair. (Courtesy of The J. T. Posey Co., Inc., Arcadia, CA)

*(continues)*

# Guidelines *(continued)*

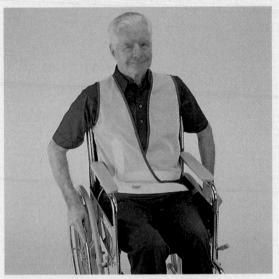

**FIGURE 8-14** A safety vest is always applied so the straps criss-cross in front. (Courtesy of The J. T. Posey Co., Inc., Arcadia, CA)

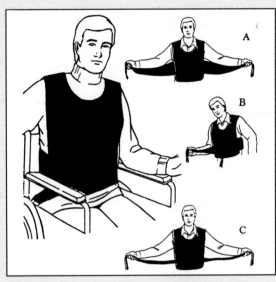

**FIGURE 8-15** Always read the manufacturer's directions for the correct application of safety devices. (Courtesy of The J. T. Posey Co., Inc., Arcadia, CA)

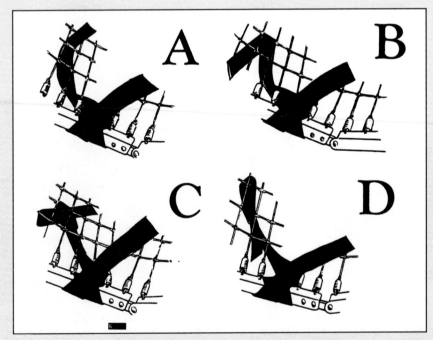

**FIGURE 8-16** Use a quick-release tie for securing the restraint. (Courtesy of The J. T. Posey Co., Inc., Arcadia, CA)

*(continues)*

## *G*uidelines *(continued)*

- Tie the device in a slip knot so that it can be released immediately in an emergency (Figure 8-16).
- Restraints applied to a resident sitting in a chair must be tied correctly and not too tightly. You should be able to insert three fingers between the restraint and the resident.
- Do not tie restraints to the stationary bed frame or side rails. Tie restraints to the mattress frame, so that the restraint will move with the resident if the bed is raised.
- The side rails should always be up when a resident is wearing a restraint in bed.

5. Check residents in restraints at least every 30 minutes and document this action.

6. Release the restraints every 2 hours and document this action.
   - Assist the resident to stand and walk if possible.
   - If the resident cannot stand, do passive range of motion exercises on all extremities.
   - Take the resident to the bathroom.
   - If the resident is incontinent, clean the resident; change clothing, chair pads, or bedding; and provide skin care.
   - Check the resident for any signs of skin breakdown or irritation and report these to the nurse.
   - Give the resident fluids and food.
   - Always place the signal light within the resident's reach.

### Preventing Accidental Poisoning

Residents who are disoriented may eat poisonous substances. Persons with dementia may eat or drink items that other residents have in their rooms, such as shaving lotion, cologne, nail polish, denture cleaning tablets, and plants. Residents may store food in their rooms until it spoils. Because of poor vision and reduced ability to taste and smell, they are unaware of spoilage. To prevent accidental poisonings:

- Keep all chemicals and cleaning solutions in locked cupboards (OSHA requirement).
- Use only nonpoisonous plants in the facility.
- The facility may provide residents with refrigerator space for perishable food items. Label containers with the residents' names, room numbers, and date. Remind residents that food is being kept for them in the refrigerator.

### Preventing Thermal Injuries

Thermal injuries (those caused by heat or cold) occur less frequently than other injuries but are still a source of concern.

- Follow procedures accurately when administering warm or cold treatments.
- Water temperature is usually regulated but check it before placing a resident in the tub or shower. Turn the hot water on last and turn it off first.
- Check food temperatures before feeding residents. Using a microwave oven to reheat food can be dangerous because of the uneven temperatures.
- Store smoking materials in a safe place and supervise residents while they smoke.

### Preventing Skin Injuries

Residents may receive **lacerations** (cuts or breaks in the skin) or skin punctures. To prevent these injuries:

- Store knives, scissors, razors, and tools in locked cupboards.
- Store needles and syringes in locked cupboards. Syringes and needles should be disposed of immediately after use in the proper sharps container.
- Clean up broken glass immediately as described earlier.

## Preventing Falls

It is estimated that each year 30% to 40% of all residents in long-term care facilities fall. To reduce falls, the environment can be altered to meet the needs of elderly persons. In Section 4 you will learn more about the changes of aging and how to adapt the environment to these changes.

1. Do not obstruct open areas with supplies and equipment. Place equipment on one side only of the hallway so residents do not need to navigate through an obstacle course.
2. Wipe up spills immediately.
3. Encourage residents to use rails along corridor walls when walking.
4. Monitor residents for signs of weakness, fatigue, dizziness, and loss of balance. Observe their actions to detect unsafe habits. Give instructions when necessary:

   • Residents who self-propel their wheelchairs need instructions on how to enter and leave elevators, how to use ramps, and reminders to use the brakes.
   • Dependent residents may benefit by learning some techniques of self-transfer. Check with the nurse to see if this is possible.

5. Provide adequate lighting in all resident areas. Avoid glare.
6. Eliminate noise and other environmental distractions. Noise can increase confusion and create anxiety even in alert individuals.
7. Do not leave residents alone in the tub or shower. All tubs and showers should have chairs so residents can remain seated throughout the procedure. Lifts for tubs minimize the risk of injuries in getting in and out of the tub. Avoid using oils that make the tub bottom slippery.
8. Check residents' clothing for fit. Loose shoes and laces, long robes, and slacks increase the risk of falling. Residents should always wear properly fitted, nonskid shoes when walking and during standing transfers.
9. Side rails are a frequent cause of falls. Many facilities leave side rails down on one side for residents who can safely transfer without help. In some situations, half-rails are more effective.
10. Care for residents' personal needs promptly. This may prevent residents from attempting unsafe transfers or ambulation.

11. Always use the correct techniques for transferring residents. Use a gait belt (transfer belt) when it is ordered. Use lift sheets when moving residents in bed to prevent skin tears from friction.

## Preventing Choking

**Aspiration** is the accidental entry of food or a foreign object into the trachea (windpipe). This causes the resident to choke. Because swallowing becomes less efficient as people age, choking occurs more often in the elderly. Residents with dementia have an increased risk of choking. To prevent incidents of choking or aspiration:

1. Be aware of residents who have problems with swallowing. Follow all instructions for giving feeding assistance to these residents.

   • Cut food into small pieces.
   • Feed slowly.
   • Offer fluids carefully between solid foods.
   • If the resident has had a stroke, place the food in the unaffected side of the mouth.
   • Make sure dentures fit well.

2. Place residents upright in good position before meals. Have them remain in this position for at least 30 minutes after eating.
3. At the end of the meal give oral care to residents who are known to keep food in their mouths. Food may remain in the mouth for several minutes after a meal and be accidentally aspirated if the resident coughs.
4. Monitor disoriented residents for placing nonedible items in their mouths. Remove such items from the environment.
5. Know how to administer the procedure for obstructed airway (see Lesson 9).

## WHEELCHAIR SAFETY

Many residents can propel their own wheelchairs. This increases their independence and allows them to move from one part of the facility to another. Whether a resident can propel a wheelchair or a care provider does it, safety measures must be followed.

1. Place the casters (smaller front wheels) in forward position for balance and stability.

   • To do this, go forward and then back up so the casters swing to the forward position.

- Remind the resident to keep the wheelchair locked when it is not moving and when the resident wishes to get up or sit down.
- The footrests must be lifted out of the way when the resident is getting in or out of the wheelchair. Footrests are usually removed if the resident can propel the wheelchair independently.

2. It is not safe for the resident in a wheelchair to attempt to pick up an object from the floor. If the resident has a reaching aid or "grabber," then small items can be picked up. The wheelchair should be moved next to the object to be picked up and the small front wheels turned forward and the large wheels locked. The resident should not attempt to pick up an item using a reaching aid by leaning over and reaching between the knees. If the resident does not have a reaching aid, the resident should be instructed to ask for assistance in picking up an object from the floor.

3. A wheelchair should never be used as a seat in a motor vehicle unless the vehicle is equipped for wheelchairs.

Procedures for manipulating curbs, ramps, and steps are not generally needed in long-term care facilities because the facilities are designed for wheelchair use. However, you must be instructed in these procedures if you will be expected to perform them.

# FIRE SAFETY

Three things are needed to start a fire: heat, fuel, and oxygen (Figure 8-17). Every staff member must know and practice the fire and evacuation plans for the facility (Figure 8-18).

1. You must know:
   - The facility fire procedure
   - Evacuation routes
   - Locations of extinguishers, fire alarms (call boxes), fire doors, and fire escapes
   - How to use fire extinguishers
2. Participate in facility fire drills.
3. Be alert to fire hazards and report:
   - Frayed electrical wires
   - Overloaded circuits

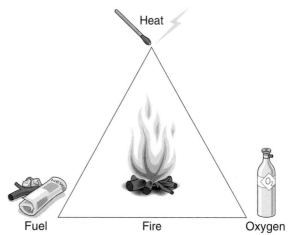

**FIGURE 8-17** The fire triangle represents the elements needed for combustion (burning).

- Improperly grounded plugs
- Accumulated clutter
- Inadequate steps to prevent fire during oxygen therapy
- Uncontrolled smoking
- Matches and cigarette lighters
- Unsafe smoking habits of staff, residents, or visitors
- Oily rags and paint rags

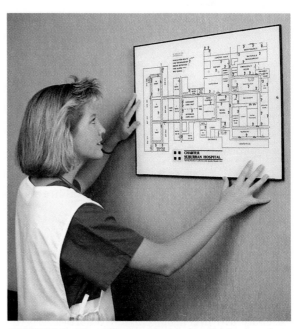

**FIGURE 8-18** All personnel should know the escape plan in the event of a fire.

**FIGURE 8-19** Remember the sequence of critical actions in case of a fire.

| | |
|---|---|
| **R** | Remove patient |
| **A** | Activate alarm |
| **C** | Contain fire |
| **E** | Extinguish (put out) fire |

4. Remember the *RACE* steps if fire occurs (Figure 8-19):
   - *Remove* all residents, staff, and other people in the immediate vicinity of the fire.
   - *Activate* the alarm and notify other staff members that a fire exists.
   - *Contain* the fire and smoke by closing all doors in the area.
   - *Extinguish* the fire, if it is very small, or allow fire department to extinguish fire.
5. Be sure that you know evacuation procedures:
   - Read evacuation plan.
   - Know the whereabouts of residents in your care.
   - Know the method of transport for residents in your care.
   - Know emergency exit routes.

Safety in the long-term care facility is the responsibility of all staff members. Teamwork prevents injuries to employees and residents.

## Fire Extinguishers

There are many different types of fire extinguishers. Each is used for a different type of fire:
- Type A extinguishers are filled with water and are used to put out paper and wood fires.
- Type B extinguishers are used for grease and oil fires.
- Type C extinguishers are used for electrical fires.
- Extinguishers marked ABC may be used on all three types of fires.

It is important that you learn:
- The location of the extinguishers
- The type of fire for which they are used
- How to use them properly. Always carefully follow the manufacturer's instructions for the use of a fire extinguisher.

Many emergency situations require rapid and effective responses from the staff. Tornadoes, hurricanes, earthquakes, floods, and bomb threats are examples of disasters that are possibilities in various parts of the country. Each facility should have its own procedures for dealing with these emergencies. You should become familiar with the procedures as quickly as possible.

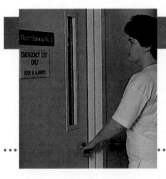

## LESSON SYNTHESIS: Putting It All Together

*Y*ou have just completed this lesson. Now go back and review the Clinical Focus. Try to see how the Clinical Focus relates to the concepts presented in the lesson. Then answer the following questions.

1. Why are residents in long-term care particularly at risk for injury due to accidents such as falls?

2. Why are fire drills carried out routinely in long-term care facilities?

3. Explain how the principles of safety applied to resident care also apply to the protection of the nursing assistant.

4. What actions can the nursing assistant take to avoid the need for restraints?

# REVIEW

**A. Select the one best answer for each of the following.**

1. The word that means adapting the environment to prevent body injury is
   a. body mechanics
   b. incident
   c. ergonomics
   d. RACE

2. One principle of body mechanics is to
   a. bend from the waist when lifting
   b. keep your feet close together when lifting
   c. use the muscles of your arms and legs for lifting
   d. keep the load as far from your body as possible

3. Material Safety Data Sheets (MSDS) are required to include information that
   a. explains whether you need personal protective equipment when using the product
   b. explains first aid measures to use if exposure occurs
   c. explains how to clean up and dispose of the product
   d. all of these

4. Which of the following residents is at risk for having an incident?
   a. Mrs. Smith who has frequency of urination because of a bladder infection
   b. Mr. James who has terminal cancer and is on bed rest
   c. Mr. Edwards who is ambulatory and has stable diabetes
   d. all of these

5. Which of the following contributes to unsafe conditions in the facility?
   a. equipment sitting in the halls
   b. chemicals in locked cupboards
   c. allowing residents to smoke only with supervision
   d. teaching residents how to use assistive devices such as canes and walkers

6. When oxygen is in use, you should not
   a. use woolen blankets on the resident's bed
   b. allow smoking in the room
   c. adjust the liter flow
   d. all of these

7. Which of the following could cause a resident to fall?
   a. taking residents to the bathroom promptly
   b. answering call lights promptly
   c. pulling the side rails up on every resident's bed
   d. monitoring residents' ambulation abilities

8. Alternatives to the use of physical restraints include
   a. appropriate activities for residents
   b. maintaining a homelike environment
   c. knowing which residents are at risk for falling
   d. all of these

9. Physical restraints may be used for residents who
   a. wander about the building
   b. are disoriented
   c. refuse to eat or take medication
   d. may harm other residents

10. Every staff member should know
    a. the facility fire procedure
    b. the location of fire extinguishers
    c. evacuation routes from the unit and building
    d. all of these

**B. Fill in the blanks by selecting the correct word or phrase from the list.**

| | |
|---|---|
| ABC | laceration |
| aspiration | mechanical lift |
| body mechanics | Material Safety |
| call light | Data Sheets |
| earthquake | (MSDS) |
| ergonomics | OSHA |
| hips and knees | physical restraints |
| incident | RACE |

11. Using your body correctly while you are working is called _____.

12. Basic rules for lifting include bend from the _____ and not from the waist.

13. An unexpected situation that can cause harm to an employee, a resident, or a visitor is called (a, an) _____.

14. Adapting the environment and using techniques and equipment to prevent body injury is called _____.

15. You should use a _____ when you need to transfer very heavy or dependent residents.

16. All residents must have access to a _____ because it may be the only way they have to summon help.

17. All manufacturers must supply _____ with the hazardous products they sell.

18. The section of the federal government that oversees employee safety is called _____.

19. A cut or break in the skin is called (a, an) _____.

20. Any device that restricts a resident's movement is called (a, an) _____.

21. _____ is the accidental entry of food or a foreign object into the trachea (windpipe).

22. The acronym used to remember the sequence of critical actions in case of fire is _____.

23. The type of extinguisher that can be used on all types of fires is the _____ extinguisher.

24. An example of a disaster involving a long-term care facility would be (a, an) _____.

# Emegencies

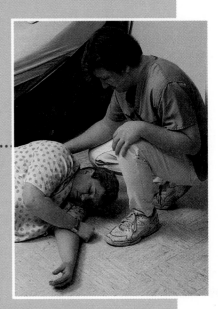

## CLINICAL FOCUS

Think about ways you can help prevent incidents

to residents as you study this lesson and meet:

Selina Lattini, who lives at the Community Nursing and Rehabilitation Center. Selina had a stroke but is able to walk with a cane. Since the stroke she receives medication for seizures but still occasionally has a seizure. She is disoriented at times and is not always able to remember recent events.

## OBJECTIVES

*After studying this lesson, you should be able to:*

- Define and spell vocabulary words and terms.
- List general measures to take in the event of an emergency.
- Describe the actions to take for the emergencies discussed in the lesson: cardiac arrest, obstructed airway, hemorrhage, falls, seizures, burns, orthopedic injuries, accidental poisoning, and fainting.

- Demonstrate the following:
  Procedure 1   Assisting the Conscious Person with Obstructed Airway—Heimlich Maneuver
  Procedure 2   Obstructed Airway, Unconscious Person
  Procedure 3   Hemorrhage
  Procedure 4   Care of Falling Resident

## VOCABULARY

**aspiration**  *(ass-pih-**RAY**-shun)*
**aura**  *(**AWE**-rah)*
**cardiac arrest**  *(**KAR**-dee ack ah-**REST**)*
**cardiopulmonary resuscitation (CPR)**  *(**kar**-dee-oh-**PUL**-moh-nair-ee ree-**sus**-ih-**TAY**-shun)*
**dislocation**  *(**dis**-loh-**KAY**-shun)*

**do not resuscitate (DNR)**  *(do not ree-**SUS**-ih-tayt)*
**emergency**  *(ee-**MER**-jen-see)*
**Emergency Medical Services (EMS)**  *(ee-**MER**-jen-see **MED**-ih-kul **SIR**-vih-sez)*
**fracture**  *(**FRACK**-shur)*

## VOCABULARY

Heimlich maneuver  (*HIGHM-lick mah-NEW-ver*)

hemorrhage  (*HEM-or-ij*)

respiratory arrest  (*RES-pih-rah-tor-ee ah-REST*)

seizure  (*SEE-zhur*)

sprain  (*sprayn*)

strain  (*strayn*)

syncope  (*SIN-koh-pee*)

## GENERAL MEASURES TO FOLLOW FOR EMERGENCIES

An **emergency** is any unexpected situation that requires immediate action. In a true emergency prompt action is needed to prevent further complications and injuries and to save the victim's life. It is important that you know the signs and symptoms of an emergency and that you are able to initiate immediate actions.

The instructions here are for emergencies in the long-term care facility. In some emergency situations the resident may be transferred by ambulance to a hospital. In other cases, the nurses will handle the emergency and the resident will remain in the facility. The following guidelines are basic actions to follow in any emergency.

## *G*uidelines for

# Responding to an Emergency

- Always remember the priorities of any emergency—the ABCs:
  - **A**irway (obstructed or unobstructed?)
  - **B**reathing (is the resident breathing?)
  - **C**irculation (is the heart beating, is there hemorrhage?)
- Stay calm. Nothing is accomplished and more problems can result if the people at the scene of an incident become flustered and agitated. If you are calm, you will be a calming influence on the resident.
- Know what to do to summon immediate help; you need to get the nurse to the scene as soon as possible. Stay with the resident and call out for help.
- Stay with the resident until the person in charge gives you permission to leave.
- Know your limitations. Be aware of what procedures nursing assistants are qualified to perform in an emergency. Never attempt a procedure unless you have received the appropriate training.
- Do not move the resident involved unless the resident is clearly in danger by staying where he or she is.
- Know the procedures to follow for emergencies. Most health care facilities have code names for various emergencies. Know what these are and how to announce a code.
- Know the procedures for activating the **Emergency Medical Services (EMS)** system. In most parts of the country this is done by dialing 911 (Figure 9-1). You will need to give the address and be able to describe what has happened (e.g., a resident was burned or has had cardiac arrest).
- Keep the person warm. Cover with blankets.
- Do not give the person any fluids or food.

*(continues)*

## $G$uidelines *(continued)*

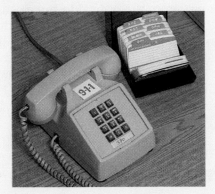

**FIGURE 9-1**  In most communities, the number for contacting EMS is 911.

- If the person starts to vomit, turn head to one side to avoid aspiration.
- If the person is conscious, assure him or her that help has been called and is on the way.
- Protect the person's privacy. Keep other residents and visitors away from the scene.

## CARDIAC ARREST

A person may stop breathing but still have a heartbeat. This is called **respiratory arrest**. If the situation is not reversed, the heart will stop beating. **Cardiac arrest** is the term used when the heart has stopped beating and respirations have ceased. When the heart and lungs are not functioning, blood and oxygen are not circulated to the brain and the rest of the body. The person is clinically dead. Permanent damage to the brain and other organs occurs within 4 to 6 minutes. Indications of cardiac arrest are:

- No response from the victim
- No breathing noted
- No pulse

**Cardiopulmonary resuscitation** or **CPR** (Figure 9-2) is a procedure used to maintain blood circulation throughout the body until the EMS can respond to the emergency. *You must never perform CPR unless you have completed an approved course.* A CPR course may be offered by your facility or the local hospital. These courses are usually sponsored through the American Heart Association or the American Red Cross. You must also know whether or not CPR is to be initiated. Many residents in long-term care facilities are very elderly and

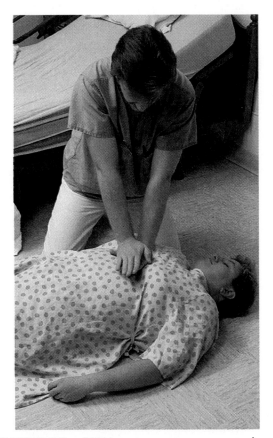

**FIGURE 9-2**  CPR is an emergency procedure that is performed only by persons who have completed an approved course.

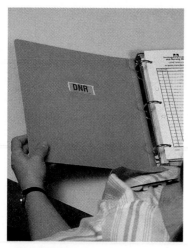

**FIGURE 9-3** DNR on a resident's chart means the resident does not wish to be resuscitated in the event of cardiac arrest.

have been ill for a long time. They are ready for death. These residents may have indicated that they do not wish to be resuscitated. The physician must write the order "**do not resuscitate (DNR)**" or "no codes" (Figure 9-3). Other residents may indicate that they wish full life support measures in the event of cardiac arrest. For these individuals, the EMS system is activated and CPR is started immediately.

## FOREIGN BODY AIRWAY OBSTRUCTION (CHOKING)

*NOTE:* If time permits, gloves should be worn for emergency procedures. Other personal protective equipment may also be needed.

---

**PROCEDURE 1**

## Assisting the Conscious Person with Obstructed Airway— Heimlich Maneuver

1. Call for help.
2. Do not attempt to interfere if the resident is coughing or is able to speak.
3. If the resident cannot speak, is not coughing, or shows the universal distress sign (Figure 9-4), take immediate action. Tell the resident you are going to help.
4. Stand behind the resident. Wrap your arms around the resident's waist.
5. Clench your fist, keeping your thumb straight (Figure 9-5).
6. Place your fist, thumb side in, against the resident's abdomen between the navel and the tip of the sternum (Figure 9-6).
7. Grasp your fist with your other hand and press your fist into the resident's abdomen with quick inward and upward thrusts (Figure 9-7).
8. Repeat the abdominal thrusts until the food or foreign object is expelled.

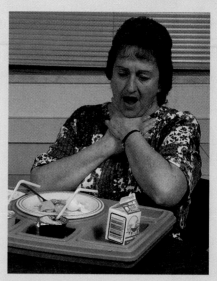

**FIGURE 9-4** Immediate action is required if the victim cannot cough or speak, or if she shows the universal distress sign.

*(continues)*

**PROCEDURE** *1* *(continued)*

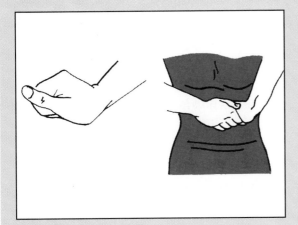

**FIGURE 9-5** Clench your fist, keeping your thumb straight.

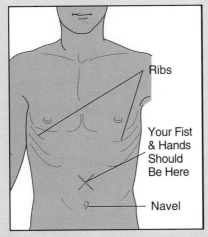

**FIGURE 9-6** Place your fist, thumb side in, against the resident's abdomen between the navel and the tip of the sternum.

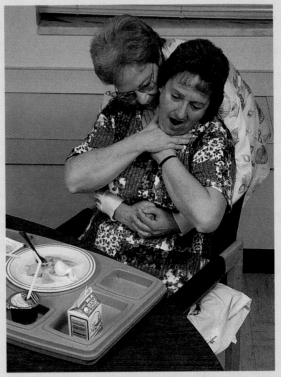

**FIGURE 9-7** Grasp your fist with your other hand and press your fist into the resident's abdomen with quick inward and upward thrusts.

If the object remains in the airway, the resident will eventually lose consciousness. If this happens, you must proceed with the procedure for obstructed airway, unconscious person.

**Aspiration** means the accidental entry of food or a foreign object into the trachea (windpipe). This causes the resident to choke. Choking occurs more readily in the elderly because the swallowing mechanism is less efficient. Aspiration can occur during vomiting. When a resident begins to vomit it is important to:

- Stay with the resident until the vomiting has ceased and you are sure the resident is out of danger.
- If the resident is in bed, turn the head to one side to allow the vomitus to drain out of the mouth instead of going into the trachea. Wipe the mouth as necessary.

**PROCEDURE 2**

# Obstructed Airway, Unconscious Person

1. If the resident has lost consciousness, place the resident on the back with face up and arms at sides.

2. Open the resident's mouth with tongue-jaw lift method and sweep deeply into the mouth to remove the foreign body, if possible (Figure 9-8). To perform tongue-jaw lift, grasp the tongue and lower jaw between your thumb and fingers and lift the jaw. To sweep, insert the index finger of your other hand deep into the resident's throat at the base of the tongue. With a hooking motion, attempt to remove the obstruction. Take care not to push the obstruction further into the throat.

3. If the foreign body cannot be removed, open the resident's airway with head-tilt/chin-lift method. First, hyperextend the neck (Figure 9-9). Then, place your hand that is closer on the resident's forehead. Apply firm pressure to tilt the head back. Place the fingertips of your other hand under the bony part of the resident's lower jaw near the chin. Lift the chin while keeping the mouth partially open.

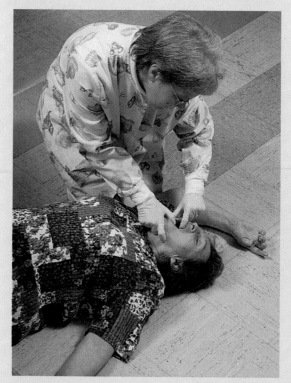

**FIGURE 9-8** Open the resident's mouth with tongue-jaw lift method and sweep deeply into the mouth with finger to remove the foreign body, if possible.

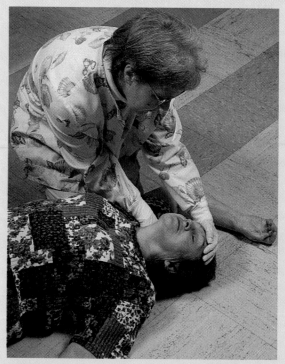

**FIGURE 9-9** If the foreign body cannot be removed, open the resident's airway with head-tilt/chin-lift method. Hyperextend the neck first.

*(continues)*

**PROCEDURE** *2* *(continued)*

Seal the resident's nose with the fingers of one hand and place the shield over the resident's mouth. In Figure 9-10 a resuscitator rather than a shield is being used. Attempt to ventilate (blow air into the resident's lungs).

4. Straddle the resident's thighs. Place heel of one hand against resident's abdomen midway between navel and xiphoid process (bottom of sternum) as in Figure 9-11.

5. Place second hand on top of first hand (Figure 9-12). Press into abdomen with quick, upward thrusts. Perform five thrusts.

6. If foreign body is still not expelled, repeat steps 2 through 6 until foreign body is expelled or until help arrives.

*NOTE:* If the foreign body is not expelled and breathing is not resumed, the resident will probably go into cardiac arrest. Take appropriate action as facility policy indicates.

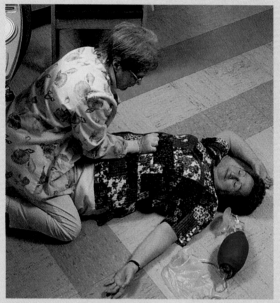

**FIGURE 9-11**  Straddle the resident's thighs. Place heel of one hand against resident's abdomen midway between navel and xiphoid process.

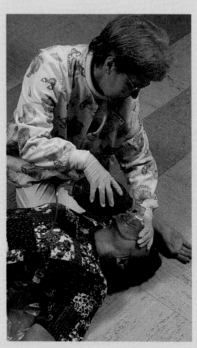

**FIGURE 9-10**  Seal the resident's mouth and nose. Attempt to ventilate.

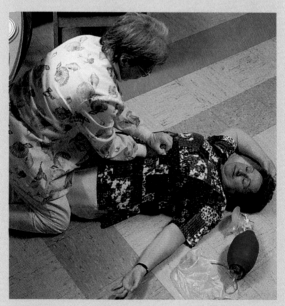

**FIGURE 9-12**  Place second hand on top of first hand.

## PROCEDURE

### 3

# Hemorrhage

Gloves should be readily available throughout the facility. Put on gloves before coming into contact with blood.

1. Call for help.
2. Identify the location of the bleeding area.
3. Apply continuous, firm, direct pressure over the bleeding area with a pad or towel or whatever is available (Figure 9-13). Elevate the area (arm or leg) above the level of the heart, if possible.

4. If seepage occurs, increase the padding and the pressure. Do not remove the saturated dressings.
5. If bleeding continues, maintain firm, direct pressure over the site, continue to elevate the extremity, and apply pressure to pulse points proximal to the injury (Figure 9-14). NEVER USE A TOURNIQUET.
6. Keep the resident warm and quiet until help arrives.

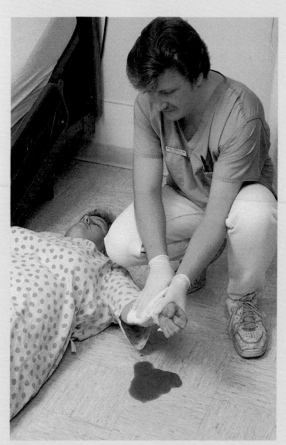

**FIGURE 9-13** Apply continuous, firm, direct pressure over bleeding area.

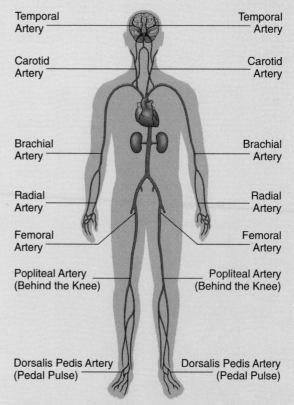

**FIGURE 9-14** If bleeding continues, maintain the direct pressure, continue to elevate extremity, and apply pressure to pulse points proximal to the injury.

• If the resident is in a chair, help the resident flex the neck to allow the vomitus to drain out of the mouth. Wipe the mouth as necessary.

When choking occurs, immediate action is necessary. There are two procedures you must know; the **Heimlich maneuver** is used for persons who are choking but are still conscious. The other procedure is for an obstructed airway in an unconscious person. You should be instructed and approved for performing these procedures.

## HEMORRHAGE

**Hemorrhage** is the rapid loss of a large amount of blood from the body. Death will occur if the hemorrhage is not stopped. Hemorrhage may be internal or external. Internal hemorrhage is suspected when the resident's:

• Pulse becomes weak, rapid, and irregular
• Blood pressure is falling
• Skin is dusky gray, cold, and clammy

Call the nurse immediately if these signs are present. Internal hemorrhage requires immediate action by the physician.

External hemorrhage is more obvious and is noted by the obvious loss of blood. Bleeding may be from an artery or from a vein. Blood coming from an artery will spurt and be bright red in color. A large amount of blood can be lost in a very short time from an artery. Blood coming from a vein will ooze out and have a bluish tinge.

## RESIDENT FALLS

Lesson 8 described measures for preventing falls. If a resident falls, you must protect both the resident and yourself.

---

**PROCEDURE 4**

## Care of Falling Resident

1. Keep your back straight, bend from the hips and knees, and maintain a broad base of support as you assist the falling resident.
2. Ease the resident to the floor, using your leg to let the person slide down gently to the floor. Protect the resident's head.
3. As you ease the resident to the floor, bend your knees and go down with the resident (Figure 9-15).
4. Call for help. *Do not attempt to move the resident until the nurse or physician has examined the resident and has given you instructions.*
5. Assist in returning the resident to bed or chair. Be sure you have adequate help.
6. Carry out procedure completion actions.
7. Record according to facility policy.

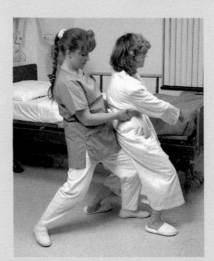

**FIGURE 9-15** Ease the resident to the floor as you bend your knees and go down with the resident.

## SEIZURES

A **seizure** or convulsion involves sudden, involuntary contractions of a group of muscles. A disturbance in consciousness and changes in behavior occur. The two types of seizures are:

- Partial seizure
  - The seizures begin in one part of the body. They may be considered simple (without disturbance in consciousness) or complex (with impairment of consciousness).
- Generalized seizure
  - Generalized seizures involve the entire body (Figures 9-16A and B).

Adult-onset seizures may occur after a brain injury, along with a brain tumor, after a stroke, and along with dementia.

### Emergency Treatment for Seizures

Seizures can occur suddenly and without warning. Some people have an aura before a seizure. An **aura** is a sensory disturbance; the person may hear a noise, smell something, or see a certain pattern. If the resident is aware of this, he or she may have time to get to a chair or to lie down. When a seizure occurs:

1. Do not leave the resident alone. Call for help.

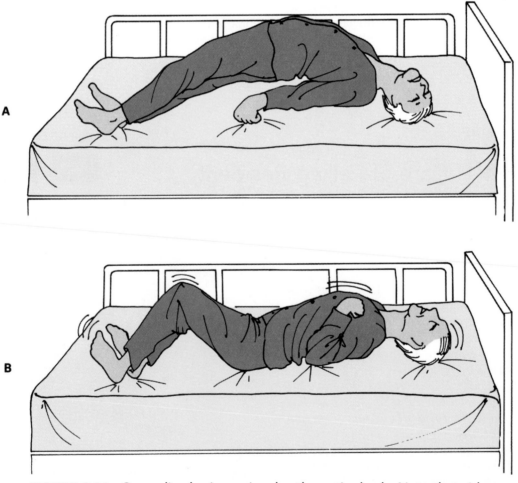

A

B

**FIGURE 9-16** Generalized seizures involve the entire body. Note that side rails should be padded and up during a seizure. The side rails are down in the figure for clarity of the view. A. Rigid posturing B. Uncontrolled movements

2. Do not restrain movements. Do not force anything into the resident's mouth. Provide privacy and keep onlookers away.
3. Protect the resident from injury. Move any objects that might cause injury.
4. Place a small pillow, folded towel, or blanket under the resident's head if the resident is on the floor.
5. Loosen clothing around resident's head.
6. Maintain open airway. Turn resident's head to the side, if possible.
7. Observe seizure. Most seizures stop on their own.
8. After movements subside, turn resident to side so fluid or vomitus can drain freely from mouth.
9. Incontinence is common after a seizure.
10. Allow the resident to rest.
11. Check for breathing and pulse. Initiate appropriate actions if either is absent.
12. Allow the resident to sleep after seizure has subsided. Position the resident on the side and observe closely while resident sleeps.
13. Note length of seizure and report.

# BURNS

Burns result in loss of skin integrity and may be caused by hot liquids or other substances, chemicals, or radiation. There is a high risk of infection with any burn. Burns may occur in the long-term care facility from:

- Spilling hot coffee, tea, or soup
- Hot water
- Careless use of smoking materials

Burns are classified as partial thickness or full thickness depending on the degree of injury. Partial thickness burns are:

- First-degree burns—involve only the top layer (epidermis) of skin. There is redness, temporary swelling and pain. There is usually no permanent scarring.
- Second-degree burns—involve both epidermis and dermis. The skin color may vary from pink or red to white or tan. Blistering, pain, and some scarring occur.

Full thickness burns are:

- Third-degree burns—involve epidermis, dermis, and subcutaneous tissue. The tissue is bright red to tan and brown. There may be no pain initially because nerve endings have been destroyed. Later, pain and scarring will result.

## Emergency Treatment for Burns

1. Call the nurse immediately.
2. If the resident's clothing is on fire, use a coat or blanket to smother the flames.
3. Cool water may be applied to lower the skin temperature and stop further tissue damage. Remove wet clothing. (Follow the nurse's instructions.)
4. Second-degree burns may require treatment at the hospital emergency room. Third-degree burns will probably require hospitalization for special treatment.

# ORTHOPEDIC INJURIES

Orthopedic injuries include injuries to bones, joints, muscles, and ligaments. These include fractures, sprains, strains, and dislocations.

## Treatment for Orthopedic Injuries

A **fracture** is a break in a bone. If you suspect a resident has suffered a fracture:

- Stay with the resident.
- Do not attempt to move the resident.
- Call the nurse immediately.

If a fracture is suspected, the EMS will be called and the resident will be transported by ambulance to the hospital for x-rays. If a fracture is present, the physician will put a cast on the affected extremity or place the resident in traction or do surgery. (This is explained further in Lesson 28.)

A **sprain** is an injury to a ligament caused by sudden overstretching. A sprained ankle may occur, for example, if a person falls and turns the ankle quickly while falling. Swelling may be noted shortly afterward.

A **strain** is excessive stretching of a muscle resulting in pain and swelling of the muscle. You may strain the muscles in your back if you use incorrect lifting and moving techniques.

A **dislocation** occurs in a joint, when one bone is displaced from the other bone. This can occur in a paralyzed arm that is allowed to hang without support. The weight of the arm pulls the upper arm bone out of position in the shoulder joint. A dislocation can also be caused by improperly lifting the resident under the arms.

If you suspect that a resident has suffered a sprain, strain, or dislocation:

- Notify the nurse at once.

You may be instructed to:

- Elevate the injured extremity.
- Apply ice packs to the area. (See Lesson 21 for instructions on application of ice packs.)

After 24 hours, you may be instructed to apply warm packs to the area.

## ACCIDENTAL POISONING

Immediate attention is needed if a resident is the victim of accidental poisoning. All potentially harmful substances must be kept in locked cupboards. However, a confused resident may obtain and ingest a harmful substance. If you suspect that this has happened:

- Call the nurse immediately.
- Try to determine what the resident has taken; save the container.

- The nurse may administer a substance that will cause vomiting. (Not all ingested poisons can be safely removed from the resident's body by vomiting.)
- Know where to find the telephone number for the regional poison control center.
- The resident may need to be transported to a hospital by ambulance.

## FAINTING

Fainting (**syncope**) is a loss of consciousness due to temporary insufficient blood flow to the brain. The attack comes on gradually with light-headedness, perspiring, and blurred vision. Fainting can occur in otherwise healthy people and may be related to emotional shock or standing in one place for a long time. Residents experiencing these symptoms should sit down in a chair or lie down before they lose consciousness. If they faint and fall, allow them to lie still unless they are in immediate danger. Recovery is usually prompt and without complications or aftereffects. Call for the nurse immediately.

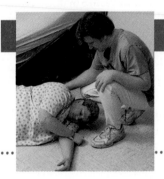

## LESSON SYNTHESIS: Putting It All Together

*Y*ou have just completed this lesson. Now go back and review the Clinical Focus. Try to see how the Clinical Focus relates to the concepts presented in the lesson. Then answer the following questions.

1. Mrs. Lattini is at high risk for falling. Her use of a cane is one risk factor. What observations should you make in regard to ambulation with a cane?

2. What steps can you take in an effort to prevent Mrs. Lattini from falling?

3. Describe what you would do in the event that Mrs. Lattini falls.

4. What can you do as a nursing assistant to ensure that you will know how to respond in the event of an emergency?

## REVIEW

**A. Select the one best answer for each of the following.**

1. If an emergency occurs in the long-term care facility, you should
   a. leave the resident where he or she is and get the nurse as quickly as possible
   b. do as much as you can and then call for the nurse
   c. call the EMS right away
   d. know your limitations

2. Indications of cardiac arrest include
   a. no pulse
   b. no breathing
   c. no response from the victim
   d. all of these

3. When a resident makes an advance directive indicating the resident does not wish to be resuscitated, the physician writes the order referred to as
   a. CPR
   b. ABC
   c. DNR
   d. EMS

4. The Heimlich maneuver should be initiated when the resident
   a. is coughing
   b. suffers cardiac arrest
   c. vomits
   d. cannot speak, is not coughing, and is conscious, or clutches the throat

5. If a resident is hemorrhaging externally you should first
   a. apply pressure directly over the wound
   b. apply pressure over the closest pressure points
   c. apply a tourniquet
   d. run for help

6. When a resident falls you should
   a. try to hold the resident in an upright position
   b. let go of the resident immediately to avoid injuring yourself
   c. ease the resident to the floor, protecting the resident's head
   d. none of these

7. If a resident has a seizure you should first
   a. place something between the resident's teeth
   b. begin CPR
   c. restrain the resident's arms and legs
   d. protect the resident from injury and allow the seizure to run its course

8. If a resident suffers a burn from hot coffee, the nurse may instruct you to
   a. apply cool water to the area
   b. apply butter or some other greasy substance
   c. hold ice cubes against the area
   d. all of these

**B. Answer each statement true (T) or false (F).**

9. T  F  The first thing to consider in an emergency are the ABCs.

10. T  F  Cardiopulmonary resuscitation is always administered when a resident has cardiac arrest.

11. T  F  If applying direct pressure to hemorrhage is not successful, you should apply a tourniquet.

12. T  F  It is common for incontinence to occur during or after a seizure.

13. T  F  If a resident ingests a poisonous substance, you should immediately force the resident to vomit.

14. T  F  You should not move a resident who has fallen until the nurse has examined the resident and given instructions.

15. T  F  Recovery from fainting is usually quick and without complications.

# LESSON
# *10*

# Infection

## CLINICAL FOCUS

Think about the causes of infections as you

study this lesson and meet:

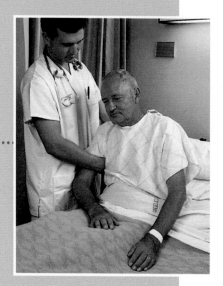

*F*ranklin Dwyer who is 66. He is HIV positive and has a history of repeated pneumonia. He also had hepatitis A and tuberculosis in his youth. Each infection was treated aggressively with medication. Now, Mr. Dwyer's CD4 count has dropped significantly and he has been diagnosed with AIDS.

## OBJECTIVES

*After studying this lesson you should be able to:*

- Define and spell vocabulary words and terms.
- Describe how infections can be introduced to the long-term care facility.
- Name five serious infectious diseases.
- Recognize the causes of several important infectious diseases.

- List the ways that infectious diseases are spread.
- List the parts of the chain of infection.
- List natural body defenses against infections.
- Explain why residents are at risk for infections.

## VOCABULARY

**antibiotic**   *(an-tih-buy-**OT**-ick)*

**antibody**   *(**AN**-tih-**bah**-dee)*

**antigen**   *(**AN**-ti-jen)*

**bacteremia**   *(**back**-ter-**EE**-mee-ah)*

**carrier**   *(**KAIR**-ee-er)*

**contagious**   *(kon-**TAY**-jus)*

**culture and sensitivity**   *(**KUL**-tyour and **sen**-sih-**TIV**-ih-tee)*

**flora**   *(**FLOOR**-ah)*

**hemoptysis**   *(he-**MOP**-tih-sis)*

**hepatitis**   *(**hep**-ah-**TYE**-tis)*

**human immunodeficiency virus (HIV)**   *(**HYOU**-man im-**MYOUN**-oh-dih-**fish**-en-see **VYE**-rus)*

**immunity**   *(im-**MYOUN**-ih-tee)*

**immunization**   *(**IM**-myou-nigh-**zay**-shun)*

**immunosuppression**   *(im-**myoun**-oh-suh-**PREH**-shun)*

# VOCABULARY

infection  *(in-**FECK**-shun)*

inflammation  *(in-flah-**MAY**-shun)*

methicillin-resistant ***Staphylococcus aureus* (MRSA)**  *(meth-ih-**SILL**-in ree-**SIS**-tant **staff**-ill-oh-**KOCK**-us **AWE**-ree-us)*

microbe  *(**MY**-krohb)*

nosocomial infection  *(noh-soh-**KOH**-mee-al in-**FECK**-shun)*

pathogens  *(**PATH**-oh-jens)*

seropositive  *(**see**-roh-**POZ**-ih-tiv)*

transmission  *(trans-**MISH**-un)*

tubercle  *(**TOO**-ber-kul)*

tuberculosis disease  *(too-**ber**-kyou-**LOH**-sis dih-**ZEEZ**)*

tuberculosis infection  *(too-**ber**-kyou-**LOH**-sis in-**FECK**-shun)*

vaccine  *(**VACK**-seen)*

vancomycin-resistant enterococci (VRE)  *(van-koh-**MY**-sin ree-**SIS**-tant **en**-ter-oh-**KOCK**-ee)*

## INFECTIOUS DISEASE

**Infections** can occur when disease-producing organisms enter the body. Infections that occur in residents while they are in the care facility are called **nosocomial infections**. Visitors, staff members, and residents can introduce infections through the spread of **microbes** (germs). This is one reason why it is so important to carry out proper handwashing techniques.

## MICROBES

Some microbes are useful and necessary to life. For example, the lower digestive tract is filled with bacteria that help in the elimination of feces. Other microbes cause disease and are called **pathogens**. They are tiny forms of life that can only be seen with a microscope. Some of the most common pathogens are:

- Bacteria
- Viruses
- Fungi (yeast and molds)
- Protozoa

### Bacteria

There are many forms of bacteria (Figure 10-1). They can cause infections in the skin, respiratory tract, urinary tract, and bloodstream. Boils and strep throat are common bacterial infections.

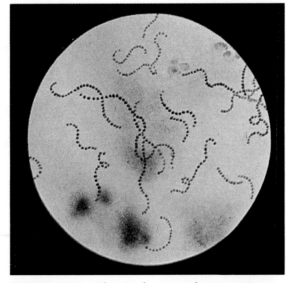

**FIGURE 10-1** This is the way the organisms (bacteria) look under the microscope. This organism causes scarlet fever and strep sore throat.

### Viruses

Viruses are smaller than bacteria. Viruses cause the common cold, flu, and many childhood diseases such as mumps, chickenpox, measles, and polio. Viruses also cause some forms of pneumonia, herpes simplex, herpes zoster (shingles), acquired immune deficiency syndrome (AIDS), and hepatitis.

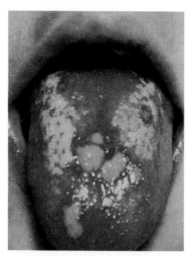

**FIGURE 10-2** The white patches on the tongue are the result of a yeast (fungus) infection. This condition is called thrush.

## Fungi

Fungi cause skin and mucous membrane infections like yeast vaginitis, athlete's foot, ringworm, and thrush (Figure 10-2).

## Protozoa

Infections due to protozoa are more rare but can affect the blood, lungs, and intestines when they occur.

## THE CHAIN OF INFECTION

Infections occur when certain conditions are met. These conditions are called the chain of infection (Figure 10-3) and include:

- Causative agent or microbe—pathogen that causes the disease
- Source—human body in which the microbe can live
- Portal of exit—manner in which the microbe leaves the body
- Method of transmission—manner in which the microbe is carried to another person
- Portal of entry—manner in which the microbe enters another person
- Susceptible host—a person who will become ill from the entry of microbes into the body

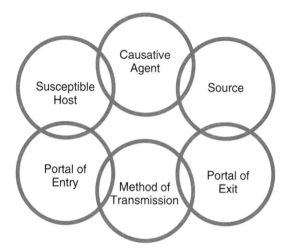

**FIGURE 10-3** The chain of infection

Microbes cause disease by entering the body through a portal of entry. They spread disease by leaving the body through a portal of exit and being transmitted to another person. They enter that person's body and can again cause disease.

Microbes enter and leave the body through body openings such as:

- Eyes, ears, nose, or mouth
- Breaks in the skin
- Penis, vagina, urinary meatus (bladder opening), or rectum

**Transmission** (spread) of infectious organisms may occur in one of three ways (Figure 10-4):

- Airborne transmission. Small particles remain suspended in the air and move with air currents or become trapped in dust, which is also carried in air currents. The resident breathes in the pathogens carried in this manner.
- Droplet transmission. Droplets are moist particles from coughing, sneezing, or talking. Pathogens are transmitted into the air with the droplets. Droplets usually travel only 3 feet from the source.
- Contact transmission is direct contact by a person with the source of the pathogens. Indirect contact occurs when a person contacts an item contaminated with pathogens, such as soiled linen.

Not all organisms are transmitted in the same way and some organisms may be transmitted in more than one way.

---

> **FIGURE 10-4** Ways in which microbes are spread from one person to others
>
> **Airborne Transmission**
> - Pathogens carried by moisture or dust particles in air; can be carried long distances
>
> **Droplet Transmission**
> Droplet Spread Within Approximately 3 Feet (No Personal Contact) of Infected Person by:
> - Coughing
> - Laughing
> - Sneezing
> - Singing
> - Talking
>
> **Contact Transmission**
> Direct Contact with Infected Person:
> - Touching
> - Sexual contact
> - Blood
> - Body fluids (drainage, urine, feces, sputum, saliva, vomitus)
>
> Indirect Contact with Infected Person:
> - Clothing
> - Dressings
> - Equipment used in care and treatment
> - Bed linens
> - Personal belongings
> - Specimen containers
> - Instruments used in treatment
> - Food
> - Water
>
> Note that pathogens can also be carried by insects and animals and passed to humans.

## Types of Infections

Infections can be:
- Local (confined to one area)—such as a boil or skin abscess
- Generalized—such as pneumonia (in the lungs)
- Systemic—widespread through the bloodstream (**bacteremia**)

People who have pathogens in their bodies, but do not show signs of disease, are called **carriers**. Carriers can transmit diseases to others. The pathogens in their bodies are not harmful to the carriers, but they may be harmful to other people.

## BODY FLORA

Different microbes live on our body surfaces. These microbes are called the normal body **flora**. The flora is not the same in all body areas. For example, the organisms making up the flora of the intestinal tract are different from those of the respiratory tract. Healthy individuals live in harmony with the normal body flora. However, the balance may be disturbed by:
- Pathogenic organisms
- Normal flora organisms that become pathogenic
- Organisms from one flora that are transferred into a different body flora
- Drugs such as antibiotics that upset the normal balance of organisms within a flora, allowing one group to flourish

You can help avoid infections in yourself by:
- Eating a healthy diet
- Getting an adequate amount of sleep daily
- Keeping your body clean and living in a clean environment
- Avoiding unhealthy habits such as smoking, drinking alcohol, or using drugs
- Learning how to cope with stress

## NATURAL BODY DEFENSES AGAINST DISEASE

Natural body defenses that can help prevent infectious diseases include:
- Tears
- Mucous membranes (the lining) of the respiratory, reproductive, and genitourinary tracts
- Intact skin
- Hydrochloric acid in the stomach
- Hair in the nose, eyelashes
- White blood cells (leukocytes) that multiply and attempt to destroy pathogenic microbes in the body

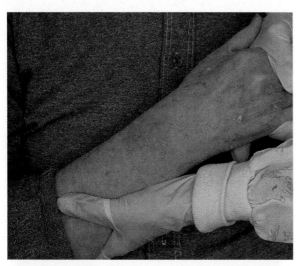

**FIGURE 10-5**   Redness, swelling, heat, pain, and loss of function are signs of the inflammatory process.

- Antibodies that develop in the blood after having an infectious disease
- **Inflammation**—a process that brings blood and white blood cells to the area of infection; a skin infection, for example, generally becomes swollen, hot, and painful, signs that inflammation is occurring (Figure 10-5).
- Temperature—an elevated temperature is believed to increase the body's ability to fight infection.

## IMMUNITY

**Immunity** is the ability to fight off disease caused by microbes. A pathogenic microbe that enters the body is an **antigen**. In response to this, the blood develops substances called **antibodies**. These antibodies provide immunity to the disease caused by that particular antigen. For example, if an individual has had antigens in the bloodstream from measles, he or she will form antibodies in the blood that prevent the occurrence of measles a second time.

### Immunosuppression

**Immunosuppression** occurs when the body's immune system is inadequate and fails to

respond to the challenge of infectious disease organisms that it normally would fight successfully. The individual becomes more likely to develop a variety of infections. A number of factors can lead to this condition, including:

- Diseases such as leukemia
- Advanced age
- Frailty
- Drug therapy
- Infection with human immunodeficiency virus (HIV)
- Injury or removal of the spleen
- Radiation therapy

## IMMUNIZATIONS

Artificial defenses called **immunizations** protect against specific pathogens. Immunization is provided by **vaccines**. These are artificial or weakened antigens that help the body develop protective antibodies before the need arises. Vaccines are available to prevent most childhood diseases such as measles, rubella (German measles), mumps, polio, diphtheria, chickenpox, whooping cough, and tetanus. Pneumonia vaccine and influenza vaccine are frequently given to elderly people. Health workers who have direct contact with residents are advised to take hepatitis B vaccine. Federal legislation requires that employers provide this vaccine without charge to employees who are considered at risk.

## SERIOUS INFECTIONS IN HEALTH CARE FACILITIES

Serious bacterial and viral infections are increasing in health care facilities as well as in the general public. Elderly and frail people are particularly susceptible to infectious diseases, as are the very young and those with compromised (poorly functioning) immune systems.

## BACTERIAL INFECTIONS

Bacteria are often the cause of serious skin, respiratory, urinary, and gastrointestinal infections in residents. If the physician suspects that a resident has a bacterial infection, a **culture and sensitivity** test may be ordered. This test can be done on urine, drainage from a wound, blood, or other body fluid. The culture tells the physician what type of microbe is causing the infection. The sensitivity tells the physician which **antibiotic** should be used to treat the infection.

When an antibiotic is prescribed, it is important to take all the medication prescribed for the stated length of time. If the person stops taking the antibiotic too soon, some of the microbes may remain and develop a resistance to the antibiotic.

Certain infectious microbes have become resistant to the antibiotics most commonly used against them. This is a serious problem in controlling infections in health care facilities. The antibiotics that are still effective often are more expensive and may have serious side effects compared to the previously preferred antibiotics. It is possible that, in time, these infectious microbes may also become resistant to these antibiotics.

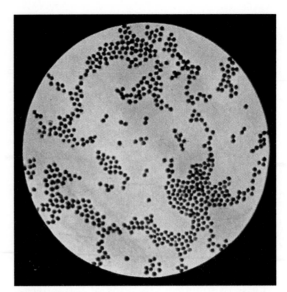

**FIGURE 10-6** Methicillin-resistant *Staphylococcus aureus* (MRSA) has developed a resistance to the antibiotic of choice for treating the infection. (Courtesy of The Centers for Disease Control and Prevention, Atlanta, GA)

## MRSA and VRE

Two groups of organisms have become resistant to two powerful antibiotics, methicillin and vancomycin. These organisms are:

- **Methicillin-resistant *Staphylococcus aureus* (MRSA)**
  Staphylococci are normally found on skin and mucous membranes. Figure 10-6 shows *Staphylococcus aureus* organisms.
- **Vancomycin-resistant enterococci (VRE)**
  Enterococci are found in the gastrointestinal tract. They are a major cause of nosocomial infections in health care facilities. Most strains are highly resistant to many antibiotics. Newer strains are resistant to vancomycin.

## Other Bacterial Infective Agents

Serious infections are also caused by the following types of bacteria:

- *Pseudomonas aeruginosa*—this organism is found in water and on other environmental surfaces. It causes urinary tract infections.
- *Escherichia coli*—bacterium commonly found in the intestinal tract where it is normally non-pathogenic. Outside the intestinal tract, however, it can cause urinary tract infections or infections in pressure ulcers.
- Streptococcus A—a bacterium that produces powerful enzymes that destroy tissue and blood cells
- Salmonella—a group of bacteria that cause mild to life-threatening intestinal infections, including "food poisoning"
- *Mycobacterium tuberculosis*—the bacterium that causes tuberculosis

## Tuberculosis

Before the development of antibiotics, tuberculosis was a widespread disease with a high fatality rate. In the 1950s, the use of antibiotics effective against tuberculosis caused the numbers of cases and deaths to drop sharply. Since 1985, the number of people infected with tuberculosis has increased, in part, because of new strains of *Mycobacterium tuberculosis* that are resistant to several antibiotics used to treat tuberculosis. There is also an increase in the number of people who are at risk for infection, including those who:

- Are HIV positive
- Are infected but fail to take their medication for the full treatment period

- Live in poverty and are malnourished
- Have immigrated to the United States from countries where tuberculosis is still common
- Have inactive tuberculosis and have grown older and experience increased disability

**Tuberculosis Infection.**  **Tuberculosis infection** occurs when the bacterium that causes the disease enters the body. The lungs are the most common site of involvement. The body usually responds to the infection by creating a barrier that prevents the spread of the pathogens to other parts of the body. This barrier is called a **tubercle**. As long as the tubercle remains intact and no other tuberculosis bacteria enter the body, the infection is called inactive or controlled. In this state the person is not **contagious** (capable of passing the infection to others). If the person is immunocompromised, the tubercle may not form and the person develops active tuberculosis disease.

**Tuberculosis Disease.**  **Tuberculosis disease** develops if the tubercle breaks down or more tuberculosis bacteria enter the body. The bacteria multiply, tissue damage increases, and the bacteria may spread to other parts of the body. As the disease progresses, the person will show one or more of the following signs and symptoms:

- Fatigue
- Loss of appetite and weight
- Weakness
- Elevated temperature in the afternoon and evening
- Night sweats
- Spitting up blood (**hemoptysis**)
- Coughing

The person with tuberculosis in the lungs can spread it to others through droplets in respiratory secretions.

**Diagnosis.**  The presence of tuberculosis bacteria in the body can be shown by:

- A sputum culture—grows the organisms from the person's lungs
- Chest x-rays—show the extent of the disease process in the lungs
- A positive skin test (Mantoux test)—shows the presence of antibodies to the tuberculosis organisms in the body

Health care providers in long-term care must undergo a skin test for tuberculosis before employment. They are then tested regularly (usually every 6–12 months) according to the degree of risk of exposure to ensure that they remain disease free.

Residents usually are skin tested once a year. Because the immune response may be weaker in the elderly, a two-step procedure of skin testing is recommended for those over 50 years of age. If the first skin test is negative, the test is repeated in 1 to 2 weeks. The second test acts as a "booster" to the test stimulus. A negative response after the second test usually indicates the person is infection free.

**Treatment.**  A person with tuberculosis is treated with a selected antibiotic or combination of antibiotics. Because many disease organisms have become more resistant to specific drugs, a combination of drugs must be used to control them. Once antitubercular drug therapy starts, the resident usually becomes noncontagious (cannot spread the disease organism) within 2 to 3 weeks. The therapy, however, continues for 6 months to 2 years.

# VIRAL INFECTIONS

Several viral infections are described in this section:

- Shingles (herpes zoster)
- Influenza
- Hepatitis
- Acquired immune deficiency syndrome (AIDS)

The viral infection herpes venereum is covered in Lesson 27.

## Shingles

Shingles (herpes zoster) occurs in people who were infected by the virus that causes chickenpox. Although the person recovered from chickenpox, the organisms did not leave the body. They remained in the body's nervous system in a nonactive state.

Years later, when the person is in a weakened condition, the organisms become active. Painful blister-like lesions develop in the skin along the paths of sensitive nerves. Eventually the lesions heal on their own. They contain infectious organisms and contact and airborne precautions should be used.

## Influenza

Influenza (or flu) is caused by a family of viruses. The infection can lead to serious consequences for elderly or frail residents. Each year new types of viruses spread rapidly by way of respiratory secretions from person to person, causing many people to become ill.

Vaccines offer some protection against influenza viruses and are often given to residents in long-term care.

Someone with the flu may experience:

- Malaise (general unwell feeling)
- Chills
- Fever
- Muscle aches and pains
- Coldlike symptoms

In addition to making the person feel ill, the viruses may lower the resident's resistance to other infectious organisms. These other organisms can cause pneumonia and other life-threatening infections. Medicines may be given that limit the effects of the viruses and antibiotics are given to combat bacterial infections that may develop.

You can help protect the residents in your care by:

- Staying healthy
- Not reporting for duty when you are ill
- Carrying out standard precautions faithfully
- Following the facility's policies regarding special precautions when a resident has a respiratory infection
- Encouraging the resident to drink fluids
- Reporting to the charge nurse when a visitor seems to be ill

## Hepatitis

**Hepatitis** is an inflammation of the liver caused by several viruses, including:

- Hepatitis A virus
- Hepatitis B virus
- Hepatitis C virus

Characteristics of these viruses are:

- Hepatitis A virus (HAV)
  - Most common
  - Transmitted by fecal-oral route
  - Vaccine being developed

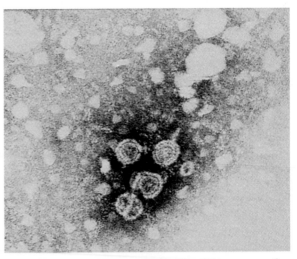

**FIGURE 10-7**  Hepatitis B virus (Courtesy of The Centers for Disease Control and Prevention, Atlanta, GA)

- Hepatitis B virus (HBV) (Figure 10-7)
  - Most serious
  - Transmitted by way of blood, sexual secretions, and fecal-oral route
  - Vaccine available for protection
- Hepatitis C virus (HCV)
  - 50% of people infected develop chronic hepatitis
  - Transmitted mainly through blood and blood products
  - Treated with alpha interferon

Any infection of the liver is serious because the liver is a vital organ. You can best protect yourself by:

- Using standard precautions (discussed in Lesson 11)
- Taking the vaccine, if available
- Practicing safe sex (using condoms)
- Not using illegal drugs
- Giving your full attention to the handling of sharps such as needles or razors

### Acquired Immune Deficiency Syndrome (AIDS)

AIDS is a viral disease. It is transmitted primarily through direct contact with the bodily secretions of an infected person. The virus that causes AIDS is the **human immunodeficiency virus (HIV)**.

The ways in which HIV is transmitted include:

- Blood to blood through:
  - Transfusion of infected blood. Note that federal regulations prohibit the use of untested and unregulated blood in the United States.
  - Treatment of hemophilia with clotting factor from infected blood
  - Needle sharing among drug users
  - Prick from a contaminated needle or sharp
  - Unsterile instruments used for procedures such as ear piercing or tattooing
- Unprotected vaginal or anal intercourse when one partner is infected
- Infected mother to infant during:
  - Pregnancy
  - Birth process
  - Nursing

**The AIDS Virus.** The AIDS virus (HIV):

- Has no known cure
- Has many variants
- Does not live for long outside the body
- Is affected by common chemicals
- Depresses the body's immune system
- Makes the infected person more susceptible to infections
- Makes the infected person more likely to experience complications such as:
  - *Pneumocystis carinii* pneumonia—a serious lung infection
  - Kaposi sarcoma—a serious malignancy affecting many body organs. Figure 10-8 shows skin lesions of Kaposi sarcoma.
  - Brain involvement leading to dementia
  - Eye involvement leading to blindness
  - Tuberculosis
  - Other opportunistic infections

**Incubation Period.** Not everyone who comes in contact with the HIV virus becomes infected. For those who are infected, there is always a period of time between contact and the start of the signs and symptoms of the infection.

- During this period the virus is in infected cells but is not active in making RNA and proteins. The body does not make antibodies to the virus.
- Most people become **seropositive** or HIV positive (show antibodies to HIV in the blood-

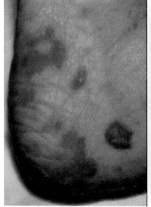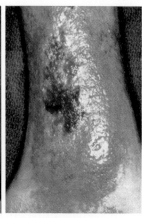

**FIGURE 10-8** HIV infection predisposes the person with AIDS to develop Kaposi sarcoma. The photographs of the heel (left) and ankle (right) show typical lesions of this type of cancer.

stream) approximately 3 months after infection. The person has HIV disease, which may progress to AIDS.

- The asymptomatic period (when no signs and symptoms are present) following infection may last months to years. AIDS does not always develop, but the person is an HIV carrier for life.

**Disease Progression.** Progression of the disease process is determined by the effect of the viruses on special protective white blood cells known as CD4 cells (T cells). Over time the number of the protective white blood cells drops. As a result, the immune system of the infected person becomes more suppressed and less able to fight infection. When the number of CD4 cells drops to a critical level (below 200 cells/mm$^3$), the person is diagnosed with AIDS.

- Symptoms of HIV infection, when they do appear, consist of:
  - Acute flulike symptoms
  - Fever
  - Night sweats
  - Fatigue
  - Swollen lymph nodes
  - Sore throat
  - Gastrointestinal problems
  - Headache
- One-fourth to one-half of people exposed to HIV show evidence of disease within 5 to 10 years of antibody development (becoming seropositive).

**Testing.** Several tests have been developed to confirm the presence of antibodies to HIV (positive for HIV infection) and to confirm the presence of AIDS.

The test for antibodies is also used to check the national blood supply. When people donate blood it is tested to be sure that it is free of HIV antibodies to protect the people who receive blood transfusions and other blood products.

**Treatment.** No specific treatment is able to cure AIDS at the present time.

- No vaccine prevents the infection from developing. However, millions of dollars are spent on research to develop a vaccine.
- Therapy is directed toward vigorously treating each infection as it appears.
- Nutritional and other forms of preventive therapy are aimed at maintaining a person with AIDS in the best health possible.
- The drug industry continues to develop drugs that slow down the disease process or reinforce the immune system. These drugs, however, do not cure the disease. At the present time there is **no** evidence that AIDS is transmitted:
  - Through kissing, touching, or hugging an HIV-infected person
  - By eating at the same table with an infected person
  - By using the same toilet seat

Nursing facilities are admitting more people in their thirties and forties who are seriously ill with AIDS. Many of these people have wasting or dementia (irreversible brain disease). This is stressful to the health care providers because it is easy to identify with the age group. It takes maturity to offer the support and care needed.

## OTHER IMPORTANT INFECTIONS ····

### Infection Caused by Fungi

Coccidioidomycosis (valley fever) is caused by *Coccidioides immitis*. It occurs primarily as a respiratory infection. It is seldom fatal in otherwise healthy people. In people with immunosuppression, however, the death rate is high. It is treated with antibiotics.

### Infection Caused by Protozoa

Two diseases caused by protozoa are becoming more common in the general public and in health facilities. Giardiasis is caused by *Giardia lamblia*, which is found in the water supplies of many communities. It causes severe diarrhea but responds to medication. Cryptosporidiosis is caused by the *Cryptosporidium* protozoa, which is found in the digestive tract of domestic animals and is transferred by contact. It causes severe diarrhea, especially in immunosuppressed people. There is no specific treatment.

## WHY THE ELDERLY IN LONG-TERM CARE ARE AT RISK FOR INFECTIONS ···············

There are several reasons why elderly people are at risk for infections.

- Residents usually have several chronic health problems. This lowers their resistance to disease.
- Body changes caused by aging make older people more susceptible to infections. They have less ability to fight disease.
- Residents may have colds or flu and spread the microbes to other residents.
- The skin of the elderly offers less protection because it is fragile and easily broken. Any break in the skin such as a pressure sore or skin tear can quickly become infected.
- Poor bladder emptying and indwelling catheters increase risk of bladder infections.
- Bowel incontinent residents are at risk for infections through accidental ingestion of feces or by contact of feces with nonintact skin (skin tears, rashes, pressure sores and ulcers).
- The ability to cough and raise secretions is reduced so the elderly have less ability to get rid of pathogens from the lungs.

The elderly are also more likely to develop serious complications from infections. A simple urinary tract infection can result in bacteremia (blood infection), causing the resident to be acutely ill. This can be fatal to the resident who has little ability to cope with additional health problems.

Infections may not be readily detected in older adults for the following reasons:

- The elderly are less likely to have an elevated temperature as a result of an infection.
- The elderly do not readily develop signs of inflammatory response, which may include pain, heat, and swelling at the site of the infection. These signs may be missing or delayed in the elderly person.
- Some elderly people do not feel pain as acutely as younger people. For example, they may feel no discomfort with a bladder infection.

Because of these factors an infection may be present in the body for several days before it is detected.

## GENERAL MEASURES TO PREVENT INFECTIONS

1. Assist residents to maintain an adequate fluid intake. This helps prevent urinary tract and respiratory tract infections and keeps the skin healthier.
2. Assist residents to maintain adequate nutritional intake. Report to the nurse when residents eat less or refuse food.
3. Assist residents to carry out exercise programs established by the nurse or physical therapist. Follow positioning schedules and orders for range of motion exercises and ambulation. This increases circulation, thus lowering the risk for pressure ulcers (a frequent source of infection). Exercise improves breathing, thereby decreasing the risk of respiratory infections.
4. Encourage residents to be outdoors to enjoy the fresh air whenever possible.
5. Regularly toilet residents who need assistance. This keeps the bladder empty and also assures residents that they will receive help when they need to urinate. Some residents hesitate to drink fluids for fear they will be incontinent.
6. When cleaning the perineal area of residents, be sure to wipe women from front to back. This prevents contaminating the urethra (bladder opening) with stool or vaginal excretions.
7. Perform catheter care as directed. Avoid opening the drainage system.

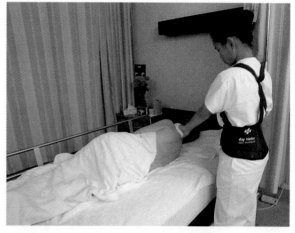

**FIGURE 10-9** Maintaining the resident's cleanliness helps prevent infectious disease.

8. Observe residents carefully and report any unusual signs or changes, such as:
   - Changes in frequency of urination or amount of urine voided
   - Complaints of pain or burning on urination
   - Changes in character of urine
   - Coughing or respiratory problems
   - Confusion/disorientation that was not present before or that has increased
   - Drainage or discharge from any body opening or skin wound
   - Changes in skin color
   - Complaints of pain, discomfort, or nausea
   - Elevated temperature
   - Red, swollen areas on body
9. Keep residents clean (Figure 10-9).
10. Staff members who have an infectious disease should not be on duty. Caring for your own health is vital in preventing illness in residents. Friends and family of residents should be advised not to visit when they do not feel well. If you notice a visitor coughing and sneezing, or otherwise obviously sick, inform your supervisor.

## OUTBREAK OF INFECTIOUS DISEASE IN A LONG-TERM CARE FACILITY

An outbreak of an infection in the facility can be serious for all residents. Unless steps are taken immediately, the infection can spread rapidly. Examples of outbreaks include:

- Influenza
- Gastroenteritis
- Hepatitis
- MRSA
- Tuberculosis
- Food-borne illnesses
- Scabies (parasites that invade the skin)

Most facilities have an action plan that is used in response to an outbreak of infection. The local health department is notified of the outbreak. The health department will assist the facility in determining the type of outbreak and its cause. All staff are informed of the characteristics of the disease and are trained in the precautions to be followed until the outbreak is over. If necessary, notices will be posted to advise visitors that the facility is closed to them for a specific length of time.

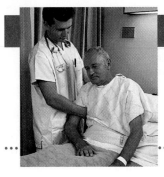

## LESSON SYNTHESIS: Putting It All Together

*Y*ou have just completed this lesson. Now go back and review the Clinical Focus. Try to see how the Clinical Focus relates to the concepts presented in the lesson. Then answer the following questions.

1. Why should Mr. Dwyer be monitored for the possibility that his tuberculosis infection will become active again?

2. Why is Mr. Dwyer's drop in white blood cell count so important?

3. What condition did Mr. Dwyer have that might have injured his liver?

4. What effect does HIV have on Mr. Dwyer's immune system?

## REVIEW

**A. Match each term (items a.–e.) with the proper definition.**

   a. antigen      d. pathogen
   b. antibody     e. vaccine
   c. inflammation

   1. _____ a body response to infection

   2. _____ term meaning a pathogenic microbe that enters the body

   3. _____ provides immunization

   4. _____ develops in the body after having an infection

   5. _____ disease-producing microbe

**B. Fill in the blanks by selecting the correct word or phrase from the list.**

   insects                reservoir
   method of              sexual contact
      transmission        sneezing
   portal of entry        susceptible host
   portal of exit         water

   6. Complete the chain of infection by naming the missing parts.
      a. _____
      b. _____
      c. _____
      d. _____

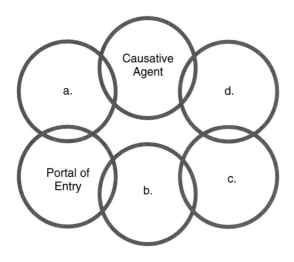

7. An example of transmission by direct contact is _____.

8. An example of direct transmission is through _____.

9. A common vehicle for the transmission of microbes is _____.

10. Vectors, such as animals and _____ also transmit disease organisms.

C. **Match the organism (items a.–e.) with the specific disease it causes.**

a. *Mycobacterium tuberculosis*  c. HBV
b. *Coccidioidomycosis*  d. HIV
 e. MRSA

11. _____ AIDS

12. _____ valley fever

13. _____ tuberculosis

14. _____ skin and wound infections by resistant *Staphylococcus aureus*

15. _____ hepatitis

D. **Select the one best answer for each of the following.**

16. A person who is infected with a pathogenic organism but does not show any signs of an infection is a (an)
a. transporter
b. harborer
c. infector
d. carrier

17. White blood cells that multiply and attempt to destroy pathogens are
a. antigens
b. phagocytes
c. antibodies
d. red blood cells

18. Which of the following is not a natural body defense?
a. antibiotic
b. hydrochloric acid in the stomach
c. hair in the nose
d. tears

19. Which is an example of a local infection?
a. pneumonia
b. septicemia
c. boil
d. AIDS

20. When a microbe can no longer be controlled or destroyed by a drug it is said to be
a. difficult
b. resistant
c. untreatable
d. noncompliant

21. A major reason residents are at risk for infection is
a. they have new chronic problems
b. aging makes them more susceptible
c. their ability to cough is strong
d. their skin is thicker and less likely to tear

22. Sonny, a nursing assistant, notices that the daughter of one of the residents is coughing and looks flushed. His best action is to
a. ask the visitor to leave
b. put a mask on the visitor
c. put a mask on the resident
d. refer the matter to the nurse

23. Juan is not feeling well this morning when he wakes up. He has an elevated temperature and is sneezing. He is due on duty at 1500. His best action is to
a. call in sick
b. go to work
c. stay home without notifying the facility
d. call a friend to go to work for him

# Infection Control

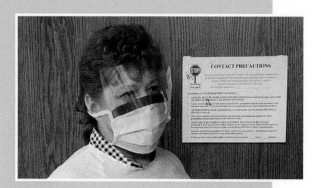

**CLINICAL FOCUS**

Think about ways you can help

residents avoid infections as

you study this lesson and

meet:

*O*scar Uritz, who is a resident in your care. He was transferred from home with a large, stage three pressure ulcer on his right ankle. He lost the use of his left side from an earlier stroke. He shared a room at the facility with Mr. Jules who also had a stroke but is ambulatory. Mr. Uritz has an MRSA infection and is now in a single room on contact isolation. The nursing assistant should wear personal protective equipment when providing care for Mr. Uritz.

## OBJECTIVES

*After studying this lesson, you should be able to:*

- Define and spell vocabulary words and terms.
- Explain the principles of medical asepsis.
- Explain the components of standard precautions.
- List the types of personal protective equipment.
- Describe nursing assistant actions related to standard precautions.
- Describe airborne precautions.
- Describe droplet precautions.
- Describe contact precautions.
- Demonstrate the following:
  Procedure 5   Handwashing
  Procedure 6   Putting on a Mask
  Procedure 7   Putting on a Gown
  Procedure 8   Putting on Gloves
  Procedure 9   Removing Contaminated Gloves

Procedure 10  Removing Contaminated Gloves, Mask, and Gown
Procedure 11  Caring for Linens in Isolation Unit
Procedure 12  Measuring Vital Signs in Isolation Unit
Procedure 13  Serving a Meal Tray in Isolation Unit
Procedure 14  Specimen Collection from Resident in Isolation Unit
Procedure 15  Transferring Nondisposable Equipment Outside of Isolation Unit
Procedure 16  Transporting Resident to and from Isolation Unit
Procedure 17  Opening a Sterile Package

# VOCABULARY

**airborne precautions** (*AIR-born pree-KAW-shuns*)

**asepsis** (*ah-SEP-sis*)

**autoclave** (*AWE-toh-klayv*)

**biohazard** (*bye-oh-HAZ-ard*)

**communicable** (*kom-MYOU-nih-kah-bul*)

**contact precautions** (*KON-tact pree-KAW-shuns*)

**contagious** (*kon-TAY-jus*)

**contaminated** (*kon-TAM-ih-nay-ted*)

**dirty** (*DER-tee*)

**disinfection** (*dis-in-FECK-shun*)

**droplet precautions** (*DROP-let pree-KAW-shuns*)

**exposure incident** (*ecks-POH-zhur IN-sih-dent*)

**isolation** (*eye-soh-LAY-shun*)

**medical asepsis** (*MED-ih-kul ah-SEP-sis*)

**occupational exposure** (*ock-you-PAY-shun-al ecks-POH-zhur*)

**personal protective equipment (PPE)** (*PER-son-al proh-TECH-tiv ee-KWIP-ment*)

**potentially infectious material** (*poh-TEN-shal-lee in-FECK-shus mah-TEER-ee-al*)

**sharps** (*sharps*)

**standard precautions** (*STAN-dard pree-KAW-shuns*)

**sterile** (*STER-ill*)

**sterilization** (*ster-ih-lie-ZAY-shun*)

**work practice controls** (*werk PRACK-tis kon-TROLS*)

---

In the last lesson you learned what infections are, some of their causes, and why residents are at risk for infections. In this lesson, you will be introduced to actions and procedures that can help prevent the transmission (spread) of infection to protect yourself, your coworkers, and those in your care.

# MEDICAL ASEPSIS

The term **asepsis** means that disease-causing pathogens and infection are not present. **Medical asepsis** means the methods by which cleanliness and freedom from pathogens are maintained:

- In your own personal hygiene
- With residents
- With equipment and supplies
- Throughout the facility

You will hear the terms "clean" and "dirty" applied to equipment and supplies used in the facility. For example, the linen you take from the linen cart is "clean." After it is carried into the resident's room, it is considered to be "dirty." If it is not used, it cannot be returned to the clean linen cart but must be placed in the laundry hamper. Once linen is in the resident's room, it is exposed to the resident's pathogens. To prevent the spread of these pathogens to other residents, the linen must be laundered. Keeping each resident's equipment and supplies separate from those for other residents is part of an action called medical aseptic technique. Articles that have come into contact with known pathogens or are exposed to potential pathogens are called **dirty** or **contaminated**. Articles that are free of pathogens are considered clean or uncontaminated.

## Maintaining Medical Asepsis

Nursing assistant actions to maintain medical asepsis include:

1. Wash your hands thoroughly and at appropriate times. (See Procedure 5.) Protect the skin on the hands by using warm water, drying thoroughly, and applying lotion if needed.
2. Treat breaks in the skin immediately by washing thoroughly, cleaning with an antiseptic, and covering. Report any breaks in the skin to your supervisor.
3. Use gloves when required.

4. Bathe or shower daily. Daily changes of clothing are necessary. Keep your hair clean and away from your face and shoulders. Keep fingernails short and clean. Do not wear rings, other than a plain wedding band.

5. Personal hygiene for residents is maintained by following bathing schedules and giving AM and PM care as required. Change clothing daily or as needed.

6. Items used for one resident are *never* used for another resident.

7. The following items should be placed in the top two drawers of each resident's bedside table and labeled with the resident's name:
   - Toothbrush and toothpaste
   - Comb and hairbrush (Figure 11-1)
   - Denture cup if resident wears dentures

8. The following items are located in the second drawer or shelf of the bedside table or in the bathroom. The are used for one resident only and are disinfected (cleaned to remove pathogens) at least once a week.
   In the second drawer you will find:
   - Emesis basin
   - Wash basin
   - Soap and soap dish

On the lower shelf you will find:
- Bedpan
- Urinal for male residents

Items such as a toothbrush, denture cup, wash basin, and emesis basin should always be placed on a separate shelf from items such as a bedpan and a urinal.

9. Disinfect bathtubs and shower chairs after each use according to facility policy (Figure 11-2). Clean items used by more than one resident, such as wheelchairs, before each use. Other equipment is cleaned regularly by the housekeeping department or as indicated by facility policy.

10. Disinfect equipment, such as a stethoscope, that is used by more than one health care provider or resident before and after each use.

11. Disinfect personal care equipment, such as bedpans, urinals, and commodes according to facility policy.

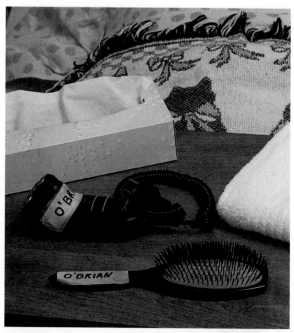

**FIGURE 11-1** Personal care items should be labeled with the resident's name and used by that resident only.

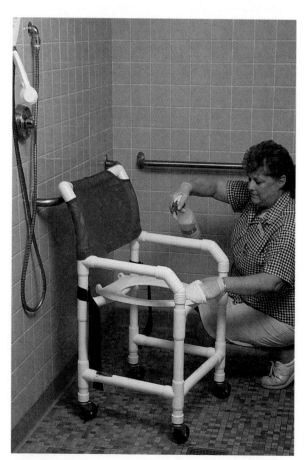

**FIGURE 11-2** Equipment should be disinfected between use by different residents.

12. Be careful when handling bedpans and urinals after use to prevent spills and splashes. Use a cover when transporting.
13. Keep food and water supplies clean. Food trays are to remain covered until they reach their destination. Remove food dishes immediately after use. Do not place used trays on cart until all clean trays have been delivered to residents.
14. Do not allow the residents to keep puddings or custards from meal trays. Bacteria multiply rapidly in these foods when they are not refrigerated.
15. Carry soiled equipment, supplies, and linens away from your uniform so that you do not spread microorganisms from resident to resident. Dispose of items according to facility policy.
16. The floor is heavily contaminated with pathogens. Do not use anything that has touched the floor without recleaning or sterilizing it first. If you are in doubt about whether an item is clean, do not use it. Any personal items that touch the floor should be disinfected before use.
17. Avoid raising dust. Vacuum cleaners, wet mops, and damp cloths are used for cleaning.
18. Do not shake linens. This scatters contaminated dust and lint. Gather or fold linens inward with the dirtiest area toward the center. Keep soiled linen hampers covered. Keep linens (even if soiled) off the floor.
19. Clean least soiled areas first and the most soiled last.
20. Keep residents' rooms as clean, bright, and dry as possible.
21. Keep work areas such as utility rooms clean. Return clean equipment to the proper storage areas after use.

## HANDWASHING

The importance of handwashing can never be overemphasized.

*Handwashing is the most important procedure you will carry out to prevent the spread of infection. It is the foundation of all preventive techniques.*

Whenever you prepare for resident care, you must wash your hands before you start. For routine care, it may not be necessary to wear gloves. For many procedures, gloves must be worn. It may be necessary to change gloves several times during the procedures for one resident. Each time gloves are removed, your hands must be washed before you touch any noncontaminated items or environmental surfaces. Hands are also washed just before you leave the room to go to another resident. When you enter the room of another resident, do not assume that your hands are still clean after being with the last resident. Wash your hands before providing care to the next resident.

---

**PROCEDURE 5**

## Handwashing

1. Check that there is an adequate supply of soap and paper towels. A waste container lined with a plastic bag should be in the area near you.
2. Turn on the faucet with a dry paper towel held between your hand and the faucet (Figure 11-3). Drop the towel in the waste container. Stand back from the sink so you do not contaminate your uniform.
3. Adjust water to a warm temperature. Wet your hands with the fingertips pointed downward (Figure 11-4).

*(continues)*

**PROCEDURE 5** *(continued)*

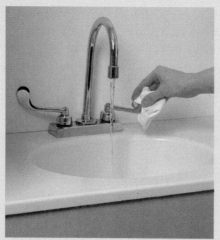

**FIGURE 11-3** A dry, clean paper towel should be used to turn faucets on and off.

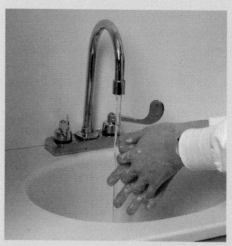

**FIGURE 11-5** Interlace the fingers to clean between them.

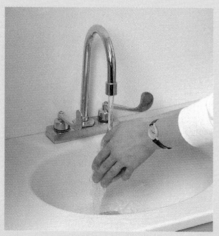

**FIGURE 11-4** Fingertips should be pointed down while washing hands.

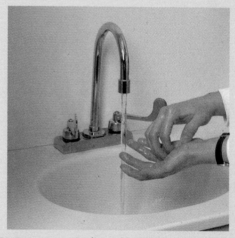

**FIGURE 11-6** Rub nails against the palms of the hands to clean under the nails.

4. Apply soap and lather over your hands and wrists and between fingers. Use friction and interlace your fingers (Figure 11-5). Work lather over every part of your hands and wrists. Clean your fingernails by rubbing them against the palm of the other hand to force soap under the nails for 10 to 15 seconds (Figure 11-6).

5. Rinse hands with your fingertips pointed down. Do not shake water from hands.
6. Dry hands thoroughly with a clean paper towel.
7. Turn off the faucet with another paper towel; drop the towel in the waste container.
8. Apply lotion to your hands.

## PROTECTING YOURSELF

As you perform your duties you may contact **potentially infectious material** such as blood or other body fluids that may contain pathogens. This is called **occupational exposure**.

Using proper medical asepsis technique and following standard precautions according to your facility policy are the best ways to limit the potential for being infected.

An **exposure incident** means that your eyes, mouth, or nonintact skin had contact with blood or other potentially infectious material. Rinse immediately with clear water. Report this at once to your supervisor and follow facility procedure.

## STANDARD PRECAUTIONS

**Standard precautions** (Figure 11-7) are the infection control actions used for all people receiving care, without regard for their condition or diagnosis. Standard precautions apply to situations in which care providers may contact:

- Blood, body fluids (except sweat), secretions, and excretions
- Mucous membranes
- Nonintact skin

Some examples of secretions and excretions are:

- Respiratory mucus (phlegm)
- Cerebrospinal fluid
- Urine

*(text continues on page 178)*

---

**STANDARD PRECAUTIONS FOR INFECTION CONTROL**

**Wash Hands (Plain soap)**
Wash after touching blood, body fluids, secretions, excretions, and contaminated items. Wash immediately after gloves are removed and between patient contacts. Avoid transfer of microorganisms to other patients or environments.

**Wear Gloves**
Wear when touching blood, body fluids, secretions, excretions, and contaminated items. Put on clean gloves just before touching mucous membranes and nonintact skin. Change gloves between tasks and procedures on the same patient after contact with material that may contain high concentrations of microorganisms. Remove gloves promptly after use, before touching noncontaminated items and environmental surfaces, and before going to another patient, and wash hands immediately to avoid transfer of microorganisms to other patients or environments.

**Wear Mask and Eye Protection or Face Shield**
Protect mucous membranes of the eyes, nose and mouth during procedures and patient-care activities that are likely to generate splashes or sprays of blood, body fluids, secretions, or excretions.

**Wear Gown**
Protect skin and prevent soiling of clothing during procedures that are likely to generate splashes or sprays of blood, body fluids, secretions, or excretions. Remove a soiled gown as promptly as possible and wash hands to avoid transfer of microorganisms to other patients or environments.

**Patient-Care Equipment**
Handle used patient-care equipment soiled with blood, body fluids, secretions, or excretions in a manner that prevents skin and mucous membrane exposures, contamination of clothing, and transfer of microorganisms to other patients and environments. Ensure that reusable equipment is not used for the care of another patient until it has been appropriately cleaned and reprocessed and single use items are properly discarded.

**Environmental Control**
Follow hospital procedures for routine care, cleaning, and disinfection of environmental surfaces, beds, bedrails, bedside equipment and other frequently touched surfaces.

**Linen**
Handle, transport, and process used linen soiled with blood, body fluids, secretions, or excretions in a manner that prevents exposure and contamination of clothing, and avoids transfer of microorganisms to other patients and environments.

**Occupational Health and Bloodborne Pathogens**
Prevent injuries when using needles, scalpels, and other sharp instruments or devices; when handling sharp instruments after procedures; when cleaning used instruments; and when disposing of used needles.

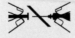

Never recap used needles using both hands or any other technique that involves directing the point of a needle towards any part of the body; rather, use either a one-handed "scoop" technique or a mechanical device designed for holding the needle sheath.

Do not remove used needles from disposable syringes by hand, and do not bend, break, or otherwise manipulate used needles by hand. Place used disposable syringes and needles, scalpels, blades, and other sharp items in puncture-resistant sharps containers located as close as practical to the area in which the items were used, and place reusable syringes and needles in a puncture-resistant container for transport to the reprocessing area.

Use resuscitation devices as an alternative to mouth-to-mouth resuscitation.

**Patient Placement**
Use a private room for a patient who contaminates the environment or who does not (or cannot be expected to) assist in maintaining appropriate hygiene or environmental control. Consult Infection Control if a private room is not available.

**FIGURE 11-7** Standard precautions (Courtesy of BREVIS Corp., Salt Lake City, UT)

# Guidelines for

## Standard Precautions

1. Wash Hands
   - When arriving for work and just before leaving for home
   - Immediately after touching blood, body fluids, mucous membranes, or contaminated articles, whether or not gloves are worn
   - Before putting on gloves and after taking them off
   - Before caring for a resident and after completing care for that resident
   - Before care procedures that may transfer pathogens from one part of the resident's body to another
   - After personal use of the bathroom
   - Before handling food
   - Using soap provided by the facility
   - Before touching your mouth, eyes, or eyeglasses
   - Before and after touching your contact lenses
   - After touching any soiled linen, clothing, equipment, or supplies

2. Wear gloves for any contact with blood, body fluids, mucous membranes, or nonintact skin, such as when:
   - Hands are cut, scratched, or have a rash
   - Cleaning up body fluid spills
   - Cleaning potentially contaminated equipment

3. Gloves are provided in resident rooms or on supply carts.

4. Carry gloves with you so they will always be available as you need them.

5. If you have an allergy to latex gloves, follow your physician's advice. Three possible options are:
   - Change to nonlatex gloves (facilities must supply them because latex allergies are not uncommon).
   - Apply a skin barrier cream to your hands before putting on latex gloves; the cream protects hands against most irritants, including latex.
   - Put on glove liners that prevent direct contact between the skin of the hands and the latex gloves.

6. Change gloves:
   - After contacting each resident
   - Before touching noncontaminated articles or environmental surfaces
   - Between tasks with the same resident if there is contact with infectious materials

7. Dispose of gloves according to facility policy.

8. Wear a waterproof gown for procedures likely to produce splashes of blood or other body fluids.
   - Remove soiled gown as soon as possible and dispose of it properly according to facility policy.
   - Wash your hands.

9. Wear a mask and protective eyewear or face shield for procedures likely to produce splashes of blood or other moist body fluids. This is to prevent contact with pathogens by your mucous membranes.

   The surgical mask covers both the nose and mouth. The mask is used once and discarded. When a mask is required, a new one is put on for each resident receiving care. If the mask becomes wet, a new one must be put on because the mask loses its effectiveness when moist.

10. Goggles or face shield helps protect the mucous membranes of the eyes from splashes or sprays of blood and other body fluids. A surgical mask must be worn with goggles and with a face shield to protect the nose and mouth.

11. When using PPE, you should:
    - Know where to obtain these items in your work area.
    - Always remove the items before leaving the work area, whether the resident's room, an isolation unit, or the utility room.
    - Place these items in the proper container for laundering, decontamination, or disposal, according to facility policy.

# *G*uidelines for

# Environmental Procedures

1. Handle all patient care items so that infectious organisms will not be transferred to skin, mucous membranes, clothing, or the environment. Reusable equipment must be cleaned and decontaminated according to facility policy before it can be used with another resident. Dispose of single-use items according to facility policy.

2. Follow facility procedures for routine care and cleaning of environmental surfaces such as beds, bedside equipment, and other frequently touched surfaces.

3. Dispose of **sharps**—needles with syringes, razors, and other sharp items—in a puncture-resistant, leakproof container near the point of use (Figure 11-8). The container should be labeled with the **biohazard** symbol (Figure 11-9) and color coded red.

4. Do not recap needles or otherwise handle them before disposal.

5. Mouthpieces or resuscitator bags should be available to minimize the need for mouth-to-mouth resuscitation if trained to use them.

6. Waste and soiled linen should be placed in plastic bags and handled according to facility policy. There are separate containers for regular waste and for biohazardous waste (waste that has contacted blood or body fluids). Containers for biohazardous waste should have the biohazard symbol (Figure 11-9), or be color coded in red (Figure 11-10). Learn your facility policy for what is biohazardous waste and follow the guidelines.

7. Wipe up blood spills immediately. Disinfect the floor according to facility policy.

   - Use disposable gloves.
   - For small spills use 1:10 dilution of bleach or disinfectant required by facility policy.
   - For larger spills use a commercial blood cleanup kit. This contains an absorbent powder that is sprinkled over the blood to absorb the spill. The blood and powder are then scooped up

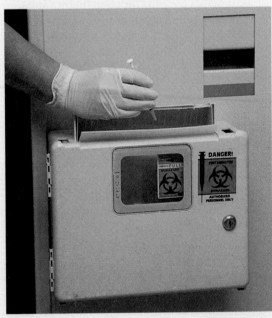

**FIGURE 11-8** Sharps must be disposed of carefully in a safety container designed specifically for this use.

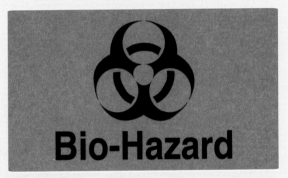

**FIGURE 11-9** This is a universal biohazard symbol used to indicate potentially infectious waste.

*(continues)*

# *G*uidelines *(continued)*

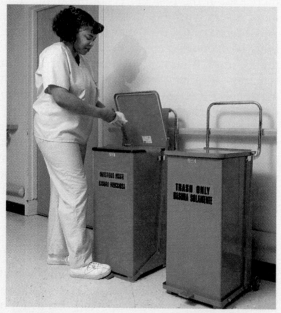

**FIGURE 11-10**   All potentially infectious materials should be disposed of in the correct waste container.

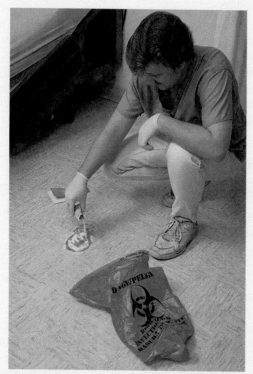

**FIGURE 11-11**   Clean all blood spills immediately using a 1 : 10 dilution of bleach or the disinfectant approved by your facility, or for larger spills, a blood spill kit. The powder absorbs the blood quickly and can be scooped up for disposal in the biohazard bag.

with the scoop provided in the kit. The material and scoop are placed in a biohazard bag for disposal (Figure 11-11).
- Use disposable cleaning cloths.
- Dispose of gloves and cleaning cloths in appropriate infectious waste receptacles.

8. Dispose of body fluids and contaminated articles according to facility policy. This includes the contents of:
   - Urinary drainage bags
   - Bedpans
   - Urinals
   - Emesis basins
   - Drainage receptacles from tracheal and gastric suction
   - Solutions returned from vaginal douches, enemas, and bladder irrigations
   - Soiled dressings
   - Incontinent pads (Chux®)
   - Vaginal pads
   - Incontinent briefs

9. Eating, drinking, smoking, applying cosmetics or lip balm, and handling contact lenses are prohibited in work areas where there may be exposure to infectious material.
10. Food and drink should not be kept in refrigerators, freezers, shelves, cabinets, or on countertops or benchtops where they may be exposed to blood or other materials that may be contaminated.
11. Do not pick up potentially contaminated broken glassware with your bare hands. Wear gloves and use a wet paper towel or brush and dust pan, tongs, or forceps. Clean and disinfect properly. Discard according to facility policy.

- Feces
- Vaginal secretions
- Semen
- Vomitus

This means that all health care workers follow specific procedures called **work practice controls** to prevent the spread of infections.

Standard precautions stress handwashing and the use of **personal protective equipment (PPE)**: gloves, gown, mask, and goggles or face shield.

# TRANSMISSION-BASED PRECAUTIONS

**Isolation** means to separate or set apart. The purpose of isolation is to separate the resident with a **communicable** or **contagious** disease (one that is readily spread to other people) to help prevent the spread of the infectious pathogens.

For residents in isolation, the proper use of precautions, known as transmission precautions, requires extra effort by all care providers, but especially nursing assistants, and is more time consuming. The fear of infection also makes working with these precautions more stressful for the care providers. Residents in isolation and their families and other visitors also feel stress.

## Psychological Aspects of Isolation

The resident in isolation fears both the disease condition requiring the isolation precautions and the practices that must be followed for these precautions to be effective. These include:

- PPE worn by all who enter the isolation unit
- Special procedures for handling waste, specimens, food, linens, and personal effects of the resident
- Restrictions on the resident's movement in the facility
- Procedures to be followed when resident is moved outside of the isolation unit
- Possible restrictions on visiting hours or number of visitors
- Need for visitors to use PPE
- Likelihood that close personal contact, such as kissing of family members, is not permitted

The resident may fear passing the infection to family and friends. If the resident does not understand the infectious process, this fear is increased. If the resident is confused, he or she may be very fearful of the PPE.

Because of the resident's fears and the possibility of decreased contact with other residents, family, and friends, the resident in isolation requires more emotional support and care. The increased time required to follow the isolation precautions, such as putting on PPE, could easily decrease the time the care providers spend with the resident at a time when the emotional attention is most needed. Nursing assistants are mindful of the resident's needs and will plan their schedules to spend the necessary time with a resident in isolation.

## Transmission-Based Isolation Precautions

Standard precautions are used with all residents regardless of their condition. When residents are known to have or are suspected of having an infectious disease, isolation precautions are used *in addition to* standard precautions. The isolation precautions used depend on the way in which the infectious pathogens are transmitted. Guidelines from the Centers for Disease Control and Prevention (CDC) indicate the specific precautions and personal protective equipment to be used based on how the disease is transmitted. The three transmission precautions are:

- Airborne precautions
- Droplet precautions
- Contact precautions

**Airborne Precautions. Airborne precautions** are used for diseases that are transmitted by air currents. The pathogens are suspended in the air or on dust particles in the air. They can travel a long distance from the source by natural air currents and through ventilation systems. Tuberculosis is a disease that requires airborne precautions. Figure 11-12 shows the required precautions.

- The resident must be in a private room with negative air pressure. This means that air is drawn into the room and leaves the room through a special exhaust system to the outside. Air from the room does not circulate directly into the facility.
- The door to the room is kept closed.

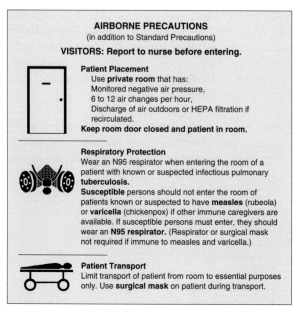

**AIRBORNE PRECAUTIONS**
(in addition to Standard Precautions)
**VISITORS: Report to nurse before entering.**

**Patient Placement**
Use **private room** that has:
Monitored negative air pressure,
6 to 12 air changes per hour,
Discharge of air outdoors or HEPA filtration if recirculated.
**Keep room door closed and patient in room.**

**Respiratory Protection**
Wear an N95 respirator when entering the room of a patient with known or suspected infectious pulmonary **tuberculosis.**
**Susceptible** persons should not enter the room of patients known or suspected to have **measles** (rubeola) or **varicella** (chickenpox) if other immune caregivers are available. If susceptible persons must enter, they should wear an **N95 respirator.** (Respirator or surgical mask not required if immune to measles and varicella.)

**Patient Transport**
Limit transport of patient from room to essential purposes only. Use **surgical mask** on patient during transport.

**FIGURE 11-12**   Airborne precautions (Courtesy of BREVIS Corp., Salt Lake City, UT)

- All care providers who enter the room must wear a high-efficiency particulate air (HEPA) filter mask (Figure 11-13). The special filters in this mask protect the care provider from the

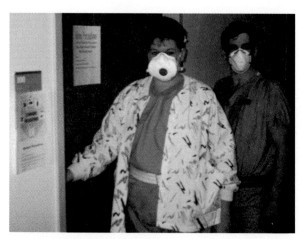

**FIGURE 11-13**   High-efficiency particulate air (HEPA) filter masks are required for care providers working with residents placed in airborne precautions. The masks are carefully fitted to each care provider. The mask must seal around the face so that all air being breathed must pass through the filters to remove the very small pathogens.

very small disease-causing pathogens. A surgical mask does not provide protection. Each care provider must be fitted with a HEPA filter mask. This ensures that air entering the mask comes through the filters only. Follow all facility policies for the use of HEPA filter masks.

- People who are not immune to measles (rubeola) or chickenpox (varicella) should not enter the room of a resident known or suspected to have either of these infections.
- If transport from the room is necessary, the resident must wear a surgical mask.

**Droplet Precautions.**   **Droplet precautions** are used for diseases that can be spread by means of large droplets in the air. A person can spread droplets containing infectious pathogens by sneezing, coughing, talking, singing, or laughing. The droplets generally do not travel more than 3 feet from the source. Influenza is an example of a disease spread by droplets.

Figure 11-14 shows the requirements for droplet precautions.

- If a resident cannot be placed in a private room, then residents requiring the same precautions can be placed together.
- The caregivers should wear surgical masks if they expect to be working within 3 feet of the resident. The door can be open if the bed is more than 3 feet from the door.
- If transport from the room is necessary, the resident must wear a surgical mask.

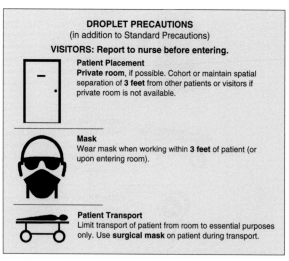

**DROPLET PRECAUTIONS**
(in addition to Standard Precautions)
**VISITORS: Report to nurse before entering.**

**Patient Placement**
**Private room**, if possible. Cohort or maintain spatial separation of **3 feet** from other patients or visitors if private room is not available.

**Mask**
Wear mask when working within **3 feet** of patient (or upon entering room).

**Patient Transport**
Limit transport of patient from room to essential purposes only. Use **surgical mask** on patient during transport.

**FIGURE 11-14**   Droplet precautions (Courtesy of BREVIS Corp., Salt Lake City, UT)

**Contact Precautions.** **Contact precautions** are used when the infectious pathogen is spread by direct or indirect contact. Direct contact occurs when the caregiver touches a contaminated area on the resident's skin or blood or body fluids containing the infectious pathogen. Indirect contact occurs when the caregiver touches items contaminated with the infectious material, such as resident's personal belongings, equipment, and supplies used in the care of the resident, contaminated linens, and so on. Examples of infections requiring contact precautions are scabies, infected pressure ulcers, and gastroenteritis.

Figure 11-15 shows the requirements for contact precautions.

• The resident should be in a private room. If this is not possible, then residents requiring the same type of isolation precautions can be

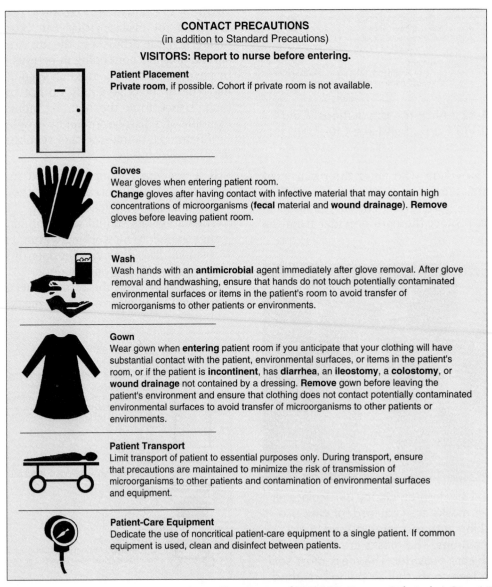

### CONTACT PRECAUTIONS
(in addition to Standard Precautions)

**VISITORS: Report to nurse before entering.**

**Patient Placement**
**Private room**, if possible. Cohort if private room is not available.

**Gloves**
Wear gloves when entering patient room.
**Change** gloves after having contact with infective material that may contain high concentrations of microorganisms (**fecal** material and **wound drainage**). **Remove** gloves before leaving patient room.

**Wash**
Wash hands with an **antimicrobial** agent immediately after glove removal. After glove removal and handwashing, ensure that hands do not touch potentially contaminated environmental surfaces or items in the patient's room to avoid transfer of microorganisms to other patients or environments.

**Gown**
Wear gown when **entering** patient room if you anticipate that your clothing will have substantial contact with the patient, environmental surfaces, or items in the patient's room, or if the patient is **incontinent**, has **diarrhea**, an **ileostomy**, a **colostomy**, or **wound drainage** not contained by a dressing. **Remove** gown before leaving the patient's environment and ensure that clothing does not contact potentially contaminated environmental surfaces to avoid transfer of microorganisms to other patients or environments.

**Patient Transport**
Limit transport of patient to essential purposes only. During transport, ensure that precautions are maintained to minimize the risk of transmission of microorganisms to other patients and contamination of environmental surfaces and equipment.

**Patient-Care Equipment**
Dedicate the use of noncritical patient-care equipment to a single patient. If common equipment is used, clean and disinfect between patients.

**FIGURE 11-15** Contact precautions (Courtesy of BREVIS Corp., Salt Lake City, UT)

placed in the same room. The door can be open.

- Gloves are put on before the caregiver enters the resident's room. Gloves are changed whenever there is contact with highly contaminated matter in the room. After removing gloves, always wash your hands before putting on a new pair of gloves. After care is completed, remove gloves and wash hands. Use a paper towel to open the door to leave the room and discard the towel in the trash container inside the room.
- Wear a gown when entering the resident's room if your uniform may contact the resident, blood or body fluids, environmental surfaces, or other items in the room. Remove the gown before leaving the room and dispose of it according to facility policy for biohazardous waste. Be careful not to touch environmental surfaces or other items with your uniform as you leave the room.
- Transport the resident from the room only when necessary. Continue precautions to minimize contamination of environmental surfaces, other residents, and health care personnel.
- Disposable equipment and supplies should be used where possible. Noncritical, nondisposable equipment should be used for one resident only. If equipment must be used for more

than one resident, it must be cleaned and disinfected between residents.

## Preparing for Isolation

To prepare a resident room for isolation do the following:

1. Place a card indicating the type of isolation precaution on the door to the resident's room.
2. Place an isolation cart outside the room, next to the door. Place in it quantities of personal protective equipment as needed:
   - Gowns
   - Masks
   - Gloves
   - Goggles or face shields
   - Plastic bags marked for biohazardous waste
   - Plastic bags for soiled linen
3. Line the wastepaper basket inside the room with a plastic bag labeled or color coded for infectious waste.
4. Place a laundry hamper in the room and line it with a yellow biohazard laundry bag.
5. At the sink, check the supply of paper towels and soap. Soap should be in a wall dispenser or foot-operated dispenser.

---

**PROCEDURE**

## *6* Putting on a Mask

1. Assemble equipment:
   - Mask
2. If gown and gloves are needed, the mask goes on first. (If a face shield is used, it is put on next.)
3. Adjust mask over nose and mouth.

4. Tie top strings of mask first, then bottom strings.
5. Replace mask if it becomes moist during procedures.
6. Do not reuse a mask and do not let the mask hang around your neck.

## PROCEDURE
### 7
# Putting on a Gown

To be effective, a gown should have long sleeves, be long enough to cover the uniform, and big enough to overlap in the back. Gowns should be waterproof.

1. Assemble equipment:
   - Clean gown
   - Paper towel
2. Remove wristwatch; place it on paper towel.
3. Wash hands.
4. If a mask and goggles or face shield are required, put them on first.
5. After tying on the mask, put on the gown outside the resident's room. Put on gown by slipping arms into sleeves (Figure 11-16A).

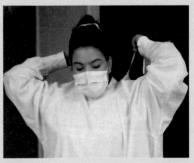

**FIGURE 11-16B** Slip fingers inside the neckband and tie gown.

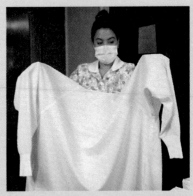

**FIGURE 11-16A** Putting on the clean cover gown before entering the resident's room. After tying on the mask, put on the gown.

6. Slip fingers of both hands under inside neckband and grasp ties in back. Secure neckband (Figure 11-16B).
7. Reach behind and overlap edges of gown. Secure waist ties (Figure 11-16C).

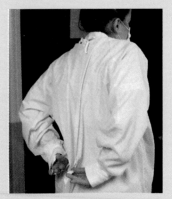

**FIGURE 11-16C** Reach behind, overlap the edges of the gown so the uniform is completely covered, and tie the waist ties.

8. Take watch into isolation unit, leaving it on paper towel.
9. Remember when using gowns:
   - A disposable gown is worn once only and is then discarded as infectious waste.
   - A cloth, reusable gown is worn once only and is then handled as contaminated linen.
   - Carry out all procedures in the unit at one time, to avoid unnecessary waste of gowns.

## PROCEDURE 8

# Putting on Gloves

1. Assemble equipment:
   - Disposable gloves in correct size
2. Wash hands.
3. If gown is required, put gloves on after gown is put on.
4. Pick up glove by the cuff and place it on the other hand.
5. Repeat with glove for other hand.
6. Interlace fingers to adjust gloves on hands.
7. Remember when using gloves:
   - Wash hands before and after using gloves.

- Remove gloves if they tear or become heavily soiled. Wash hands and put on a new pair.
- Gloves are used whenever there is the possibility of contact of body fluids, blood, secretions, or excretions with mucous membranes or nonintact skin.
- Change gloves between residents and wash hands.
- Discard gloves immediately after removing, in biohazardous waste receptacle.

## PROCEDURE 9

# Removing Contaminated Gloves

1. Grasp cuff of one glove on the outside with the fingers of the other hand (Figure 11-17A).

2. Pull cuff of glove down, drawing it over the glove and turning the glove inside out (Figure 11-17B). Pull glove off hand.

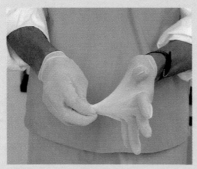

**FIGURE 11-17A** Removing contaminated gloves. With fingers of one hand, grasp glove of other hand.

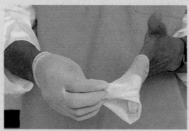

**FIGURE 11-17B** Pull the glove down over the hand and the fingers and remove it. The glove is inside out with the contaminated side inside.

*(continues)*

**PROCEDURE 9** *(continued)*

3. Hold the glove with the still-gloved hand.
4. Insert two fingers of the ungloved hand under the cuff of the glove on the other hand (Figure 11-17C).
5. Pull the glove off inside out, drawing it over the first glove.

6. Drop both gloves together into the biohazardous waste receptacle (Figure 11-17D).
7. Wash hands. Dry with a paper towel and discard towel in proper container. Use a dry towel to turn off water faucet. Discard towel.

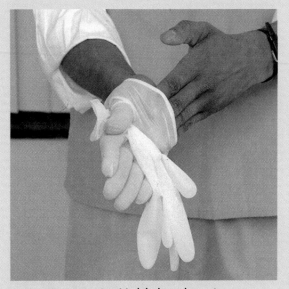

**FIGURE 11-17C** Hold the glove just removed in the gloved hand. Insert two fingers of the ungloved hand inside the cuff of the other glove.

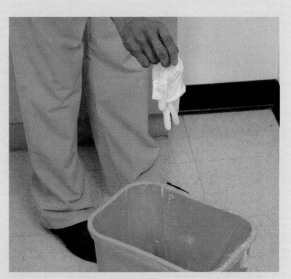

**FIGURE 11-17D** Pull the glove down over the hand and glove and then pull both gloves off, holding the inside (noncontaminated side of glove). Discard the gloves in the receptacle for contaminated trash.

**PROCEDURE 10** Removing Contaminated Gloves, Mask, and Gown

1. Assemble equipment:
   - Biohazardous waste receptacle for disposable items
   - Waste receptacle for gown if it is not disposable
   - Paper towels

*(continues)*

**PROCEDURE** *10*   *(continued)*

2. Follow Procedure 9 for removing contaminated gloves.
3. Undo waist ties of gown (Figure 11-18A).

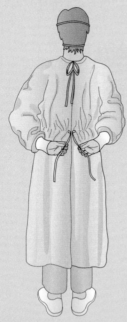

**FIGURE 11-18A**   Remove gloves. Wash hands and then untie waist tie of gown.

4. Turn faucets on with clean paper towel. Discard towel.
5. Wash hands and dry with clean paper towel.
6. Hold clean, dry paper towel to turn off faucet.
7. Remove goggles if used. Dispose of according to facility policy.
8. Remove mask:
   - Undo bottom ties first, then top ties (Figure 11-18B).
   - Holding top ties, dispose of mask in appropriate waste receptacle.
9. Undo neck ties and loosen gown at shoulders (Figure 11-18C).
10. Slip fingers of dominant hand inside cuff of other hand without touching outside of gown (Figure 11-18D).

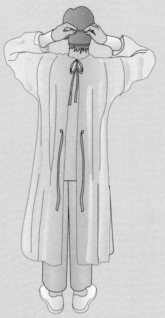

**FIGURE 11-18B**   Remove mask by untying top ties first and then bottom ties. Holding mask by ties, place it in the receptacle for contaminated trash.

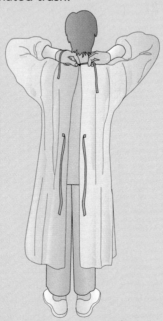

**FIGURE 11-18C**   Untie neck ties of gown.
*(continues)*

**PROCEDURE 10** *(continued)*

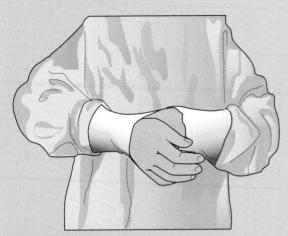

**FIGURE 11-18D** Slip fingers of one hand inside the cuff of the other hand. Pull gown down over the hand. Do not touch the outside of the gown with either hand.

**11.** Using gown-covered hand, pull the gown down over the dominant hand (Figure 11-18E) and then off both arms.

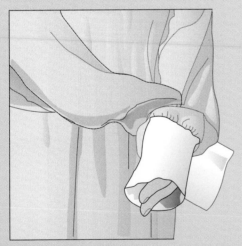

**FIGURE 11-18E** Using the gown-covered hand, pull the gown down over the other hand.

**12.** As the gown is removed, fold it away from the body with the contaminated side inward and then roll it up (Figure 11-18F). Dispose of contaminated gown in appropriate receptacle.

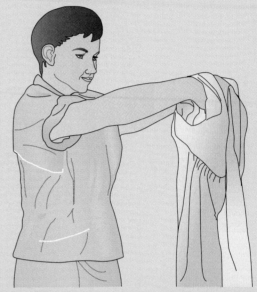

**FIGURE 11-18F** Pull the gown down off the arms being careful that the hands do not touch the outside of the gown. Hold the gown away from your uniform and roll it up with the contaminated side inside. If gown is disposable, place it in the receptacle for contaminated trash. If gown is not disposable, place it in laundry hamper for contaminated linens.

**13.** Undo mask and dispose of in appropriate container.
**14.** Wash hands.
**15.** Remove watch from paper towel. Hold clean side of paper towel, and dispose of towel in wastepaper receptacle.
**16.** Use paper towel to grasp handle to door as you leave resident's room. Discard paper towel in appropriate receptacle before you leave the unit.

**PROCEDURE**

# 11 Caring for Linens in Isolation Unit

1. Assemble linen required and place on chair or stand outside isolation unit.
2. Wash and dry hands.
3. Outside the isolation unit, put on PPE as required by type of transmission precautions.
4. Once inside the isolation unit, place clean linen on a chair.
5. Identify the resident and explain what you plan to do.
6. Provide privacy.
7. Allow resident to help as much as possible.
8. Raise bed to comfortable working height.
9. Remove soiled linen from bed by starting at the edges and working toward the center. Roll the linen toward the center with the soiled side inside.
10. Handle soiled linen as little as possible. Pick up the linen from the bed and hold it away from your uniform and gown (if used).
11. Place soiled linen in a meltaway laundry bag (a bag that dissolves in the wash water in the laundry), or follow facility policy.
12. Place meltaway bag in laundry hamper lined with biohazard plastic bag, or follow facility policy. Bag should be labeled as biohazardous material for laundry.
13. Secure bag and route soiled linen to laundry according to facility policy.
14. If gloves are heavily contaminated from the soiled linens, remove gloves and dispose of in appropriate receptacle. Wash hands, dry, and put on a clean pair of gloves. Then remake resident's bed with the clean linens.
15. Carry out all procedure completion actions.

You may remove your PPE after you have finished all tasks in the resident's room. Follow the instructions in Procedures 9 and 10.

**PROCEDURE**

# 12 Measuring Vital Signs in Isolation Unit

*Note:* Equipment to measure vital signs in isolation should be dedicated to the resident, meaning that the equipment will remain in the room with the resident. If the equipment must be shared with other residents, it must be cleaned and disinfected before use with another resident.

1. Before entering the isolation unit:
   - Wash hands.
   - Remove wristwatch and place it on a clean paper towel.
   - Put on PPE as required by the type of transmission-based precautions used.

*(continues)*

**PROCEDURE 12** *(continued)*

2. Pick up the paper towel with the watch. Enter the isolation unit.
3. With the watch still on the paper towel, place it where you can see it during the procedures.
4. Identify the resident and explain what you plan to do.
5. Provide privacy.
6. Allow resident to help as much as possible.
7. Raise bed to comfortable working height.
8. Using the equipment dedicated to the resident, measure vital signs.
9. Note the readings on a paper towel so you do not forget them.
10. Clean and store the equipment used according to facility policy.
11. Carry out all procedure completion actions.
12. Remove and discard PPE according to facility policy.
13. Wash hands, dry, and pick up watch.
14. Handling only the clean side of the paper towel, discard it in the appropriate receptacle.
15. Pick up your notes. Use a paper towel to open the door and leave the isolation unit. Discard paper towel before you leave the unit.

**PROCEDURE 13** Serving a Meal Tray in Isolation Unit

1. Before entering the isolation unit:
   - Wash hands.
   - Obtain the meal tray for the resident. Check the meal card on the tray and check that the correct menu is provided.
   - Ask for the assistance of another member of the team.
   - Place the tray on the isolation cart.
   - Put on PPE as required by the type of isolation precautions used.
2. Enter the isolation room and identify the resident.
3. Explain what you plan to do.
4. Provide privacy.
5. Allow resident to help as much as possible.
6. Raise the bed to comfortable working height.
7. Pick up the meal tray that remains in the room. Make sure the tray is clean.
8. Return to the door and open it. The team member assisting holds the meal tray while you carefully transfer items to the isolation tray.
9. Place isolation meal tray on overbed table. Prepare resident for the meal.
10. Check resident's identification band against the meal tray card.
11. Assist resident with food preparation and feeding as needed.
12. When the resident finishes, note how much food and liquid have been eaten. Uneaten food (except bones) is flushed in the toilet.
13. All disposable items (bones, dishes, eating utensils, covers, plastic wrap, foil,

*(continues)*

**PROCEDURE** *13*   *(continued)*

napkins, cups, cartons) are placed in the appropriate waste receptacle.

**14.** Reusable dishes may be handled as follows:

- Use a paper towel open door to isolation unit.
- Prop door open with your foot. Transfer dishes to a tray held by another assistant outside the door.
- Assistant outside the room covers the dishes and returns the tray to the food cart.

*Note:* CDC no longer *requires* the use of disposable dishes on transmission-based precautions.

**15.** Clean meal tray and store in the isolation unit.

**16.** Carry out all procedure completion actions.

**17.** Remove PPE and discard in the appropriate receptacle.

**18.** Wash hands.

**19.** Use paper towel to open door to leave the isolation unit.

---

**PROCEDURE** *14*   Specimen Collection from Resident in Isolation Unit

**1.** Outside the isolation unit, assemble equipment:

- Clean specimen container and cover
- Paper towel
- Biohazard bag for specimen container (Figure 11-19)
- Two completed labels, one for the specimen container and one for the specimen bag

*Note:* The specimen bag may have a preprinted block on the bag that can be completed with the required information. In this case, a second label is not needed.

**2.** Place the equipment on the isolation cart while you put on the PPE.

**3.** The biohazard bag for specimen transport remains outside the isolation unit.

**4.** Carry the specimen equipment into the isolation unit. Place container and cover on a paper towel.

**5.** Identify resident and explain what you plan to do.

**6.** Provide privacy.

**7.** Allow resident to help as much as possible.

**8.** Raise bed to comfortable working height.

**9.** Place specimen into container without touching the outside of the container.

**10.** Cover the container and apply label.

**11.** Clean equipment used to obtain the specimen according to facility policy.

**12.** Carry out all procedure completion actions.

**13.** Remove personal protective equipment as described in Procedures 9 and 10.

**14.** Wash hands.

**15.** Use a paper towel to pick up specimen container. Use another paper towel to open door to leave isolation unit.

*(continues)*

**PROCEDURE** *14* *(continued)*

**16.** Outside the unit, gather the towel in your hands so the edges do not hang loosely. Place the specimen container in the biohazard transport bag, being careful not to allow the paper towel to touch the outside of the transport bag.

**17.** Discard the paper towels in the appropriate receptacle.
**18.** Follow facility policy for the transport of the specimen.
**19.** Wash hands.

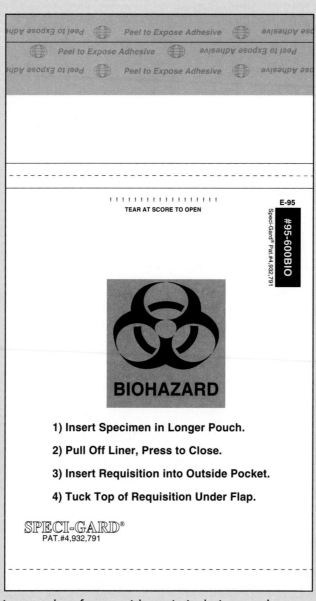

**FIGURE 11-19** Specimens taken from residents in isolation can be transported in specimen bags marked with the biohazard symbol.

**PROCEDURE**
**15**

# Transferring Nondisposable Equipment Outside of Isolation Unit

1. Nondisposable equipment used with a resident in transmission-based precautions may be dedicated to that resident; that is, the equipment remains in the isolation unit and is used only by that resident. Cleaning as required is done in the room by the nursing assistant or the housekeeping staff according to facility policy.
2. If the equipment must be used for other residents, it must be removed from the isolation unit and disinfected or sterilized before use with another resident.
3. Before leaving the isolation unit, clean the equipment with a disinfectant.
4. Place the equipment in a biohazard plastic bag.
5. Follow Procedure 10 for removing contaminated gloves, mask, and gown.
6. Pick up the bag containing the equipment and leave the isolation unit.
7. Once outside the unit, follow facility policy for the disinfection or sterilization of the equipment.
8. Some equipment may be terminally (finally and completely) cleaned with disinfectant in the resident's unit when isolation is discontinued.

**PROCEDURE**
**16**

# Transporting Resident to and from Isolation Unit

1. Wash your hands.
2. Assemble equipment:
   * Transport vehicle (wheelchair or stretcher)
   * Clean sheet
   * Mask for resident, if isolation precautions require it
3. Notify department to which resident is to be transported that resident from isolation unit is being transported.
4. If the resident is to be transported by stretcher, ask for assistance in moving the resident to the stretcher. Two other care providers will be needed.
5. Cover transport vehicle with clean sheet. Do not let the sheet touch the floor.
6. Wash your hands.
7. Put on PPE as required by type of precautions being used. If other care providers are needed to move the resident onto a stretcher, they also must put on PPE.
8. Wheel transport vehicle into isolation unit.
9. Identify resident. Explain what you plan to do.
10. Provide privacy.
11. Allow resident to help as much as possible.
12. If resident is to be transported by wheelchair, the bed must be in the lowest horizontal position. For transport by stretcher, raise the bed to the same height as the stretcher.

*(continues)*

## PROCEDURE *16* (continued)

13. Assist the resident into the wheelchair or onto the stretcher.
14. Put mask on resident, if required.
15. Wrap resident in sheet, if required. Make sure sheet does not touch the floor.
16. Remove PPE and wash hands. Open door and take resident out of isolation unit (Figure 11-20).
17. To return resident to isolation unit, place wheelchair or stretcher near wall of room as you put on PPE.
18. Enter the isolation unit, unwrap resident from sheet and remove mask, if used.
19. Assist resident from wheelchair or stretcher (with help of other caregivers) and return to bed.
20. Carry out procedure completion actions.
21. Place sheet in laundry hamper for contaminated linens and discard mask in receptacle for biohazardous trash.
22. Remove PPE and wash your hands.
23. Remove transport vehicle from isolation unit. Follow facility procedure for cleaning and storing vehicle used with resident in isolation.
24. Report completion of procedure: transport of resident in isolation to another department and back to isolation unit.

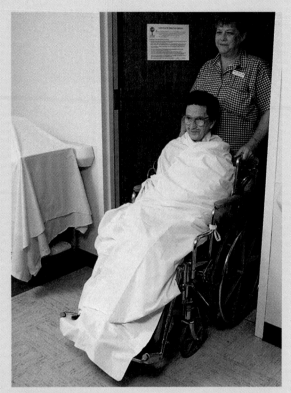

**FIGURE 11-20** This resident is leaving her room where contact precautions are in effect and is to be transported to another area of the facility.

## DISINFECTION AND STERILIZATION

**Disinfection** is the process of eliminating harmful pathogens from equipment and instruments. A chemical called a disinfectant is used for this procedure. You may be required to disinfect personal care items such as wash basins, bedpans, and urinals. You may also use disinfectants to clean wheelchairs and other furniture items. Items are usually washed before they are disinfected. The procedure for disinfecting depends on the chemicals that are used. Follow the directions of the facility for use of disinfec-

tants. Wear disposable gloves and a gown for completing these procedures. You may also need a face shield. Wear PPE that is appropriate to the procedure.

**Sterilization** removes all microorganisms from an item. This process can be completed in an **autoclave**, which uses steam and pressure to kill organisms. Gas sterilization is also used in some health care facilities. Sterilization procedures are used for all nondisposable equipment that is exposed to potentially infectious materials. Equipment to be sterilized is wrapped in special material. Strips on the packaging material turn a particular color when the package is ster-

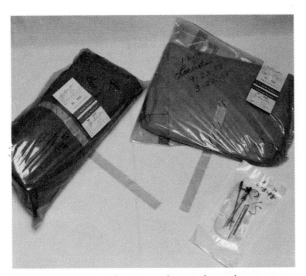

**FIGURE 11-21** These packages have been sterilized with steam or gas. The strips below each package show how they look before sterilization. The strips shown on the packages have changed color because they have been sterilized.

ilized (Figure 11-21). Do not use the package if the strip has not turned the appropriate color. Do not use a sterilized package that has been accidentally opened.

## STERILE PROCEDURES

Surgical asepsis is the means by which the environment is maintained free of microorganisms, both pathogens and nonpathogens. In procedures where surgical asepsis is used, equipment and supplies must be **sterile**. In other words, items used in the procedure must go through a sterilization process.

In most facilities, nursing assistants are not expected to carry out procedures requiring sterile techniques. If you are responsible for sterile procedures, you should first be given thorough training. Your responsibilities may include opening sterile packages such as gloves.

---

**PROCEDURE 17**

## Opening a Sterile Package

1. Wash your hands.
2. Assemble equipment:
   - Sterile package
3. If color code has not changed, or seal does not look intact, do not consider article sterile. *If you have any doubt about sterility, consider item unsterile and inform the nurse.*
4. Touch only outside of package. Only sterile surfaces contact other sterile surfaces. Never reach over a sterile field.
5. Commercially prepared products will be sealed. If package is in poor condition or discolored, do not consider item sterile. Discard item.

6. Place package, fold side up on a flat, clean surface.
7. Remove tape.
8. Unfold flap farthest away from you by grasping outer surface only between thumb and forefinger (Figure 11-22A).
9. Open right flap with right hand using same technique (Figure 11-22B).
10. Open left flap with left hand using same technique (Figure 11-22C).
11. Open final flap (nearest you) (Figure 11-22D). Touch only the outside of flap. Be careful not to stand too close. Do not allow uniform to touch flap as it is lifted free. Be sure the flaps are pulled open completely to prevent them from folding back over sterile items.

*(continues)*

**PROCEDURE** *17* *(continued)*

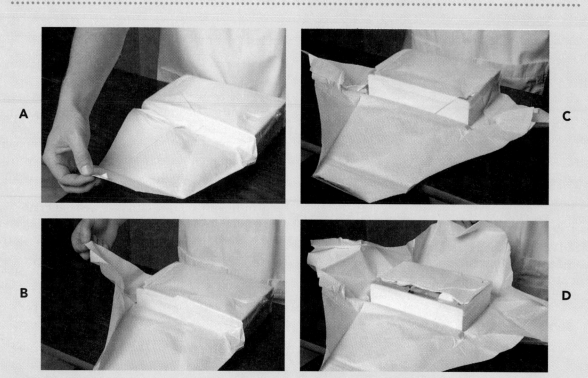

**FIGURE 11-22** Opening a sterile package. A. Open the top flap away from you; handle only the outside. B. Open the right side. Do not touch the inside of the folded-over portion. C. Open the left side, drawing the left flap to the side. D. Without reaching over the sterile field, open the side toward you.

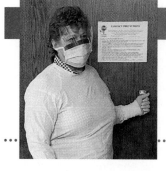

## LESSON SYNTHESIS: Putting It All Together

*Y*ou have just completed this lesson. Now go back and review the Clinical Focus. Try to see how the Clinical Focus relates to the concepts presented in the lesson. Then answer the following questions.

1. What kind of precautions are in use for Mr. Uritz?

2. How is MRSA spread?

3. Why is this resident in a private room?

4. When Mr. Uritz is in his room, is it necessary to keep the door shut?

## REVIEW

**A. Fill in the blanks by selecting the correct word or phrase from the list.**

communicable      sterile
disinfectants      work practice
medical asepsis      controls

1. The process of making an environment pathogen free is known as _____.

2. An article is _____ when there are no living organisms present.

3. _____ are procedures to prevent the spread of infections in the work area.

4. An easily transmitted disease is called _____.

5. Chemicals that destroy pathogens on articles are called _____.

**B. Answer each statement true (T) or false (F).**

6. T   F   Items for one resident may be used by another resident.

7. T   F   Food trays should remain covered until they are delivered to the resident.

8. T   F   Laundry dropped on the floor may be used as long as there is no visible dirt.

9. T   F   Soiled linens may be placed on the floor until all the linen is gathered together and put in the laundry hamper.

10. T   F   Hands need not be washed after gloves are removed as long as there are no tears in the gloves.

11. T   F   Gloves are always used when handling bedpans and urinals.

12. T   F   Occupational exposure means coming in contact with potentially infectious material as you work.

13. T   F   Standard precautions require the wearing of gloves for any contact with blood or body fluids.

14. T   F   The biohazard symbol is a green square with a line through it.

15. T   F   A used razor may be disposed of by dropping it in the waste basket.

**C. Select one best answer for each of the following.**

16. Housing and caring for a person with an infection is known as
   a. segregation
   b. isolation
   c. sequestration
   d. separation

17. To remove PPE after caring for a resident on isolation precautions, you should
   a. remove the gown first
   b. remove the gloves first
   c. remove the mask first
   d. remove PPE in any order

18. If a nursing assistant is sensitive to latex gloves
   a. gloves need not be worn
   b. wear the latex gloves anyway
   c. ask the supervisor for nonlatex gloves
   d. put powder in the gloves

19. The basic foundation of medical asepsis is
   a. handwashing
   b. wearing goggles
   c. wearing a mask
   d. wearing a gown

20. If there is an exposure incident you should
   a. ignore the situation
   b. report it at once to the supervisor
   c. call the doctor
   d. tell other nursing assistants

# Characteristics of the Long-Term Care Resident

## LESSONS

*12* The Long-Term Care Resident

*13* The Psychosocial Aspects of Aging

*14* The Physical Effects of Aging

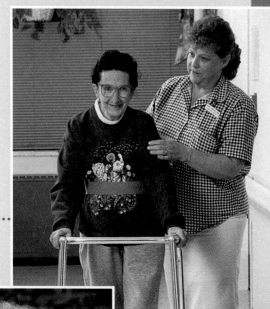

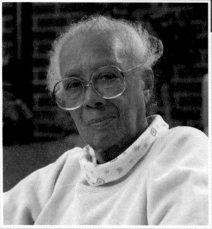

# The Long-Term Care Resident

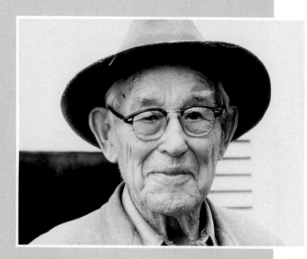

## CLINICAL FOCUS

Think about how stereotypes and myths about the elderly and those who live in long-term care make it difficult to recognize the uniqueness of each person as you study this lesson and meet:

*S*am Jacobzinski, age 84, who was admitted to Riverview Skilled Care Facility in acute cardiac failure 4 years ago. There was little hope for his recovery, but Sam fooled everyone. He recovered and was transferred to your facility where he has been a resident ever since. He is alert and involved in facility activities, acting as the Resident Council president. He uses a motorized wheelchair and makes a daily round of visits to other residents. Periodically he "overdoes it" and needs bed rest, but even then his spirit is felt throughout the unit.

## OBJECTIVES

*After studying this lesson, you should be able to:*

- Define and spell vocabulary words and terms.
- List four reasons why residents are admitted to long-term care facilities.
- List three facts about the over-65 population.

- Describe five facts to remember when caring for younger adults.
- Recognize the stereotypes and myths of aging.
- Describe three facts about the aging process.
- Identify the unique needs of younger residents in long-term care facilities.

# VOCABULARY

chronic disease  (**KRON**-ick dih-**ZEEZ**)

developmental disability  (dee-vel-op-**MEN**-tal dis-ah-**BILL**-ah-tee)

disability  (dis-ah-**BILL**-ah-tee)

impairment  (im-**PAIR**-ment)

instrumental activities of daily living (IADL)  (**in**-strew-**MEN**-tal ack-**TIV**-ih-tees of **DAY**-lee **LIV**-ing)

myth  (mith)

self-care (functional) deficit  (self-kair [**FUNK**-shun-al] **DEF**-ih-sit)

stereotype  (**STEH**-ree-oh-type)

trauma  (**TRAW**-mah)

value system  (**VAL**-you **SIS**-tum)

## ILLNESS AND DISABILITY

The residents are in the long-term care facility for several reasons. Many have a chronic illness or a **disability.** A disability occurs when there is an impairment that interferes with the individual's ability to perform the activities normal for a person of that age. A disability is present if any adult is unable to perform the activities of daily living. An **impairment** is a loss or abnormality of the body structure and function. The damage to brain cells in Alzheimer's disease, for example, interferes with the person's ability to perform activities of daily living. A disability or impairment could be the result of:

1. Chronic disease
   A **chronic disease** is one that begins slowly and is expected to continue for a long time, perhaps for life. Some chronic diseases are progressive, which means the symptoms will increase in severity as time goes on. Examples of chronic diseases are:
   - Arthritis
   - Neurologic disorders such as multiple sclerosis, Parkinson's disease (Figure 12-1), Huntington's disease, or Alzheimer's disease
   - Heart or lung disease
   - Diabetes
   - Illnesses with acute onset that have chronic aftereffects, such as stroke

2. Trauma
   **Trauma** refers to injuries received in an accident. These accidents may result in brain

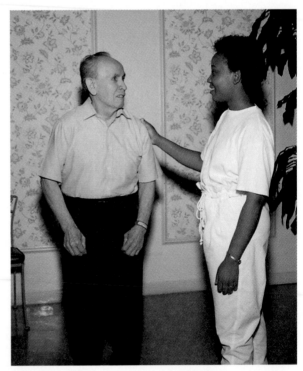

**FIGURE 12-1** Note the typical bent posture in this front view of a resident with Parkinson's disease.

injuries, spinal cord injuries, multiorgan damage, or amputation of one or more extremities. The injuries may prevent the individual from being independent.

3. Developmental disabilities
   A **developmental disability** is a permanent condition that is present at birth or occurs

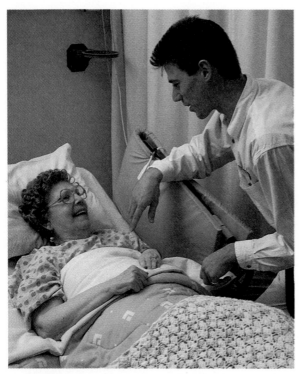

**FIGURE 12-2**  This woman has had a developmental disability since birth.

before the age of 21. Developmental disabilities limit the ability to care for oneself in an independent way (Figure 12-2). This topic is discussed further in Lesson 31.

4. Acquired immune deficiency syndrome (AIDS) An increasing number of persons with AIDS are being cared for in long-term care facilities. This disease makes the individuals more susceptible to other infections and diseases. Admission generally occurs when the person is in the terminal stages of disease and needs continual care.

5. Many long-term care facilities have residents with cancer. Sometimes they are receiving treatments specific for the cancer (chemotherapy or radiation). Other residents may be in the terminal stage of the illness.

6. A growing number of residents in long-term care are admitted directly from hospitals for additional care after surgery or illness or for rehabilitation after fractures or strokes. These residents generally stay for a short time, with stays ranging from several weeks to several months. The goal is to return these

residents to their homes or to another facility where more independent living is possible. In many facilities these residents are cared for in the subacute care unit (see Lesson 33).

Most residents in long-term care facilities are women because women have a longer life expectancy than men. The older a person gets, the greater the chance that a chronic illness will develop. Most residents have multiple health problems. A resident may be admitted because of a stroke, but also have diabetes and a heart problem. Because of the health problems, residents have **self-care (functional) deficits**. This means they are unable to care for themselves in one or more areas of activities of daily living (ADL) (Figure 12-3). The activities of daily living include:

• Personal grooming and hygiene
• Bathing
• Dressing and undressing
• Eating
• Toileting
• Mobility

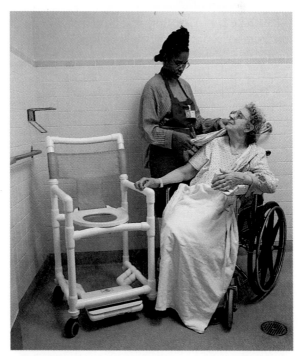

**FIGURE 12-3**  This resident needs assistance in completing her activities of daily living.

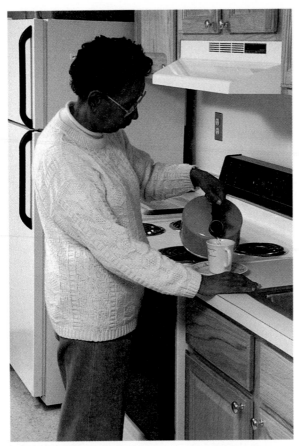

**FIGURE 12-4** Cooking is an example of an instrumental activity of daily living.

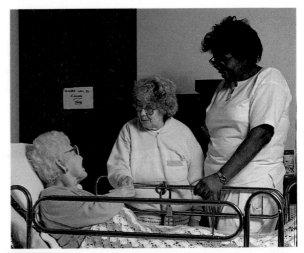

**FIGURE 12-5** This elderly woman makes an important contribution to society by visiting residents in long-term care facilities.

There are also **instrumental activities of daily living (IADL)** (Figure 12-4). The IADL include activities such as:

- Managing a household
- Managing money
- Driving a car

## THE PROCESS OF NORMAL AGING

Aging is a natural process and is not a result of disease. The term *gerontology* means the study of aging. It is used to describe a specialty area for health care providers. For example, a nurse working with older adults is a gerontologic nurse. You may also hear the word *geriatrics*. Geriatrics refers to the diagnosis and treatment of disorders that occur with aging. Although there are expected changes of aging, no disorders are unique to the aged population. The word *gerontology* is preferred because it emphasizes health and aging rather than illness.

Aging is a progressive process that begins at birth and continues until death. It is a normal process experienced by all human beings. During the life span, a unique person of value emerges and makes contributions to society. When elderly, this same person of value needs and deserves respect, support, and care. The elderly make many contributions to society (Figure 12-5).

Here are some facts about aging from the U.S. Bureau of the Census:

- Persons 65 years or older make up 12.7% of the population of the United States.
- Since 1990, this age group has increased by 7% as compared to an increase of 4% for the under-65 population.
- There are 146 women for every 100 men in the over-65 age group.
- In 1993, persons reaching age 65 had an average life expectancy of an additional 17.3 years.

## STEREOTYPES AND MYTHS

**Stereotypes** of people are rigid ideas about people as a group. A stereotype may partly be true, or it may be true for some people, but all members of a group are never totally alike. For example, many elderly people are hearing impaired, but not all of them. Beliefs of this kind that are not even partly true are **myths**.

Imagine someone asking you to describe a cat if you had only seen two small, black, short-haired cats in your life. You would undoubtedly say that cats are small, black, and short-haired. As you know, this does not even begin to describe the different cats throughout the world. Describing all cats with one narrow set of characteristics establishes a stereotype for cats; it is only partly true. It is easy to form stereotypes, because limited experience tends to make us think that everyone in a certain group has the same characteristics as the few people we know in that group.

## The Dangers of Stereotyping

Stereotypes about the elderly are limiting to both the people who believe them and to the elderly themselves. This is true for several reasons.

- *Stereotyping does not consider the uniqueness of the individual.* Although they have certain characteristics in common, the elder members of society have developed from their own special life experiences. This makes each person different, in some ways, from all others.
- *Stereotyping may make people devalue themselves because they see themselves as a reflection of what others think.* If people are treated with respect, they feel respectable and behave in respectable ways. If people are viewed as helpless and unable to make their own decisions, some may lose confidence in their ability to handle their own affairs and will become increasingly dependent on others.

It is unwise and unfair to take stereotypes at face value. It is especially important for those who work in long-term care facilities to realize that the people in their care are not representative of all people in the age group.

You can help residents by:

- Resisting the temptation to stereotype
- Accepting them as individuals
- Giving them as much control over their lives as possible
- Supporting their efforts to remain as independent as possible
- Treating all residents with respect and courtesy

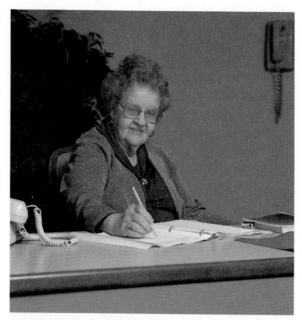

**FIGURE 12-6**   Age alone does not determine a person's abilities or activities.

## Myths

A *myth* is an untruth that some people believe. It is a myth that age alone causes the diseases that are often associated with elderly residents. Although many elderly residents have cancer, heart disease, diabetes, or strokes, younger people also have these conditions.

Another myth is that age alone determines the value of the contributions a person can make to society. Many people make their most valuable contributions to society in their later years. Civic groups and charities could not survive without the involvement of older people (Figure 12-6).

## Commonly Held Beliefs

- *As people age, they experience the same characteristic changes in the structure and function of their bodies.* This stereotype is partly true. Aging is usually shown by graying of the hair, diminished eyesight, and slower reaction times. The rate and type of changes due to aging are different for different people. In general, the functioning of the body is slowed but is still adequate to meet the needs of the older life-style.
- *Older people are incompetent and unable to make correct judgments and decisions.* This is

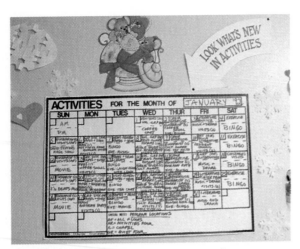

**FIGURE 12-7**   Activities can provide opportunities for acquiring new skills and information.

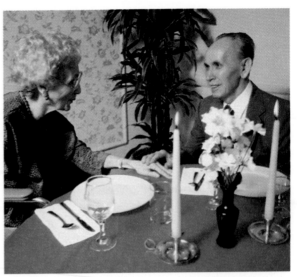

**FIGURE 12-8**   Older people have the same emotional needs as younger people.

a myth. Sensory losses occur with aging, but most older people remain mentally sound until they die. They manage their own affairs, can learn new skills, and process new information (Figure 12-7).

- *Older people are unhappy, without focus in their lives, and have little interest in sex.* In general, the older population is no less and no more content with life than younger people. They fill their lives with activities suitable to their needs. Their views of life in later years are usually a reflection of the attitudes they had in younger years. They are still sexual beings and can express sexual feelings and fulfill sexual needs (Figure 12-8).
- *Old people are sent to nursing homes because society does not want to be bothered with them.* Compared to the general population, a small number of people over 65 years live in long-term care facilities. The percentage increases with age. For persons aged 64 to 74 years, only 1% live in these facilities. This number increases to 6% for persons 75 to 84 years and to 24% for persons over 85 years. Admission to a long-term care facility is often a difficult decision for the individual and the family. The decision is usually based on the fact that the person needs the type of care available only in the long-term care facility.
- *Being "old" is determined solely by the number of years a person has lived.* This is not necessarily true. The term *old* is subjective and rela-

tive and has a great deal to do with a person's outlook on life. To a child 5 years old, someone of 35 years is old.

## Myths Versus Facts About the Aged

The first list is made up of myths about the aged. The second is based on facts. Note that the facts in List 2 are true for most elderly people in general, but not all of them.

LIST 1: MYTHS Many people believe that *all* older persons:

- Cannot care for themselves
- Are unable to learn
- Have no interest in life
- Are neglected by family, friends, and society
- Are living in poverty
- No longer contribute to society
- Have no interest in sexuality
- Become "old" at a certain age, such as 65
- Are incompetent to make decisions

LIST 2: FACTS It is true, in general, that the elderly:

- Have sensory losses (changes in vision and hearing)
- Have changes in sleep patterns
- Have slower sexual responses
- Are more prone to certain chronic conditions
- Undergo postural changes
- Have less efficient elimination

- Have less tolerance to glucose
- Experience physical changes such as graying of the hair and drying of the skin

### Positive Stereotypes

Many stereotypes are negative, but some may be positive. For example, some positive stereotypes are that older people:

- Are more peaceful
- Are wiser and more self-confident
- Have a well-developed **value system** and know what is important to them
- Have more time to do the things that are important to them

Even these stereotypes do not apply to all the residents in your care.

## THE YOUNGER RESIDENT IN THE LONG-TERM CARE FACILITY··········

You may care for younger people in the long-term care facility. These young people may be there because of injuries from accidents, birth defects, or disease. Common reasons for admission are:

- Traumatic brain injuries
- Spinal cord injuries
- Developmental disabilities
- Chronic diseases (Figure 12-9)
- AIDS

The health care team must recognize that although the needs of all humans are the same, regardless of age, the ways in which individuals meet these needs may vary with age.

Young residents have the same needs as other persons their age. Their natural development has often been interrupted during a critical

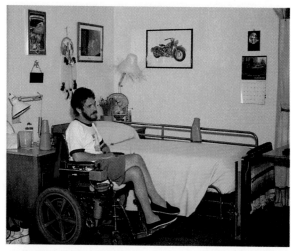

**FIGURE 12-9**   Multiple sclerosis is an example of a chronic disease that may affect a younger person.

stage of life. Some of them may have been unable to complete their education, to experience a career, to marry, or to have children. Others may have a spouse and young children at home. It is often difficult for these residents to adapt to and accept the change in their life-style.

Adjustment to a long-term care facility may be more difficult for the younger resident. Young people have had fewer years in which to accumulate the resources for dealing with crises. Their lives have been interrupted and they still have more years of living ahead of them. Because of improved medical technology, young persons with a chronic disease or disability can expect to live almost as long as they would have without the disease or disability.

Opportunities for continuing their education may be provided. Vocational training may be a part of the care plan for some younger residents.

# *G*uidelines for

## Caring for Younger Residents

Remember when caring for younger residents that:

1. Many younger residents may be your peers. You will need to learn how to have empathy (putting yourself in the other person's place) without becoming emotionally involved to the extent that you cannot remain objective.

2. They may be frustrated and angry because their lives have been interrupted; they may never have the opportunity to marry, have a family, or earn a living.

3. Sexual feelings are at the most intense level during young adulthood. These feelings do not decrease just because the person is in a long-term care facility. Residents may act out these feelings. Discuss these situations with the nurse so that you are prepared to handle them. Like all residents, they need to have privacy and an opportunity for intimacy with a companion, whether a spouse or "significant other."

4. If the young resident has children, try to provide a place where the family can visit together without interruption.

5. Socialization with other people of the same age is essential to the continuing development of the individual. Younger residents may not wish to be constantly with the elderly residents. If there are several younger residents in a facility, they may enjoy age-related activities together.

6. Emotional problems such as depression may be present in residents of any age. These problems must be addressed by the interdisciplinary health care team.

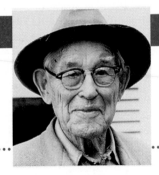

## LESSON SYNTHESIS: Putting It All Together

*Y*ou have just completed this lesson. Now go back and review the Clinical Focus. Try to see how the Clinical Focus relates to the concepts presented in the lesson. Then answer the following questions.

1. How does Sam indicate his desire to stay an active participant in life?

2. How does Sam compare with the common stereotypes and myths about aging?

3. What situations might lead to a younger person entering a long-term care facility?

4. What needs do nursing assistants have to meet that are the same for the elderly and for young residents in long-term care? What needs must nursing assistants meet that are different for the elderly and young residents?

# REVIEW

**A. Select the one best answer for each of the following.**

1. Residents are admitted to long-term care facilities because they
   a. are old
   b. need health care
   c. have no loved ones
   d. have no other place to live

2. A chronic disease
   a. results from an injury
   b. comes on suddenly and is usually cured
   c. is a form of cancer
   d. begins slowly and is expected to continue for a long time

3. The need to receive long-term health care because of trauma may be due to
   a. spinal cord injury
   b. heart attack
   c. stroke
   d. dementia

4. The aging process begins
   a. during middle age
   b. after age 65 years
   c. at birth
   d. all of these

5. Instrumental activities of daily living include
   a. bathing
   b. toileting
   c. eating
   d. household management

6. Myths many people believe are that all older persons
   a. are unable to learn
   b. have no interest in sexuality
   c. are incompetent to make decisions
   d. all of these

7. It is generally true that older persons
   a. become very forgetful
   b. become incontinent
   c. usually have sensory losses
   d. all of these

**B. Match each term with the correct definition.**

a. injury received in accident
b. permanent condition present at birth or occurs during childhood
c. one that begins slowly and is expected to last a long time
d. loss or abnormality of the structure or function
e. inability to perform activities normal for one's age
f. an untruth that some people believe
g. rigid ideas about a group of people

8. _____ impairment

9. _____ disability

10. _____ trauma

11. _____ chronic disease

12. _____ developmental disability

13. _____ myth

14. _____ stereotype

**C. Answer each statement true (T) or false (F).**

15. T  F  A developmental disability is always present at birth.

16. T  F  Parkinson's disease is an example of a chronic illness.

17. T  F  The inability to feed one's self is an example of a self-care deficit.

18. T  F  There are more men over age 65 than women over age 65.

19. T  F  The over-65 population is the fastest growing age group.

20. T  F  Stereotypes are true generalizations about specific types of groups.

**D. Indicate which of the following is myth (M) and which is stereotype (S) regarding residents of advanced age.**

21. S   M   Age alone causes diseases.

22. S   M   All older people have gray/white hair.

23. S   M   Only people who are young are of value to society.

24. S   M   Elderly people are always more peaceful.

25. S   M   Eyesight diminishes in all elderly people.

26. S   M   All elderly people are unable to manage their own affairs.

27. S   M   All elderly people have little interest in sex.

28. S   M   Reaction time is prolonged in all of the elderly.

29. S   M   Being old is only determined by the number of years lived.

30. S   M   All elderly people have less energy.

31. S   M   All elderly people live in poverty.

32. S   M   All elderly people are self-confident.

# *13*

# The Psychosocial Aspects of Aging

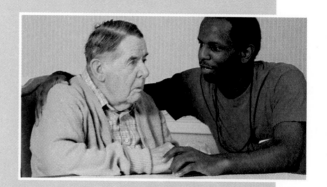

## CLINICAL FOCUS

Think about how you can assist residents in meeting their psychosocial needs as you study this lesson and meet:

**M**r. Warner, age 87, who has been a resident of your facility for 2 years since his wife of 51 years died. During that time you have come to know him well. He is in a wheelchair but his mind is still very clear. He confides to you one morning that he really misses "having a woman" and wishes that he had a way to relieve his sexual tension. The staff is sensitive to his needs.

## OBJECTIVES

*After studying this lesson, you should be able to:*

- Define and spell vocabulary words and terms.
- Identify the needs common to all human beings.
- Describe the developmental tasks of older adults.
- List the ways in which you can help residents feel safe and secure.

- List the ways in which you can help residents fulfill psychosocial needs.
- Describe how you can assist a resident to maintain sexuality.
- Discuss the challenges to adjustment faced by residents.
- Recognize signs of stress reaction.
- Describe actions to take when residents display unusual behaviors.

## VOCABULARY

**amulet** *(AM-you-let)*

**compensation** *(kom-pen-SAY-shun)*

**defense mechanism** *(dee-FENS MECK-ah-niz-em)*

**denial** *(dih-NIGH-al)*

**deteriorate** *(dee-TER-ee-or-ayt)*

**developmental tasks** *(dee-vel-op-MEN-tal tasks)*

**manipulative behavior** *(mah-NIP-you-lah-tiv bee-HAY-vyour)*

## VOCABULARY

masturbation  (*mass-tur-BAY-shun*)           rationalization  (*rash-un-al-ih-ZAY-shun*)

personality  (*per-son-AL-ih-tee*)            self-esteem  (*self-es-TEEM*)

projection  (*proh-JECK-shun*)                suppression  (*suh-PRESH-un*)

rapport  (*rah-POOR*)                         talisman  (*TAL-iss-man*)

## Basic Human Needs

Basic human needs are those activities required by all people to live their lives satisfactorily. Basic human needs are the same for all people, at all ages.

Abraham Maslow and Erik Erikson were two leaders in the study of human behavior. They made valuable contributions to our understanding of basic needs and how people satisfy them.

Maslow described three groups of basic needs (Figure 13-1):

- Physical needs
- Safety and security needs
- Psychosocial needs

He found that the order in which needs are satisfied is based on their importance to survival.

Physical needs are satisfied first. Safety and security needs are next in importance to survival. Only after these needs are satisfied can the psychosocial needs (emotional needs) be considered.

### Physical Needs

The most basic human needs relate to the physical functioning of our bodies. These needs must be met to maintain life:

- Oxygen
- Water
- Food
- Sleep
- Activity
- Elimination
- Sexuality

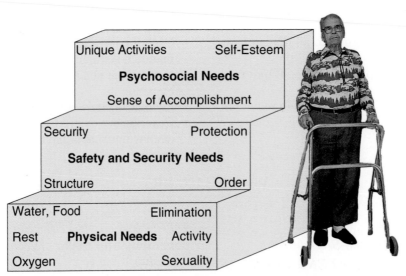

**FIGURE 13-1** People meet needs in order of their importance to survival. Physical needs must be satisfied first.

Illness can make meeting these needs a challenge for the resident and the caregiver. Residents may require assistance in meeting physical needs for a number of reasons:

1. There is a physical limitation, such as:
   - Paralysis of an arm or leg
   - Visual impairment
   - Arthritis
   - Lung or heart problems
2. The resident is disoriented and unable to follow instructions.

The nursing staff is responsible for helping residents meet their physical needs. Nursing assistants have an important role in helping residents meet their basic needs.

## Safety and Security Needs

Residents who do not feel safe will experience fear. Living in a state of fear prevents an individual from achieving psychosocial well-being. You can help residents feel safe by:

- Being dependable and trustworthy
- Being kind and considerate
- Providing care promptly, gently, and safely
- Helping the residents maintain a life-style structured to their choice
- Protecting their possessions from theft
- Letting residents know that the facility is protected against fire and other disasters

## Psychosocial Needs

The psychosocial needs of the elderly are the same as those at any age. There is a need to:

- Love and be loved
- Be treated with respect and dignity
- Feel needed
- Feel important as an individual

When residents first enter a long-term care facility, they often feel depressed and frightened. They are in a strange environment and they fear that they will lose all privacy and control of their own lives.

Elderly residents have fewer opportunities to satisfy their psychosocial needs. Most are aware that their bodies are failing, that they are separated from family and friends, and that they may be dependent on others for meeting even basic needs. All of these factors are major threats to emotional security.

Most residents react to these threats by relying on actions that have been successful for them in past years. Some residents may move backward in their emotional responses and use less satisfactory means to deal with the problems. Others may be so overwhelmed by the changes that they become withdrawn, disoriented, or depressed.

You can help residents meet their psychosocial needs if you:

- Treat each resident as an individual with specific characteristics and needs.
- Give the resident choices whenever possible (Figure 13-2).
- Honor the residents' identities. Call residents by the name they choose. Allow them to reflect their identity by the way they dress, the way they arrange their rooms, and the activities they choose.
- Allow residents to do as much as possible for themselves. Encourage their independence to the level their conditions permit.
- Respect the residents' rights.

The way each resident satisfies psychosocial needs depends on personality. **Personality** is the sum of the ways we react to the events in our lives. Personality is gradually formed through life's experiences.

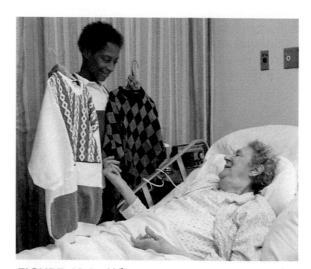

**FIGURE 13-2** Whenever necessary, assist the resident but allow her to make her own decisions.

**FIGURE 13-3** Erickson's list of the tasks of personality development from infancy through old age

| Growing Stage | Task |
| --- | --- |
| Infancy | Learning to trust |
| Early childhood years | Recognizing identity as part of a family unit |
| School years | Skill development; constructive activities |
| Adolescent years | Developing identity as an individual |
| Young adulthood | Forming intimate relationships, raising a family |
| Middle years | Carrying out one's chosen work |
| Old age | Integrating life's experiences |

Erikson suggests that as we mature from infancy to old age, we pass through several developmental stages. During each stage, certain tasks must be accomplished. These are called **developmental tasks** (Figure 13-3).

The developmental tasks specific to older adults are just as important as those for younger people. They include the need to:

- Adjust to decreased abilities such as physical limitations caused by the aging process
- Integrate life experiences through reminiscing
- Accept the onset of chronic illness
- Accept one's place in the community structure
- Adapt to possible changes in social and financial security
- Recognize and accept that life is limited
- Act as a role model for others

Nursing assistants can play an important role in helping residents accomplish the developmental tasks by:

- Allowing residents to talk about their experiences and feelings
- Creating an atmosphere of acceptance where the residents are not judged

If these stages are interrupted and not completed because of illness, the individual may display behavior that is inappropriate for the age and the culture we live in.

## CULTURAL INFLUENCES

The residents you care for may come from different cultures. More complete care is given if nursing assistants are sensitive to the cultural influences on a resident's behavior. People from the same culture usually share similar values, customs, clothing, and food preferences. Cultural values and customs are passed from generation to generation and are the foundation for accepted behavior. Cultural influences play an important role in how a person views and reacts to illness.

Each culture may have its own belief system and religious faith. An understanding of some of the major belief systems will help you assist your residents to meet their needs. Always remember that you are caring for an individual within a cultural framework (Figure 13-4).

## SPIRITUALITY

Spirituality is the part of a person that gives a sense of wholeness by fulfilling the human need to feel connected with the world and to a power greater than self. Spirituality and religion (an organized system of belief) are products of the individual's cultural background and experience. Spiritual values form the guiding principles that people may use to determine right or wrong.

Facing death, coping with loss, and accepting life as it really is are all spiritual tasks for the elderly.

A person's spiritual feelings play an important part in helping him or her through crises and stress periods. Spiritual feelings are personal, are expressed in different ways, and may or may not be associated with a specific religion (Figure 13-5).

**FIGURE 13-4** Belief systems related to health/illness

| Culture | Some Countries of Origin | Related Concepts | Health Care Provider | Cause of Illness | Methods of Treatment |
|---------|--------------------------|------------------|----------------------|------------------|----------------------|
| European Americans | Germany, England, France, Poland, Italy, Scandinavia | Illness is not superficial but can be influenced by poor health practices. Disease is treatable and sometimes curable. | Physician | • Punishment for sins <br> • Self-abuse; outside forces such as germs | Diet, exercise, home remedies, medication, surgery, religious rituals, wearing amulets |
| Asian Americans | Hawaii, Philippines, Korea, Japan, China, Laos, Vietnam, Cambodia | Body has two energy forces: yang which is cold and yin which is hot (hot and cold do not refer to temperature). Hot conditions are treated with cold foods and treatments. Cold conditions are treated with hot foods and treatments. | Traditional Healers | • Imbalance between the positive (yang) energy and the negative (yin) energy that are found in the body <br> • Over-exertion | Herbs, hot foods for conditions associated with yin and cold foods for conditions associated with yang conditions, home remedies and folk medicines |
| Hispanic Americans | Spain, Cuba, Mexico, Puerto Rico, Spanish-speaking countries in Central and South America | Body contains four humors (fluids) that need to be balanced. Illness develops from imbalance. Humors are blood (hot, moist), phlegm (cold, moist), black bile (cold, dry), yellow bile (hot, dry). | Native Healers (Jerbero, Curandera) | • Punishment from God for sins | Candles, prayers, wearing medals, hot and cold foods to restore balance of humors |

*(continues)*

**FIGURE 13-4** *(continued)*

| Culture | Some Countries of Origin | Related Concepts | Health Care Provider | Cause of Illness | Methods of Treatment |
|---|---|---|---|---|---|
| Native Americans | Over 170 tribes of American Indians, Eskimos (Inuit, etc) | Spiritual powers control body's energy. Harmony must exist between body, mind and spirit. Illness results when harmony is disrupted. | Medicine man, Shaman | • Violation of taboo<br>• Attack by witch or evil spirits<br>• Do not believe in germ theory | Sandpainting to diagnose condition and determine treatment<br>Elaborate rituals<br>Carrying medicine bundles<br>Masks worn to hide from evil spirits |
| African Americans | Africa, Haiti, Jamaica, Dominican Republic | Body, mind and spirit must be in harmony for health. Life is a process rather than a state. Illness can occur if self-care is not taken. | Folk Practitioners, Root Workers | • Punishment from God<br>• Spirits and demons | Prayer, diet, home remedies, wearing copper and silver bracelets, wearing talismans and amulets |

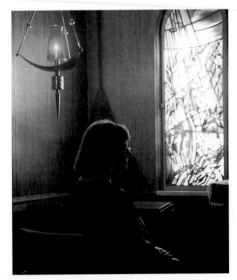

**FIGURE 13-5** Spiritual needs must be respected and supported.

## RELIGION

Religion is not the same as spirituality although spiritual people are frequently religious. Religion is a formal system that includes rituals and ceremonial acts that are an outward expression of faith (Figure 13-6). Many religions have objects of special significance, ranging from **amulets** (protective charms), **talismans** (engraved stones, rings, or other objects to ward off evil), copper or silver bracelets, and religious medals, to holy books such as the Bible, Koran, and Torah. You must be careful to handle all items having religious significance with respect and to protect them from damage or loss.

Residents may wish to talk to you about their beliefs or may need help in carrying out certain practices or rituals. Be open to discussions with

**FIGURE 13-6** Some common belief systems (religious)

| Religion | Belief in a Diety | Value of Prayer | Belief in Hereafter | Special Practices or Symbols |
|---|---|---|---|---|
| Protestant | Yes | Important | Yes | Baptism, Holy Communion, Cross, Bible |
| Roman Catholic | Yes | Important | Yes | Baptism, Holy Communion, Eucharist, Anointing the sick, Reconciliation, Bible, Medals, Pictures of Saints, Rosaries, Crucifix, Statues of Saints |
| Orthodox Judaism | Yes | Important | Yes | Torah, yarmulka (cap), tallith, menorah |
| Hinduism | Yes (many forms) | Important | Yes | No sacraments |
| Buddhism | Yes | Important | Yes | No sacraments |
| Moslems (Islam) | Yes | Important | Yes | Koran prayer rug |

Within the framework of each belief system there are individual differences in the depth of belief and extent of practice.

the resident even if you do not share the same beliefs. The nursing assistant supports the resident's spirituality and religious practices by:

- Being a willing listener
- Respecting the resident's belief system
- Never trying to convert the resident to your belief system
- Respecting religious symbols
- Not interrupting during religious rituals
- Reading aloud resident's favorite passages from religious books such as the Bible, Talmud, Koran, or Book of Mormon, for example
- Providing privacy during prayers and meditation and when clergy visits

## SEXUALITY

Sexuality is a lifelong characteristic that defines the maleness or femaleness of each person. This definition may be different for each person. All individuals are sexual beings.

Being old or disabled does not decrease human sexuality. However, our society tends to define sexuality as youth, beauty, and physical agility. Applying this definition, older people would not be considered sexual beings.

The human person within the aging body does not change. Although the hair is gray, the skin is wrinkled, and the body not so agile, the person inside still has the basic human need to love and to be loved. When this need is not met, **self-esteem** decreases. (Self-esteem is how one feels about oneself.) With low self-esteem, human beings do not feel good about themselves.

As people age it becomes more difficult to share love. Relationships that provided love, affection, and friendship may be lost through death or geographic distance. In addition, not all people understand that older people are still interested in and capable of sexual expression and experience. Some caregivers ignore these needs or pretend they do not exist. Others feel that there is something wrong or childish about residents who want to express their sexuality.

## Sexual Expression

Sexual expression may take many forms. Sexual intercourse, genital and nongenital caressing, tender communications, **masturbation** (self-stimulation), and mental imaging (fantasizing) are examples of ways that people satisfy their sexual needs.

**Sexual Intercourse.** Sexual intercourse is desired and can be achieved by many older couples. Before sexual intercourse actually occurs, there is an excitement phase. This phase is brought about by sexual thoughts or physical caressing. Erection occurs as the tissues of the penis fill with blood and the penis becomes firm and enlarged. During this phase, the vagina becomes moist. The excitement reaches a plateau of arousal and is then followed by orgasm (climax) and a release of sexual tension.

- In the woman, the sexual sensations are centered in the vagina, uterus, rectum, and clitoris.
- In the man, they are associated with ejaculation (release of semen).

Orgasm for both men and women is a series of pleasurable muscular contractions that are strong initially and gradually slow and stop.

Men must wait a while before repeating intercourse, but women may experience another orgasm very soon if stimulated adequately.

Sexual intercourse has psychological and physical benefits because it meets sexual needs and is good physical exercise. Even those with severe physical limitations can have successful sexual experiences.

**Self-Stimulation.** Remember that masturbation is the act of stimulating oneself sexually. Many men and women find this sexual outlet satisfying. It is a common way of gaining comfort when stressed and when other sexual opportunities are not available (Figure 13-7).

You may feel uncomfortable when you notice such an activity, but you must remember that the appropriate response is to:

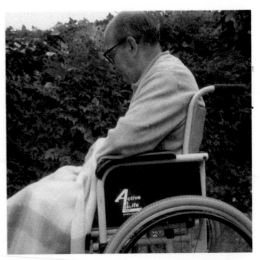

**FIGURE 13-7** Self-stimulation is one way some elderly people reduce built-up sexual tension.

- Treat the situation calmly
- Draw the curtains to provide privacy or move the resident to a more private area
- Not criticize or make fun of the resident

## Helping Residents Express Their Sexuality

Health care providers now recognize that the elderly have sexual needs and that satisfying these needs often has beneficial results. Many facilities are revising their procedures to allow couples living in the facility to express their sexuality without fear of interruption by staff or other residents. Some facilities now provide a secure area where a spouse living outside the facility can have a sexual relationship with the spouse living in the facility in privacy and without fear of embarrassment.

## Nursing Assistant Actions

Nursing assistants can help residents maintain their sexuality. First, however, you must think honestly about your own sexuality and your attitude regarding the sexuality of the elderly people in your care. These feelings may influence your actions. You can help residents if you:

1. Help them to maintain their appearance and look their best. Give sincere compliments to

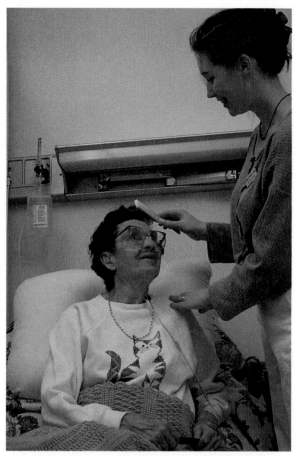

**FIGURE 13-8**   Sincere compliments assure residents that they are still worthy of respect.

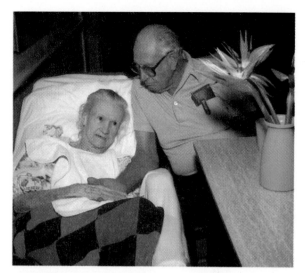

**FIGURE 13-9**   Provide privacy for residents and spouses when spouses are visiting.

residents about their appearance. This assures them of their attractiveness (Figure 13-8).

2. Use touch frequently. Touch is the only sense that does not usually diminish with aging and yet it is the sense most likely to be neglected and deprived. Remember, however, to use touch according to the cultural preferences of the resident. Some cultures consider the casual touch of a nonfamily member as rudeness or as an improper sexual advance.
3. Support friendships among residents. Treat all relationships with dignity and respect.
4. Residents who are mentally competent have the right to do in private whatever is pleasing to them both unless there are medical reasons to prevent it.
5. Always knock before entering a room. If you accidentally interrupt sexual activity, leave the room and quietly shut the door.

6. Provide privacy for residents and visiting mates. They have a need to talk and to hold each other (Figure 13-9). Some couples may wish to continue a sexual relationship.
7. Provide privacy for a resident who is masturbating.
8. Protect the rights of residents who do not want to be a partner in sexual activity.

The health care staff is responsible for protecting residents who are mentally incompetent or physically unable to protect themselves from sexual advances. Care providers, visitors, and other residents cannot be allowed to sexually abuse residents. Report any observations of potential sexual abuse to your supervisor immediately.

## MAJOR CHALLENGES TO ADJUSTMENTS

Each phase of life brings with it challenges to be met and adjustments to be made. The challenges that develop personality often come as the result of a major life crisis. Three crises older people are likely to experience are:

• Loss of a loved one (spouse or companion)
• Living with illness and disability
• Loss of independence

For many people, these events occur in close succession, and the stress can be overwhelming.

## Loss of a Loved One

A person who loses a loved one faces major psychological adjustments. This is a time of great uncertainty at any age. It is particularly difficult when one is old, with failing health and limited resources. Many important decisions about the future must be made at a time when loneliness, confusion, and grief are at a peak.

When a spouse dies, the surviving spouse may sense a loss of identity or place in social situations. If able, he or she will eventually adjust to a new life alone. Although family and friends can help in the process, it is the individual who must face the loss and make the adjustment.

Sometimes a pet is a beloved member of the family to an elderly person. The loss of the pet through death can also require major psychological adjustments similar to those experienced when a human family member dies. Most facilities do not allow personal pets. The person who leaves a pet behind to enter a long-term care facility also feels a great sense of loss as well as guilt about leaving the pet. The separation is painful for the resident.

Having someone to confide in can help the elderly person work through the grief and adjustment period. The nursing assistant who has good **rapport** (sympathetic and understanding relationship) with the resident can help fill this role (Figure 13-10).

Giving the resident the opportunity to talk about lost loved ones helps to put feelings and memories into a proper perspective. Working through feelings gives the resident a sense of strength and better understanding of himself.

## Chronic Illness

Many older people must adjust to the changes caused by aging and the problems associated with a chronic illness.

Some people try to deny these changes. They become angry when they realize they cannot control the changes going on in their bodies. Over time, most people adjust to and accept their limitations. Eventually they accept that life does not go on forever and that death is inevitable.

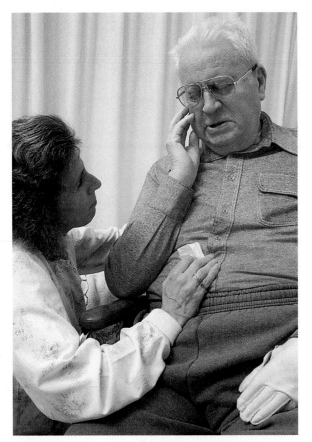

**FIGURE 13-10** The nursing assistant can help residents work through a period of grieving.

## Loss of Independence

The third crisis involves the loss of independence that comes with the move to a long-term care facility. Dependency is natural for a child but not for a mature adult. The emotional distress before admission is high. Making the decision to enter a long-term care facility is never easy for the family or the person involved. It may require separation from loved ones, personal possessions, and pets. A person's sense of independence is threatened just by knowing that this type of care and support is necessary.

The anxiety and stress levels may be even higher once the person is admitted to the facility. New surroundings, new people, a room shared with another resident, and new procedures and rules now define the resident's world. Feelings of fear and frustration grow as the resident comes to know the degree to which independence is

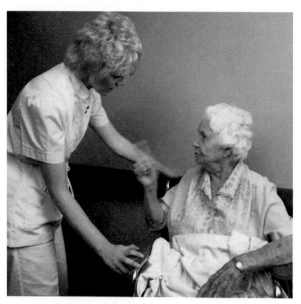

**FIGURE 13-11**   Residents may become frustrated with the changes occurring in their lives.

sacrificed (Figure 13-11). The calm manner, caring attitude, and patience of the nursing assistant are vital factors in helping the new resident adjust to life in the facility.

## USING DEFENSE (COPING) MECHANISMS

Making positive psychological adjustments in later life depends to a large extent on how well the developmental tasks of earlier life periods were mastered and how the personality was formed. The ways of adjusting that a person used successfully through life become part of the person's **defense** (or coping) **mechanisms**.

Residents will react to situations using defense mechanisms that worked for them in the past. Residents may use defense mechanisms to protect their self-esteem. The use of defense mechanisms is harmful only when they become the major way of dealing with stressful situations. If this occurs, a mental health professional may counsel the resident. Here are some definitions for common defense mechanisms:

1. **Suppression:** refusing to recognize a painful thought, memory, feeling, or impulse.

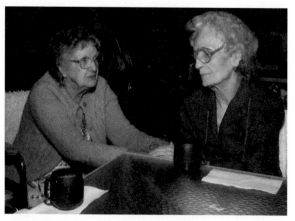

**FIGURE 13-12**   Treat relationships between residents with respect.

A person who has been abused, for example, may refuse to admit the memory of the abuse.
2. **Projection:** attributing one's own unacceptable feelings, thoughts, and actions to others. For example, a resident may tell you the bed is wet because you did not bring the bedpan on time. The resident is blaming you rather than admitting that she is incontinent.
3. **Denial:** pretending that a problem does not exist. For example, a resident is in denial when he or she talks about going home but there is little realistic chance that this will occur. This is different from similar expressions in dementia.
4. **Rationalization:** giving false but believable reasons for a situation. A resident may be rationalizing when he or she tells you that he or she must stay in bed all day because there was too much noise to sleep the night before.
5. **Compensation:** making up for a situation in some other way. A woman who received much satisfaction from caring for a husband and children may compensate for this loss by caring for and protecting other residents (Figure 13-12).

## MEETING RESIDENTS' PSYCHOSOCIAL NEEDS

It is important to see each resident as a whole person. The psychological needs of each resident must be recognized and met. Unmet psychological needs have a great effect on physical needs and status. For example, if psychological needs go unmet, the resident may become depressed and refuse to cooperate in therapy. Such a refusal may start a physical and emotional decline that rules out any chance of the resident returning home and could lead to death.

Nursing assistants can do much to help the residents meet their needs. If the residents' rights are respected at all times, you will be helping the residents to fulfill their psychosocial needs.

1. Remember that emotional needs cannot be fulfilled unless the residents' physical and safety needs are first met.
2. New residents must adjust to living in the long-term care facility. Help them to:
   * Develop trust in staff members
   * Meet other residents
   * Adapt to the routine of the facility
   * Adjust to having less personal space. You must respect the space that is theirs
   * Adjust to the loss of a home and many personal belongings
   * Use their own personal possessions, such as clothing or books
   * Display family photos and mementos
   * Find activities that have meaning and contribute to the resident's sense of self-worth
3. Always give residents the opportunity to be as independent as possible. Allow choices whenever possible.
4. Attend to the residents' comfort. Report complaints of pain or signs of anxiety immediately.
5. Explain procedures and routines to residents; notify your supervisor if the resident does not understand procedures and routines.
6. Listen carefully to everything residents say.
7. Recognize that each resident is an individual with likes and dislikes.
8. Answer signal lights promptly.
9. Treat all residents as adults.
10. Help residents feel loved and accepted by:
    * Accepting each resident in a nonjudgmental manner
    * Using touch appropriately to indicate your acceptance of the person

11. Help residents feel positive self-esteem and respect from others by:
    * Calling them by the names/titles of their choice
    * Learning about them, their families, and their histories
12. Unless they choose not to, residents should have the opportunity to contribute to facility life. These activities must be voluntary and written into the care plan so no violation of the resident's rights occurs. Activities may include:
    * Visiting other residents who may have no family and few visitors
    * Sharing their knowledge of a hobby with other residents
    * Working on the facility newsletter
    * Creating items for a facility craft sale
    * Delivering mail to other residents
    * Stuffing envelopes for mailings
    * Caring for nursing home pets such as birds or fish
    * Serving on the Residents' Council
    * Playing the piano or leading singing groups
    * Leading current events groups

## STRESS REACTIONS

When defense mechanisms are inadequate, stress reactions develop and can take several forms. Examples are:

* Chronic complaining without reason
* Agitation
* Restlessness
* Sleeplessness
* Depression
* Withdrawal

Some residents may just give up and begin to **deteriorate** physically and mentally. This means their condition weakens. Others may become combative in an attempt to assert themselves.

## REACTIVE BEHAVIORS

Residents display reactive behaviors when they are not able to meet their psychosocial needs.

They are frustrated by their lack of control and use these behaviors in an attempt to satisfy the unfulfilled needs and to ease anxieties. Some reactive behaviors include:

- Demanding behavior—expressing excessive wants or needs
- Manipulative behavior—directing the actions of others for one's own purposes
- Maladaptive behavior—abnormal responses

### Demanding Behavior

Demanding behavior occurs when residents make unreasonable requests for service, special meals, or special treatment. For example, a resident may ask to be repositioned every 10 to 15 minutes.

Try to learn and appreciate the factors that are causing the behavior. Demands and complaints are often due to the residents' feelings about their loss of control over their lives. Give the residents as much personal control as possible and offer choices.

Listen to the resident and be sensitive to body language. The resident may feel more secure if caregiving is consistent, with all staff members completing procedures in a consistent manner. Try to talk with the resident at times other than when care is needed. Do not take the resident's behavior personally.

### Manipulative Behavior

Residents who develop devious methods to get staff members to do what residents want them to do are using **manipulative behavior**.

Residents may become manipulative in an attempt to control their lives. They may try to develop a special relationship with you. If the resident with manipulative behavior compliments you, accept the compliment graciously and in a matter-of-fact manner. Do not allow the compliments to influence your judgment or cause you to show favoritism to the resident. The resident with manipulative behavior may voice criticisms of other staff members to you. Avoid agreeing with critical comments. If the resident persists in the comments, tactfully tell the resident to talk to the nurse or social worker about the problems.

Do not falsely label a resident as manipulative. Compliments may be sincere and the resident may have real problems with another staff member. Relay concerns to the nurse if the behavior becomes a pattern.

All staff members should treat the resident in a consistent manner. Develop a sense of trust with the resident. Do not make promises you cannot keep; respond to requests promptly.

### Maladaptive Behaviors

Maladaptive behaviors are abnormal behaviors. These behaviors may be noted when a resident is unable to function smoothly with staff, other residents, and perhaps family. Depression and disorientation are examples of maladaptive behaviors. These situations require assessment and planning by members of the interdisciplinary team. Interventions by a mental health professional or psychiatrist are often necessary. However, you can also help residents with maladaptive behaviors.

**Depression.**   Depression is a serious condition that requires professional treatment. If you are caring for any residents who are suffering from depression:

1. Stress the resident's worth and assist him or her in using available support systems.
2. Do not pity the resident. This validates depressed feelings.
3. Make sure the resident has eyeglasses and hearing aids if these are needed. Residents who cannot see or hear well may not interact successfully with others. This often causes the resident to withdraw.
4. Provide the resident with activities that help him think beyond himself.
5. Avoid tiring activities.
6. Use simple language and speak slowly.
7. Encourage and assist the resident to participate in activities involving physical exercise.
8. Monitor intake, elimination, and sleep patterns. Depression may cause major changes in these functions.
9. Monitor skin condition. Depression often results in less movement, increasing the risk for skin breakdown.

Be alert for the potential for suicide. Watch for and report:

1. A change in response or mood
2. Withdrawal or secretiveness
3. Sudden loss of a support system

4. Refusal of medications, food, fluids, or nursing care
5. Sudden interest or disinterest in religion
6. Attempts to obtain scissors, knives, or other dangerous objects
7. Statements about "ending it all," "killing myself," or "nothing to live for"
8. An inability to complete simple tasks without a physical reason

9. Deep preoccupation with something that they cannot explain

**Disorientation.** Residents who are disoriented do not know one or all of the following:

- The time of day, day of the week, month, year
- Where they are: facility, city, state
- Who they are

This is discussed in more detail in Lesson 29.

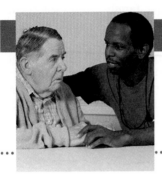

## LESSON SYNTHESIS: Putting It All Together

*Y*ou have just completed this lesson. Now go back and review the Clinical Focus. Try to see how the Clinical Focus relates to the concepts presented in this lesson. Then answer the following questions.

1. What factors make it more difficult for the resident in long-term care to meet sexual and psychological needs?

2. How does the attitude of the staff help or hinder the expression and satisfaction of psychosocial needs of residents?

3. What ways do residents have to indicate that their needs are not being met? Do they always act directly?

4. What losses do you think Mr. Warner has suffered that have contributed to his level of stress? Are these stresses common to many older residents in long-term care?

## REVIEW

**A. Fill in the blanks by selecting the correct word from the list.**

deterioration     self-esteem
personality     sexuality
masturbation

1. The sum of the ways we react to the events in our lives: _____

2. A lifelong characteristic that describes the maleness or femaleness of a person:

   _____

3. Gradual weakening of physical and mental abilities: _____

4. Feelings about oneself: _____

5. Self-stimulation for sexual pleasure:

   _____

**B. Select the one best answer for each of the following.**

6. A resident who uses her call bell repeatedly even though she frequently does not require immediate attention is showing
   a. loss of independence
   b. manipulative behavior
   c. demanding behavior
   d. depression

7. When caring for a resident who is depressed the nursing assistant should
   a. show pity
   b. engage the resident in many activities to produce fatigue so the resident will sleep
   c. stress the resident's problems so he understands you care
   d. use simple language and speak slowly

8. According to Maslow, which human needs must be met first?
   a. psychological needs
   b. social needs
   c. security needs
   d. physical needs

9. Helping the residents maintain a lifestyle structured to their choices helps meet the residents'
   a. psychological needs
   b. social needs
   c. security needs
   d. physical needs

10. A nursing assistant helps residents meet psychological needs by
    a. selecting the residents' clothing
    b. making sure the door is always open during care
    c. protecting residents' possessions from theft
    d. calling residents by a name of their choice

11. Which of the following is a physical need?
    a. to be treated with kindness
    b. to be loved
    c. elimination
    d. to feel needed

12. People of the same culture tend to
    a. look alike
    b. have the same life experiences
    c. share similar values and customs
    d. share the same faith

13. Spirituality
    a. is an organized system of beliefs
    b. gives an individual a sense of wholeness
    c. is a type of religion
    d. is present at birth

14. The nursing assistant can promote self-esteem in a resident by
    a. being respectful and touching the resident as little as possible
    b. ignoring what the resident says because the elderly tend to ramble
    c. giving sincere compliments
    d. insisting that residents contribute by serving on the Residents' Council

15. A resident is withdrawn and secretive and has suddenly shown an interest in religion. You report this to the nurse because you suspect the resident is
    a. manipulative
    b. demanding
    c. angry
    d. depressed

C. **Answer each statement true (T) or false (F).**

16. T   F   At each stage of human development, the individual has certain tasks to complete.

17. T   F   Cultural values affect the residents' response to illness.

18. T   F   People lose interest in sexual activity as they become older.

19. T   F   When a spouse dies, the surviving spouse may feel a loss of identity.

20. T   F   If a resident is depressed, it is important to provide him with activities that help him think beyond himself.

D. **Match each defense mechanism (items a.–d.) with the correct example.**

a. projection          c. compensation
b. denial              d. rationalization

21. _____   Mr. Brooks spills a glass of water and explains that it happened because the glass was too close to the edge of the overbed table.

22. _____   Miss Alcott wants to stay in her room because, she says, the other residents do not like her.

23. _____ Mrs. Jones spends most of her time out of bed helping other residents, even when they do not want or need the help.

24. _____ When the nursing assistant tries to talk to Miss Anderson about her incontinence (she had wet the bed the night before), Miss Anderson says, in a tone of injured innocence, "Why, I don't know what on earth you are talking about!"

25. _____ Mr. Ramirez tells everyone how much his family loves him and that they would visit him more often if they lived closer. You know that his family lives in the same town as the facility and that they have transportation.

## E. Clinical Situation

Mr. Williams is 85 and confined to a wheelchair. He has been a resident in your facility for years. He came to the facility after his wife of 50 years died. He never tires of describing how happy they were. Recently the staff has noticed that he has occasionally been masturbating alone in his room. Answer the following questions by circling yes (Y) or no (N).

26. Y  N   Are Mr. Williams' actions abnormal for a man his age?

27. Y  N   Should the staff try to stop his actions?

28. Y  N   Do you think Mr. Williams is trying to meet a basic human need?

29. Y  N   If Mr. Williams acted this way in front of others, would you leave him in their presence?

30. Y  N   Will masturbating cause Mr. Williams harm?

# The Physical Effects of Aging

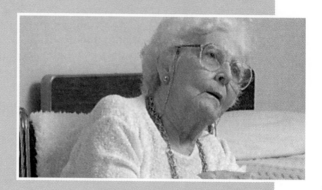

## CLINICAL FOCUS

Think about how the natural aging process affects the residents in your care as you study this lesson and meet:

Vera Clemmons, who is 91. She is forgetful and has a tendency to ramble, yet she can hold a sensible conversation. She enjoys watching television game shows and competing with the contestants. She has diabetes, has suffered at least two episodes of transient cerebral ischemia, and has fallen. A broken hip 5 years ago makes ambulation difficult and she uses a wheelchair for transportation. She often complains of vaginal itching. Her urine output is diminished. When she stands, her vertebral column is flexed. She takes great pride in her beautiful white hair; she keeps her glasses polished and carefully close at hand when not on. Her major complaint is that she just wishes that "they could make the food taste like my mother did."

## OBJECTIVES

*After studying this lesson, you should be able to:*

- Define and spell vocabulary words and terms.
- Describe current theories of aging.
- Identify four expected physical changes that occur in normal aging.

- List five common functional changes that occur in the aging process.
- Describe three considerations required for giving care related to the physical and functional changes of aging.

## VOCABULARY

**functional changes** (*FUNK-shun-al CHAYN-jez*)

**senescent changes** (*seh-NES-ent CHAYN-jez*)

# THE PROCESS OF NORMAL AGING

Aging is a process that begins before birth and continues until death. People age at different rates. During the life span, a unique person of value emerges. As people age, they deserve respect, support, and care. The elderly continue to make valuable contributions to society. They:

- Assist younger family members
- Volunteer many hours of service to the community
- Serve as role models and share life experiences

There are over 31 million people 65 years or older in this country—12.5% of the U.S. population. The number will continue to rise as the "baby boom" generation of Americans reaches retirement age. It is estimated that by 2030 over 21% of the U.S. population will be 65 years and older. Of this group, about 10% to 15% will be physically challenged by health problems. The number of Americans this age is 10 times larger than it was in 1900.

Most elderly people are able to remain independent. They live in their own homes or in homes they share with others. Only 5% of the elderly require long-term nursing care. Some may require temporary care in a nursing facility while they recover from surgery or an acute illness. Then they return to their own homes.

People over the age of 65 are called older adults. There are subgroupings within the older adult group. Some commonly used terms for these subgroups are:

- Mature stage—people between 65 and 75 years
- Old-old—people between 75 and 85 years
- Frail elderly—people over 85 years (this group has the fastest rate of growth)

# THEORIES OF AGING

No one fully understands the complex series of changes that occur in aging. Several theories (ideas) about the aging process are being investigated:

1. The rate of aging is inherited and is "built into" our personal genetic code. Thus, if a person's parents and grandparents lived many years, then the person can expect an equally long life.
2. Cells of the body are programmed to reproduce a specific number of times. Toward the end of the cycle the reproductions become less perfect and the cells are less functional.
3. As people age, the body produces smaller amounts of the chemicals that control body activities. This means that fewer protective substances are available and there is greater susceptibility to disease.
4. There is a close relationship between a person's mental and emotional health and the rate of aging.

# ABOUT AGING

Some general conclusions about aging can be stated.

- Aging is progressive and universal.
- No diseases are specific to aging.
- Aging and disease are not the same thing.
- As people age, not all functional changes are related to disease. Interest, personal and financial resources, family structure, genetics, attitude, and life-style all play a part. Elements of life-style that contribute to the aging process include smoking, misuse of chemicals such as alcohol or drugs, type of diet, and exercise.
- A wider range of what is considered "normal" function exists among older people than among younger people. A greater variability occurs among older people in their physical abilities, sizes, and characteristics compared to younger groups.
- All older adults are not alike. People in their sixties, seventies, eighties, and nineties are all different.

# CHANGES CAUSED BY AGING

Normal aging changes are called **senescent changes**. These changes occur in every body system, but not at any specific time or at any specific rate (Figure 14-1). Some changes are more obvious than others. Aging is both a physical and psychological process. One person may feel and act old at 60, and another may be spry at 80. Both

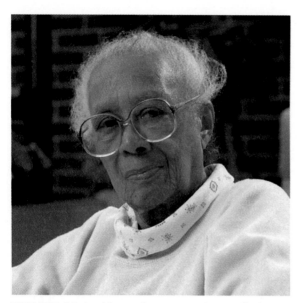

**FIGURE 14-1**   Note the many signs of aging.

will usually show some physical evidence of their ages. In general, with increasing age:

- The body's systems become less effective.
- This results in **functional changes**; that is, the ability to carry out activities of daily living decreases.
- The risk of acquiring a disease and disability increases.

Most older adults have at least one chronic health condition and many have several. Some of the most common conditions are

- Arthritis
- Hypertension
- Heart disease
- Hearing impairments
- Vision impairment

Normal aging changes are listed in Figure 14-2. Some of these changes are usually seen in all older adults. For example, hair begins to turn gray, the skin becomes dry, wrinkles develop, and posture changes.

## Functional Changes

Functional changes may occur as people age. Consider these changes as you care for your residents.

1. Changes in the muscles and joints result in slower movements and decreased flexibility.

| **FIGURE 14-2**   Senescent changes | |
|---|---|
| **Body System** | **Physical Changes of Aging** |
| Integumentary | • Hair loses color and becomes thinner<br>• Skin dries, is less elastic, and wrinkles develop<br>• Skin is fragile and tears easily<br>• Bruises easily (senile purpura common)<br>• Fingernails and toenails thicken<br>• Sweat glands do not excrete perspiration as readily<br>• Oil glands do not secrete as much oil<br>• There is increased sensitivity to cold<br>• Skin discolorations (age spots) become more common |
| Nervous | • Problems with balance<br>• Temperature regulation is less effective<br>• Sensation of pain decreases<br>• Deep sleep is shortened, more awakenings during the night<br>• Brain cells are lost but intelligence remains intact unless disease is present<br>• Decreased sensitivity of nerve receptors in skin (heat, cold, pain, pressure) |

*(continues)*

**FIGURE 14-2** *(continued)*

| Body System | Physical Changes of Aging | Body System | Physical Changes of Aging |
|---|---|---|---|
| Senses | • More difficult to see close objects<br>• Night vision may decrease<br>• Cataracts (clouding of the lens of the eye) are more common<br>• Side vision and depth perception diminish<br>• Hearing diminishes in most elderly persons<br>• Smell receptors and taste buds are less sensitive so foods have less taste | Digestive | • Primary taste sensations of salt, sweet, and sour decrease<br>• Constipation increases<br>• Flatulence increases<br>• Movement of food through the digestive system slows |
| Musculoskeletal | • Less muscle strength<br>• Less flexibility<br>• Slower movements<br>• Arthritis and osteoporosis common<br>• Body becomes more stooped | Cardiovascular | • Blood vessels less elastic, more narrowed<br>• Heart may not pump as efficiently leading to decreased cardiac output and circulation |
| Respiratory | • Breathing capacity lessens | Endocrine | • Decrease in levels of estrogen, progesterone<br>• Hot flashes, nervous feelings<br>• Higher levels of parathormone and thyroid-stimulating hormone<br>• Weight gain<br>• Insulin production less efficient<br>• Diabetes mellitus |
| Urinary | • Kidneys decrease in size<br>• Urine production is less efficient<br>• Emptying bladder completely may become more difficult<br>• Stress incontinence may develop | Reproductive | *Females:*<br>• Ovulation and menstrual cycle cease<br>• Vaginal walls are thinner and drier<br>*Males:*<br>• Scrotum less firm<br>• Prostate gland may enlarge |

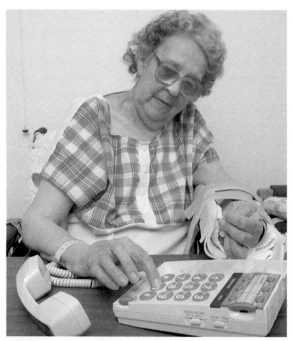

**FIGURE 14-3**   The large numbers on the telephone help the resident remain independent.

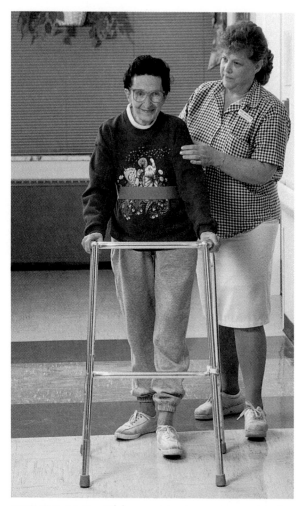

**FIGURE 14-4**   Older residents may need help to remain physically active. The walker provides support and stability, giving the resident more confidence in walking.

Residents will take longer to accomplish an activity. Less flexible fingers mean that residents may need help to open and close things, to write, to dial a telephone (Figure 14-3) and to button clothing.

2. Residents have a greater risk of falling because of loss of balance when walking or moving from a sitting to a standing position. Encourage residents to use handrails and to move carefully, without haste. Exercise helps to decrease the loss in flexibility and increase bone density. Be sure that residents have the necessary aids to help them keep their mobility (Figure 14-4).

3. Changes in the urinary system may make it more difficult to empty the bladder completely. This puts the older adult at risk for bladder infections. Providing adequate fluids is important in preventing such infections. Older adults generally have to go to the bathroom more often than younger people. Provide privacy and help the residents assume a comfortable position when you help them to the toilet.

4. Changes in the intestinal tract lead to loss of muscle tone and slower peristalsis, resulting in constipation. Flatulence is more common.

Provide the residents with adequate fluids and food. Help them to remain physically active.

5. Visual changes mean that most older adults need to wear glasses for reading. Make sure glasses are clean and readily available. Evening hours can be hazardous because of poor lighting and shadows. Position lights for maximum illumination. Do not turn corridor lights lower in evening hours. Older adults may also be more sensitive to glare so lights should not be shining directly into their eyes. Use indirect lighting whenever possible.

6. Hearing loss is common as people age. They may not respond as quickly because they do

not hear you. They may act irritated when they hear only part of a conversation or instruction. Be patient and repeat the message using only the essential words.

7. The senses of taste and smell influence one another. Loss of appetite may occur when the ability to taste and smell decreases. Taste buds lose their sensitivity, especially for salt and sugar. As a result, older adults may use more sugar and salt in an attempt to add more flavor to foods.

8. Changes in the cardiovascular system mean the elderly may tire more easily with exertion. As a result, they require more time to complete an activity. More time for resting between activities may be needed. Circulation may be impaired. Residents should be cautioned to sit with the legs uncrossed and to change positions slowly to avoid postural hypotension.

9. The sex drive in men and women may last throughout life. However, decreased estrogen production in women means there is less vaginal moisture. This may make sexual intercourse uncomfortable or painful. Men may need more time to attain an erection during sexual activity. More time may also be needed for ejaculation to occur.

The changes described here occur slowly, over many years. Because they take place so gradually, people compensate for many of these changes; that is, they learn to deal effectively with the changes.

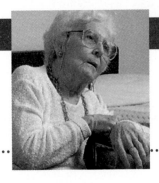

## LESSON SYNTHESIS: Putting It All Together

*Y*ou have just completed this lesson. Now go back and review the Clinical Focus. Try to see how the Clinical Focus relates to the concepts presented in the lesson. Then answer the following questions.

1. The description and picture of Vera Clemmons present what signs of aging?

2. Would you say the changes that she is experiencing are caused by aging or disease?

3. How do changes caused by aging or disease, or a combination, alter the older person's chances for injury and trauma?

4. How might Vera Clemmons be described in a particular age group?

5. Does society still view Vera Clemmons as having value?

## REVIEW

**A. Fill in the blanks by selecting the correct word or phrase.**

frail elderly          senescent
functional             theory

1. One _____ of aging is that it is due to an inherited factor.

2. _____ changes cause organs to become less able to do their job.

3. Aging changes are also known as _____ changes.

4. People who are over 85 years are sometimes called the _____.

**B.** **Answer each statement true (T) or false (F).**

As people age:

5. T   F   The female menstrual cycle ceases.

6. T   F   The male prostate gland tends to shrink.

7. T   F   The blood vessels relax and widen.

8. T   F   Insulin production becomes less efficient.

9. T   F   Night vision is more difficult.

10. T   F   Hair loses color.

11. T   F   Oil glands produce more oil.

12. T   F   Heat sensitivity decreases.

13. T   F   The body becomes more erect.

14. T   F   Breathing capacity decreases.

**C.** **Select the one best answer for each of the following.**

15. The elderly are at greater risk for falls because
    a. they tend to be constipated
    b. of decreased flexibility
    c. of decreased appetite
    d. of increased sensitivity to cold

16. The elderly are more likely to suffer skin injuries because
    a. fingernails grow longer
    b. wrinkles develop
    c. the skin becomes drier and more fragile
    d. fluid intake is inadequate

17. Changes in the urinary system mean the elderly need to
    a. void more often
    b. empty the bladder less often
    c. limit liquid intake
    d. eat more fiber

18. Changes in the cardiovascular system mean that when you care for the older adult, you should remember to
    a. encourage vigorous exercise
    b. allow more rest time between activities
    c. have residents breathe deeply before exercise
    d. continue exercise even if fatigue develops

19. Older adults may add more sugar and salt to their food than younger people because
    a. the food served has no flavor
    b. they are fussy eaters
    c. taste buds are less sensitive
    d. they cannot see as well

**D.** **Complete each statement.**

20. Name three chronic conditions commonly seen in older adults.

21. State three theories of aging.

22. In the next 30 years what is expected to happen to the population of older adults?

# SECTION
# 5

# Meeting the Residents' Basic Needs

## LESSONS

**15** Care of the Residents' Environment

**16** Caring for the Residents' Personal Hygiene

**17** Meeting the Residents' Nutritional Needs

**18** Meeting the Residents' Elimination Needs

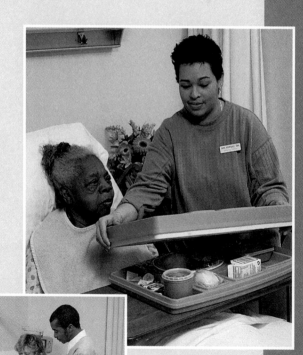

# LESSON
# *15*

# Care of the Residents' Environment

**CLINICAL FOCUS**

Think about how controlling the environment for the resident contributes to the resident's sense of well-being and comfort as you study this lesson and meet:

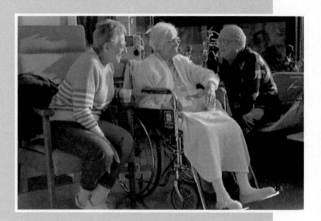

*E*dith Curry, a resident who is 96 and constantly complains of feeling cold. She has congestive heart failure and non–insulin-dependent diabetes mellitus. She also suffers from chronic respiratory infections. She shares a room with two other residents whose grandchildren visit and the noise bothers her. She reads but requires extra lighting. She becomes disoriented during the early evening hours. When out of bed in a wheelchair, she enjoys watching television. On warm days, she likes to sit on the sheltered and enclosed patio.

## OBJECTIVES

*After studying this lesson, you should be able to:*

- Define and spell vocabulary words and terms.
- State three components of the resident's environment.
- Name four ways in which a safe, comfortable, and pleasant environment can be maintained for the resident.

- Describe two actions to be taken at the beginning and end of each resident care procedure.
- Demonstrate the following:
  Procedure 18 Unoccupied Bed: Changing Linens
  Procedure 19 Occupied Bed: Changing Linens

# VOCABULARY

draw sheet    *(draw sheet)*

environment    *(en-**VIRE**-on-ment)*

mitered corner    *(**MY**-terd **KOR**-ner)*

occupied bedmaking    *(**OCK**-you-pyed **BED**-may-king)*

procedure    *(proh-**SEE**-zhur)*

square corner    *(skwair **KOR**-ner)*

unoccupied bedmaking    *(un-**OCK**-you-pyed **BED**-may-king)*

## RESIDENT ENVIRONMENT

The resident's **environment** is the surroundings in which the resident now lives. Anything that is part of the environment affects the resident's sense of comfort, happiness, and security. The environment includes:

- Physical surroundings
- People who interact with the resident
- Quality of care given
- General atmosphere of the facility and staff

Nursing assistants have a responsibility for maintaining a safe, clean, and pleasant environment for the residents (Figure 15-1).

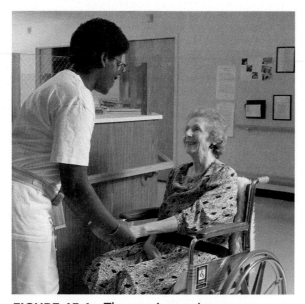

**FIGURE 15-1** The nursing assistant contributes greatly to the friendly and comfortable environment that creates a pleasant atmosphere.

The resident's sense of well-being is a reflection of how the resident believes he or she is being treated. Residents respond positively when they are treated with respect, are viewed as persons with value, exercise some control over their lives, and experience some personal independence. Negative feelings result when residents feel neglected, unimportant, unworthy, and powerless. A warm and friendly atmosphere promotes the well-being of both residents and health care providers.

## PERSONAL SPACE

Personal space is the area immediately around a person's body. The boundaries of personal space are viewed differently by different cultures and by individuals within a culture. For example, people of some Asian cultures stand very close to each other when speaking. People of other cultures are uncomfortable and feel threatened if someone stands too close. Eye contact is another factor that defines personal space. Some cultures, such as some Native American groups, view eye contact as rude and a personal space violation (Figure 15-2).

For a resident in a long-term care facility, personal space is often extended to include personal articles and the room in which the resident lives. You can show respect for a resident's personal space by:

- Making sure a resident's personal articles are not placed in another resident's area when a room is shared.
- Allowing the resident to arrange personal possessions as desired as long as safety is not an issue. Do not rearrange the resident's personal possessions without permission. Residents are

**FIGURE 15-2**   Personal space is interpreted differently by people of different cultures.

| Culture | Definition of Personal Space | Eye Contact |
|---|---|---|
| American | About 3 feet | Yes |
| Asian | Close, no contact | No |
| African | Close | Yes |
| European | Distant | Yes |
| Native American | Distant | No |
| Hispanic | Close | Yes |

encouraged to keep a favorite chair or chest, as space permits. Moving these items can upset the resident. Because the residents become used to the placement of furniture in the room, moving furniture may cause accidental injury.

- Treating personal belongings with respect. Residents are encouraged to keep blankets, spreads, pillows, plants, photos, and mementos of family and their lives before their admission to the facility. These reminders help residents make the transition to living in the facility.

Note that residents are not usually allowed to keep certain items in their rooms because these items are a safety hazard. Items that are not permitted vary from state to state. Some of these items include:

- Uncovered food
- Perishable food
- Matches and lighters
- Razor
- Knife
- Medications
- Cigarettes
- Alcohol

Check the facility regulations for items residents are not allowed to keep in their rooms.

- Being sensitive to the clues the resident gives you about how the resident views personal space

- Knocking before entering the room
- Speaking before drawing back a privacy curtain
- Closing privacy curtains before carrying out procedures
- Explaining procedures and asking permission before starting the procedure
- Being patient with residents and treating each as a person of value

## RESIDENT UNIT

The resident's immediate environment is the unit or room where the resident lives. This room is often shared with another resident. The most important item in the room for the resident's comfort is the bed. Although many residents can be dressed and up for the day, some residents must remain in bed. The comfort and safety of the bed are important considerations for all residents.

### Beds

The typical bed is adjustable and can be raised in height to make giving care easier. At the end of care, the bed is lowered to make it easier and safer for residents to get into and out of the bed. The back and foot of the bed can be raised to different positions for comfort and therapeutic reasons. Beds are usually provided with adjustable side rails.

Electric control of the bed positions is used in many facilities, but some manually, crank-operated beds may still be used. If the bed has cranks to change positions, be sure they are returned to the nonuse position so that no one will be injured by hitting them. The wheels of the bed should be locked to prevent the bed from rolling. If the bed has large wheels, they should be turned inward to prevent tripping over them.

## EXTENDED RESIDENT ENVIRONMENT

All facility employees are responsible for ensuring that safety, physical comfort, and a spirit of well-being are maintained throughout the extended resident environment, which includes the:

- Dining room
- Bathing area
- Activity area
- Therapy rooms
- Lounges
- Lobby
- Dayroom

To achieve these conditions the following factors must be managed:

- Cleanliness and order
- Adequate air circulation
- Proper temperature
- Adequate lighting
- Noise control
- Odor control

## Cleanliness and Order

Dust and dirt, crumbs from food, and dirty dishes and glasses are contaminated by microbes that can contribute to the spread of disease. Food left in the residents' rooms may attract insects such as cockroaches and ants. The food can also cause unpleasant odors. Remove all dishes as soon as the resident finishes a meal or nourishment. Clean up any spills and crumbs immediately. Remember that residents are not usually allowed to store food in their rooms. Some facilities permit candy in the room if it is sealed or in a closed container.

Routine cleaning of the environment is done by housekeeping personnel. However, nursing assistants are responsible for a safe and orderly environment and are expected to keep the resident areas neat. Clutter is a safety hazard and often is disturbing to the older adult. Return all equipment to its proper place as soon as you finish using it. Move equipment carefully to avoid hitting walls and furniture.

## Adequate Air Circulation

Everyone feels refreshed when fresh, clean air is available. Most facilities have central controls to manage ventilation. Some facilities have controls in each resident room so ventilation can be controlled to meet individual needs.

Circulating air may produce drafts. Blankets, screens, and curtains are used to control the flow of air to meet the residents' comfort needs.

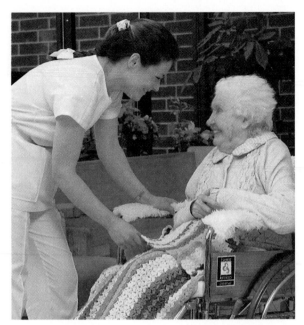

**FIGURE 15-3** A lap robe provides comfort and protects the resident's dignity if she is wearing a dress.

## Temperature Control

Older adults often prefer warmer temperatures than do younger people. The facility temperature is usually controlled at 70° to 72° Fahrenheit. A resident may use a lap robe, sweater, or shawl for comfort and to protect dignity when wearing a dress (Figure 15-3).

## Adequate Lighting

*Make sure there is adequate lighting for resident and staff safety.* This is especially important at dusk and during the night. The light level can be controlled by adjusting the overbed light, any lamps that may be in the room, and the room light (Figure 15-4). The overbed light usually has more than one level of brightness. The cord for controlling the overbed light should be within reach of the resident whenever the resident is in bed or sitting near the bed. A night light near the floor will not disturb the resident at night and is an added safety feature. Lights must be left on in the hallways and on stairways at night. Bright sunlight can be controlled using curtains and shades.

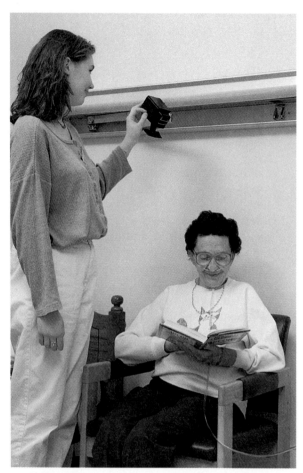

**FIGURE 15-4**  The best lighting is indirect lighting.

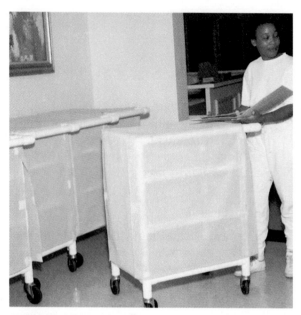

**FIGURE 15-5**  Handle equipment carefully to control noise and position according to facility policy to prevent clutter.

## Noise Control

Loud noises are disturbing to most people. Older adults are often more sensitive to noise and find a noisy environment upsetting. Noisy equipment, banging trays, loud radios or televisions, ringing telephones, squeaking wheels, and loud or excited voices all add to the noise level in the facility. Health care providers can make the environment more pleasant by controlling noise when they work (Figure 15-5). Many surveyors will write a deficiency for too much noise in the facility.

## Odor Control

Odors can be a problem in a long-term care facility unless everyone makes an effort to control them. Odors should be eliminated, not cov-

ered up. Residents who are incontinent must be cared for immediately. Soiled pads, garments, and linens must be placed in covered containers and handled according to facility policy.

Bedpans, urinals, commodes, and emesis basins should be emptied, cleaned, and disinfected immediately after use, or as dictated by facility policy. Utility rooms and dining areas must be cleaned regularly.

Nursing assistants have a major responsibility for influencing the environment in which the residents live. Each day you will care for the residents' belongings and ensure that the resident unit and other areas are safe and clean.

## CRITICAL PROCEDURE ACTIONS ·····

Caring for residents safely means you must perform tasks in a manner specified by facility policy. Such tasks are called **procedures**. As you continue your study, you will learn the procedures for many nursing assistant tasks. You have already learned several emergency care and infection control procedures, including handwashing. The procedures that follow give you

# *G*uidelines for

# Ensuring a Safe and Comfortable Environment

The nursing assistant makes important contributions to maintaining a safe and comfortable resident environment.

*Follow all infection control guidelines and use standard precautions for the care of all residents.*

### Cleanliness

1. Remove dishes immediately after use and clean up crumbs and spills.
2. Check that resident is not storing food in the room. If food is permitted, check that it is wrapped or in a closed container.
3. Clean overbed table after use; use disinfectant, if necessary.
4. If the floor is soiled with blood or body fluids, call housekeeping for immediate cleanup, or follow facility policy.
5. Pick up resident clothing and place in laundry hamper if soiled or hang in closet.
6. Each time you enter the room, check it for cleanliness and order.
7. Provide a bag for used tissues and change it often.
8. Empty wastebaskets if full and reline with a plastic bag (this is usually done by housekeeping, but a basket may become full before the scheduled change).
9. Try to keep dresser and table tops uncluttered, but remember that the resident has the right to display personal items and to expect that they will not be disturbed. Ask permission to clean around them when necessary.

### Noise

1. Exercise care in using and moving equipment to keep the noise level down.

2. Speak in a conversational tone of voice. Call out to other staff members only if the resident has had an incident, you cannot leave the resident, you cannot reach the call button, and you need assistance; otherwise, walk to another staff member to talk.
3. Keep radio and television volumes at a reasonable level on a station desired by the resident.
4. Close door to resident room, and tell resident why you are doing so, if cleaning or construction is underway in the hallway or a nearby room.

### Odor

1. Control odors by caring for incontinent residents immediately.
2. Follow facility policy for handling of clothing and bed linens soiled by feces, urine, vomitus, respiratory secretions, wound drainage, or food spills.
3. Empty bed pans, urinals, and commodes promptly. Clean and disinfect after each use or according to facility policy.

### Other Environmental Concerns

1. Be aware of residents' needs for ventilation and air circulation, temperature control, and adequate lighting; assist resident as necessary to ensure comfort.
2. Check that all equipment used by the resident is in good repair and safe to use.
3. Be sensitive to residents' wishes relating to cultural preferences and accommodate them as much as possible without violating facility policy.

step-by-step directions for performing tasks that involve personal care of residents.

Certain steps must be done before you perform the actual resident care procedure. These steps are called beginning procedure actions. When the resident care procedure is completed, another series of steps, called procedure completion actions, must be done (Figure 15-6).

| FIGURE 15-6   Beginning procedure actions and procedure completion actions | |
|---|---|
| **Beginning Procedure Actions** | **Rationale** |
| 1. Assemble equipment needed and take to resident's room. | 1. Improves the efficiency of the procedure. Means you do not have to leave the resident. |
| 2. Knock on the resident's door and identify yourself by name and title. | 2. Respects the resident's right to privacy. Notifies the resident who is giving care. |
| 3. Identify the resident by checking the identification bracelet. | 3. Ensures that you are caring for the correct resident. |
| 4. Ask visitors to leave the room and advise where they may wait. | 4. Respects the resident's right to privacy. Shows hospitality to visitors by advising them where to wait. |
| 5. Explain what you are going to do and how the resident can assist. Answer questions about the procedure. | 5. Informs the resident of what is going to be done and what is expected. Gives the resident an opportunity to get information about the procedure and the extent of resident participation. |
| 6. Provide privacy by closing the door, privacy curtain, and window curtain. | 6. Respects the resident's right to privacy. All three should be closed even if the resident is alone in the room. |
| 7. Wash your hands. | 7. Applies the principles of standard precautions. Prevents the spread of microorganisms. |
| 8. Apply gloves if contact with blood, moist body fluids, secretions, excretions, or nonintact skin is likely. | 8. Applies the principles of standard precautions. Protects the care provider and resident from transmission of pathogens. |
| 9. Apply a gown if your uniform will have substantial contact with linen or other articles contaminated with blood, moist body fluids (except sweat), secretions, or excretions. | 9. Applies the principles of standard precautions. Protects your uniform from contamination with bloodborne pathogens. |
| 10. Apply a gown, mask, and eye protection if splashing of blood or moist body fluids is likely. | 10. Applies the principles of standard precautions. Protects the care provider's mucous membranes, uniform, and skin from accidental splashing of bloodborne pathogens. |
| 11. Raise the bed to a comfortable working height. | 11. Prevents back strain and injury caused by bending at the waist. |
| 12. Lower the side rail on the side where you are working. | 12. Provides an obstacle-free area in which to work.   *(continues)* |

**FIGURE 15-6** *(continued)*

| Procedure Completion Actions | Rationale |
|---|---|
| 1. Check to make sure the resident is in good alignment. | 1. All body systems function better when the body is correctly aligned. The resident is more comfortable when the body is in good alignment. |
| 2. Remove gloves. | 2. Prevents contamination of environmental surfaces from the gloves. |
| 3. Raise the side rail. | 3. Resident's right to a safe environment. Prevents accidents and injuries. |
| 4. Remove other personal protective equipment, if worn, and discard according to facility policy. | 4. Prevents unnecessary environmental contamination from used gloves and protective equipment. |
| 5. Wash your hands. | 5. Applies the principles of standard precautions. Prevents the spread of microorganisms. |
| 6. Return the bed to the lowest horizontal position. | 6. Resident's right to a safe environment. Prevents accidents and injuries. |
| 7. Open the privacy and window curtains. | 7. Privacy is no longer necessary unless preferred by the resident. |
| 8. Leave the resident in a position of comfort and safety with the call signal and needed personal items within reach. | 8. Prevents accidents and injuries. Ensures that help is available. Eliminates the need to call or reach for needed personal items. |
| 9. Wash your hands. | 9. Although the hands were washed previously, they have contacted the resident and other items in the room. Wash them again before leaving to prevent potential transfer of microorganisms to areas outside the resident's unit. |
| 10. Inform visitors that they may return to the room. | 10. Courtesy to visitors and resident. |
| 11. Report completion of the procedure and any abnormalities or other observations. | 11. Inform the nurse that your assigned task has been completed so further resident care can be planned and you can be reassigned to other duties. Notifies the nurse of abnormalities and changes in the resident's condition for further assessment. |
| 12. Document the procedure and your observations. | 12. Ongoing progress and care given is documented. Provides a legal record. Provides a record of what has been done, for other members of the interdisciplinary team. |

# BEDMAKING ············

You will learn two basic methods of making the resident's bed:

- **Unoccupied bedmaking** (when the resident is not in the bed)—see Procedure 18
- **Occupied bedmaking** (when the resident is in the bed)—see Procedure 19

The following linens are used to make the resident's bed:

- Sheets, top and bottom (the bottom sheet may be contoured or have elastic edges to fit over the edges of the mattress)
- Pillowcases, usually two although more may be required if several pillows are used to position and support the resident in bed
- **Draw sheet** or lift sheet, a small sheet or a regular top sheet folded in half and placed sideways across the bed to cover the area between the resident's upper back and thighs
  - The sides of the draw sheet may or may not be tucked under the mattress.
  - The draw sheet can be changed frequently without changing the rest of the bed linen if the bottom sheet is not soiled.
  - The draw sheet can be used to lift the resident to change position in bed (in this case, the edges of the draw sheet would not be tucked under the mattress).
- Underpad (protective pad) may be placed on top of the bottom sheet or draw sheet to provide additional protection. Underpads may be disposable, paper-type pads with a moisture-resistant layer that are placed under the resident and changed when soiled. Other types of reusable moisture-resistant materials can also be used.
- Blanket
- Spread (when the resident is out of bed, the spread is usually placed on the bed and covers the pillows)

Bed linens that are not soiled by blood, body fluids, body secretions or excretions, or spilled food are changed according to a schedule set by the facility. All soiled linens are changed immediately.

---

## *G*uidelines for

# Handling Linens and Making the Bed

### Handling Linens

1. Wash hands and use gloves as required; other personal protective equipment may be required.
2. Laundry hampers placed in the hallway should be at least two rooms away from clean linen carts.
3. Clean linen cart is always covered; replace covers after removing required linen.
4. Take only the linens you need into the resident's room.
5. Linens that touch the floor are considered dirty and placed in the laundry hamper; they are not used.
6. Avoid contact between the linens and your uniform (for both clean and soiled linens).
7. Unused linen is never returned to the clean linen cart; it is placed in the laundry hamper.
8. As soiled linen is removed from the bed, keep the soiled areas on the inside and fold or roll the linen toward the center.
9. Never shake soiled bed linens because microbes will be released into the air.
10. Soiled linen is never placed on environmental surfaces in the room, such as overbed table, chair, or floor; soiled linens are placed in the appropriate laundry hamper (follow facility policy).
11. Fill laundry hampers no more than two-thirds full.
12. Many facilities do not permit laundry hampers or barrels to be taken into the resident's room. Soiled linen may be placed in a plastic bag or a pillowcase in the room. Make a cuff at the top of the bag or open end of the pillowcase and place the cuff

*(continues)*

## $G$uidelines *(continued)*

over the back of the chair. When the bag or case is two-thirds full, secure the top and place it in the hamper in the hallway.

13. Laundry hampers or barrels are returned to utility room after use, or as directed by facility policy.

**Making the Bed**

1. Use proper body mechanics at all times to prevent back injury.
2. Work on one side of the bed at a time to complete removing soiled linen and placing clean linen (see Procedures 18 and 19).
3. Make sure the bottom sheet and draw sheet (if used) are smooth and unwrinkled (wrinkles in bed linens can lead to skin breakdown, especially for residents who remain in bed).
4. Follow the care plan for the positioning of the head and foot of the bed, the number of pillows to be used, and the need for pillows for positioning.

---

**PROCEDURE**
**18**
# Unoccupied Bed: Changing Linens

1. Carry out the beginning procedure actions (Figures 15-6 and 15-7).

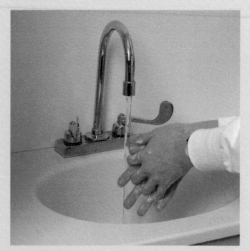

**FIGURE 15-7** Remember to start and end each procedure by washing your hands.

2. Assemble equipment:
   - Disposable gloves (if linens are soiled with blood or body fluids, secretions, or excretions)
   - Pillowcases
   - Spread
   - Blankets, as needed
   - Two large sheets (90 × 109) (substitute one fitted, if used)
   - Draw sheet, for selected residents
   - Laundry hamper (Figure 15-8)

3. Lock bed wheels so the bed will not roll and place chair at the side of the bed.
4. Raise bed to comfortable working height.
5. Arrange linens on chair in order in which they are to be used. Make a cuff at the top of a plastic bag or pillowcase. Place the cuff over the back of the chair and use the bag or case for the disposal of soiled linen.

*(continues)*

**PROCEDURE** *18* *(continued)*

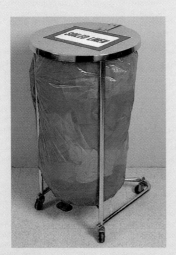

**FIGURE 15-8**  If facility policy permits, take a laundry hamper or barrel into the room with you.

6. Remove soiled linen as follows:
   a. Loosen the bedding on one side of the bed by lifting the edge of the mattress with one hand and drawing the linens out with the other.
   b. Remove the pillow from the bed. Grasp pillow with one hand. Using the other hand, gather the pillowcase and pull it back over the pillow so it is inside out. Place pillow on chair and put pillowcase in bag for soiled linen.
   c. If the spread is clean and to be reused, fold it lengthwise by bringing the far edge toward the near edge. Fold it once more from the center lengthwise. Then fold the spread from top to bottom and place it over the back of the chair.
   *Note:* If the spread is soiled, it must be handled as the sheets are handled.
   d. Gather the top sheet by folding the edges inward so that the dirtiest side is on the inside. Place sheet in bag.
   e. Gather up the draw sheet (if used) by folding the dirtiest side inward. Place draw sheet in bag.

   f. Repeat process with the bottom sheet. Before putting the linen in the hamper or pillowcase, remember to check it for items such as dentures, eyeglasses, hearing aids, equipment, supplies, syringes, and so on. Remove the items and follow facility policy for cleaning, disinfection, storage, or disposal. Mattresses have a plasticized top for protection against soiling. If the top of the mattress is wet from the linens, wipe dry using a disinfectant. Secure top of plastic bag or pillowcase and place in hamper in hallway. Remove gloves and dispose of properly, wash hands, dry, and put on fresh gloves, if required.
7. Position mattress to head of bed by grasping handles on mattress side.
8. Work from one side of the bed until that side is completed, and then go to the other side of the bed.
9. Place bottom sheet lengthwise on mattress with fold at center of bed. Be sure the smooth side (hemside) is up and the narrow hem is even with the foot of the mattress (Figure 15-9A). See Figure 15-9B if a fitted bottom sheet is used.

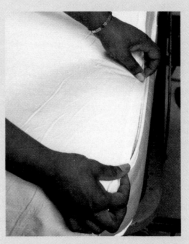

**FIGURE 15-9A**  Place flat bottom sheet even with end of mattress at foot of bed.

*(continues)*

**PROCEDURE 18** *(continued)*

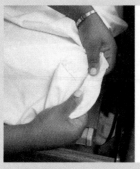
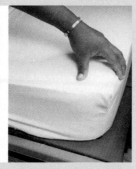

**FIGURE 15-9B** If a fitted bottom sheet is used, fit it properly and smoothly around the corner of mattress.

10. Tuck 12 to 18 inches of sheet smoothly over the top of the mattress.
11. Make a **mitered** (Figure 15-10) or **square corner**.

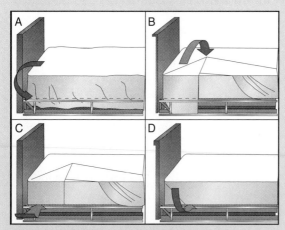

**FIGURE 15-10** Making a mitered corner A. The sheet is hanging loose at the side of the bed. B. Pick up the sheet about 12 inches from the head of the bed to form a triangle. Pull back toward the bed to smooth out the sheet and lay triangle on bed. C. Tuck in sheet at head of bed. D. Pick up triangle and place other hand at edge of bed near head to hold edge of sheet in place. Bring triangle over edge of mattress and tuck smoothly under mattress. Tuck in the rest of the sheet along the side of the mattress. Make sure sheet is smooth.

12. Tuck in the sheet on one side, keeping it straight. Work from the head to the foot of the bed. If a fitted sheet is used, adjust it over the head and bottom ends of the mattress.
13. Unfold the top sheet and place wrong side up, top hem even with the upper edge of the mattress, and center fold on the center of the bed. Tuck in sheet at the bottom of the bed, as shown in Figures 15-11A–C.

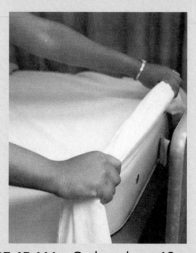

**FIGURE 15-11A** Gather about 12 to 18 inches of top sheet at bottom of bed.

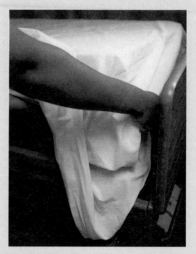

**FIGURE 15-11B** Face foot of bed and lift mattress with near hand.

*(continues)*

**PROCEDURE** *18* *(continued)*

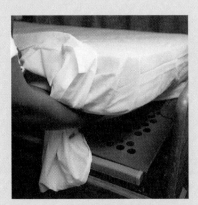

**FIGURE 15-11C** Using other hand bring sheet smoothly over end of mattress.

14. Spread blanket over the top sheet and foot of mattress. Keep blanket centered.
15. Tuck top sheet and blanket under mattress at the foot of the bed as far as the center only and make a mitered or square corner (Figure 15-12A–C).

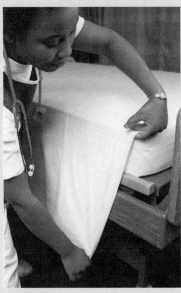

**FIGURE 15-12A** Make the square (box) corner following the steps of Figure 15-10A–C. Then, holding the corner with one hand, grasp the bottom of the sheet and pull it straight down until fold is even with the edge of the mattress.

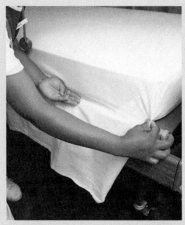

**FIGURE 15-12B** Holding the square corner in place, tuck sheet under mattress.

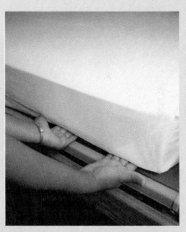

**FIGURE 15-12C** Finished square corner should look like this.

16. Place spread with top hem even with head of mattress.
17. Unfold to foot of bed.
18. Tuck spread under mattress at the foot of one side of bed (Figure 15-13) and make mitered or square corner.
19. Go to other side of bed and fanfold the top sheet, blanket, and spread to the center of the bed to work with lower sheets and pad.

*(continues)*

**PROCEDURE** *18* *(continued)*

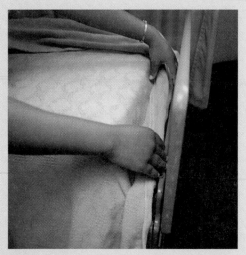

**FIGURE 15-13A** Gather top sheet and spread together and smooth evenly over end of mattress.

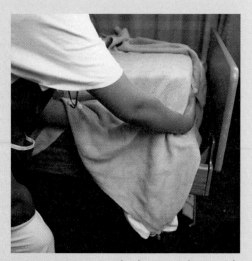

**FIGURE 15-13B** Tuck sheet and spread under mattress together.

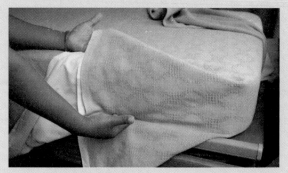

**FIGURE 15-13C** Continue as in the procedure for a mitered corner.

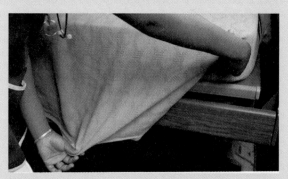

**FIGURE 15-13D** Slide finger to the end to make a smooth edge.

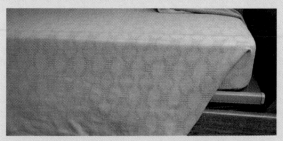

**FIGURE 15-13E** The completed top bedding. The procedure is repeated on the other side.

20. Tuck bottom sheet under head of mattress and make mitered or square corner. Working from top to bottom, smooth out all wrinkles and tighten sheet as much as possible, or adjust fitted bottom sheet smoothly and securely around mattress corners.

21. Tuck in top sheet and blanket.
22. Fold top sheet back over blanket, making an 8-inch cuff.
23. Tuck in spread at foot of bed and make a mitered or square corner.
24. Bring top of spread to head of mattress.

*(continues)*

**PROCEDURE 18** *(continued)*

25. Insert pillow in pillowcase properly. Be sure corners of pillows are in corners of pillowcases.
26. Place pillow at head of bed with open end away from the door.
27. Spread is brought up to cover pillow.
28. Lower bed to lowest horizontal position.

29. Replace bedside table parallel to bed. Place chair in assigned location. Place overbed table over the foot of the bed opposite the chair.
30. Wash hands.
31. Perform procedure completion actions.
32. Report completion of task.

**PROCEDURE 19** Occupied Bed: Changing Linens

1. Carry out each beginning procedure action.
2. Assemble equipment:
   - Disposable gloves (if linens are soiled with blood, body fluids, secretions, or excretions; gown is required if there may be contact between your uniform and soiled linens.)
   - Draw sheet, for selected residents
   - Two pillowcases
   - Two large sheets (or one large sheet and one fitted sheet)
   - Laundry hamper
3. Place bedside chair at the foot of the bed.
4. Arrange bed linen on chair in the order in which it is to be used.
5. The bed should be flat with wheels locked, unless otherwise indicated. Raise to working horizontal height.
6. If bed linens are soiled with blood or body fluids, wash hands and put on disposable gloves.
7. Loosen the linens on one side by lifting the edge of the mattress with one hand and drawing bedclothes out with the other.
8. Adjust mattress to head of bed. If resident's condition permits, have resident

bend knees, grasp side rails or headboard of bed with hands, and pull on frame as you draw mattress to the top (Figure 15-14) or have another person help from the opposite side.

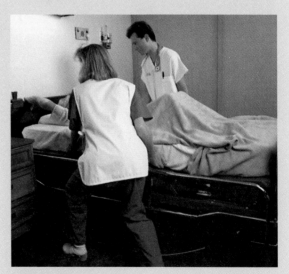

**FIGURE 15-14** The resident grasps the head of the bed and pushes in with the heels while two nursing assistants pull mattress to head of bed.

*(continues)*

## PROCEDURE *19* *(continued)*

9. Remove covers, except for top sheet, one at a time. Fold to bottom and pick up in center. Place over the back of chair.
10. Place a clean sheet over top sheet. Have the resident hold the top edge of the clean sheet, if possible. If not, tuck the sheet beneath the resident's shoulder.
11. Slide out the soiled top sheet, from top to bottom. Place in hamper.
12. Ask the resident to roll toward you and assist if necessary. Move one pillow with the resident. Pull up side rail for safety.
13. Go to the other side of the bed. Fanfold the draw sheet, if used, and the bottom sheet close to the resident (Figure 15-15).
14. Place a clean bottom sheet on the bed so that the narrow hem comes to the edge of the mattress at the foot and the length-wise center fold of the sheet is at the center of the bed.
15. Tuck top of clean bottom sheet under the head of the mattress.
16. Make a mitered or square corner. Tuck side of bottom sheet under mattress, working toward the foot of the bed.
17. Position clean draw sheet if used. Tuck it under the mattress. If used, place protective underpad on top of draw sheet.
18. Ask the resident to roll toward you and assist as needed. Move the pillow with the resident.
19. Raise side rail for safety.
20. Go to the other side of the bed. Remove soiled linen by rolling the edges inward.
21. Keep soiled linen away from your uniform, and place in hamper, plastic bag, or pillowcase.
22. Complete the bed as an unoccupied bed. Some residents prefer not to have the blanket, top sheet, or spread tucked in.
23. Turn resident on back. Place clean case on pillow. Replace pillow. If other pillows are used for positioning, change pillowcases each time bed linens are changed, or according to facility policy.
24. Remove and dispose of gloves (if used) according to facility policy. Wash hands.
25. Adjust bed position for the resident's comfort.
26. Be sure side rails are up and secure, if needed. Lower bed to lowest horizontal position.
27. Replace bedside table and chair.
28. Make sure call signal and fresh water are within reach of resident.
29. Carry out each procedure completion action.
30. Report completion of task.

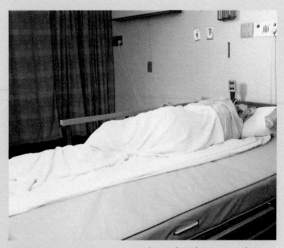

**FIGURE 15-15** Note that the bottom linen is flat and the resident is positioned on far side of the bed.

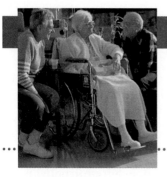

## LESSON SYNTHESIS: Putting It All Together

You have just completed this lesson. Now go back and review the Clinical Focus. Try to see how the Clinical Focus relates to the concepts presented in the lesson. Then answer the following questions.

1. What actions could you take to increase Edith Curry's comfort when the grandchildren of her roommates visit?

2. How should the environment be adjusted to increase safety during evening hours?

3. How can you help Mrs. Curry to be comfortable when she is sitting on the patio area and the sun is shining in?

4. How does a well-made bed, properly positioned, contribute to the safety and well-being of the resident?

## REVIEW

**A. Match each term (items a.–e.) with the proper definition.**

  a. side rails      d. mitered corner
  b. draw sheet     e. unoccupied bed
  c. environment

  1. _____ half-sheet

  2. _____ bed without a resident

  3. _____ sheet tucked in at a 45° angle

  4. _____ safety feature on beds that can be regarded as a restraint

  5. _____ surroundings in which the resident lives

**B. Select the one best answer for each of the following.**

6. Most facilities regulate the room temperature to approximately
  a. 60–62°
  b. 64–66°
  c. 70–72°
  d. 78–80°

7. A positive atmosphere is created when
  a. radios play loudly
  b. residents are treated with respect
  c. odors are covered up
  d. equipment is out of place

8. Which of the following is not usually permitted to be stored in the resident's room?
  a. uncovered food
  b. books
  c. radio
  d. pictures

9. To ensure privacy you should
  a. arrange resident's belongings to please yourself
  b. enter rooms without knocking
  c. close curtains around bed before carrying out procedures
  d. leave curtains open around a resident receiving care if only her roommate is present

10. Underpads
  a. are half-sheets
  b. reduce pressure
  c. can be easily changed when soiled
  d. are also called draw sheets

## C. Answer each statement true (T) or false (F).

11. T  F  Adjustable beds provide for resident comfort and therapeutic positioning.

12. T  F  Bed linens are completely changed every day even if they are not soiled.

13. T  F  A draw sheet is a half-sheet placed over the bottom sheet.

14. T  F  When making an unoccupied bed, make one side completely before going to the opposite side.

15. T  F  It is important that the bottom sheet be smooth.

16. T  F  When making a bed, linens should be arranged on a chair in the order in which they are to be used.

17. T  F  The mattress should be positioned to the top of the bed before clean linen is applied.

18. T  F  If the linen is soiled with blood, the nursing assistant should wear gloves when making the bed.

19. T  F  The occupied bed should be left in a high horizontal position with the side rails down.

20. T  F  Side rails should be checked for security when up in place.

21. T  F  If a crank is left protruding it can cause an injury.

22. T  F  Beds should be raised to a comfortable working height before linens are changed.

23. T  F  The nursing assistant is responsible for maintaining a safe and comfortable environment for the resident.

24. T  F  Side rails must be up and secured for all residents, regardless of condition.

25. T  F  When stripping soiled linen from a bed, the linens should always be gathered so the dirtiest part is inside.

# Caring for the Residents' Personal Hygiene

## CLINICAL FOCUS

Think about ways you can assist residents in meeting their personal hygiene needs as you study this lesson and meet:

*M*ary Mandell, one of your residents, who is a charming lady, full of stories about growing up on an Oklahoma cattle ranch. She is right-handed. A stroke 2 years ago left her paralyzed on the right side. She is up in a wheelchair most of the day, and a small reddened area has developed over her sacrum.

## OBJECTIVES

*After studying this lesson, you should be able to:*

- Define and spell vocabulary words and terms.
- Name the parts and functions of the integumentary system.
- Review changes in the integument due to aging.
- Describe common skin conditions affecting the long-term care resident.
- Identify factors that contribute to skin breakdown.
- List actions that prevent skin breakdown.
- Explain the use of comfort and positioning devices.
- Demonstrate the following:
  Procedure 20 Backrub
  Procedure 21 Bed Bath
  Procedure 22 Tub Bath or Shower

Procedure 23 Partial Bath
Procedure 24 Female Perineal Care
Procedure 25 Male Perineal Care
Procedure 26 Daily Hair Care
Procedure 27 Shaving Male Resident
Procedure 28 Hand and Fingernail Care
Procedure 29 Foot and Toenail Care
Procedure 30 Assisting Resident to Brush Teeth
Procedure 31 Cleaning and Flossing Resident's Teeth
Procedure 32 Caring for Dentures
Procedure 33 Assisting with Special Oral Hygiene
Procedure 34 Dressing and Undressing Resident

# VOCABULARY

**axilla** *(ack-**SILL**-ah)*

**bridging** *(**BRIJ**-ing)*

**caries** *(**KAIR**-eez)*

**constricting** *(kon-**STRICK**-ting)*

**cuticle** *(**KYOU**-tih-kul)*

**decubiti** *(dee-**KYOU**-bih-tie)*

**dentures** *(**DEN**-churz)*

**dermis** *(**DER**-mis)*

**dilating** *(die-**LAY**-ting)*

**dry sterile dressing (DSD)** *(dry **STER**-ill **DRESS**-ing)*

**epidermis** *(ep-ih-**DER**-mis)*

**friction** *(**FRICK**-shun)*

**genitalia** *(**jen**-ih-**TAIL**-ee-ah)*

**halitosis** *(**hal**-ih-**TOH**-sis)*

**integumentary system** *(in-**teg**-you-**MEN**-tair-ee **SIS**-tem)*

**lesions** *(**LEE**-zhuns)*

**oil gland** *(oil gland)*

**oral hygiene** *(**OR**-al **HIGH**-jeen)*

**perineal care** *(**pair**-ih-**NEE**-al kair)*

**pore** *(por)*

**pressure ulcer** *(**PRESH**-zhur **UL**-sir)*

**pubic** *(**PYOU**-bick)*

**receptor** *(ree-**SEP**-tor)*

**senile lentigines** *(**SEE**-nile len-**TIJ**-ih-nees)*

**shearing** *(**SHEER**-ing)*

**skin tear** *(skin tair)*

**subcutaneous tissue** *(sub-kyou-**TAY**-nee-us **TISH**-you)*

**sweat gland** *(swet gland)*

---

The **integumentary system** consists of the skin, oil and sweat glands of the skin, hair, nails, teeth, and the environmental sense organs. The teeth are formed from the tissues of the integument (body shell) but also make a major contribution to the digestive system.

The outermost layers of the skin make up the **epidermis** (Figure 16-1). Under the epidermis is the **dermis**, and under the dermis is the **subcutaneous tissue** that attaches the skin to the muscles.

## EPIDERMIS

The epidermis consists of dead outer cells that are constantly shed as new cells move upward from the dermis. There are no blood vessels in the epidermis, so injury to this level does not produce bleeding. Nerve endings reach into this outer covering. The nerves form sense organs that keep us in contact with changes in the environment. Nerve endings called **receptors** receive information about temperature, pressure, and pain.

## DERMIS

The dermis contains blood vessels, nerve fibers, and two kinds of glands:

- **Sweat glands**
- **Oil glands**

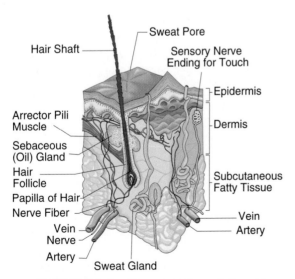

Sweat Pore
Hair Shaft
Sensory Nerve Ending for Touch
Epidermis
Dermis
Arrector Pili Muscle
Sebaceous (Oil) Gland
Hair Follicle
Subcutaneous Fatty Tissue
Papilla of Hair
Nerve Fiber
Vein
Vein
Artery
Nerve
Artery
Sweat Gland

**FIGURE 16-1**   Cross section of the skin

## Sweat Glands

The sweat glands produce perspiration that reaches the skin surface through tubes or ducts that end in openings called **pores**. Heat from deep in the body is brought to the skin by blood vessels. This heat is transferred to the perspiration. At the skin surface, the perspiration and the heat are lost through the pores to the air. The heat of the body is controlled by changes in the size of the blood vessels in the skin.

- **Dilating** (enlarging) blood vessels bring more heat to the body surface.
- **Constricting** (narrowing) blood vessels bring less heat to the body surface.

## Oil Glands

Oil glands lubricate and keep flexible the hairs found in the skin. Hair covers almost all the body surfaces except for the palms of the hands and the soles of the feet.

## SKIN FUNCTIONS

The skin has many functions that are critical to the well-being of the body:

- Protection—forms a continuous membranous covering and regulates body temperature
- Storage—stores fat and vitamins
- Elimination—loses water, salts, and heat through perspiration
- Sensory perceptions—contains nerve endings that keep us aware of environmental changes

## SKIN CHANGES CAUSED BY AGING

### Common Changes in the Aging Skin

As people age, changes occur in the integumentary system (Figure 16-2). These changes include:

1. Sweat glands decrease in activity.
2. Loss of elasticity and fatty tissue causes wrinkling. The eyelids tend to droop.
3. The skin is drier as oil gland secretions decrease.
4. Areas of pigmentation seem more pronounced. In light-skinned people, the skin

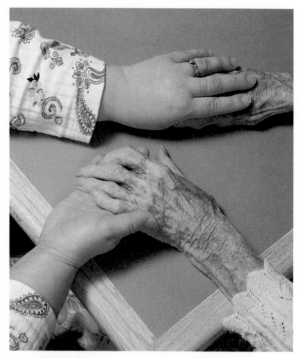

**FIGURE 16-2**   Look carefully at the skin of the hands of the nursing assistant and the resident. Note the aging changes in the skin of the resident.

becomes more sallow or yellow and less pink. Skin tabs and moles are more common.

5. The hair loses its color, becoming first gray and then white. Less oil causes the hair to become drier and duller. The amount of hair, especially in men, diminishes.
6. Nails on both fingers and toes thicken, becoming more brittle and likely to split.
7. Peripheral blood vessels weaken. These are more easily seen under the thinned epidermis. Small hemorrhages occur due to the weakness of the blood vessels. Peripheral circulation to the skin decreases so that general skin nutrition is less satisfactory.
8. Loss of teeth may result in the need for **dentures** (artificial teeth).

### Injury and Healing

The skin is exposed to the environment and is constantly in danger of trauma and infection. The skin of the older adult is fragile because of aging changes. Injuries to the skin of older adults are slower to heal. Compared to younger people, the skin receives less blood flow and, as a result, fewer nutrients to help the healing process.

Caution is always required when caring for the elderly to prevent injury to the skin. Bathing, dressing, positioning, and bedmaking (occupied bed) are all situations in which the elderly may experience skin injuries if the nursing assistant is not careful.

## SKIN LESIONS

Changes in the structure of the skin are called **lesions**. The lesions may be caused by the aging process, disease, trauma, or wear. It is the nursing assistant's responsibility to observe the residents carefully. Observations about the condition of the skin and changes in the skin are important. Any changes noted should be reported immediately and described accurately. The following types of lesions are discussed: skin cancer, senile lentigines, skin breakdown, and pressure ulcers.

### Skin Cancer

Cancers of the skin are fairly common in the older individual. Be sure to report any changes you note in the size or shape of a wart or mole or indications of inflammation (redness) around the area of a wart or mole. Skin cancer can also appear as an area of darkened pigmentation in the skin. Skin that has been exposed to the sun for long periods of time over the years is susceptible to skin cancer. The earlier any changes noted are reported, the earlier treatment can begin.

### Senile Lentigines

Areas of skin pigmentation seem to become more pronounced with advancing years. **Senile lentigines** (Figure 16-3) are sometimes called liver spots although they are not related to liver function. They are thought to be a response to environmental exposure. They appear as yellowish or brownish spots on exposed skin surfaces.

A professional evaluation may be needed to determine if a lesion is a relatively harmless senile lentigine or an early indication of skin cancer.

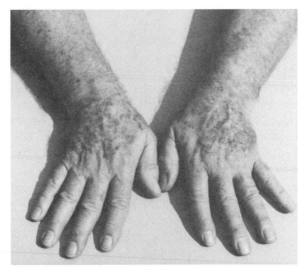

**FIGURE 16-3** Senile lentigines

### Skin Breakdown

Friction, shearing, and pressure are common causes of skin breakdown. **Friction** occurs when the skin moves against a firm or rough surface, including bed linens, wheelchair parts, a crutch or brace, or tubing, such as a nasogastric tube or urinary catheter (Figure 16-4). Friction also occurs when parts of the body rub together, for example, ankles or knees rubbing against each other. The rubbing action may cause skin abrasions that can lead to deeper tissue injury.

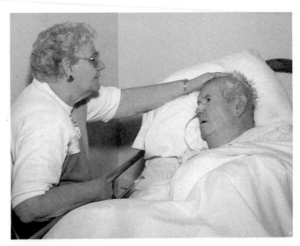

**FIGURE 16-4** The rubbing of nasal catheters, nasogastric tubes, or urinary catheters can cause skin breakdown.

**Shearing** occurs when the skin moves in one direction while the structures under the skin, such as the bones, remain fixed or move in the opposite direction. This can happen when residents are dragged rather than lifted up in bed, when positions are changed, or when residents slide down in bed or in a wheelchair (Figure 16-5). Blood vessels become twisted and stretched causing the tissues being served to lose essential oxygen and nutrients, leading to breakdown. In addition, shearing may cause actual tears in fragile skin. These **skin tears** are painful, a portal of entry for infectious pathogens, and commonly lead to further breakdown.

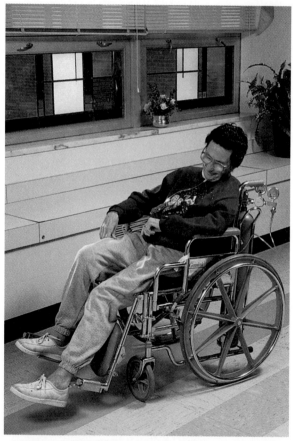

**FIGURE 16-5** Shearing can occur when the resident's position is poorly supported. As the resident slides down in bed or in a chair, the skeleton remains stationary while the skin slips, causing tension both on the skin and underlying blood vessels, leading to tissue damage.

When pressure is put on tissues for a long time, skin breakdown can occur. The tissues are usually trapped between a bony prominence such as the heel, hip bone, or sacrum and the source of the pressure. The pressure causes the collapse of tiny blood vessels. Skin surfaces receiving less nourishment through the damaged vessels quickly break down.

## Pressure Ulcers

Skin breakdown may progress to the formation of deep, painful lesions called **pressure ulcers** (also known as **decubiti**). They are a serious problem, especially for older adults. Residents are assessed by the interdisciplinary team for the probability of developing pressure ulcers. A care plan is developed with specific actions to prevent the formation of pressure ulcers. In some facilities, this activity is performed by a nurse who is specially trained in skin and wound care.

**Factors Leading to Breakdown.** Pressure ulcers can frequently be prevented by conscientious care and attention. Nursing assistants must be alert to the factors that contribute to their formation, including:

- Impaired circulation due to pressure
- Prolonged contact with moisture
- Prolonged contact with excretions/secretions
- Poor nutrition and debilitation
- Dehydration
- Shearing forces and friction
- Immobility
- Incontinence

**Signs of Tissue Breakdown.** Tissue breakdown is described and classified in four stages. Unless action is taken the damage is progressive.

1. Stage one: The intact skin surface shows redness or blue-gray discoloration over a pressure point, which does not disappear when the pressure is removed (Figure 16-6). In darker-skinned people, the area may seem drier, and under pressure, become darker or purplish in color, and feel warm to the touch.
2. Stage two: The reddened skin is accompanied by an abrasion, blisters, or a shallow

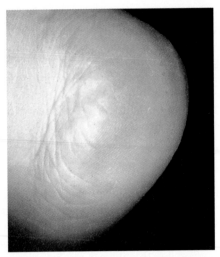

**FIGURE 16-6** First indication of tissue damage (stage one) is redness and heat over a pressure point, such as this heel. (Courtesy of Emory University Hospital, Atlanta, GA)

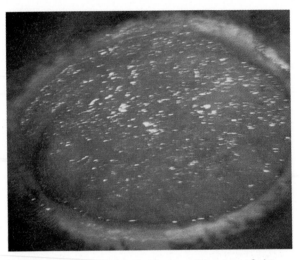

**FIGURE 16-8** In stage three, all layers of skin have been destroyed. A deep crater has been formed. *Note:* Photo shows right hip. (Courtesy of Emory University Hospital, Atlanta, GA)

crater (Figure 16-7). The epidermis alone or the epidermis and dermis may be involved. The area around the site is reddened.

3. Stage three: The deeper subcutaneous tissues break down and a deep crater is formed (Figure 16-8).
4. Stage four: The deeper tissues of muscles and bones are involved. At this stage, residents experience fluid loss and pain and are at great risk for infection (Figure 16-9).

**Actions to Take When Breakdown Occurs.** Residents with existing skin breakdown may be admitted to the long-term care facility from home or another health care facility. At other times, despite careful preventive care, skin breakdown occurs. In these situations, the nursing assistant actions include:

- Performing the actions listed in the guidelines to prevent further breakdown
- Following the care plan exactly

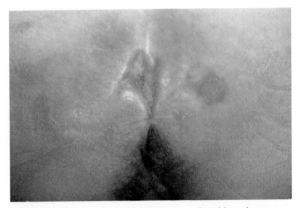

**FIGURE 16-7** Stage two is marked by destruction of the epidermis and partial destruction of the dermis. *Note:* The area shown is the sacrum. (Courtesy of Emory University Hospital, Atlanta, GA)

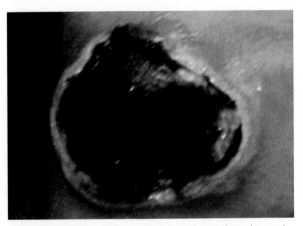

**FIGURE 16-9** This pressure ulcer developed over the hip of a resident. It involves deep tissues (stage four). (Courtesy of Emory University Hospital, Atlanta, GA)

# *G*uidelines for
# Preventing Skin Breakdown

Nursing assistant actions are vital in identifying potential causes of breakdown and taking steps to eliminate or minimize them.

1. Carefully inspect the resident's skin during care and report findings to the nurse.
2. Bathe resident regularly. Handle the skin gently and use a mild cleansing agent. Avoid hot water and do not scrub the skin. Dry thoroughly by patting the skin with the towel. Closely inspect potential pressure or friction areas.
3. Immediately remove feces, urine, or moisture of any kind, including perspiration, from the resident's skin. Prolonged contact is irritating to the skin. Keep the skin clean and dry.
4. Use underpads or briefs that are moisture absorbent to help keep the resident dry.
5. Use lotion on dry skin areas but do not use on broken skin. Pat lotion on skin gently; do not rub vigorously.
6. Encourage good nutrition and adequate fluid intake.
7. Change position of in-bed resident at least every 2 hours to reduce pressure in any one area. Some residents may need repositioning more often than others. The care plan for each resident must be followed carefully. The turning schedule will be posted in the care plan and in the room. Figure 16-10 shows an example of the sequence of turns.

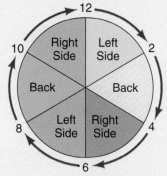

**FIGURE 16-10** Example of a turning schedule with a position change every 2 hours

8. Keep bed linens wrinkle free.
9. Encourage residents sitting in geri-chairs or wheelchairs to raise themselves or change position to relieve pressure every 15 minutes. If the resident is not able to do so, assist the resident in repositioning at least every hour.
10. Check for improperly fitted or worn braces, shoes, and restraints that may rub the skin.
11. Check nasogastric tubes and urinary catheters to be sure they are positioned so they do not irritate the skin. Keep nasal and urinary openings clean and free of drainage. These areas must be checked frequently and carefully.
12. Do passive range of motion exercises twice daily.
13. Use a turning sheet to help move dependent residents in bed. Some residents may be able to help reposition themselves in bed by using a trapeze. Do not drag the resident over the bed linens.
14. Do not elevate the head of the bed too high. This may cause shearing of tissues as the resident slides down in bed. An elevation of no more than 30° is recommended for residents at risk for pressure ulcers.
15. Separate body areas likely to rub together, especially over bony prominences, by using pillows or foam wedges, according to the care plan.
16. For residents sitting in geri-chairs or wheelchairs, use foam, gel, or air cushions to reduce pressure on buttocks and sacrum.
17. For residents in bed, relieve pressure on heels by supporting feet off the bed.
18. Use special pressure-reducing mattresses or alternating-pressure mattresses for residents in bed.
19. Report signs of infection, such as fever, odor, drainage, inflammation, or bleeding to the nurse.

- Reporting indications of infection such as fever, odor, drainage, bleeding, and changes in size
- Keeping the area around the breakdown clean and dry
- Assisting with whirlpool baths, if ordered, to keep the area clean

The nurse or physician may perform other procedures to care for areas of skin breakdown. For example:

- The area may be covered with a **dry sterile dressing (DSD)**. Holding a DSD in place without causing additional injury is not easy. The skin of older adults may be sensitive to regular tape. In this case, silk tape, paper tape, cellophane tape or other hypoallergenic tape may be used. To prevent injury when removing the tape before a dressing change, a saline solution is applied to loosen the tape.
- Residents may be placed on alternating-pressure mattresses or pressure-reducing mattresses or beds.
- In some facilities, the open lesions are packed loosely with gauze soaked in a wound gel. The gel keeps the lesions moist, breaks down dead cells, and promotes healing.
- The area may be protected and kept moist by using special dressings. They have a clear plastic covering that permits air to reach the tissues as well as keeping them moist to promote healing. The dressing must extend beyond the wound edge. It is held in place with a frame of either paper or silk tape. The dressing must be changed every 3 to 5 days unless there is leakage or according to facility policy.
- The wounds may be cleaned by the nurse or physician with saline solution and debrided (dead tissue removed) using instruments and proteolytic enzymes.
- Antiseptic sprays, antibiotic ointments, and dressings are used to control infection.
- Surgery may be needed to close the ulcerated area in severe cases.

Residents are encouraged to participate to whatever extent is possible in their own care. Attentive nursing care is essential in preventing skin breakdown. Remember that it is far easier to prevent pressure ulcers than to heal them.

**Blood Circulation to Tissues.** Ensuring adequate circulation to tissues is a major factor in preventing skin breakdown. This can be accomplished by:

- Positioning the resident properly
- Using mechanical aids
- Providing backrubs
- Performing active or passive range of motion exercises

The most common sites for skin breakdown are shown in Figure 16-11.

**Positioning.** Five basic in-bed positions are used to relieve pressure as the resident's condition permits. Each position must be supported for comfort. The nursing assistant must remember that all residents may not be able to assume the full range of positions because of disabilities such as arthritis, contractures, or breathing limi-

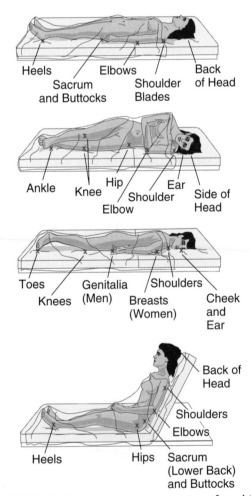

**FIGURE 16-11** Most common sites for skin breakdown

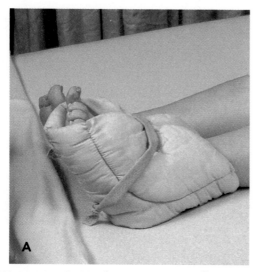
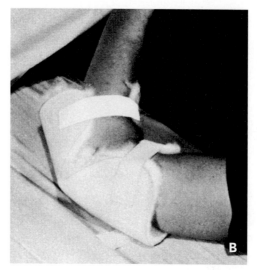

**FIGURE 16-12**   A. Heel protector  B. Elbow protector  (Courtesy of J. T. Posey Company, Arcadia, CA)

tations. Residents who sit in geri-chairs or wheelchairs for long periods of time must also change position to relieve pressure.

Residents with special problems require extra care when they are positioned in bed. For example:

- Be sure the resident can breathe properly.
- Remember that a fractured hip is never rotated over the unaffected leg.
- If the resident had a stroke, elevate the weak arm to reduce edema.
- Always maintain proper body alignment.
- The resident with a recent stroke is turned on the unaffected side.

The five basic positions residents assume in bed are:

- Supine position
- Semisupine position
- Lateral position
- Semiprone position
- Fowler's position

These positions are described fully and illustrated in Lesson 22 on restorative care.

## Mechanical Aids

Mechanical aids are used to reduce pressure. Examples are

- Sheepskin pads (or artificial sheepskin)
- Foam pads and pillows

- Protectors for areas such as heels and elbows (Figure 16-12) that are subject to friction as the resident moves in bed
- Bed cradles (foot cradles)
- Alternating pressure mattresses
- Flotation mattresses
- Pillows
- Gel-filled mattresses

**Sheepskin Pads (or Artificial Sheepskin).** These absorb moisture and reduce friction when placed under the resident (Figure 16-13).

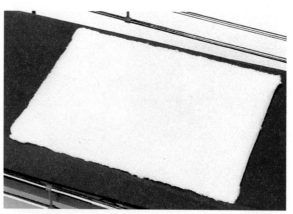

**FIGURE 16-13**   A soft, synthetic fleece pad takes pressure off the back (Courtesy of J. T. Posey Company, Arcadia, CA)

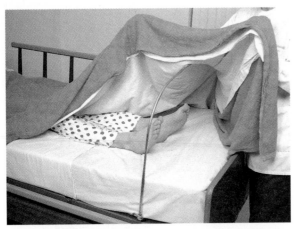

**FIGURE 16-14** A bed cradle keeps the sheet and blanket from putting pressure on the feet.

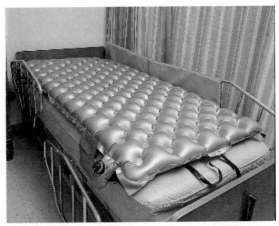

**FIGURE 16-16** Mattress filled with water helps to minimize pressure points on the body.

**Foam Pads and Pillows.** These are used to bridge areas to reduce pressure. Watch residents for signs of disorientation that might be caused by the feeling of weightlessness. Adequate fluid intake to prevent urinary stasis must be provided and conscientious range of motion exercises must be carried out. Rubber or hard doughnut-shaped pads may not be effective. Although they shield the affected areas, they create pressure by their own shape.

**Bed (Foot) Cradles.** These devices can lift the weight of bedding but must be carefully posi-

tioned and may be padded, because injury can occur if the resident strikes them (Figure 16-14).

**Alternating-Pressure Mattress (Air Mattress).** This type of mattress (Figure 16-15) is used in some facilities. Air pressure is reduced in a different area of the mattress on an alternating basis. The pressure alteration reduces pressure against the body so that no skin area is continuously subjected to pressure.

**Flotation Mattress.** This mattress (Figure 16-16) is a water bed with controlled temperature. The weight of the resident's body displaces water to the extent that pressure is consistently equalized against the skin. Sheets should not be tucked tightly over the flotation mattress because this will restrict the function of the mattress.

**Special Equipment.** Specialized beds or overlays are available for residents who need continuous pressure relief. One type of bed is the Clinitron® bed (Figure 16-17). It is filled with a sandlike material. Warm, dry air circulates through the material to maintain an even temperature and support the body evenly.

**Gel-Filled Mattress.** The gel in this type of mattress has a consistency similar to body fat. It allows for a more equal distribution of body weight by conforming to the body contours.

**Pillows.** Pillows are used in a technique called **bridging**. In bridging, body parts are supported by pillows in such a way that spaces are left to relieve pressure on specific areas.

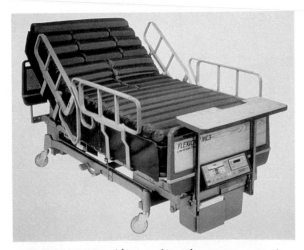

**FIGURE 16-15** Alternating air pressure mattress overlay. Alternating air pressure in the mattress cells changes pressure points against the resident's skin and gently massages the skin. (Courtesy of Hill-Rom, Charlestown, SC)

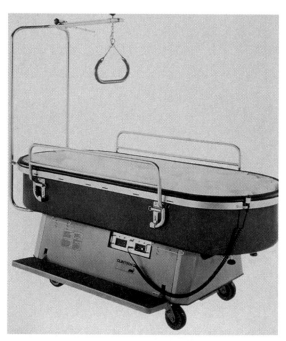

**FIGURE 16-17**  Clinitron® air fluidized mattress (Courtesy of Support Systems International, Inc., Charleston, SC)

Each of these aids reduces pressure but nothing can take the place of nursing observation and care.

## BACKRUB

Regular back care is given after the bath. It may also be given after the use of the bed pan or after changing a resident's position. When performed properly, with long, smooth strokes, it stimulates the resident's circulation and aids in preventing skin breakdown. It is also soothing and refreshing. (See Procedure 20.)

## BATHING RESIDENTS

A complete bath two or three times a week will maintain cleanliness. Too frequent bathing can lead to skin dryness and itching. Many facilities require a daily partial bath. Incontinent residents are bathed as often as necessary.

---

**PROCEDURE**
## *20* Backrub

1. Carry out each beginning procedure action.
2. Assemble equipment:
   - Disposable gloves
   - Basin of water (105°F)
   - Bath towel
   - Soap and lotion
3. Put up far side rail.
4. Place lotion in basin of water to warm (Figure 16-18).
5. Put on disposable gloves if resident has open lesions.
6. Turn the resident on his or her side with back toward you.
7. Expose and wash back, dry carefully. This step is not necessary if backrub is given after a bath.

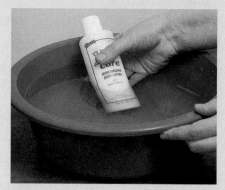

**FIGURE 16-18**  Before the backrub, the bottle of lotion can be placed in a basin of warm water for several minutes so the lotion will not be cold when applied to the resident's back.

*(continues)*

**PROCEDURE 20** *(continued)*

8. Pour a small amount of lotion into one hand.
9. Apply to skin and rub with gentle but firm strokes. Give special attention to all bony prominences (Figure 16-19).

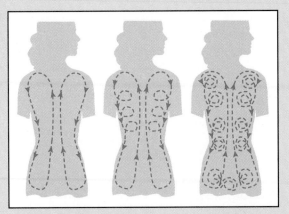

**FIGURE 16-20** Strokes to be used during the backrub

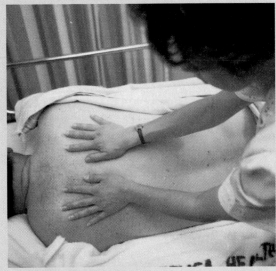

**FIGURE 16-19** Use long, smooth strokes as you apply the lotion.

10. Begin at base of spine:
    • With long, soothing strokes rub up the center of back, around the shoulders, and down sides of back and buttocks (Figure 16-20, left).
    • Repeat previous step four times, using long, soothing upward strokes and circu-

lar motion on downstroke (Figure 16-20, middle).
    • Repeat, but on downward stroke rub in small circular motions with palm of hand. Include areas over coccyx (over base of spine) (Figure 16-20, right).
    • Repeat long, soothing strokes on muscles for 3 to 5 minutes (Figure 16-20, left).
    • Dry area well.
    • If redness on pressure areas is noted, report to nurse. Straighten and tighten bottom sheet and draw sheet.
11. Change resident's gown if needed.
12. Replace equipment.
13. Carry out each procedure completion action.

Bathing may be performed as:
• Complete bed bath
• Partial bed bath
• Perineal care
• Tub bath
• Shower bath
• Whirlpool bath

During bathing, special attention should be given to skin areas that touch, including:
• Between the legs
• Under the arms
• Under the breasts
• Under the scrotum
• Between the buttocks

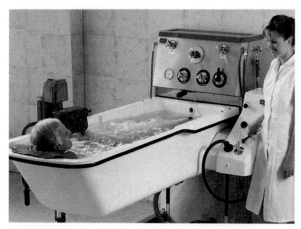

**FIGURE 16-21**  This tub is a whirlpool tub in which the water circulates around the resident's body to give a mild therapeutic massage that helps tone muscles and relieve tension. (Courtesy of Arjo-Century, Inc.)

- Around the anus
- For obese people, under folds of skin or fat

Gently sponge and pat these areas dry. Follow facility policy for the use of talcum or cornstarch.

A partial bath, bed bath, and tub and shower bath are all ways to meet resident needs for cleanliness. The most stimulating form of bathing for residents is a therapeutic bath that is given in a whirlpool tub (Figure 16-21). The whirlpool bath is beneficial for the resident because:

1. The temperature of the water can be regulated to an optimum 97°F.
2. The movement of the water stimulates circulation.
3. Being surrounded by warm circulating water is relaxing and invigorating.

## Safety Issues

General safety issues must be considered when giving a tub or shower bath:

- The tub or shower must be clean before and after use (Figure 16-22).
- Be sure that there is adequate help.
- Check that all safety aids such as hand rails, shower seats, and hydraulic lifts are in good repair and proper working order.

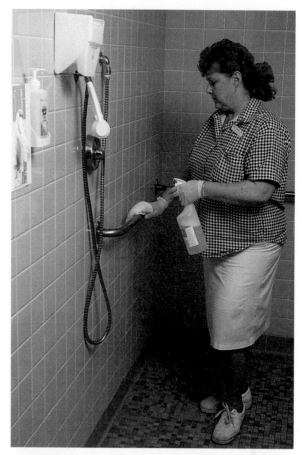

**FIGURE 16-22**  The shower is cleaned with a disinfectant before and after each use.

- Wipe up all water spilled on the floor immediately to prevent falls.
- Keep the temperature of the room comfortable and the area free of drafts.
- Wear gloves if there may be contact with open lesions or body fluids.
- Observe the skin for any changes or irregularities. Do not disturb or injure any warts or moles. Report anything unusual.
- Protect resident from fatigue by transporting resident to and from the tub room and carrying out the bathing procedure as efficiently as possible.
- Use good body mechanics to protect yourself and the resident.
- Use a bath thermometer to be sure the temperature of the water is correct. If a bath thermometer is not available, test the water with your wrist. (See Procedures 21 and 22.)

## PROCEDURE
## 21  Bed Bath

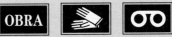

1. Carry out each beginning procedure action.
2. Assemble equipment (Figure 16-23).
   - Disposable gloves
   - Bed linen
   - Bath blanket
   - Laundry bag or hamper
   - Bath basin
   - Bath thermometer
   - Soap and soap dish
   - Washcloth
   - Face towel
   - Two bath towels
   - Facility gown or the resident's clothes

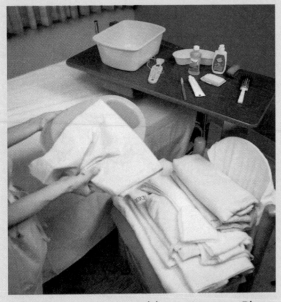

**FIGURE 16-23** Assemble equipment. Place bed linens on chair next to bed and remaining items (except bedpan) on overbed table. If used, bedpan or urinal will be removed from bedside stand, used, cleaned immediately, and returned to stand.

- Lotion
- Equipment for oral hygiene
- Nail brush, emery board, and orangewood stick (if available)
- Brush and comb
- Bedpan and cover or urinal

3. Close the door and windows to prevent chilling the resident.
4. Close privacy curtain.
5. Put towels and linen on chair in order of use.
6. Place laundry hamper so that it is convenient.
7. Offer bedpan or urinal. Put on gloves if resident wants to use bedpan or urinal. Empty and clean before proceeding with bath. Return to storage. Remove gloves and discard according to facility policy. Wash hands.
8. Put on disposable gloves.
9. Lower the back of bed and side rails on side you are working. Be sure opposite side is up.
10. Loosen top bedclothes. If blanket is to be reused, remove it from bed, fold it, and place it over the back of the chair. Otherwise, place bath blanket over top bedclothes and remove top bedclothes by sliding them out from under the bath blanket. Place in laundry hamper.
11. Leave one pillow under resident's head. Place other pillow on chair.
12. Remove resident's nightwear and place in laundry hamper.
13. Fill bath basin two-thirds full with water at 105°F.
14. Assist resident to move to the side of the bed nearest you.
15. Fold face towel over upper edge of bath blanket to keep blanket dry.

*(continues)*

**PROCEDURE *21* (continued)**

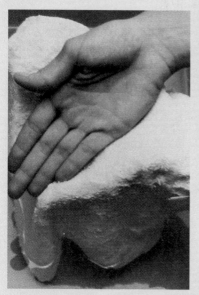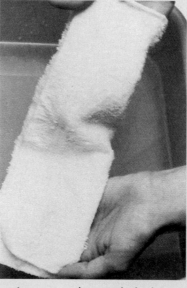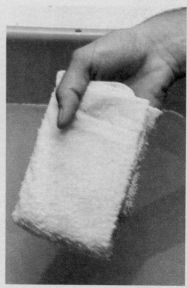

**FIGURE 16-24**   To make a bath mitt, wrap the washcloth around one hand. Then bring the free end back over palm and tuck in the end. Thumb is free to hold washcloth in place. *Note:* If gloves are used in the procedure, make the bath mitt over the glove.

16. Form a mitten by holding washcloth around hand (Figure 16-24). Wet washcloth; wash eyes, using separate corners of cloth for each eye. Do not use soap near eyes.
17. Rinse washcloth and apply soap if resident desires. Squeeze out excess water.
18. Wash and rinse resident's face, ears, and neck (Figure 16-25). Use towel to dry.
19. Expose resident's far arm. Protect bed with bath towel placed under arm. Wash, rinse, and dry arm and hand. Be sure **axilla** (armpit) is clean and dry. Apply deodorant if resident agrees. Repeat for other arm.
20. If necessary, care for hands and nails as follows:
    a. Wash each hand carefully. Rinse and dry. Push back cuticle (base of fingernails) gently with towel while wiping the fingers. Be sure to dry the areas between the fingers.

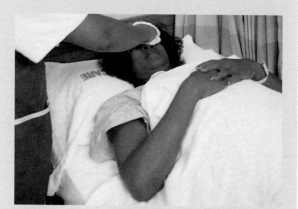

**FIGURE 16-25**   Wash face carefully, doing eyes separately. Do not use soap on washcloth when cleaning around eyes.

    b. Clean under nails with orangewood stick and shape with emery board. Be careful not to file nails too close. If resident is diabetic, inform the nurse if nail care is needed.

*(continues)*

## PROCEDURE *21* *(continued)*

21. Discard used bath water and refill basin two-thirds full with water at 105°F.
22. Put bath towel over resident's chest, and then fold blanket to waist. Under towel, wash with soap, rinse, and dry chest. Rinse and dry under breasts of female resident. Wash carefully to avoid irritating skin.
23. Fold bath blanket down to **pubic** area. Wash with soap, rinse, and dry abdomen. Replace bath blanket over abdomen and chest. Slide towel out from under bath blanket.
24. Ask resident to flex far knee if possible. Fold bath blanket up to expose thigh, leg, and foot. Protect bed with bath towel, and put bath basin on towel. Place resident's foot in basin (Figure 16-26). Wash and rinse leg and foot. When moving leg, support leg properly.

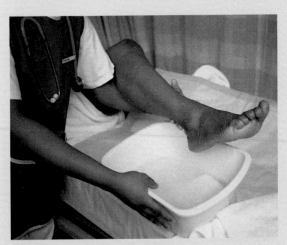

**FIGURE 16-26** Support leg and place the foot in the basin.

25. Lift leg and move basin to other side of bed. Dry leg and foot. Dry well between toes.
26. Repeat for other leg and foot. Take basin from bed before drying leg and foot.
27. Care for toenails as necessary. File nails straight across. Do not round edges. Do not push back the cuticle because it is

easily injured and infected. Apply lotion to feet of resident with dry skin, except between toes. Observe toenails carefully so that you can report condition of nails to nurse. If resident is diabetic, inform nurse if toenail care is needed.
28. Discard used bath water and refill basin two-thirds full with water at 105°F. Several water changes are suggested in this procedure, but you may need to change water more often.
29. Help resident to turn on side away from you and to move toward center of bed. Place towel lengthwise next to resident's back. Wash, rinse, and dry neck, back, and buttocks. Use long, firm strokes when washing back.
30. A backrub is usually given at this time. (See Procedure 20.)
31. Place towel under buttocks and upper legs. Place washcloth, soap, basin, and bath towel within convenient reach of resident. Instruct resident to wash **genitalia**, assisting if necessary. (You must assume responsibility for this procedure if resident has difficulty. Residents often are reluctant to acknowledge the need for help. Wear gloves when assisting.) When assisting female resident, always wash from front to back, drying carefully. When assisting male resident, carefully wash and dry penis, scrotum, and groin area. If male is uncircumcised, gently push foreskin back and carefully wash and dry penis. Then gently pull foreskin down when you are finished.
32. Help resident to turn on back. Remove gloves (if used) and discard according to facility policy. Wash your hands.
33. Carry out range of motion exercises as ordered.
34. Cover pillow with towel and comb or brush hair. Oral hygiene is usually given at this time. (See procedures later in this lesson.)

*(continues)*

**PROCEDURE *21* (continued)**

**35.** Place used towels and washcloth in hamper.
**36.** Provide clean gown.
**37.** Clean and replace equipment, according to facility policy.
**38.** Change bed linen, following occupied bed procedure. Put soiled linen in laundry hamper.

**39.** Remove and discard disposable gloves according to facility policy. Wash your hands.
**40.** Raise side rails if required.
**41.** Carry out each procedure completion action.

**PROCEDURE**
## *22* Tub Bath or Shower

**1.** Carry out each beginning procedure action.
**2.** Assemble equipment:
  - Disposable gloves
  - Soap
  - Washcloth
  - Two to three bath towels
  - Bath blanket
  - Resident's gown, robe, and slippers
  - Bath thermometer
  - Chair or stool
  - Bath mat
**3.** Take the supplies to the bathroom and prepare it for the resident. Make sure tub is clean.
**4.** Fill tub one-third full with water at 105°F or adjust shower flow. Use your elbow to test the water temperature if a shower is being given. The water should feel comfortably warm.
**5.** Assist resident to bathroom and help him or her with robe and slippers.

**6.** Help resident undress. Give the resident a towel to wrap around midriff. Cover resident with bath blanket when going to and from bath or shower.
**7.** Assist resident into tub or shower. For the resident's safety, the bottom of the tub and the shower floor are covered with a nonskid surface. In addition, a tub chair or a shower chair can be provided so the resident can sit safely while bathing.
**8.** Put on disposable gloves if there are open lesions.
**9.** Wash resident's back. Observe skin for signs of redness or breaks. If resident's condition permits, allow resident to assist as much as possible in the procedure. Give resident the choice of washing genitalia. If you assist with this part of the procedure, put on gloves. On completion, remove gloves and discard according to facility policy. Wash your hands.

*(continues)*

**PROCEDURE 22** *(continued)*

10. If resident shows any signs of weakness, remove plug and let water drain out, or turn off shower. Allow resident to rest until feeling better before making any attempt to assist him or her out of tub or shower. Keep resident covered with bath towel to avoid chilling.
11. If resident wants a shampoo and you have permission to do so:
    - Ask resident to hold washcloth over eyes.
    - Pour small amount of water on hair (enough to wet hair thoroughly).
    - Use a small amount of shampoo to lather hair.
    - Massage scalp gently.
    - Rinse hair with warm water.
    - Repeat lathering, massaging, and rinsing, if necessary.
    - Towel hair dry.
12. Hold bath blanket around resident when he or she is stepping out of tub or shower. A resident may choose to remove wet towel under bath blanket.
13. Assist resident to dry, apply deodorant, dress, and return to unit.
14. Put on gloves and clean bathtub. Remove gloves and discard according to facility policy. Wash your hands. Put supplies away.
15. Carry out each procedure completion action.

## Partial Bath

A partial bath is cleaning of the hands, face, axilla, buttocks, and genitals. It is very refreshing. Many residents will be able to help with the bath process and, whenever possible, should be encouraged to do so. (See Procedure 23.)

**PROCEDURE 23    Partial Bath**

1. Carry out each beginning procedure action.
2. Assemble equipment:
   - Disposable gloves
   - Bed linen
   - Bath blanket
   - Bath thermometer
   - Soap and soap dish
   - Washcloth
   - Face towel
   - Bath towel
   - Gown or robe
   - Laundry bag or hamper
   - Bath basin
   - Lotion
   - Equipment for oral hygiene
   - Nail brush, orangewood stick, and emery board

*(continues)*

**PROCEDURE 23** *(continued)*

- Brush, comb, and deodorant
- Bedpan or urinal and cover
- Paper towels or bed protector

3. Close the door and any windows to prevent chilling resident.
4. Put towels and linen on chair, in order of use. Place laundry hamper so that it is convenient.
5. Put on disposable gloves.
6. Offer bedpan or urinal. Empty and clean before proceeding with bath. Remove gloves and discard according to facility policy. Wash hands and put on pair of new gloves.
7. Elevate head rest, if permitted, to comfortable position.
8. Loosen top bedclothes. Remove and fold blanket and spread and place over back of chair. Place bath blanket over top sheet and remove sheet by sliding it out from under bath blanket.
9. Leave one pillow under resident's head. Place other pillow on chair.
10. Assist resident to remove gown and place gown in laundry hamper. Wrap bath blanket around resident.
11. Place paper towels or bed protector on overbed table.
12. Fill bath basin two-thirds full with water at 105°F and place on overbed table.

13. Push overbed table comfortably close to resident.
14. Place towels, washcloth, and soap on overbed table within easy reach.
15. Instruct resident to wash as much as he or she is able and that you will return to complete the bath.
16. Place call bell within easy reach. Ask resident to signal when ready.
17. Remove gloves and discard according to facility policy. Wash hands and leave unit.
18. Wash hands and return to unit when resident signals. Put on a new pair of gloves.
19. Change bath water. Bathe those areas the resident could not reach. Make sure the face, hands, axilla, buttocks, back, and genitalia are washed and dried.
20. Give a backrub with lotion.
21. Assist the resident in applying deodorant and fresh gown.
22. Cover pillow with towel and comb or brush hair. Assist with oral hygiene if needed.
23. Clean and replace equipment according to facility policy.
24. Change bed linen, following occupied bed procedure. Discard soiled linen in laundry hamper.
25. Remove and dispose of gloves according to facility policy.
26. Carry out each procedure completion action.

## Perineal Care

**Perineal care** is the cleaning of the area between the resident's legs. Keeping this area clean is especially important when residents are unable to control bladder and bowels. Excreta left on the skin is unpleasant and uncomfortable. If left unattended, it can lead to skin breakdown.

Perineal care may be performed as part of general bathing or as a separate procedure as needed. (See Procedures 24 and 25.)

**PROCEDURE**

## 24 Female Perineal Care

1. Carry out each beginning procedure action.
2. Assemble equipment:
   - Disposable gloves
   - Bath blanket or topsheet
   - Bedpan and cover
   - Liquid soap
   - Basin with warm water (105°F)
   - Bath thermometer
   - Bed protector
   - Washcloth and towel
3. Lower side rail on side where you will be working. Be sure opposite side rail is up and secure.
4. Remove bedspread and blanket. Fold and place on back of chair.
5. Resident is to be on back. Cover resident with bath blanket and fanfold sheet to foot of bed.
6. Put on disposable gloves.
7. Ask resident to raise hips while you place bed protector underneath resident.
8. Offer bedpan to resident. If used and resident is on intake and output, record amount. Then empty and clean the bedpan before continuing with the procedure. Remove gloves and discard according to facility policy. Wash hands and put on a new pair of gloves.
9. Position bath blanket so only the area between the legs is exposed.
10. Ask resident to separate her legs and flex knees. *Note:* If resident is unable to spread legs and flex knees, turn the resident on her side with legs flexed. This position provides easy access to the perineal area.
11. Wet washcloth, make mitt, and apply a small amount of liquid soap. *Note:* Heavy soap application may be difficult to rinse off completely. Soap residue is irritating.

12. Use one gloved hand to stabilize and separate the vulva (Figure 16-27). With the other gloved hand, proceed as follows.
    a. Bring soaped washcloth in one downward stroke along the far side of outer labia to perineum.
    b. Rinse washcloth, remake mitt, and rinse area just cleaned.
    c. Repeat steps a and b, washing and rinsing inner far labia.
    d. Repeat steps a and b, washing and rinsing inner near labia.
    e. With gloved hands, separate labia. Clean and rinse inner part of vulva to perineum.
    f. Dry washed area with towel.

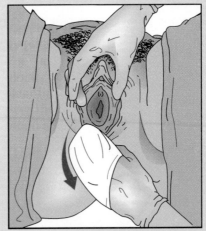

**FIGURE 16-27** Spread the vulva with one hand. With the washcloth in the other hand, start at the front and stroke downward along the outer labia.

13. Turn resident away from you. Flex upper leg slightly if permitted.
14. Make a mitt, wet, and apply soap lightly.

*(continues)*

**PROCEDURE 24** *(continued)*

15. Expose anal area. Wash area, stroking from perineum to coccyx (front to back) (Figure 16-28).

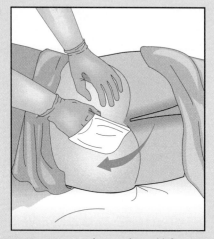

**FIGURE 16-28**   With one hand lift up on the buttocks to expose the rectal area. Wipe from the perineum back toward the anus.

16. Rinse well in the same manner.
17. Dry carefully.
18. Return resident to back.
19. Remove and dispose of bed protector according to facility policy.
20. Cover resident with sheet.
21. Remove and dispose of gloves according to facility policy. Wash hands.
22. Remove, fold, and store bath blanket according to facility policy.
23. Replace top covers, tuck under mattress, and make mitered corners. (Resident may prefer that the top covers not be tucked in.)
24. Put up side rail.
25. Put on gloves. Empty water, clean equipment, and dispose of or store, according to facility policy.
26. Remove gloves and discard according to facility policy. Wash hands.
27. Carry out each procedure completion action.

**PROCEDURE 25**   Male Perineal Care

1. Carry out each beginning procedure action.
2. Assemble equipment:
   - Disposable gloves
   - Bath blanket
   - Bath thermometer
   - Urinal and cover
   - Soap, washcloth, and towel
   - Plastic bag
   - Bed protector or bath towel
   - Ordered solution (if other than water)
3. Fill basin with warm water at approximately 105°F.
4. Lower side rail and position bed protector (or towel) under resident's buttocks.
5. Fanfold blanket and spread to foot of bed.
6. Cover resident with bath blanket and fanfold sheet to foot of bed.
7. Put on disposable gloves.

*(continues)*

**PROCEDURE** *25* *(continued)*

8. Offer bedpan or urinal. If used and resident is on intake and output, record amount. Then empty and clean the bedpan or urinal before continuing with the procedure. Remove gloves and discard according to facility policy. Wash hands and put on a new pair of gloves.

9. Have resident flex and separate knees. *Note:* If the resident is unable to spread legs and flex knees, the perineal area can be washed with the resident on the side with legs flexed. This position provides easy access to the perineal area.

10. Draw bath blanket upward to expose perineal area only.

11. Make a mitt with washcloth and apply a small amount of soap. *Note:* Heavy soap application may be difficult to rinse off completely. Soap residue is irritating.

12. Grasp penis gently with one hand and wash. Begin at the meatus and wash in a circular motion toward the base of the penis (Figure 16-29).

13. If resident is not circumcised, draw foreskin back (Figure 16-30). Be sure entire penis is washed. Rinse thoroughly.

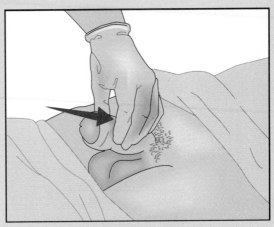

**FIGURE 16-30** If the resident is not circumcised, gently push the foreskin back so the glans can be washed. Once the penis is washed and dried, the foreskin is returned to its normal position.

14. Wash scrotum. Lift scrotum and wash perineum.
15. Rinse washcloth, remake mitt, and rinse area just washed.
16. Dry washed area with towel. Reposition foreskin if necessary.
17. Turn resident away from you. Flex upper leg slightly if permitted.
18. Make a mitt, wet, and apply soap lightly.
19. Expose anal area. Wash area, stroking from perineum to coccyx.
20. Rinse well in the same manner.
21. Dry carefully.
22. Return resident to back.
23. Remove and dispose of bed protector according to facility policy.
24. Cover resident with sheet.
25. Remove and dispose of gloves according to facility policy. Wash hands.

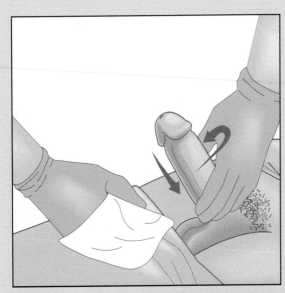

**FIGURE 16-29** Grasp penis gently with one hand. With the other hand, wipe in a circular motion from the glans (head) down to the base of the penis.

*(continues)*

**PROCEDURE** *25* *(continued)*

26. Remove, fold, and store bath blanket, according to facility policy.
27. Replace top covers, tuck under mattress and make mitered corners. (Resident may prefer that the top covers not be tucked in.)
28. Put up side rail.

29. Put on gloves. Empty water, clean equipment, and dispose of or store, according to facility policy.
30. Remove gloves and discard according to facility policy. Wash hands.
31. Carry out each procedure completion action.

## DAILY HAIR CARE

Neat, attractively arranged hair contributes to a feeling of being well groomed. Daily hair care is part of the morning care but should be done whenever it is needed to keep the resident groomed. Residents should be encouraged to take care of their hair and choose the style they prefer.

In many facilities, barbers and beauticians visit once a week to cut, wash, and style the hair of residents who desire the service. Often there is a charge for the service. Normally the residents are prescheduled for their hair care. Some residents may have standing appointments every week or every 2 weeks. The nursing assistant should know which residents have hair appointments. The hair would not be washed just before the appointment.

The hair should be combed and brushed each morning. Tangles can be loosened by sectioning the hair with a comb or brush, working with one section at a time. Grasp the hair near the scalp to reduce pulling (Figure 16-31). Start combing or brushing tangles out starting at the ends and working toward the scalp. Braiding long hair after brushing can help reduce tangles. Tangles can be reduced in wiry, dry hair by using conditioner and keeping the hair short or in braids.

Some residents prefer to have their hair washed in the tub or shower. Be sure you have specific instructions. When assisting with a shampoo in the tub or shower, you must:

- Protect resident's eyes
- Towel dry the hair thoroughly

When a resident must remain in bed and a shampoo is ordered, it can be given using a

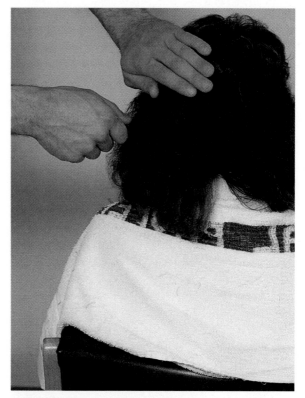

**FIGURE 16-31**  To remove tangles from long hair, divide the hair into sections. Work with one section at a time. Hold hair near the scalp to reduce pulling and start combing at the end of the hair, working toward the scalp.

shampoo tray and pitchers of water to wet and rinse the hair. The water is collected in a pail or bucket placed on the floor next to the bed. The water is collected in the shampoo tray and drains into the pail (Figure 16-32).

**PROCEDURE**

## *26*    Daily Hair Care

**OBRA**

1. Carry out each beginning procedure action.
2. Assemble equipment:
   - Towel
   - Comb and brush
3. Ask resident to move to the side of bed nearest you, or resident may sit in chair if permitted. If a resident is sitting up, put a towel around her shoulders.
4. Cover pillow with towel.
5. Part or section hair and comb with one hand between scalp and end of hair.
6. Brush carefully and thoroughly.
7. Have resident turn so hair on back of head may be combed and brushed. If hair is snarled, work section by section to unsnarl hair, beginning near ends and working toward scalp.
8. Complete brushing and arrange attractively. Braid long hair to prevent repeated snarling.
9. Clean and replace equipment according to facility policy.
10. Carry out each procedure completion action.

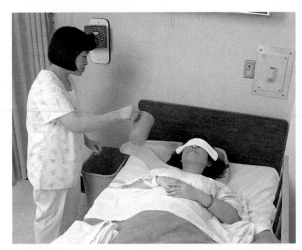

**FIGURE 16-32** The shampoo tray collects the water used to wet and rinse the hair and directs it into a bucket or pail on the floor next to the bed when a shampoo is given.

## FACIAL HAIR

Men feel better groomed when they are shaved regularly (Figure 16-33). This procedure is usually done during the morning care. For safety, use an electric razor or rotary razor.

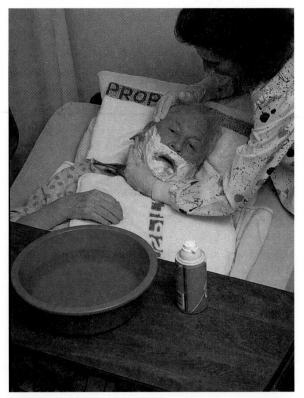

**FIGURE 16-33** Shaving is part of the daily routine for most men.

**FIGURE 16-34**   Special shaving precautions

- Wear disposable gloves.

- Use the resident's own shaving equipment if possible. Otherwise, use disposable, one-use safety razors.

- If the resident is receiving anticoagulants, a special procedure may be required. For example, an electric razor provides the greatest safety. Check with your supervisor for the proper procedure.

- If oxygen is being given, it may be possible to discontinue it during this procedure. Consult your supervisor and follow facility policy.

Refer to Figure 16-34 for safety considerations for shaving.

Older women have an increase in the growth and coarseness of hairs on the chin and upper lip. Many women find this distressing. Tweezers can be used to remove some of the hairs, but a more permanent method is to have the hairs removed professionally with an electric needle. Some women may require a shave. In some facilities nursing assistants are not permitted to shave women residents. Be sure to check the policy of your facility.

**PROCEDURE**

## *27*   Shaving Male Resident

1. Carry out each beginning procedure action.
2. Assemble equipment:
   - Disposable gloves
   - Electric shaver or safety razor
   - Shaving lather or preshave lotion for electric razor
   - Basin of water (105°F)
   - Face towels
   - Mirror
   - Washcloth
   - Aftershave lotion
3. Put on gloves.
4. Raise the head of the bed. Place equipment on overbed table.

5. Place one face towel across resident's chest and one under head.
6. Moisten face and apply lather (or preshave lotion).
7. Starting in front of ear:
   a. Hold skin taut and bring razor down over cheek toward chin (Figure 16-35).
   b. Repeat until lather on cheek is removed and area has been shaved. Rinse frequently.
   c. Repeat on other cheek.
   d. Use firm short strokes. Shave in direction of hair growth.
   e. Rinse razor frequently.

*(continues)*

**PROCEDURE 27** *(continued)*

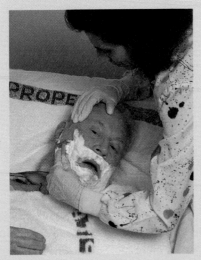

**FIGURE 16-35** Hold the skin with one hand. Using short strokes, bring razor down over cheek toward chin. Start near the ear. Rinse the razor often in basin.

8. Lather neck area and stroke up toward the chin. Rinse and repeat until all lather is removed.
9. Wash face and neck and dry thoroughly.
10. Apply aftershave lotion if desired.
11. If the skin is nicked, apply pressure directly over the area and then apply an antiseptic and Bandaid. Report incident to nurse.
12. Clean and replace equipment. Dispose of razor according to facility policy. Remove head of electric razor. Use razor brush to remove clippings. Store according to facility policy. Remove and dispose of gloves according to facility policy.
13. Carry out each procedure completion action.

## HAND AND FINGERNAIL CARE

Fingernails are routinely cleaned during the morning care. Use a soft brush and orangewood stick to gently clean under the nails. Fingernail care can also be carried out as a separate procedure. Soak the hands in warm soapy water. Creams can be used to soften the **cuticles**, which can then be gently pushed back with a towel. When cutting the fingernails, follow the curve of the finger and then file any rough edges. Be careful not to injure the corners of the fingers when cutting the nails.

Some facilities do not permit nursing assistants to perform nail care on diabetic residents.

**PROCEDURE 28**

# Hand and Fingernail Care

*Note:* Check with nurse and nursing care plan to learn if this procedure is permitted for the resident or if it is to be modified because of the resident's condition.

This procedure can be carried out independently or can be modified and added to the bath procedure.

*(continues)*

**PROCEDURE 28** *(continued)*

1. Carry out each beginning procedure action.
2. Assemble equipment:
   - Basin with water at 105°F
   - Bath thermometer
   - Soap
   - Bath towel and washcloth
   - Lotion
   - Plastic protector
   - Nail clippers
   - Nail file
   - Orangewood stick
   - Nail polish (optional)
3. Elevate head of bed, if permitted, and adjust the overbed table in front of resident. If resident is allowed out of bed, assist to transfer to a chair and position overbed table waist-high across lap.
4. Place plastic protector on overbed table.
5. Fill basin with warm water at approximately 105°F using bath thermometer to test temperature. Place basin on overbed table.
6. Use a soft brush or orangewood stick to clean under nails.
7. Instruct resident to put hands in basin and soak for approximately 5 minutes. Place towel over basin to help retain heat. Add warm water if necessary. Remember to remove the resident's hands before adding water.
8. Wash hands. Push cuticles back gently with washcloth. (A cream may be used to soften the cuticles first.)
9. Dry hands with towel.
10. Use nail clippers to cut fingernails straight across. Do not cut below tips of fingers. Keep nail cuts on protector to be discarded.
11. Shape and smooth fingernails with nail file. Apply polish to nails if the resident desires.
12. Pour small amount of lotion in your palms and gently smooth on resident's hands.
13. Empty basin of water. Gather equipment, clean, and store according to facility policy.
14. Return overbed table to foot of bed. If resident has been sitting up for the procedure, assist into bed.
15. Carry out each procedure completion action.

# FOOT AND TOENAIL CARE

Residents should be given routine foot care, including bathing, massage of the feet, and attention to the toenails. Proceed carefully:

- Dry feet carefully after soaking in warm water.
- Give special attention to drying between the toes.
- Carefully inspect the feet and apply lotion to dry areas. Pat, rather than rub, lotion on skin.
- Check the resident's toenails. If the nails are thick or curved and need trimming, inform the nurse.

Some residents may require the services of a podiatrist for foot care. The podiatrist will care for the toenails of residents who have poor circulation or diabetes or those whose nails are deformed.

Part of good foot care includes being sure that the resident's shoes fit well and are securely laced so that they offer optimum support.

*Note:* Be sure to check with the nurse and the nursing care plan to learn if this procedure is permitted for the resident. In some cases, this procedure may be modified according to the resident's condition.

## PROCEDURE 29

# Foot and Toenail Care

1. Carry out each beginning procedure action.
2. Assemble equipment:
   - Basin
   - Soap
   - Bath mat
   - Bath thermometer
   - Lotion
   - Nail brush
   - Disposable bed protector
   - Bath towel and washcloth
   - Orangewood stick
3. If permitted, assist resident out of bed and into chair.
4. Place bath mat on floor in front of resident. Fill basin with warm water (105°F). Put basin on bath mat.
5. Remove slippers and allow resident to place feet in water. Cover with bath towel to help retain heat.
6. Soak feet approximately 20 minutes. Add warm water as necessary. Lift feet from water while warm water is being added.
7. At end of soak period, wash feet with soap.
8. Rinse and dry. Note any abnormalities such as corns or calluses.
9. Remove basin, covering feet with towel.
10. Use orangewood stick to gently clean toenails. If nails are long and need to be cut, report this fact to the nurse. Follow facility policy.
11. Pour lotion into palms of hands. Hold hands together to warm lotion and apply gently to feet.
12. Assist resident with socks or stockings and shoes if ambulatory. Otherwise, return resident to bed.
13. Make resident comfortable.
14. Gather equipment, clean, and store according to facility policy. Leave unit neat.
15. Carry out each procedure completion action.

## ORAL HYGIENE

The elderly need good **oral hygiene** just as much as younger people. Regular cleansing by brushing (Figure 16-36) and flossing should be carried out routinely three times daily when the resident has any teeth of his or her own. Visits by a dentist can help maintain existing dental function. Older people can develop dental **caries** (cavities) just as readily as younger people. Regular cleaning helps make the breath fresh and eliminates **halitosis** (bad breath). Improved appetite can also result. (See Procedures 30 and 31.)

### Dentures

Many residents wear dentures. Care of dentures includes:

- Cleaning dentures daily under cool running water
- Storing dentures in a safe place when out of the resident's mouth
  In addition, you will care for the resident by:
- Cleaning and checking the resident's mouth daily for signs of irritation
- Checking resident's lips for cracking and dryness
- Applying creams, petroleum jelly, or glycerin to lips for excessive dryness

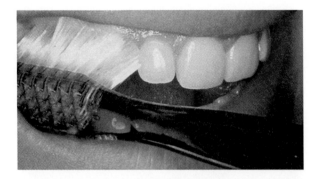

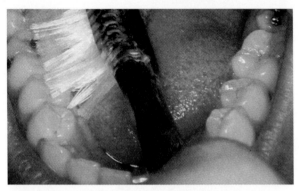

**FIGURE 16-36A** Place the head of the toothbrush beside the teeth, with the bristle tips at a 45° angle against the gumline. Move the brush back and forth in short (half-a-tooth-wide) strokes several times, using a gentle scrubbing motion. Brush the outer surfaces of each tooth, upper and lower, keeping the bristles angled against the gumline. (Toothbrushing photos and descriptions complements of American Dental Association)

**FIGURE 16-36B** Use the same method on the inside surfaces of all teeth, still using short back-and-forth strokes.

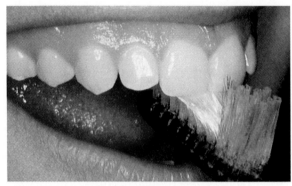

**FIGURE 16-36D** To clean the inside surfaces of the front teeth, tilt the brush vertically and make several gentle up-and-down strokes with the "toe" (the front part) of the brush.

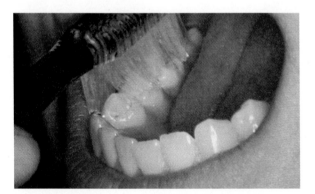

**FIGURE 16-36C** Scrub the chewing surfaces of the teeth.

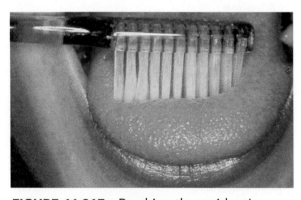

**FIGURE 16-36E** Brushing the resident's tongue will help freshen breath and clean the mouth by removing bacteria.

Many residents have partial plates, which are removable but attached by small metal clips. Partial plates should be given the same care as full dentures.

Dentures should be stored in a denture cup inside the bedside stand when not in use. Some residents prefer storing dentures dry while most prefer to store dentures in a special solution. If

## PROCEDURE 30
## Assisting Resident to Brush Teeth

1. Carry out each beginning procedure action.
2. Assemble equipment:
   - Disposable gloves
   - Emesis basin
   - Toothbrush
   - Toothpaste
   - Glass of cool water
   - Mouthwash (if permitted)
   - Hand towel
   - Bed protector
   - Dental floss
3. Elevate head of bed. Help resident into comfortable position.
4. Lower side rails and position overbed table across resident's lap.
5. Cover table with protector and place equipment on table (Figure 16-37).
6. Place towel across resident's chest.
7. Be prepared to help as resident brushes and flosses teeth. Use gloves if you do assist.
8. After resident has brushed teeth, push overbed table to foot of bed.
9. Gather equipment, clean, and store according to facility policy. Place soiled linen in proper receptacle.
10. Remove disposable gloves, if used, and discard gloves according to facility policy.
11. Lower head of bed. Help resident to assume comfortable position and adjust bedding.
12. Raise side rails.
13. Carry out each procedure completion action.

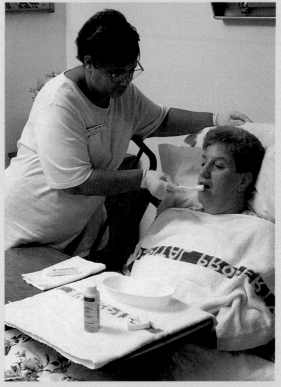

**FIGURE 16-37** Equipment for oral hygiene is assembled and placed on the resident's overbed table.

in doubt, store dentures in water when out of the mouth to keep them moist and prevent cracking. (See Procedure 32.)

Residents who are unconscious still require oral hygiene. Premoistened swabs may be used, followed by glycerine and lemon. Because the resident cannot participate, the staff must carry out this procedure for the resident. (See Procedure 33.)

## PROCEDURE 31

# Cleaning and Flossing Resident's Teeth

1. Carry out each beginning procedure action.
2. Assemble equipment:
   - Disposable gloves
   - Emesis basin
   - Toothbrush
   - Toothpaste
   - Glass of cool water
   - Mouthwash (if permitted)
   - Hand towel
   - Bed protector
   - Dental floss
3. Elevate head of bed. Help resident into a comfortable position.
4. Lower side rails and position overbed table across resident's lap.
5. Place protector on overbed table and arrange equipment on table.
6. Place towel across the resident's chest.
7. Put on disposable gloves.
8. Place toothpaste on moistened toothbrush.
9. Clean all surfaces of each tooth. Use a sweeping motion working from gumline to tip of tooth.
10. Have resident rinse mouth into emesis basin.
11. Select a piece of dental floss about twelve inches long. Wrap ends of dental floss around middle fingers, leaving center area free (Figure 16-38).
12. Ask resident to open his or her mouth. Gently insert floss between each tooth down to, but *not into*, gumline.
13. Ask resident to rinse mouth using emesis basin.
14. Wipe resident's face dry with towel.
15. Push overbed table to the foot of bed.

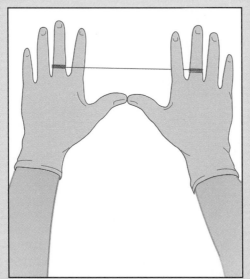 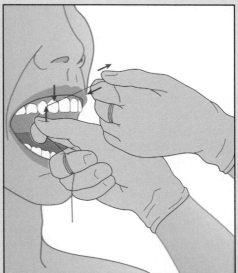

**FIGURE 16-38**   Floss is wrapped around the middle fingers (left). The proper method of using the floss to clean between the teeth (right).

*(continues)*

**PROCEDURE *31* (continued)**

16. Gather equipment, clean, and store according to facility policy. Place soiled linen in proper receptacle.
17. Remove and discard gloves according to facility policy.

18. Position resident comfortably. Be sure that water and call bell are close at hand.
19. Raise and secure side rails.
20. Carry out each procedure completion action.

**PROCEDURE**
**32**
## Caring for Dentures

OBRA

1. Carry out each beginning procedure action.
2. Assemble equipment:
   - Disposable gloves
   - Tissues
   - Emesis basin
   - Tongue depressor
   - Brush
   - Toothpaste or tooth powder
   - Mouthwash, if permitted
   - Gauze squares
   - Applicators
   - Denture cup
3. Apply disposable gloves.
4. Allow resident to clean dentures if he or she is able to do so. If resident cannot, give tissue to resident and ask him or her to remove dentures. Assist if necessary. *To remove upper dentures:* Grasp dentures firmly, ease downward and then forward, and remove from the mouth. *To remove lower dentures:* Grasp dentures firmly, ease upward and then backward, and remove from the mouth.
5. Place dentures in denture cup padded with gauze squares. Take to bathroom or utility room.

6. Place a paper towel or washcloth in the bottom of the basin to protect the dentures. Add a small amount of cool water.
7. Dentures may be soaked in a solution with a cleansing tablet before brushing, if necessary.
8. Put toothpaste or tooth powder on brush. Hold dentures and brush until all surfaces are clean (Figure 16-39).

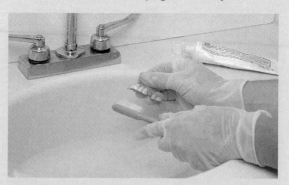

**FIGURE 16-39** Place a paper towel or washcloth on the bottom of the sink and partially fill with water. Place toothpaste or denture cleaning paste on the brush and hold the dentures over the sink while you brush them clean. Rinse with warm water. Never use hot water on dentures.

*(continues)*

**PROCEDURE 32** *(continued)*

9. Rinse dentures thoroughly under cool or warm running water. Never use hot water. Rinse denture cup.
10. Place fresh gauze squares in denture cup with clean cool water unless instructed otherwise.
11. Place dentures in cup and take them to bedside.
12. Assist resident to rinse mouth with mouthwash, if permitted. Otherwise use water. Hold mouth open gently with wooden tongue depressor. Clean gums and tongue with applicators moistened with mouthwash or use foam "toothettes."
13. Use tissue or gauze to hand wet dentures to resident. Insert if necessary.
14. Clean and replace equipment according to facility policy.
15. Remove and dispose of gloves according to facility policy.
16. Carry out each procedure completion action.

**PROCEDURE 33** Assisting with Special Oral Hygiene

1. Carry out each beginning procedure action.
2. Assemble equipment:
   - Disposable gloves
   - Emesis basin
   - Bath towel
   - Plastic bag
   - Premoistened applicators
   - Tissues
   - Tongue depressor
   - Water-based lubricant for lips
3. Put on disposable gloves.
4. Cover pillow with towel and turn resident's head to one side. Place emesis basin under resident's chin.
5. Gently pull down on chin to open mouth.
6. Using premoistened applicators, wipe gums, teeth, tongue, and inside of mouth (Figure 16-40).

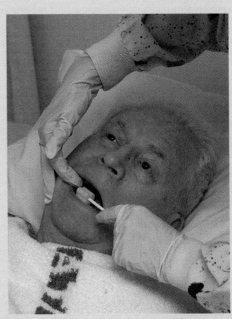

**FIGURE 16-40** Using premoistened applicators, wipe gums, teeth, and tongue.

*(continues)*

---

**PROCEDURE 33** *(continued)*

7. Discard used applicators in plastic bag.
8. Using clean applicators, apply lubricant to lips. Place used applicators in plastic bag.
9. Clean and replace equipment.

10. Remove and discard gloves according to facility policy.
11. Carry out each procedure completion action.

---

## DRESSING RESIDENT

Residents are encouraged to wear their own clothes because it contributes to their sense of identity. If residents are not confined to bed they dress after morning care every day.

Some residents will be able to dress themselves with assistance; those who are totally dependent will have to be dressed by the staff. It is part of your responsibility to see that the clothing is clean and neat and in good repair. You should remember to:

- Whenever possible, allow the resident to choose the clothing to be put on. The clothing should be lightweight but provide adequate warmth. Do not offer too many choices because that may confuse the resident.

- Encourage resident to participate, in the dressing or undressing procedure, to the extent of ability.

The resident who requires complete help is easiest to dress in bed. Residents who can help themselves may wish to sit in a chair with clothing placed nearby. You can help by:

- Arranging the clothing in the order that it will be put on.
- Being prepared to assist with shoes and stockings even for residents who can do much themselves. Bending over to adjust shoes and stockings can result in dizziness and loss of balance.
- Removing clothing from unaffected or strongest side first if the resident has difficulty moving one side or is paralyzed.

---

**PROCEDURE 34** ## Dressing and Undressing Resident

1. Carry out each beginning procedure action.
2. Select appropriate clothing and arrange in order of application. Encourage resident to participate in selection.
3. Cover resident with bath blanket and fan-fold top bedclothes to foot of bed.

4. Elevate head of bed to sitting position.
5. Assist resident to comfortable sitting position.
6. Remove night clothing, keeping resident covered with bath blanket. Remove from strong side first and then from weaker side. Place in laundry hamper.

*(continues)*

**PROCEDURE 34** *(continued)*

7. If the resident wears a bra, slip straps over resident's hands (weak side first), move straps up arms, and position on shoulders. Adjust breasts in cups of bra. Then hook bra in back (assist resident to lean forward so bra can be fastened).

8. For an undershirt, or any garment that slips on over the head:
   a. Gather undershirt and place it over the resident's head.
   b. Grasp resident's hand and guide it through the arm hole by reaching into the arm hole from the outside.
   c. Repeat procedure with opposite arm.
   d. Assist resident to lean forward, and adjust undershirt so it is smooth over upper body.

9. Alternate procedure for slipover garments:
   *Note:* Garment must be large enough or made of stretchy fabric for this procedure.
   a. Place garment front side down on resident's lap with bottom opening facing the resident.
   b. Put resident's hands into bottom of garment and, one at a time, into the sleeve holes.
   c. Pull the sleeves up as far as possible on the resident's arms and pull hands through at wrist if it is a long-sleeved garment. The garment should now be high on the resident's chest.
   d. Gather up the back of the garment with your hand and slip the garment over the resident's head.
   e. Smooth the garment down and position it comfortably about the resident's body. Adjust sleeves and shoulders as needed.

10. Shirts or dresses that fasten in the front:
    a. Insert your hand through sleeve of garment and grasp hand of resident, drawing sleeve over your hand and resident's.
    b. Adjust sleeve at shoulder.
    c. Assist resident to sit forward. Arrange clothing across back.
    d. Gather sleeve on opposite side by slipping your hand in from the outside.
    e. Grasp resident's wrist and pull sleeve of garment over your hand and resident's hand. Draw upward and adjust at shoulder.
    f. Button, zip, or snap garment.

11. Underwear or slacks:
    a. Facing foot of bed, gather resident's underwear from waist to leg hole.
    b. Slip underwear over one foot at a time. Pull underwear up legs as high as possible.
    c. Assist resident to raise buttocks and draw garment over buttocks and up to waist. If resident cannot raise buttocks, assist resident to roll first to one side as you pull up the garment and then the other side. Adjust garment until it is comfortable.
    d. Fasten garment if required.

12. Socks or knee-high (or thigh-high) stockings:
    a. Roll sock or stocking with heel in back and place over toes.
    b. Draw sock up over foot and adjust until smooth. Pull stockings smoothly up to knee or thigh.
    c. Repeat for other foot.

13. Pantyhose:
    a. Gather pantyhose and adjust over toes and feet. Draw up legs as high as possible.
    b. Draw over hips as described in step 11c. Adjust until comfortable at waist.

14. Shoes:
    a. Slip shoe on, using shoe horn if necessary.

*(continues)*

**PROCEDURE 34** *(continued)*

b. Be sure shoe is fastened securely (Velcro tabs or ties). If the shoes tie, be sure that ends of shoelaces do not drag on the floor. The shoes should be fastened tight enough to prevent them from slipping off the resident's feet but not so tight that circulation is impaired.

c. Shoes should have rubber soles for better traction. Leather soles slide easily on tile and linoleum floors.

15. To undress, reverse order of steps.
16. Carry out each procedure completion action.

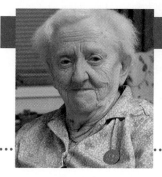

## LESSON SYNTHESIS: Putting It All Together

*Y*ou have just completed this lesson. Now go back and review the Clinical Focus. Try to see how the Clinical Focus relates to the concepts presented in the lesson. Then answer the following questions.

1. Do older persons really care about how they look? What relationship does appearance have to self-esteem?

2. What danger does Mary Mandell face because of sitting in a wheelchair for so many hours?

3. What evidence is there to concern the staff and what steps must be taken?

4. How can the nursing assistant help Mary Mandell feel that she still has some control over her personal hygiene?

## REVIEW

A. Match each term (items a.–e.) with the proper definition.

a. caries
b. pressure ulcer
c. lesions
d. dentures
e. skin tears

1. _____ skin breakdown due to prolonged pressure over bony prominences

2. _____ artificial teeth

3. _____ changes in skin structure

4. _____ small breaks in the skin

5. _____ dental cavities

B. Brief answers

6. Name five factors that contribute to skin breakdown.

7. List three ways you can encourage adequate circulation to tissues.

8. Briefly describe each of the four stages of pressure ulcer development.

9. Name five basic positions that are routinely used to ensure that pressure is not prolonged on any body part.

10. List five ways to relieve pressure on body parts.

**C. Fill in the blanks by selecting the correct word or phrase from the list.**

| | |
|---|---|
| dentures | senile lentigines |
| diabetes | skin tears |
| friction | strong |
| oral hygiene | turning schedule |
| pressure ulcers | weak |
| sacrum | |

11. Liver spots are more properly called _____.

12. Small breaks that occur in fragile skin are called _____.

13. When body parts rub together _____ results, which may cause tissue damage.

14. Skin breakdown may progress to the formation of deep, painful lesions called _____.

15. For residents who are confined to bed, a _____ is followed to relieve pressure on body parts.

16. One of the most common sites for skin breakdown is the _____.

17. Generally, nursing assistants are not allowed to perform nail care, especially toenail care, on residents with _____.

18. The process of cleaning teeth, the tongue, and the inside of the mouth is called _____.

19. Artificial teeth are known as _____.

20. When dressing a resident with a weakness on one side due to a stroke or other condition, clothing is applied to the _____ side first. Clothing is removed from the _____ side first.

**D. Select the one best answer for each of the following.**

21. Which of the following is not a function of the skin?
    a. perception of sensations
    b. regulation of body temperature
    c. protection of structures under the skin
    d. production of insulin

22. Which of the following is a characteristic of the aging skin?
    a. skin glands produce more oil
    b. fingernails and toenails thin
    c. sweat glands increase activity
    d. circulation to the skin decreases

23. Shearing of tissues is most likley to occur when the resident
    a. is resting on her abdomen
    b. is positioned with the head of the bed elevated
    c. is walking around
    d. is resting flat on her back in bed

24. Select the best position for the resident considering the condition given.
    a. Position the resident with respiratory problems flat in bed.
    b. Position the resident who has had a recent stroke by turning her on the affected side.
    c. Position the resident who has had a recent stroke by turning her on the unaffected side.
    d. Position the resident who has a fractured hip by rotating her over the unaffected leg.

**E. Clinical Experience**

25. Janine was assisting Mrs. Docker with her tub bath when Mrs. Docker said she felt dizzy. What action should Janine take?

26. Carl is giving foot care to Mr. Dobrinski. The toenails are long and thick. What action should Carl take?

27. Chris is shaving Mr. Gates who moves suddenly. A small nick is made by the razor in the skin. How should Chris handle this situation?

28. Mrs. Marks has long curly hair that frequently tangles. How can Holly, her nursing assistant, care for Mrs. Marks' hair during morning care to reduce the amount of tangles?

# Meeting the Residents' Nutritional Needs

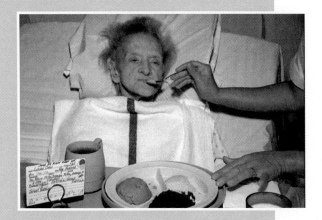

## CLINICAL FOCUS

Think about how food is processed by the body and how you can help residents meet their nutritional needs as you study this lesson and meet:

*M*rs. Hartley, a Christian Scientist, who is 92 and almost blind. Although she can make out light and dark, everything is blurred and shadowy. She has a cold and wants to rest in bed instead of going to the dining room to eat. Nursing assistants are serving trays and assisting residents to eat. Mrs. Hartley has dentures and an order for a soft diet. The nursing assistant serving trays notes that Mrs. Hartley seems listless and her skin is dry.

## OBJECTIVES

*After studying this lesson, you should be able to:*

- Define and spell vocabulary words and terms.
- Identify the parts and function of the gastrointestinal system.
- Review changes in the digestive system as they relate to the aging process.
- Name the six classes of nutrients.
- List the functions of each class of nutrients.
- Name the six food groups.
- List four diets commonly provided in long-term care facilities.
- Name six therapeutic diets ordered in long-term care facilities.
- Measure intake properly using the metric system.
- State ways the nursing assistant can promote adequate nutrition.

- Assist the resident who can feed herself or himself.
- Feed the dependent resident.
- Provide between meal feedings.
- Provide the resident with fresh water.
- List alternate ways of delivering nutrition.
- Briefly describe seven gastrointestinal disorders.
- Demonstrate the following:

| | |
|---|---|
| Procedure 35 | Measuring and Recording Fluid Intake |
| Procedure 36 | Assisting the Resident Who Can Feed Self |
| Procedure 37 | Feeding the Dependent Resident |

# VOCABULARY

anus *(AY-nus)*

carbohydrate *(kar-boh-HIGH-drayt)*

colon *(KOH-lon)*

constipation *(kon-stih-PAY-shun)*

cubic centimeter (cc) *(KYOU-bick SEN-tih-mee-ter)*

defecation *(def-eh-KAY-shun)*

dehydration *(dee-high-DRAY-shun)*

digestion *(die-JEST-shun)*

diverticuli *(die-ver-TICK-you-lie)*

diverticulitis *(die-ver-tick-you-LIE-tis)*

duodenum *(dew-oh-DEE-num)*

dyspepsia *(dis-PEP-see-ah)*

dysphagia *(dis-FAY-jee-ah)*

edema *(ee-DEE-mah)*

enzymes *(EN-zighms)*

esophagus *(eh-SOF-ah-gus)*

fats *(fats)*

feces *(FEE-cees)*

fiber *(FYE-ber)*

flatulence *(FLAT-you-lens)*

gastritis *(gas-TRY-tis)*

gastrointestinal tract *(gas-troh-in-TES-tih-nal trackt)*

gastrostomy (G) tube *(gas-TROS-toh-mee toob)*

hemorrhoids *(HEM-oh-royds)*

hernia *(HER-nee-ah)*

hiatal hernia *(high-AY-tal HER-nee-ah)*

high density *(high DEN-sih-tee)*

hyperalimentation *(high-per-al-ih-men-TAY-shun)*

intake and output (I&O) *(IN-tayk and OUT-put)*

ileum *(ILL-ee-um)*

inguinal hernia *(ING-gwih-nal HER-nee-ah)*

jejunum *(jeh-JOO-num)*

metric system *(MET-rick SIS-tum)*

milliliter (mL) *(MILL-ih-lee-ter)*

mineral *(MIN-er-al)*

nasogastric (NG) tube *(nay-zoh-GAS-trick toob)*

obesity *(oh-BEES-ih-tee)*

pharynx *(FAR-inks)*

protein *(PROH-tee-in)*

regularity *(reg-you-LAIR-ih-tee)*

rupture *(RUP-chur)*

therapeutic *(ther-ah-PYOU-tick)*

total parenteral nutrition (TPN) *(TOH-tal pah-REN-ter-al new-TRISH-un)*

vitamin *(VYE-tah-min)*

water *(WOT-er)*

## THE DIGESTIVE SYSTEM

The digestive system processes the foods eaten, releasing simple nutrients that are needed by the body. There are six nutrients: vitamins, minerals, water, fats, proteins, and carbohydrates. The nutrients pass through the wall of the intestine into the bloodstream; they are carried in the blood to where they are used by the body cells.

Chemicals (**enzymes**) help break down or digest the food, and the nondigestible portion of what is eaten is eliminated from the body as solid waste called **feces**. This process is called a bowel movement (BM) or **defecation**.

The digestive system (Figure 17-1) is also called the **gastrointestinal tract**. It is a tube about 30 feet long, stretching from the mouth to the end opening called the **anus**. The walls of the tube are made of smooth muscle and the entire tract is lined with mucous membrane. The digestive system consists of the true digestive organs:

- Mouth (Figure 17-2)
- **Pharynx**
- **Esophagus**

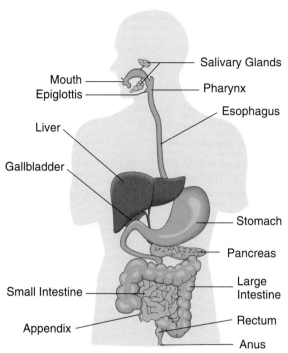

Mouth
Epiglottis
Salivary Glands
Pharynx
Esophagus
Liver
Gallbladder
Stomach
Pancreas
Small Intestine
Large Intestine
Appendix
Rectum
Anus

**FIGURE 17-1**  The digestive system

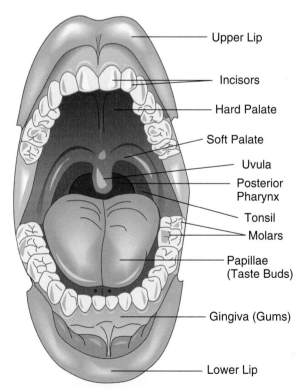

Upper Lip
Incisors
Hard Palate
Soft Palate
Uvula
Posterior Pharynx
Tonsil
Molars
Papillae (Taste Buds)
Gingiva (Gums)
Lower Lip

**FIGURE 17-2**  The mouth

- Stomach
- Small intestine
- Large intestine

The true digestive organs receive the help of other organs in breaking food into simpler substances. These organs are called accessory organs and include the:

- Tongue
- Salivary glands
- Teeth
- Liver
- Pancreas
- Gallbladder

The liver produces bile, which is stored in the gallbladder. The pancreas produces digestive enzymes as well as the hormones insulin and glucagon. The tongue and teeth mechanically break down the food and direct it toward the rest of the tract.

## THE DIGESTIVE PROCESS

The process of **digestion** is both mechanical and chemical. Foods are broken up and moved along the tract by rhythmic muscular contractions. At the same time, digestive enzymes and bile are mixed with the food. The digestive enzymes from the stomach, pancreas, and small intestine (Figure 17-3) together with bile chemically break the foods into simple nutrients:

- Proteins are changed to amino acids.
- Carbohydrates are changed to simple sugars like glucose.
- Fats are changed to fatty acids and glycerol.

The undigestible portion of food is moved along in the intestines and finally excreted from the body as feces.

### Mouth

Digestion begins in the mouth. The teeth and tongue break the food into smaller pieces, mix it with saliva, and form a rounded mass of food. The food is swallowed into the pharynx and moves down the esophagus into the stomach.

The tongue is a skeletal muscle covered with taste buds. It:

- Pushes the food between the teeth
- Propels the food backward to aid swallowing
- Assists in speech

**FIGURE 17-3** Enzymes and digestion

| Organ | Important Enzymes | Food Acted On |
|---|---|---|
| Salivary glands | Salivary amylase | Starches |
| Stomach | Pepsin<br>Lipase<br>Renin (infants) | Proteins<br>Fats<br>Milk protein |
| Pancreas | Lipase<br>Amylase<br>Trypsin | Fats<br>Starches<br>Proteins |
| Small intestine | Lactase<br>Sucrase<br>Maltase<br>Peptidase | Lactose (sugar)<br>Sucrose (sugar)<br>Maltose (sugar)<br>Protein |

Salivary glands secrete saliva. It contains an enzyme, salivary amylase, to start carbohydrate digestion. Saliva:

- Moistens food for easier swallowing
- Amounts to about 1½ quarts daily in the average adult. The amount of fluid varies with the person and may be altered by specific health problems.

Teeth mechanically break up the food. They:

- Number 32 in the adult
- May be replaced by dentures when lost

The pharynx is a common passageway for:

- Food to the esophagus
- Air to the trachea

The gag reflex normally occurs if food begins to go into the trachea instead of the esophagus. This causes coughing and clearing of the airway.

## Stomach

The stomach begins protein digestion by the action of the enzyme pepsin and hydrochloric acid (HCl). It:

- Holds the food about 4 hours
- Churns and mixes the gastric juice with the food to form a liquid

## Small Intestine

The small intestine is about 20 feet long and is coiled in the abdominal cavity. It is divided into three parts:

- **Duodenum**
- **Jejunum**
- **Ileum**

The small intestine is attached by the duodenum to the stomach and by the ileum to the large intestine.

**FIGURE 17-4** Basic nutrients and their functions

| Nutrient | Form Used | Function |
|---|---|---|
| Complex carbohydrates | Glucose | Supply blood sugar—primary energy for body |
| Proteins | Amino acids | Build and repair tissues |
| Fats | Fatty acids<br>Glycerol | Supply stored energy<br>Needed to benefit from fat-soluble vitamins |
| Water | Water | Needed to carry on body chemistry |
| Vitamins | Fat-soluble—A,D,K,E<br>Water-soluble—B,C | Act as co-enzymes in promoting body activities |
| Minerals | Calcium, phosphorus, potassium, sodium, and traces of others | Important in formation of body tissues and body chemistry |

The small intestine produces a fluid containing digestive enzymes and receives:

- Food from the stomach
- Bile from the liver and gallbladder to begin fat breakdown
- Pancreatic fluid from the pancreas, which completes the breakdown of:
    - Proteins to amino acids
    - Carbohydrates to simple sugar (glucose)
    - Fats to fatty acids and glycerol

Most of the digestion and absorption of nutrients occurs in the small intestine. Figure 17-4 shows the functions of the basic nutrients and the forms in which they are used in the body.

As food moves slowly through the small intestine, the simple nutrients pass through the wall of the intestine and into the bloodstream where they are carried to the liver for more action before being used by the body cells.

Once released from foods, the following nutrients can be absorbed directly:

- Water
- Vitamins
- Minerals

### Large Intestine

The large intestine is called the **colon**. It extends from the end of the small intestine to the rectum, which ends in the anus. It is not as long as the small intestine. Its main purpose is to carry the unused food out of the body, but some vitamins and water are absorbed through the colon walls. A muscle holds the anus closed and can be voluntarily relaxed to permit defecation.

## AGING CHANGES

As the body ages some changes take place in the digestive process.

- The flow of enzymes is somewhat decreased.
- The muscular walls of the tract lose some tone and strength so that movement along the tract is slower.
- The gag reflex that prevents food from slipping into the trachea is not as active, so choking is possible.
- Absorption of nutrients is slower.

Figure 17-5 is a summary of the changes in the digestive process that are the result of aging.

**FIGURE 17-5**  Changes in the digestive system caused by aging

- Decreased taste buds
- Reduced digestive enzymes
- Thicker saliva
- Tongue more sensitive
- Movement of food not as efficient
- More **flatulence** (gas production)
- Less effective gag reflex
- Poorer tolerance to some foods
- Slower absorption of nutrients
- Decreased chewing/poor dentures
- Weaker muscular walls
- **Constipation** (difficult defecation) more common

Some older persons find they may not tolerate foods they previously enjoyed.

## NUTRIENTS

Nutrients provide us with essential materials to:

- Build and repair tissues
- Perform body functions
- Provide energy for the work the body does

It takes energy to perform activities such as walking or getting in and out of bed. Even when a person is quiet and inactive, energy is needed for the heart to beat and for the kidneys to produce urine. These are examples of vital body activities that sustain life.

Energy is supplied by the nutrients in the foods we eat. The amount of energy from nutrients is measured in units of heat called calories. When not enough nutrients are eaten, the body gradually uses up its stored supply and becomes depleted; illness follows.

## Classes of Nutrients

There are six classes of nutrients. Many foods contain more than one nutrient. The basic nutrients are:

- Carbohydrates
- Fats
- Proteins
- Vitamins
- Minerals
- Water

**Carbohydrates** are the primary source of immediate body energy. One gram of carbohydrates provides 4 calories of energy. Many foods contain this nutrient. Fruits, vegetables, breads, cereal, and pasta products are good sources. Carbohydrate foods supply the body with **fiber**. Fiber helps maintain **regularity** (bowel activity).

**Fats** provide energy and are found in both plant and animal foods. One gram of fat provides 9 calories of energy. Sources of fats include butter, meat, nuts, egg yolks, and vegetable oils.

**Proteins** are essential for tissue building and repair. One gram of protein provides 4 calories. Foods rich in protein include meats, fish, poultry, eggs, beans, nuts, and lentils.

**Vitamins** and **minerals** regulate body processes. The different kinds of vitamins are represented by letters. Vitamins A, D, K, and E are fat soluble and are found in fatty foods as well as in fruits and vegetables. Vitamins B and C are water soluble and are found in fruits, vegetables, and whole grain products. The minerals include sodium, potassium, calcium, and iron.

**Water** is essential to life. Each person needs to take in about 2½ quarts (2½ liters or 2,500 milliliters [mL]) of water in some form daily. (In certain circumstances, under a doctor's order, water intake may be limited.) Water is consumed in drinks such as plain water, tea, coffee, and other beverages. Water is also taken in with foods such as fruits and vegetables that have high water content.

# FOOD GROUPS

Food can be classified into six food groups. Adequate selections from each group ensure proper nutrition. The six food groups are the:

- Bread, cereal, rice, and pasta group
- Fruit group
- Vegetable group
- Milk, yogurt, and cheese group
- Meat, poultry, fish, dry beans, eggs, and nuts group
- Fats, oils, and sweets group

In 1990, the United States Department of Agriculture (USDA) revised the guidelines for healthy nutrition. The guidelines explained the food groups from which selections could be made. They also named the number of servings that should be taken from each group. The report emphasized that for most adult Americans:

- The overall calories should be decreased.
- Sugars and salts should be used in moderation.
- Fats, oils, and cholesterol (animal fat) should be limited.
- Alcohol, if consumed at all, should be used in moderation.

## Food Guide Pyramid

In 1992, the USDA presented the Food Guide Pyramid. This is the official visual guide to help people understand the new written guidelines (Figure 17-6).

Look carefully at the pyramid. You will see that the bread, cereal, rice, and pasta group is at the base of the pyramid. Selections from this group should make up the biggest part of the diet. Fats, oils, and sweets are at the very small top of the pyramid, meaning that these foods should be only a very small part of the total diet.

Selections must be made from each group in the amounts indicated because important nutrients for the body's well-being are found in each group.

## The Bread, Cereal, Rice, and Pasta Group (6–11 Servings Daily)

This food group provides:

- Carbohydrates for energy
- Vitamins such as vitamin B
- Minerals such as iron
- Roughage or fiber

Members of this group generally have little fat and provide fiber. The fiber adds bulk, which helps to satisfy appetite and promotes bowel activity and elimination. Whole grains and enriched products provide the richest source of fibers and nutrients. Making varied selections ensures that different types of fibers will be included in the diet.

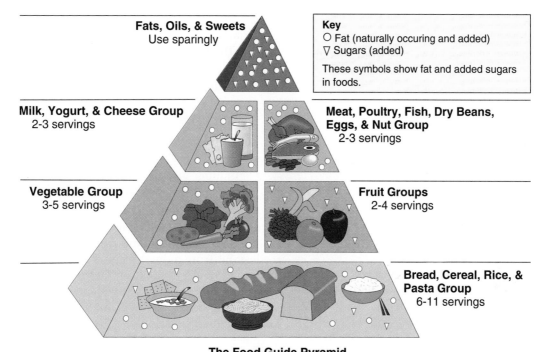

**The Food Guide Pyramid**
A guide to daily food choices

**FIGURE 17-6** The Food Guide Pyramid illustrates the fundamentals of healthy nutrition. (Courtesy of USDA)

Examples of single servings from this group are:

- 1 slice of bread
- ½ bun, or bagel, or English muffin
- 1 ounce of ready-to-eat cereal
- ½ cup of cooked cereal, rice, or pasta

## The Fruit Group (2–4 Servings Daily)

This food group provides:

- Vitamins
- Minerals
- Fiber
- Carbohydrates

Include melons, berries, and citrus fruits regularly. Citrus fruits are a good source of vitamin C, which must be replaced daily. Fruits may be served as juices and make good desserts.

Examples of single servings from this group are:

- 1 medium apple, orange, or banana
- ½ cup small or diced fruit
- ¾ cup fruit juice

## The Vegetable Group (3–5 Servings Daily)

This food group provides:

- Vitamins such as A and C and folic acid
- Minerals
- Carbohydrates
- Fiber

Include dark green leafy and deep yellow vegetables often. Dried beans and peas may be counted as either a vegetable serving or may be substituted for 1 ounce of meat. Dried beans and peas provide the nutrients of the vegetables and contain some of the important proteins found in meat.

Starchy vegetables, such as potatoes, provide complex carbohydrates as well as other nutrients and should be considered as part of the vegetable selections.

Fruits and vegetables can be made easier to chew by:

- Cooking
- Chopping

- Dicing
- Pureeing

Examples of single servings from this group are:

- 1 cup raw, leafy vegetables
- ½ cup dry beans or peas
- ½ cup other vegetables

## The Milk, Yogurt, and Cheese Group (2–3 Servings Daily)

This food group provides:

- Protein for tissue building and repair
- Minerals such as calcium and phosphorus
- Vitamins such as A, B, and D

Low-fat milk and yogurt provide the same essential nutrients without as many calories from fat.

One serving of milk has about the same amount of calcium as:

- 1 cup of yogurt
- 2½ slices of cheese
- 1 cup of pudding
- 2 cups of cottage cheese

Examples of single servings from this group are:

- 1 cup milk
- 1 cup yogurt
- 1½ ounces cheese
- 1 cup pudding
- 2 cups cottage cheese

## The Meat, Poultry, Fish, Dry Beans, Eggs, and Nuts Group (2–3 Servings Daily)

This food group provides:

- High-quality protein
- Vitamins such as D and B
- Minerals such as iron and zinc
- Fats

The amount of fat in this food group can be reduced by:

- Preparing properly, for example, baking rather than frying
- Choosing lean cuts of beef and poultry
- Removing poultry skin because the fat immediately under it adds to the total calories if eaten

An example of a single serving from this group is:

(Total intake = 6 ounces)

- ½ cup dry beans or peas = 1 ounce meat serving

## The Fats, Oils, and Sweets Group

This food group provides:

- Energy
- Vitamins such as A and D

These nutrients can be obtained from other food sources that will not raise the calorie level as high. It is recommended that less than 30% of the daily calories come from fat sources. Eating less fat from animal sources will help lower the cholesterol and the total fat in the diet. High levels of cholesterol and other fats in the blood can cause serious health problems. Therefore, use fats and oils sparingly.

## Sugars and Salt

Added sugar and salt may make food pleasing to the taste but often mask the natural flavors of the foods. Sugar and salt should be used in moderation.

Sugars left in the mouth favor bacterial growth, contributing to dental cavities. Many so-called sweets, such as desserts and candy, provide calories but little nourishment.

Salt (sodium chloride) is widely found in food. Therefore, a varied diet will provide adequate amounts of salt for health. It should not be necessary to add it to the cooking process or at the table. Salt does increase the pleasure of eating for many people, but it should be used in moderation.

## Alcoholic Beverages

Alcoholic beverages add nothing to the diet but calories and are not essential to a healthy diet. Because of the potential for addiction, injuries due to impaired behavior, and birth defects, it is wise to avoid routine consumption of alcoholic beverages.

If alcohol is consumed, it should be done moderately. At present, moderate drinking is considered to be:

- No more than 2 drinks per day for men
- No more than 1 drink per day for women

Count as one drink:

- 12 ounces of regular beer
- 5 ounces of wine
- 1½ ounces of distilled spirits (80 proof)

# NUTRITIONAL STATUS

Eating to meet nutritional needs is one of major activities of daily living. Elderly people who live independently may prepare foods that satisfy their appetites, yet do not meet basic nutritional needs.

**Obesity** (the condition of being overweight) and **dehydration** (inadequate fluid level in the body) are problems for more than 20% of older persons. Obesity is taking in more calories than the body needs. Dehydration is often due to inadequate water intake or excessive water loss.

Easy-to-chew, high-calorie foods may provide energy in excess of body needs; the extra energy is stored as fat. Although the person's appetite is satisfied by these foods, they do not necessarily provide the nutrients needed. Essential vitamins, minerals, and proteins may be lacking.

# DIETS

Some residents may need to have their diets modified because of health problems. Special diets are based on the food groups described

## BUILDING CULTURAL AWARENESS

- Remember that food may have an important relationship to cultural practices.
- Learn the cultural dietary preferences of the residents in your care.
- Check with the nurse if food is brought in by the family to be sure it is permitted on the resident's diet.
- Report to the nurse if the resident is not eating because of cultural preferences.

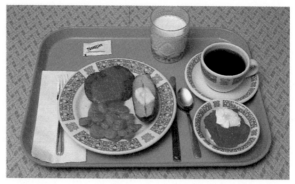

**FIGURE 17-7** Well-balanced, smaller servings are more appealing to the elderly appetite.

previously, but consistency and method of preparation may be altered.

## Standard Diets

Four standard diets are offered in long-term care facilities. They are the:

1. Regular diet
2. Mechanical soft diet
3. Pureed diet
4. Clear liquid diet

**Regular Diet.** The regular diet is prepared for most residents. It includes varied selections from the food groups. It is rich in vitamins and minerals and provides adequate bulk and balanced calories (Figure 17-7).

**Mechanical Soft Diet.** The mechanical soft diet is based on the regular diet but includes liquids and semisolid foods that are more easily chewed and digested (Figure 17-8).

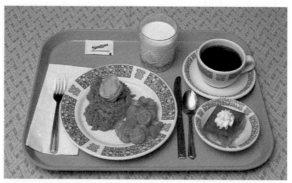

**FIGURE 17-8** The mechanical soft diet is easy to chew and digest.

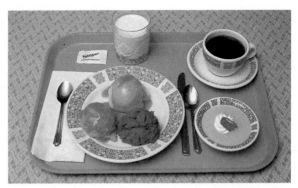

**FIGURE 17-9** The pureed diet includes foods from each of the food groups. The foods have been placed through a blender.

**Pureed Diet.** The pureed diet meets nutritional needs with foods that can be put into semiliquid or liquid form at room temperature (Figure 17-9). It may be given to residents with diseases of the intestinal tract or those who are unable to chew because of infection, stroke, or lack of teeth.

**Clear Liquid Diet.** The clear liquid diet is usually prescribed when a resident is ill and needs to have fluids replaced. This diet is not given for prolonged periods because it does not provide adequate nutrition. Milk is not included in the clear liquid diet because the liquids must be clear (that is, you can see through them), but broths and filtered fruit juices are permitted.

## Therapeutic Diets

**Therapeutic** diets, also called special diets, are prepared for residents with specific needs (Figure 17-10). They include the:

1. Diabetic diet
2. Low sodium diet
3. Low fat diet
4. Calorie restricted diet
5. High protein diet
6. Low residue diet

The diabetic diet is usually a carefully balanced diet for residents who have diabetes mellitus and who must restrict concentrated sugar (for example, candy or pastry) in their diet. They may eat only foods on their diet, but they must eat everything that is ordered for them. It is important that you report the exact amounts of foods eaten by the diabetic resident because their medication is calculated based on food intake.

The low sodium diet is prescribed for the resident with a heart condition or one who retains fluids. The low fat diet limits the amounts of fats in the diet and is served to residents who have gallbladder, cardiovascular, or liver disease. The

| **FIGURE 17-10** Summary of therapeutic diets | |
|---|---|
| Diabetic | Amounts of carbohydrates, fats, and proteins are balanced and prescribed. Concentrated sweets are restricted. |
| Low Sodium (Sodium Restricted) | Amounts of sodium specifically prescribed, such as 500 mg sodium. Sodium-rich foods such as milk and bacon or salted nuts are excluded. |
| Low Fat | Foods with high fat content are restricted, such as whole milk and eggs. Eliminates use of fats in preparation of food. |
| Calorie Restricted | Limits the number of calories while ensuring an adequate intake of nutrients. |
| High Protein | High in protein, iron, and vitamins, served in six small meals per day. Hot, spicy foods excluded. |
| Low Residue | Roughage, fresh fruits, and vegetables (except bananas and potatoes), nuts, and whole grains are limited. |

calorie restricted diet is given to residents in need of weight control. The high protein diet is provided for residents who are underweight and poorly nourished and when diseases such as cancer make unusual nutritional demands.

The low residue diet is served to residents who need to limit roughage intake. It is given when residents have lower bowel problems such as colitis and diarrhea.

Remember, special diets are *therapeutic*, which means they are used as *treatments*. Always check to be sure that the resident receives the right tray.

A progressive diet is ordered for many residents after digestive upset, as their conditions permit. The usual progression is:

- Ice chips/sips of water
- Clear liquids
- Full liquids
- Soft or light diet
- Regular diet

## PERSONAL DIETARY PRACTICES

Some people have personal dietary preferences because of their religious beliefs or cultural heritage. Figure 17-11 shows common dietary restrictions for several religious groups.

Foods that are popular and eaten by most people in an area are called *ethnic foods* (Figure 17-12). Often, the ethnicity of the food relates to the way the food is prepared and the seasoning used. Some foods are so satisfying that they have become part of menus all over the world.

Once people have lived in an area for some time they tend to adjust their diets to the food of the area. However, older people and those who are newly arrived to an area may find that it is not easy to adjust. The adjustment is made more difficult when the person is placed on a therapeutic diet.

The dietitian is the best guide in planning diets that conform with dietary needs and ethnic preference.

As a nursing assistant, your close attention, observations, and understanding of your residents can provide valuable information in guiding the planning and preparation of satisfying diets. Make sure your team leader knows if residents are not eating because of their preferences for foods familiar to them.

## INTAKE AND OUTPUT (I&O)

The amount of fluid taken into the body and the amount of fluid lost should be just about equal. The **intake and output (I&O)** is frequently measured and recorded. Imbalances in intake and output can result in fluid imbalances such as **edema** (water retention) and dehydration.

### Intake

Intake includes everything taken in that is liquid at room temperature. For example, included in the intake fluids are:

- Water or tea
- Gelatin, junket, pudding, ice cream
- Fluids given directly into a vein (IV)
- Fluids given by nasogastric tube or gastric tube

### Output

The output includes all fluids lost. This includes:

- Urine
- Perspiration
- Blood
- Diarrhea
- Vomiting
- Wound drainage

### Calculating Fluid (Liquid) Intake (Output is covered in Lesson 18)

Calculating oral fluid intake is the responsibility of the nursing assistant. To do this correctly, you must know:

- The amount of fluid the container holds when full
- How to calculate the amount of fluid the resident drank from the container

The containers used include cups, glasses, soup bowls, water pitchers, milk cartons, ice cream cups, and gelatin and pudding cups. There are many types of containers and facilities do not all use the same kinds. Your facility will have a chart listing the sizes (amount of fluid the con-

**FIGURE 17-11** Religious dietary practices

| Restricted Food | Faith | | | | | | | | | |
|---|---|---|---|---|---|---|---|---|---|---|
| | Christian Science | Roman Catholic | Latter Day Saints (Mormons) | Seventh Day Adventist | Some Baptist | Greek Orthodox (On Fast Days) | Jewish Orthodox | Moslem Islam | Hinduism | Buddhism |
| Coffee | • | | • | • | • | | | | | |
| Tea | • | | • | • | • | | | | | |
| Alcohol | • | | • | • | • | | | • | | |
| Pork/Pork Products | | | | • | | | • Also shellfish | • | | |
| Caffeine-containing Foods | | | • | • | | | | | | |
| Dairy Products | | | | | | • | Certain holy days | | | |
| All Meats | | 1 hour before communion, Ash Wed., Good Friday | | | | Fasting from meat and dairy prod on Wed/Fri during Lent and other holy days | Forbids the serving of milk and milk prod with meat. Regulates food prep. Forbids cooking on the Sabbath. | Fasting during Ramadan during day, feasting at night. | Some are vegetarians. | Meat must be blessed and killed in special ways. Some sects are vegetarians. |

| FIGURE 17-12    Ethnic dietary preferences | | |
|---|---|---|
| **The Netherlands**<br>Smoked fish<br>Rich pastry<br>Cheese<br>Lamb<br>Shellfish<br>Dairy products | **Germany**<br>Smoked meat<br>Fruit<br>Beans<br>Pickled vegetables | **Italy**<br>Pasta<br>Olives (oil)<br>Tomatoes<br>Meat, poultry<br>Parmesan cheese<br>Anise, tarragon, oregano,<br>   bay leaves, basil, spices |
| **The Near East**<br>Lamb<br>Rice<br>Poultry<br>Cracked wheat foods<br>Fish<br>Lemon juice, garlic<br>Spices<br>Perfumed sweets | **South Africa**<br>Bredie (stew of meat/fish<br>   and vegetables/chilies)<br>Pickled/curried fish<br>Corn as porridge<br>Corn on cob<br>Cloves, garlic, cinnamon<br>Spices | **Southeast Asia**<br>Rice<br>Hot, dry curries<br>Chili<br>Shell fish<br>Soy sauce<br>Garlic, citronella<br>Spices |

tainer can hold when full) of the containers used in the facility.

Fluids can be measured using either a standard system (ounce, pint, quart) or the **metric system** (milliliter or cubic centimeter). A comparison of these measurements follows. Note that the abbreviation for milliliter is mL.

| | | |
|---|---|---|
| drop (gtt) | = .06 mL | |
| teaspoon (tsp) | = 5 mL | |
| tablespoon (tbsp) | = 15 mL | |
| ounce (oz) | = 30 mL | |
| pint (pt)   = 16 oz | = 480 mL | |
| quart (qt)   = 32 oz | = 2 pt = 960 mL | |
| gallon (gal) = 128 oz | = 4 qt = 8 pt = 3,840 mL | |

You cannot actually measure what is gone from the container. Therefore, your calculation will be an estimate. It is important that the estimate be as accurate as possible. In facilities, fluid is recorded in **cubic centimeters (cc)** or **milliliters (mL)**. These measurements are the same amount. The preferred measurement is mL, but many facilities still use cc. All liquids and all foods that become liquid at room temperature (ice cream, sherbet, gelatin) are recorded as fluid intake. All fluids taken with meals and between meals are recorded.

To simplify the calculation, some facilities consider a pint to be 500 mL, a quart 1,000 mL, and a gallon 4,000 mL. Some containers may be marked in ounces. The amount measured in ounces must be converted into mL. For example, a can of soda may be marked as 12 ounces. This equals 360 mL (12 × 30 mL where 30 mL is the same as 1 ounce).

To calculate intake when the resident has finished drinking:

- Pick up the container and hold it at eye level.
- Determine whether $\frac{1}{4}$, $\frac{1}{3}$, $\frac{1}{2}$, $\frac{2}{3}$, or $\frac{3}{4}$ of the container of liquid has been consumed. Remember that containers are not filled to the top when full.
- Look at the facility's chart to see how much that type of container holds when it is full (Figure 17-13).
- Calculate the intake by multiplying the amount consumed times the amount the container holds when it is full.

Examples:

1. A juice glass holds 120 mL when full. The resident has consumed half of the juice. The intake is calculated: $\frac{1}{2}$ × 120 (2 into 120) = 60 mL intake.

**FIGURE 17-13** Average container amounts

| |
|---|
| Water glass = 6 oz = 180 mL |
| Styrofoam cup = 6 oz = 180 mL |
| Juice glass (small) = 4 oz = 120 mL |
| Juice glass (large) = 8 oz = 240 mL |
| Full water pitcher (1 qt) = 32 oz = 960 mL |
| Coffee or tea pot = 10 oz = 300 mL |
| Coffee cup = 5 oz = 150 mL |
| Milk carton = 8 oz = 240 mL |
| Soup bowl (small) = 6 oz = 180 mL |
| Soup bowl (large) = 10 oz = 300 mL |
| Gelatin = 4 oz = 120 mL |
| Ice cream cup = 5 oz = 150 mL |
| Creamer = 1 oz = 30 mL |

2. A water glass holds 180 mL when full. The resident has consumed $\frac{3}{4}$ of the water. The intake is calculated: $\frac{3}{4} \times 180$ (take 4 into 180 = 45) and multiply 45 times 3 which equals 135 mL intake.
3. An ice cream cup holds 150 mL when full. The resident has consumed all of the ice cream. Intake is recorded as 150 mL.
4. A soup bowl holds 180 mL when full. The resident has consumed $\frac{2}{3}$ of the soup. The intake is calculated: $\frac{2}{3} \times 180$ (take 3 into 180 = 60) and multiply 60 times 2. The intake is 120 mL.

When calculating fluids for a meal you may need to calculate the separate quantities, add them, and record the total intake for the meal. For example:

| | |
|---|---|
| $\frac{2}{3}$ carton of milk | = 160 mL |
| 1 small orange juice | = 120 mL |
| $\frac{1}{2}$ cup coffee | = 75 mL |
| $\frac{1}{3}$ glass water | = 60 mL |

Total breakfast intake: 415 mL

A special form for recording I&O may be kept at the bedside to be used each day. Fluids taken in and lost are listed on the I&O sheet in the resident's health record.

## PROCEDURE 35 Measuring and Recording Fluid Intake

1. Carry out each beginning procedure action.
2. Assemble the following:
   - Intake and output record at bedside
   - Graduated pitcher
   - Pen for recording
3. Record intake on the I&O record at the bedside (Figure 17-14) by listing all fluids taken in. Total intake includes:
   - The amount of liquid the resident takes with meals
   - The amount of water and other liquids taken between meals
   - All other fluids given by mouth, intravenously, or by tube feeding. How these fluids are taken should also be recorded.
4. Copy information on the resident's chart from the bedside I&O record, according to facility policy. Report low intake to the nurse. The average person should take in between 2,000 and 3,000 mL (cc) daily.

*(continues)*

PROCEDURE *35* *(continued)*

### INTAKE AND OUTPUT

Room: 103 B          Name: Simon, Grace                         Date: _____

Instructions: Record all I and O

| 2300-0700 | | 0700-1500 | | 1500-2300 | |
|---|---|---|---|---|---|
| Intake | Output | Intake | Output | Intake | Output |
| | | | | | |
| | | | | | |
| | | | | | |
| | | | | | |
| | | | | | |
| | | | | | |
| | | | | | |
| Total | | Total | | Total | |

Drinking Glass.........200 mL   Full Water Pitcher....950 mL   Milk Carton..............236 mL   Jello...........................90 mL
Styrofoam Cup........200 mL   Coffee or Teapot.....300 mL   Soup Bowl...............250 mL   Ice Cream Cup..........90 mL
Juice Glass (small)..100 mL   Coffee Cup.............150 mL   Soup Bowl (small)...100 mL   Creamer....................50 mL
Juice Glass (large)..250 mL

FOLEY CATHETER DRAINAGE: (Circle the following when applicable)

Color:     Yellow     Amber     Brown     Red

Appearance:     Cloudy     Clear     Sediment     Mucous     Bloody          24 hour INTAKE_____

Abdomen Distended     Catheter Irrigated     Catheter Changed               24 hour OUTPUT_____

**FIGURE 17-14**  An intake and output chart becomes part of the resident's record.

## Ensuring Proper Nutrition······

Meals and supplements for residents are carefully planned by a dietitian to meet their needs. In general, the elderly diet must:

- Be lower in calories
- Be lower in fat
- Be rich in vitamins and minerals
- Contain plenty of fluid
- Include bulk to promote regularity
- Be provided in smaller, more frequent portions

The diet for the elderly should contain adequate levels of all nutrients except calories. Calorie content must be decreased because the elderly are generally less active. Coarse foods are avoided because the lining of the mouth of older adults is thinner and easier to injure. Vegetables and fruits that are cooked and chopped may be easier to chew and to digest. They are included for their nutrient and fiber value. They may be lightly steamed to keep their nutrients.

Some elderly may have lower levels of hydrochloric acid in the stomach, making the absorption of some minerals more difficult.

Vitamin and mineral supplements may be added to the general diet.

Small servings are more appealing, especially when inactivity causes poor appetites. Many facilities serve several (four or five) small meals instead of three larger meals. The evening meal is usually lighter to promote comfortable sleeping. A bedtime snack of graham crackers and milk may help with sleep.

Remember that adequate water is essential. Liquids should be included in meals and as planned supplements three times each day—morning, afternoon, and early evening. Fluids are offered whenever the opportunity arises. Each time you provide care to the resident, offer water or some other desired liquid.

In some individual cases, the physician may order that fluids be limited.

# NURSING ASSISTANT RESPONSIBILITIES

Nursing assistants have a personal responsibility for providing good nutrition for themselves so they will stay healthy and have the energy to do their work. They also play an important role in helping residents to meet their nutritional needs.

It is important that each nursing assistant know and understand:

- The nutrients and amounts needed for health
- The importance of adequate water to prevent dehydration
- Ways diets can be modified to meet individual health needs

Mealtime is a busy time in the long-term care facility. The nursing assistant has a major responsibility to see that it goes smoothly and pleasantly. You will:

- Make sure the area is pleasant and odor free.
- Assist residents to reach the dining room.
- Serve trays.
- Help residents needing assistance in eating.
- Always be sure the resident receives the proper diet (standard or therapeutic) by checking the tray card.
- Be sure foods are served at the proper temperature.
- Make sure that used trays are not returned to serving cart until all clean trays have been served.
- Keep food trays covered until served.
- Housekeeping carts and laundry hampers should be out of the corridor when food is served or kept at least two room widths away from the food cart when it is placed in the corridor.
- Place the food cart against the wall when it is

brought into the dining room.
- Doors to the food cart should be closed until the trays are served.

Eating may be one of the few generally enjoyable activities left to the elderly. In addition to meeting nutritional needs, meals should also be sensually and socially satisfying. Large dining areas permit residents to eat together and promote a social atmosphere. The meals are prepared by the dietary staff in large kitchens and brought to the dining area on tray carts (Figure 17-15).

In many facilities, special evening meals are organized so that residents who are able will dress up and eat in a restaurant-like atmosphere. Dining tables are set up home style and dinner is not served on trays.

This activity meets both social and nutritional needs and is greatly appreciated by residents.

## Assisting with Feeding

If residents can go to the dining room:

- Assist them to the toilet before mealtimes.
- Help them wash their hands.
- Help them into the dining room.

Wheelchairs and geri-chairs can be rolled into the dining room if residents cannot walk. Some residents may remain in their wheelchairs. Other residents will transfer to dining room chairs. After washing your own hands, help serve the trays and assist as necessary (Figure 17-16).

- Cut meat into small bite-size pieces. Allow resident time to chew thoroughly.
- Pour liquids. Do not fill containers too full. Cool hot drinks with milk or water to prevent burns.
- Butter bread and cut into small pieces.
- Unfold and position napkin or towel over clothing.

## Feeding the Resident

Even when a resident is confined to bed or must be fed, you can make the experience more pleasant if you:

- Position the resident comfortably.
- Remove all unpleasant things from sight.
- Never hurry the resident.
- Allow the resident to help as much as possible.
- Identify the food offered.

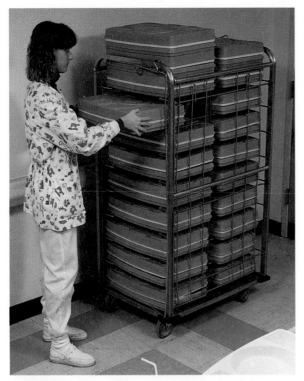

**FIGURE 17-15**   Residents' diets are prepared in the dietary department. The nursing assistant takes the marked tray from the tray cart to serve to the resident.

- Follow the resident's preference, offering liquids frequently.
- Talk with the resident in an unhurried manner about subjects of interest.

*Note:* Carry extra straws with you during mealtimes. It can save you steps.

If the resident has difficulty seeing:

- Make sure there is as much light as possible.
- Describe the arrangement of the foods on the place, relating them to the face of a clock.
- Explain placement of other items on the tray so the resident can feed self as much as possible.

When preparing to assist an in-bed resident to eat, remember to carry out the beginning procedure actions. Before delivering a food tray, wash your hands and recheck the tray for correct resident and diet. Place the tray on the overbed table and position the resident in a sitting position, if permitted, or on the unaffected side if he or she has had a stroke. Place a napkin or towel on the resident's lap or under the chin.

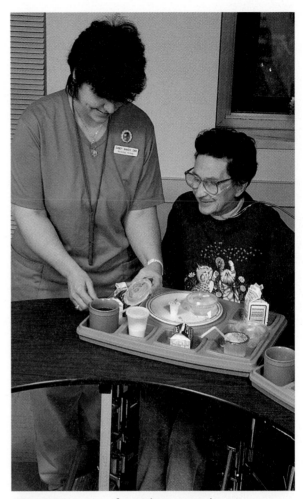

**FIGURE 17-16**   If residents need assistance, nursing assistants help them eat.

Prepare food as necessary, such as cutting it into small pieces. Feed small amounts slowly; avoid having the resident talk or laugh during feeding. After feeding, be sure the resident is left clean and comfortable. Help to perform oral hygiene.

## Use of Food Thickeners

If the resident has difficulty swallowing, commercial food thickeners may be added to the diet. The type and amount of thickener is usually ordered by the speech therapist. The nursing assistant adds the thickener at the time of feeding. When adding thickener, the nursing assistant must be sure that the:

- Correct thickener is added
- Correct amount of thickener is added

PROCEDURE

*36*

# Assisting the Resident Who Can Feed Self

OBRA

1. Carry out each beginning procedure action.
2. Assemble equipment:
   - Bedpan/urinal
   - Wash water
   - Oral hygiene items
   - Tray of food
3. Offer bedpan/urinal. (If used, follow steps in Procedure 38 in Lesson 18.)
4. If permitted, elevate head of bed or assist resident out of bed.
5. Clear overbed table and position in front of resident (Figure 17-17A). Remove unpleasant equipment from sight. Remove sources of odors.

6. Provide water, soap, and towel to wash resident's hands and face (Figure 17-17B).

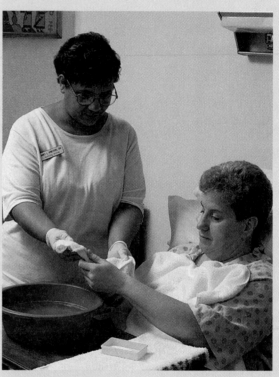

**FIGURE 17-17B**  Give resident water to wash hands.

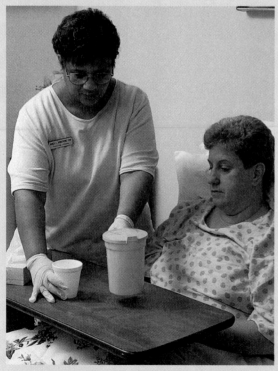

**FIGURE 17-17A**  Clear off overbed table to make room for food tray.

7. Assist with oral hygiene if desired.
8. Wash your hands. Obtain tray from dietary cart.
9. Check the diet with the dietary card and with the resident's identification band (Figure 17-17C).
10. Place tray on overbed table and arrange food in a convenient manner.
11. Assist in food preparation as needed (Figure 17-17D). Encourage resident to do as much as possible.

*(continues)*

**PROCEDURE** *36* *(continued)*

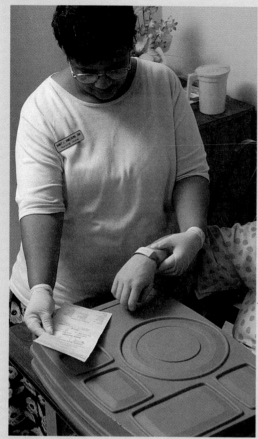

**FIGURE 17-17C** Check resident's arm band against the tray card to ensure the resident is getting the right diet.

12. Remove tray as soon as resident is finished. Be sure to note what the resident has and has not eaten.
13. Record fluids on intake record, if necessary.

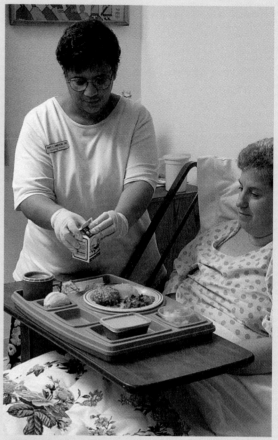

**FIGURE 17-17D** Assist resident in food preparation as needed.

14. Push overbed table out of the way.
15. Help to perform oral hygiene to clean teeth or dentures and mouth.
16. Carry out each procedure completion action.

• Thickener is added according to the manufacturer's instructions

When using food thickeners, follow the procedure for feeding the dependent resident. (See Procedure 37.) Be sure to allow enough time so the resident is not rushed. Direct the food and liquids toward the unaffected side of the mouth. Feed with the tip of the spoon that is not more than one-half full.

**PROCEDURE 37**

# Feeding the Dependent Resident

1. Carry out each beginning procedure action.
2. Assemble equipment:
   - Bedpan/urinal
   - Wash water
   - Oral hygiene items
   - Tray of food
3. Offer bedpan or urinal. (If used, follow steps in Procedure 38 in Lesson 18.)
4. Provide oral hygiene if desired.
5. Remove unnecessary articles from the overbed table.
6. Elevate head of bed. Assist resident into a sitting or upright position with head slightly bent forward. If resident is out of bed, position resident in chair in an upright position with feet flat on the floor.
7. Place napkin, bib, or towel under resident's chin (Figure 17-18A).

8. Obtain tray and check diet with the dietary card and resident's identification band.
9. Place tray on overbed table (Figure 17-18B). Sit down facing the resident so you are at eye level. The environment should be quiet and calm.

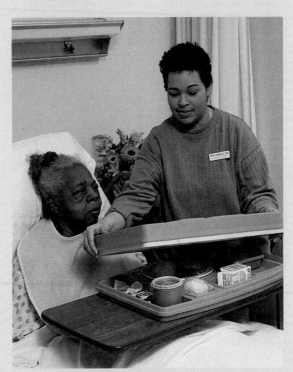

**FIGURE 17-18B** Uncover the food and place it on the overbed table.

10. Butter bread and cut meat. Do not pour hot beverage until resident is ready for it. Be sure, however, that the beverage is cool enough to drink before offering it to the resident.
11. Use different drinking straws for each fluid or use a cup. Thick fluids are more easily controlled by using a straw.

*(continues)*

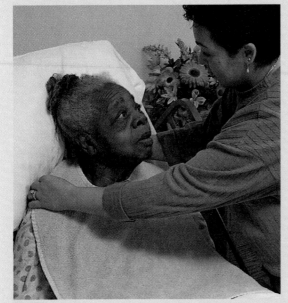

**FIGURE 17-18A** Place a towel or bed protector under the resident's chin

**PROCEDURE *37* (continued)**

12. Holding spoon at a right angle:
    - Give solid foods from point of spoon (Figure 17-18C).
    - Alternate solids and liquids.
    - Rotate the offerings of food to give variety.
    - Describe or show resident what kind of food you are giving.
    - If resident has had a stroke, direct food to unaffected side of mouth and check for food stored in affected side.
    - Test hot foods by dropping a small amount on the inside of your wrist before feeding them to the resident.
    - Never blow on the resident's food to cool it.
    - Never taste the resident's food.
    - Do not hurry the meal.
13. Allow resident to hold bread or assist to the extent possible.
14. Use napkin to wipe resident's mouth as often as necessary.
15. Remove tray as soon as resident is finished. Make sure you note what the resident has or has not eaten.
16. Provide oral hygiene.
17. Carry out each procedure completion action.

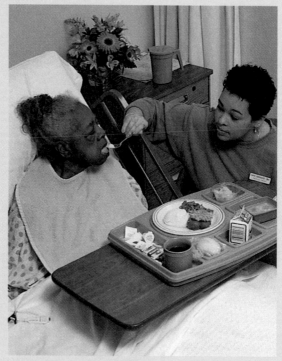

**FIGURE 17-18C** Give solid foods from the tip of the spoon.

## Choking

Choking is always a danger when feeding dependent or elderly residents because their swallowing ability is not always effective. All health care providers working with the elderly should know how to do abdominal thrusts for choking victims (Heimlich maneuver). Be especially careful with dry, grainy foods such as bran or corn bread because these are more difficult to swallow. Put such foods in milk or give in small amounts followed by liquid. Care of the choking resident is covered in Lesson 8.

## NOURISHMENTS AND SUPPLEMENTS

Nourishments are tasty refreshments residents enjoy between meals. Supplements are liquids or foods ordered by the physician to improve the nutritional status of the resident. Supplements are often given to increase weight. It is important that all ordered supplements are served in a timely manner and not be allowed to sit on the table for long periods of time.

Nursing assistants may be asked to serve nourishments or supplements, encourage residents to eat or drink them, and assist as necessary. If this is your assignment, be sure that you:

- Wash your hands before serving nourishments or supplements.
- Follow the dietary instructions carefully.
- Check that the right nourishment or supplement is given to the right resident.
- Allow a choice of nourishments if possible.
- Assist the resident if help is needed.
- Serve supplements at scheduled times. If they are served too close to meal time, the resident may feel too full to eat.
- Do not offer nourishments or supplements to residents who are not scheduled to receive them.
- If a resident asks for a supplement or a different supplement, check with your supervisor.
- Do not allow partially eaten nourishments or supplements to remain in the residents' rooms. Most nourishments or supplements are served in disposable containers.
- Record the nourishment or supplement served and the amount consumed according to facility policy. Record fluids on the intake form if required.

## PROVIDING WATER

Water in adequate amounts is essential to normal body functioning. Most older adults need to consume about 2,000 to 3,000 mL or 2 to 3 quarts of liquid each day. If the body is functioning properly, the amount of fluids taken in will be balanced by the amount lost.

Dehydration (inadequate fluid level in the body) develops when fluid intake is not adequate. In addition, some drugs cause excessive amounts of fluids to be lost from the body. It is important to recognize the signs of dehydration (Figure 17-19). All signs of dehydration must be reported immediately so corrective actions can be taken.

Many residents do not take in enough fluids. This is especially true when they feel ill, have a fever, or have a decreased appetite. An essential task of nursing assistants is to remind and

| **FIGURE 17-19** Signs of dehydration |
|---|
| • Confusion |
| • Decreased urine output |
| • Increased temperature |
| • Decreased energy level |
| • Constipation |
| • Thirst |
| • Dry skin |
| • Restlessness |

encourage residents to drink water or other fluids frequently. Follow these guidelines for the residents in your care:

- Always follow the care plan for each resident for fluid intake. Some residents may be on limited intake because of their medical conditions and should not be offered fluids.
- For other residents be sure fresh water is within reach. Keep pitchers full. Some residents may request that ice be added to the water.
- Remind the resident to drink whenever you have contact with the resident.
- A resident who has a fever requires careful monitoring of fluid intake.
- Increase attention to fluid intake during hot weather.
- If residents cannot drink unaided, offer fluids frequently and assist as needed.
- If a resident is on intake, record the amount of fluid consumed each time the resident drinks. If this is not possible, the amount of water left in a pitcher can be measured before the pitcher is refilled. The amount left is subtracted from the total amount of water in the pitcher originally.
- Fluid intake over 24 hours is usually consumed during the day and evening shifts (0700 to 2300). It is important for nursing assistants on these shifts to encourage residents to drink adequate fluid.

The procedure for changing water is outlined in the facility procedure manual. Be sure you know the requirements for changing water, especially the steps to prevent the spread of infection. For example, if pitchers are taken to a central area to be refilled, be sure each resident receives her pitcher and not one belonging to another resident. Pitchers must be covered before being taken back to the residents' rooms and remain covered in the room.

# ALTERNATE METHODS OF FEEDING

There are several alternate ways to provide nutrition to a resident. They include:

- Enteral feedings
  - Nasogastric tube (NG tube) feedings
  - Gastrostomy tube (G tube) feedings
- Total parenteral nutrition (TPN)

## Enteral Feeding

A **nasogastric (NG) tube** is a small tube introduced into the nose and through the pharynx and esophagus and into the stomach by the physician or nurse. A **gastrostomy (G) tube** is a small tube surgically placed directly into the resident's stomach (Figure 17-20A). Feedings may be introduced through the gastrostomy or nasogastric tube using a syringe or feeding pump.

Tube feedings require special training and are performed by the nurse. Commercially prepared formula or liquid food is introduced directly into the tube (Figure 17-20B). The head of the bed must be elevated at 45°, or according to facility policy, during the feeding and for 30 minutes after. Great care must be taken to ensure that the tubes are properly positioned and are not pulled out or moved even slightly. You must inform the nurse if:

- You find the tube in the bed
- The resident complains of discomfort

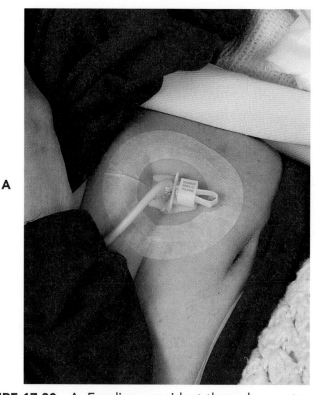
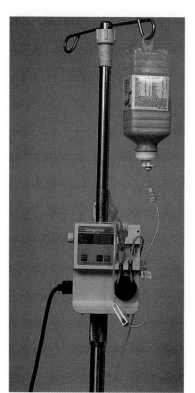

**FIGURE 17-20**  A. Feeding a resident through a gastrostomy tube B. using a feeding pump and prepared liquid nutrients

- The resident is coughing or choking
- The resident feels nauseated or vomits or retches

Other actions the nursing assistant can take include:

- Not permitting tension on the tubes
- Being alert for kinks in tubing
- Reporting signs of irritation near the tube entrances
- If food is given by pump, informing the nurse if:
  - The alarm goes off
  - The bag holding the solution is empty
  - The resident is coughing or choking

Nursing assistant actions relating to the resident who receives tube feedings are listed in Figure 17-21.

### Total Parenteral Nutrition (TPN)

**Total parenteral nutrition (TPN)** or **hyperalimentation** is a technique in which **high density** (concentrated) nutrients are introduced into a large vein such as the subclavian vein or the superior vena cava. The nurse manages TPN.

# DISORDERS OF THE DIGESTIVE SYSTEM

### Constipation

Constipation is a common problem for the elderly. Hard, difficult to expel feces is a sign of constipation. This can be very uncomfortable for the resident and can cause bleeding if hemorrhoids are present. Regular bowel movements are aided by:

- Enough fluid intake to lubricate the colon and soften the feces
- Adequate fiber in the diet to act as bulk to promote intestinal activity
- Regular exercise to promote muscle tone
- Regular toileting opportunities

### Dysphagia

**Dysphagia** (difficult swallowing) may be caused by decreased saliva production, paralysis due to a stroke, or obstructions such as malignancy of the esophagus. The resident with dysphagia can

**FIGURE 17-21** Nursing assistant actions to help residents receiving tube feedings

The nursing assistant:

- Keeps head of bed elevated at 45° during feeding and for $\frac{1}{2}$ hour after feeding.
- Checks taping of tubes. If taping is loose, inform the nurse.
- Reports any retching (straining to, but not vomiting), nausea, or vomiting immediately.
- Checks tubing for kinks. Be sure the resident is not lying on tubing.
- Ensures end of tube is closed between feedings.
- Provides frequent mouth hygiene.

more easily consume thick liquids and pureed foods than solid foods. If the difficulty is prolonged, it may be necessary to provide nourishment directly into the stomach or through hyperalimentation.

### Hernias

A **hernia** occurs when a structure such as the intestine pushes out of its normal body position. Hernias are also known as **ruptures**. These may develop as the intestines push through a weakened area in the abdominal wall.

There are different kinds of hernias, depending on location. Two types of hernias are common in elderly persons:

- **Inguinal hernias**
- **Hiatal hernias**

**Inguinal Hernia.** This is a protrusion of the intestines through the wall in the groin area. It is felt as a small lump, especially when the resident strains.

**Hiatal Hernia.** In a hiatal hernia, the stomach pushes upward into the thoracic cavity, through the normal opening that allows the esophagus to pass through the diaphragm to the stomach. Signs and symptoms of hiatal hernia are:

* Dysphagia
* Pain and pressure in the chest as food and gastric fluid become trapped in the esophagus

The hydrochloric acid in the trapped gastric fluid can be very irritating, causing inflammation and ulceration of the esophagus.

Hiatal hernias tend to be a chronic problem. Residents feel better when they:

* Eat smaller meals
* Eat sitting up

They also feel more comfortable sleeping when the head of the bed is slightly raised. Antacids are sometimes ordered to overcome the acidity and reduce discomfort. Residents should avoid lying flat after meals.

## Inflammation

Inflammation anywhere along the gastrointestinal tract can cause distress and the possibility of tissue breakdown and the formation of ulcers. Inflammation of the stomach (**gastritis**) can lead to **dyspepsia** (indigestion). A combination of overeating, foods that are too spicy, and natural aging changes can cause gastric distress. Also, ulcerations in the colon can cause blood in the stool and painful defecation.

## Diverticulosis

**Diverticuli** are small, weakened areas in the wall of the colon. These areas form small pockets. Seeds and other hard food particles sometimes become trapped, causing inflammation (**diverticulitis**). When the diverticuli become inflamed, the resident complains of constipation and pain and is more susceptible to infection.

Usually diverticuli are multiple and the condition is then called diverticulosis. Residents who have diverticulosis feel best when:

* A bland diet is eaten
* Weight is controlled
* Constipation is avoided

Sometimes part of the bowel must be removed to correct the problem.

## Malignancy

Malignancies, or cancers, of the digestive system occur frequently in older people. Cancers may occur anywhere along the tract, but commonly occur in the lower colon. Because the lumen of the large intestine is fairly big, cancer can grow inside the colon for a relatively long time before it becomes large enough to cause an obstruction or change the character of the feces.

## Hemorrhoids

**Hemorrhoids** are varicose veins of the rectum. Their presence can make defecation painful, and they sometimes bleed. Regularity and keeping feces soft to avoid straining are important in preventing complications.

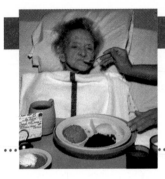

## LESSON SYNTHESIS: Putting It All Together

*Y*ou have just completed this lesson. Now go back and review the Clinical Focus. Try to see how the Clinical Focus relates to the concepts presented in the lesson. Then answer the following questions.

1. Why is it especially important for Mrs. Hartley to receive proper nutrition and hydration at this time?

2. What kind of supplemental nourishments might be beneficial for her and when might you offer them?

3. From your observations, what might you suspect about Mrs. Hartley's level of hydration?

4. What beverage would you not serve to this resident?

## REVIEW

**A. Match each term with the proper definition**

a. digestive system    f. flatulence
b. defecation    g. gastritis
c. digestion    h. nasogastric tube
d. dehydration    i. hyperalimentation
e. enzymes    j. obesity

1. _____ chemicals that help digest foods

2. _____ inflammation of the stomach

3. _____ bowel movement

4. _____ the condition of being overweight

5. _____ feeding tube

6. _____ total parenteral nutrition

7. _____ gastrointestinal tract

8. _____ gas

9. _____ excessive water loss

10. _____ mechanical and chemical process that breaks down food

**B. Identify the parts of the digestive system by inserting the correct number of each part.**

_____ appendix     _____ mouth
_____ colon     _____ pharynx
_____ esophagus     _____ rectum
_____ gallbladder     _____ small intestine
_____ liver     _____ stomach

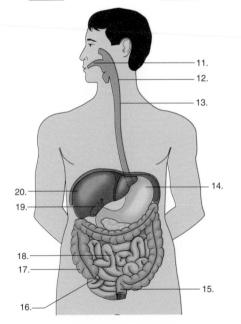

**C.  Indicate which of the following changes are associated with aging by circling yes (Y) or no (N).**

21.  Y   N   More sensitive taste

22.  Y   N   Thinner saliva

23.  Y   N   Reduced digestive enzymes

24.  Y   N   More rapid absorption of nutrients

25.  Y   N   Poorer tolerance to some foods

**D.  Select the one best answer for each of the following.**

26.  The primary source of energy for the body is
   a.  fat
   b.  minerals
   c.  carbohydrates
   d.  proteins

27.  Which basic nutrient is essential for tissue building and repair?
   a.  fats
   b.  carbohydrates
   c.  minerals
   d.  proteins

28.  Vitamins B and C are found in
   a.  beef
   b.  fruits and vegetables
   c.  eggs
   d.  vegetable oils

29.  How much water should be taken in daily?
   a.  1 pint
   b.  3 glasses
   c.  2 cups
   d.  2 to 3 quarts

30.  Cottage cheese belongs in which food group?
   a.  vegetable group
   b.  fruit group
   c.  milk, yogurt, and cheese group
   d.  meat, poultry, fish, dry beans, eggs, and nut group

31.  Which of the four common diets prepared for long-term care residents includes liquids and semisolid foods that are more easily chewed and digested?
   a.  pureed
   b.  clear liquid
   c.  regular
   d.  mechanical soft

32.  Which food is likely to be restricted on a low fat diet?
   a.  apples
   b.  whole milk
   c.  bananas
   d.  white fish

33.  Which food is excluded from a low sodium diet?
   a.  potato
   b.  bacon
   c.  whole grain cereal
   d.  carrot

34.  Which food may be included on a low residue diet?
   a.  celery
   b.  orange
   c.  banana
   d.  bran flakes

**E.  Match the therapeutic diet (items a.–e.) with the specific requirements.**

a.  diabetic          d.  calorie restricted
b.  low sodium        e.  high protein
c.  low fat

35.  _____  prescribed for resident with heart condition or one who retains fluid

36.  _____  served to residents who are underweight or poorly nourished

37.  _____  served to residents with cardiovascular, gallbladder, or liver disease

38.  _____  carefully balanced, concentrated carbohydrates restricted

39.  _____  given to residents who need weight control

**F. Determine the resident's intake using the chart in Figure 17-14. The resident has consumed:** mL

40. ⅔ of a drinking glass of water _____
41. ¾ of a small glass of orange juice _____
42. ⅔ of a small glass of apple juice _____
43. ½ of a water pitcher _____
44. ¾ of a water pitcher _____
45. ⅓ of a cup of coffee _____
46. ¼ of a carton of milk _____
47. ¾ of a dish of gelatin _____

Total intake _____

**G. On the chart provided below, make a record of the resident's intake and output for an 8-hour period.**

| 48. | 0730 | urine | 300 mL |
| | 0800 | orange juice | 90 mL |
| | | coffee | 120 mL |
| | 0930 | water | 60 mL |
| | 1130 | tea | 120 mL |
| | | soup | 120 mL |
| | 1300 | urine | 400 mL |
| | 1315 | water | 80 mL |
| | 1500 | cranberry juice | 100 mL |
| | 1515 | vomitus | 120 mL |
| | 1620 | tea | 120 mL |
| | | sherbet | 120 mL |
| | 1730 | urine | 300 mL |
| | 1800 | water | 150 mL |
| | 2100 | ginger ale | 100 mL |
| | 2130 | urine | 300 mL |
| | 2200 | water | 90 mL |

---

**INTAKE AND OUTPUT**

Room: _____  Name: _____  Date: _____

Instructions: _____

| Intake | Output | Intake | Output | Intake | Output |
|--------|--------|--------|--------|--------|--------|
| | | | | | |
| | | | | | |
| | | | | | |
| | | | | | |
| | | | | | |
| | | | | | |
| Total | | Total | | Total | |

Drinking Glass.........200 mL  Full Water Pitcher....950 mL  Milk Carton..............236 mL  Jello...........................90 mL
Styrofoam Cup........200 mL  Coffee or Teapot.....300 mL  Soup Bowl...............250 mL  Ice Cream Cup..........90 mL
Juice Glass (small)..100 mL  Coffee Cup.............150 mL  Soup Bowl (small)...100 mL  Creamer....................50 mL
Juice Glass (large)..250 mL

FOLEY CATHETER DRAINAGE: (Circle the following when applicable)

Color:  Yellow  Amber  Brown  Red

Appearance:  Cloudy  Clear  Sediment  Mucous  Bloody

Abdomen Distended  Catheter Irrigated  Catheter Changed

24 hour INTAKE_____

24 hour OUTPUT_____

**H. Match the metric amounts with their approximate equivalents.**

a. 500 mL      d. 3,840 mL
b. 0.06 mL      e. 1,000 mL
c. 30 mL

49. _____ 1 minim

50. _____ 1 quart

51. _____ 1 gallon

52. _____ 1 pint

53. _____ 1 ounce

**I. Show your understanding of fractions by completing the following problems.**

54. $\frac{1}{2} + \frac{1}{2} =$ _____

55. $\frac{2}{3} + \frac{1}{3} =$ _____

56. $\frac{1}{4} + \frac{1}{4} =$ _____

57. $\frac{3}{4} + \frac{1}{4} =$ _____

58. Your resident drinks $\frac{2}{3}$ of her juice. The glass held 120 mL. How much juice did she drink? Show how you determined your answer.

59. You picked up an empty coffee cup when your resident finished eating. How much did he drink if the cup held 150 mL and you filled it twice? Show how you determined your answer.

60. Your resident consumed a bowl of soup that contained 300 mL. How many ounces of soup did your resident consume? Show how you determined your answer.

**J. Clinical Experiences**

Read the clinical experiences and answer the questions about each long-term care resident.

Amelia Drage, age 92, spent her life as a homemaker. She contributed many hours to civic organizations. Her current frail condition requires assistance in feeding. She is on a soft diet and receives nourishments.

61. The best combination of foods for her soft diet is
   a. coleslaw and milk
   b. toast and fresh fruit salad
   c. chicken and cottage cheese
   d. garden salad and eggs

62. When feeding her, remember
   a. do not remove equipment such as the emesis basin
   b. allow her to help herself as much as possible
   c. taste foods first to be sure they are not too hot
   d. offer the bed pan following the meal

63. When serving her nourishments
   a. offer a full meal since she is so frail
   b. leave the used dishes and glasses at the bedside because someone else can pick them up
   c. do not record the nourishments
   d. follow the dietary instructions carefully using the nourishment list as a guide

Russell Barnes, age 82, has a large obstructing tumor of the esophagus. He is unable to take nourishment by mouth and transfer it to his stomach because of the tumor. A commercial nutritional formula is provided for him through a feeding tube. He has a gastrostomy tube in place.

64. The gastrostomy tube is in Mr. Barnes's
   a. esophagus
   b. pharynx
   c. stomach
   d. colon

65. When taking care of Mr. Barnes you note the tube is out of place and lying in the bed. You should
   a. throw the tube away as it probably is not needed
   b. notify the nurse immediately
   c. reinsert the tube so you will be ready for the next feeding
   d. leave the tube alone because the nurse can take care of it when she checks the resident

66. Your care of Mr. Barnes following a feeding includes
    a. elevating the head of the bed at 40° for one-half hour
    b. allowing him to lie on the tube
    c. keeping the bed flat for one-half hour
    d. keeping the end of the tube open between feedings

Joe Spando is 78 years old and has chronic obstructive pulmonary disease, a hiatal hernia, and diverticulosis. He was a jockey as a young adult and smoking was a way of life. Even now he insists on his smoking time, which he enjoys under supervision.

67. Mr. Spando's hiatal hernia means that his
    a. intestines protrude through the wall in the groin area
    b. colon is inflamed
    c. rectum has varicose veins
    d. stomach protrudes up into the thoracic cavity

68. This resident probably suffers from
    a. painful defecation
    b. dysphagia
    c. blood in his stool
    d. pain in his rectum

69. He will probably be most comfortable if he
    a. eats while lying down
    b. eats three big meals a day
    c. sits up after meals
    d. sleeps with the head of the bed flat

## LESSON
# 18
# Meeting the Residents' Elimination Needs

### CLINICAL FOCUS

Think about how you may help a

resident meet elimination needs as

you study this lesson and meet:

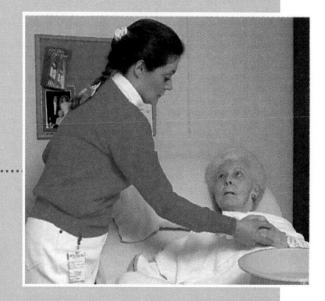

Jessica Beebe, age 79, who has been assigned to your care. She seems listless, complaining of an upset stomach and cramps. She refused breakfast and you note some fecal soiling on the bedding. When you ask her about her last bowel movement, she cannot remember. You report the situation to the charge nurse who examines Ms. Beebe for fecal impaction. It is decided that Ms. Beebe will benefit from a soapsuds enema.

## OBJECTIVES

*After studying this lesson, you should be able to:*

- Define and spell vocabulary words and terms.
- Identify ways people eliminate wastes.
- Identify the parts and functions of the digestive system.
- Identify the parts and function of the urinary tract.
- Review changes in the urinary system as they relate to the aging process.
- Describe common urinary system conditions affecting the long-term residents.
- Collect and care for urine and stool specimens.
- Measure and record fluid output.
- Demonstrate the following:
  Procedure 38 Giving and Receiving the Bedpan

Procedure 39 Giving and Receiving the Urinal

Procedure 40 Assisting With the Use of the Bedside Commode

Procedure 41 Assisting Resident to Use the Bathroom

Procedure 42 Checking for Fecal Impaction

Procedure 43 Giving an Oil-Retention Enema

Procedure 44 Giving a Soapsuds Enema

Procedure 45 Giving a Commercially Prepared Enema

Procedure 46 Inserting a Rectal Suppository

Procedure 47 Inserting a Rectal Tube and Flatus Bag

# OBJECTIVES

Procedure 48  Giving Routine Stoma Care (Colostomy)
Procedure 49  Collecting a Stool Specimen
Procedure 50  Routine Drainage Check
Procedure 51  Giving Indwelling Catheter Care
Procedure 52  Disconnecting the Catheter
Procedure 53  Measuring and Recording Fluid Output
Procedure 54  Emptying a Urinary Drainage Unit

Procedure 55  Emptying Leg Bag
Procedure 56  Connecting Catheter to Leg Bag
Procedure 57  Collecting a Routine Urine Specimen
Procedure 58  Collecting a Clean-Catch Urine Specimen
Procedure 59  Applying a Condom for Urinary Drainage

# VOCABULARY

**anuria**   *(ah-NEW-ree-ah)*
**bladder**   *(BLAD-der)*
**Bowman's capsule**   *(BOH-manz KAP-syoul)*
**catheter**   *(KATH-eh-ter)*
**colon**   *(KOHL-on)*
**colostomy**   *(koh-LAHS-toh-mee)*
**condom**   *(KON-dum)*
**constipation**   *(kon-stih-PAY-shun)*
**continent**   *(KON-tih-nent)*
**cystocele**   *(SIS-toh-seel)*
**diarrhea**   *(die-ah-REE-ah)*
**distended**   *(dis-TEN-ded)*
**dysuria**   *(dis-YOU-ree-ah)*
**emesis**   *(EM-eh-sis)*
**enema**   *(EN-eh-mah)*
**excreta**   *(ecks-KREE-tah)*
**fecal impaction**   *(FEE-kal im-PACK-shun)*
**glomerulus**   *(gloh-MER-you-lus)*
**hematuria**   *(hem-ah-TOO-ree-ah)*
**ileostomy**   *(ill-ee-OS-toh-me)*
**incontinence**   *(in-KON-tih-nens)*
**indwelling catheter**   *(IN-dwell-ing KATH-eh-ter)*
**meatus**   *(mee-AY-tus)*

**micturition**   *(mick-too-RISH-un)*
**nephron**   *(NEF-ron)*
**nocturia**   *(nock-TUR-ee-ah)*
**oliguria**   *(ol-ih-GYOU-ree-ah)*
**ostomy**   *(OS-toh-mee)*
**prostate gland**   *(PROS-tayt gland)*
**rectocele**   *(REC-toh-seel)*
**renal calculi**   *(REE-nal KAL-kyou-lee)*
**retention**   *(ree-TEN-shun)*
**sepsis**   *(SEP-sis)*
**septicemia**   *(sept-tih-SEE-mee-ah)*
**specimen**   *(SPES-ih-men)*
**sphincter**   *(SFINK-ter)*
**stoma**   *(STOH-mah)*
**stool**   *(stool)*
**suppository**   *(sup-POZ-ih-toh-ree)*
**uremia**   *(you-REE-mee-ah)*
**uremic frost**   *(you-REE-mick frost)*
**ureter**   *(you-REE-ter)*
**urethra**   *(you-REE-thrah)*
**urinalysis**   *(you-rih-NAL-ih-sis)*
**urination**   *(you-rih-NAY-shun)*
**voiding**   *(VOYD-ing)*

# INTRODUCTION

The human body produces waste products continuously. Eliminating waste products regularly is one of the basic human needs.

Waste products (**excreta**) that must be eliminated (excreted) include:

- Solid wastes
  - Feces from the digestive tract
- Liquid wastes
  - Urine from the urinary system
  - Perspiration (water and salts) from the skin
  - Water in the feces
  - Water from the lungs
- Gaseous wastes
  - Carbon dioxide ($CO_2$) from the lungs

In Lesson 17 you learned how nutrients are processed from foods. The undigested portion of the food (roughage or bulk) continues to move through the colon to the anus where it leaves the body as feces.

In this lesson you will learn ways to:

- Help residents maintain regular elimination
- Assist residents who need special help in eliminating wastes
- Care for residents as they eliminate solid wastes from the digestive system and liquid wastes from the urinary system

A resident who is **continent** is able to control the elimination of waste products. **Incontinence** is the inability to predict and control elimination. Therefore, an incontinent resident has no control over elimination. Incontinence leads to emotional and physical problems that hinder social interaction.

# THE CONTINENT RESIDENT

Nursing assistant responsibilities in helping continent residents to meet their elimination needs (Figure 18-1) include:

- Being aware of the resident's need to reach the proper facilities in time
- Being observant so that you can be available to help the resident reach the toilet or commode. Answer call bells promptly for residents who use a bedpan. Be ready to assist them when they are finished.

**FIGURE 18-1**  Nursing assistant actions when assisting with elimination procedures

When assisting with elimination procedures:

- Wear disposable gloves.

- Wash hands immediately before and after procedure.

- Provide privacy.

- Make resident as comfortable as possible during elimination procedures.

- Ensure safety.

- Immediately answer call light as resident may be finished.

- Always noting and reporting the frequency and character of the excreta

# EQUIPMENT TO ASSIST ELIMINATION

Residents are encouraged to use regular bathroom facilities if their conditions permit. They may need help to reach the toilet in time and with their clothing.

Several devices can make it easier and safer for residents to achieve more independence in elimination. An elevated toilet seat (Figure 18-2) means the resident does not have to bend as much compared to a regular toilet seat. Grab bars on the wall next to the toilet help stabilize the resident when sitting down and getting up. They also help stabilize the resident in the proper position for toileting. Proper positioning makes it easier for the resident to void. The preferred position for women is to sit upright with the feet flat on the floor. Men may prefer to stand.

A commode or portable toilet (Figure 18-3) may be left in the room for convenience, but the container must be emptied and cleaned after

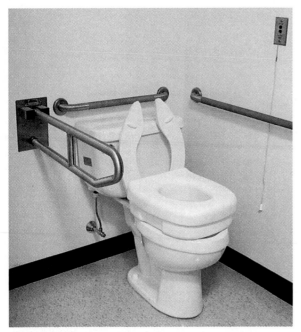

**FIGURE 18-2** An elevated toilet seat promotes independent toileting.

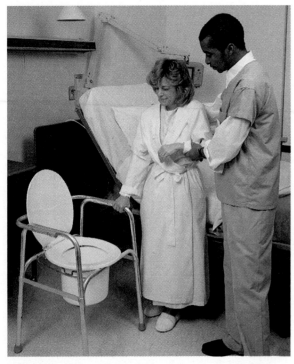

**FIGURE 18-3** A bedside commode allows the resident to assume the best seated position for elimination.

each use and the cover closed. A commode with a rolling base and support arms may be placed over the toilet for security. The wheels of this type of commode must be locked once it is in place. Residents in bed who can be placed on a commode probably will be more comfortable and have a more natural elimination than when using a bedpan.

Often, a bedpan must be used (Figure 18-4). The resident may be more comfortable if the bedpan is placed on the edge of the bed and the resident sits with the feet resting on a chair. For comfort, the bedpan can be padded and the resident supported by pillows. Always make sure the resident is safely and comfortably supported.

Bedpans are not comfortable in any position when left in place for any length of time. An orthopedic bedpan (fracture pan) is used when it is difficult for the resident to move. This type of bedpan is preferred for the resident who does not get out of bed.

As you provide care, remember to perform all beginning and ending procedure actions. Always follow the principles of medical asepsis.

- Apply principles of standard precautions when handling, emptying, and cleaning bedpans, urinals, and commodes.
- Wash hands before and after applying disposable gloves.
- Cover bedpans and urinals and close the covers of commodes after use until emptied.
- Avoid contamination of environmental surfaces with gloves.

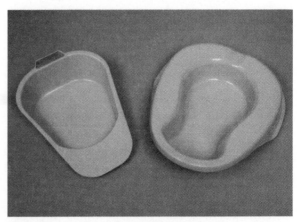

**FIGURE 18-4** (Left) Orthopedic (fracture) bedpan; (Right) regular bedpan

- Encourage residents to perform perineal care after toileting, or assist as necessary.
- Restrict use of bedpan or urinal to specific resident; each resident has a personal bedpan or urinal that is stored in the bedside stand.

### Safety Precautions

Following certain precautions can help prevent incidents during toileting.

- Be sure that resident knows how to use emergency signal in the bathroom and can reach it when using the toilet.

- Encourage resident to use grab bars for support.
- Lock wheels of commode after positioning it over toilet.
- Be sure resident is positioned comfortably on toilet before leaving. Do not leave a resident who is confused or disoriented.
- Do not restrain resident on the toilet or commode.
- Provide as much privacy as possible.
- Answer call bell promptly (resident may have completed toileting).

---

**PROCEDURE**

## 38 Giving and Receiving the Bedpan

1. Carry out each beginning procedure action.
2. Assemble equipment:
   - Disposable gloves
   - Bedpan and cover
   - Basin
   - Washcloth
   - Toilet tissue
   - Soap
   - Towel
3. Lower the head of the bed if necessary.
4. Put on gloves.
5. Take the bedpan and tissue from the bedside stand.
   - Place the bedpan on the bedside chair. Never place it on the bedside stand or overbed table.
   - Put the remainder of the equipment on the bedside table.
6. Place bedpan cover at the foot of the bed. *Note:* Never carry or allow a used bedpan to sit uncovered. If a bedpan cover is not available, cover the bedpan with a towel, pillowcase, or paper towels.

7. Fold top bed covers back at a right angle. Raise the resident's gown. If the resident is thin or has a pressure sore, consult the nurse for the appropriate action. The nursing care plan may have specific instructions for such cases. For example, it may be necessary to pad the bedpan with a folded towel or take some other action.
8. Ask resident to flex knees and rest weight on heels, if able.
9. Help the resident to raise buttocks by:
   - Putting one hand under the small of the resident's back and lifting gently and slowly with one hand.
   - With the other hand, place the bedpan under the resident's hips.
   - If the resident is unable to raise the buttocks, two assistants may be needed to lift the resident.
   - The bedpan may also be placed by rolling the resident to one side, positioning the bedpan against the buttocks and rolling the resident back on it (Figure 18-5).

*(continues)*

## PROCEDURE *38* *(continued)*

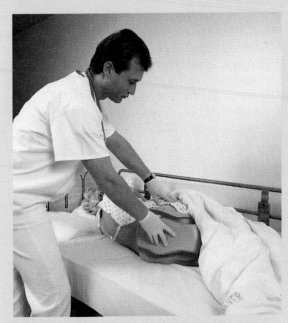

**FIGURE 18-5** Roll resident away from you while supporting resident with one hand on resident's hip. Place bedpan against resident's buttocks with other hand. Then roll resident back onto bedpan.

- Alternatively, if a trapeze is in place over the bed, place the bedpan under the resident as the resident lifts self using the trapeze.
- The resident's buttocks should rest on the rounded shelf of the regular bedpan. The narrow end should face the foot of the bed.

10. Remove gloves and dispose of properly. Wash hands. Replace top bedcovers. Raise the head of the bed to a comfortable height.
11. Make sure the toilet paper and signal cord are within easy reach of the resident. Leave the resident alone unless contraindicated in the nursing care plan.

*Note:* If a specimen is to be taken, instruct the resident that toilet tissue is not to be placed in the bedpan. In this case, the nursing assistant will clean the resident and provide perineal care.

12. Watch for resident's signal.
13. Answer the resident's call signal immediately. Wash hands and put on disposable gloves. Use a paper towel to turn faucet on and another one to turn faucet off.
14. Fill the basin with warm water (105°F) and place next to soap, washcloth, and towel on overbed table.
15. Remove bedpan from under resident.

- Ask the resident to flex knees and rest weight on heels. Place one hand under the small of the back and lift gently to help raise the buttocks off bedpan. Take the bedpan with the other hand. Cover it and place it on the chair.

16. Assist the resident to a clean area of the bed, if necessary. Provide perineal care.

- If the resident is unable to raise the buttocks, two assistants may be needed to lift. Otherwise, roll the resident off the pan to the side and remove the pan. Lift and move carefully. Hold the pan firmly with one hand.

17. Change linen or protective pads as necessary. Replace bedclothes.
18. Assist the resident to wash hands after the procedure.
19. Take the bedpan to the bathroom or utility room and observe contents. Measure, if required.
20. Empty bedpan.

*(continues)*

**PROCEDURE 38** *(continued)*

**21.** Turn faucet on holding a paper towel in the hand. Rinse with cold water and disinfectant. Rinse, dry, and return bedpan to storage in resident's bedside stand.

**22.** Remove gloves and discard according to facility policy. Wash hands.

**23.** Carry out each procedure completion action.

---

**PROCEDURE 39**

# Giving and Receiving the Urinal

**1.** Carry out each beginning procedure action.

**2.** Assemble equipment:
- Disposable gloves
- Urinal and cover (Figure 18-6)
- Basin
- Soap
- Washcloth
- Towel

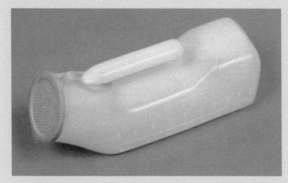

**FIGURE 18-6**   Male urinal with cover

**3.** Put on gloves, Lift the top bedcovers and place the urinal under the covers so the resident may grasp the handle. Instruct resident to place his penis in the urinal opening. If he cannot do this you must place the urinal in position and ensure the penis is placed in the opening.

**4.** Remove gloves and dispose of them properly. Wash hands. Make sure the signal cord is within easy reach of the resident. Leave the resident alone if possible. Watch for his signal.

**5.** Answer the resident's signal immediately. Wash hands. Use a paper towel to turn on faucet. Fill a basin with warm water (105°F), and place next to the soap, washcloth, and towel, so resident can wash and dry hands.

**6.** Put on gloves. Ask the resident to hand the urinal to you. Cover it. Rearrange bedclothes if necessary.

**7.** Take the urinal to the bathroom or utility room and observe the contents. Measure, if required. Do not empty urinal if anything unusual (such as blood) is observed. Rather, save the contents of the urinal for your supervisor's inspection.

**8.** Empty the urinal. Use a paper towel to turn on the faucet and another paper towel to turn the faucet off. Rinse with cold water and clean with warm soapy water. Rinse, dry, and cover urinal. Remove gloves and dispose of them properly. Wash hands.

**9.** Place urinal inside resident's bedside table. Clean and replace other articles.

**10.** Carry out each procedure completion action.

## PROCEDURE 40 — Assisting with the Use of the Bedside Commode

 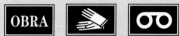 

1. Carry out each beginning procedure action.
2. Assemble equipment:
   - Disposable gloves
   - Portable commode
   - Toilet tissue
   - Basin
   - Washcloth
   - Soap
   - Towel
3. Position commode beside bed, facing head. Lock wheels and open lid. Be sure receptacle is in place under seat.
4. If bed and side rails are elevated, lower side rail nearest you and place bed in lowest horizontal position. Make sure bed wheels are locked.
5. Put on gloves.
6. Assist resident to sitting position. Swing resident's legs over edge of bed.
7. Assist resident to put on robe. Put shoes on resident. Assist resident to stand. If needed, use a transfer belt.
8. Support resident with hands on either side of the belt. Remember to use proper body mechanics. Pivot resident to the right and lower to commode. Do not restrain the resident on the commode.
9. Leave call bell and tissue within reach.
10. Remove gloves and discard according to facility policy. Wash hands.
11. When resident signals return promptly. Wash hands and put on gloves. Use a paper towel to turn on the faucet and another paper towel to turn the faucet off. Fill the basin with warm water (105°F). Bring basin to bedside along with soap, towel, and washcloth.
12. Assist resident to stand. Wipe anal area or perineum if required.
13. Allow resident to wash and dry hands. Remove gloves and dispose of according to facility policy. Wash hands.
14. Assist resident to return to bed. Adjust bedding and pillows for comfort.
15. Leave signal cord within easy reach.
16. Put on gloves. Remove receptacle from commode and cover. Close lid of commode.
17. Take receptacle to bathroom. Note contents and measure if required.
18. Empty and clean receptacle per facility policy. Replace in commode. Remove and dispose of gloves properly.
19. Put commode in proper place. If it remains in the room, place it out of the way.
20. Carry out each procedure completion action.

## PROCEDURE 41 — Assisting Resident to Use the Bathroom

1. Answer call bell promptly.
2. Carry out each beginning procedure action.
3. Assist resident to toilet. Shut door for privacy.

*(continues)*

**PROCEDURE 41** *(continued)*

4. Help resident position himself with the back of his legs against the toilet and facing you.
5. Assist as needed to:
   - Lift skirt or gown
   - Undo belt and lower trousers
   - Lower underwear
6. Assist resident to sit comfortably on toilet with feet flat on floor.
7. Place call bell within reach of the resident.
8. Adjust clothing to cover resident as much as possible or place towel over lap.
9. Leave toilet tissue close at hand. Indicate your willingness to return and assist resident to clean genital/anal area after toileting.
10. Leave resident alone if safe. Do not leave a resident who is confused, disoriented, or weak.
11. Return immediately when resident signals.
12. Wash hands. Put on disposable gloves. Assist resident to stand. (Gather up skirt with one hand to keep clean.)
13. Clean genital/anal area as needed.
14. Remove gloves and discard according to facility policy. Wash hands.
15. Help resident redress.
16. Note contents of toilet and flush.
17. Help resident wash and dry hands.
18. Wash your hands.
19. Assist resident to a comfortable area with call bell and water close at hand.
20. Carry out each procedure completion action.

## ELIMINATION FROM THE LOWER DIGESTIVE TRACT

Solid wastes are eliminated through the lower digestive tract or large intestine (**colon**) (Figure 18-7). The colon is divided into the:

- Ascending colon—located up the right side of the abdomen
- Transverse colon—wastes are moved through it to the opposite side
- Descending colon—located down the left side of the body
- Rectum in the pelvis and the anal opening to the outside of the body

Digested food leaves the stomach in liquid form and enters the small intestine. Here water and some vitamins are absorbed. As the wastes move into the large intestine, they have changed to the more solid form known as feces. The more water the body needs, the more is absorbed from the wastes and the harder the feces become. Normal feces should be brown in color and formed but soft.

Bowel movements are recorded in the resident's record. Observe the bowel movement and report anything unusual about the feces (also known as **stool**).

- Infections and some medications, such as antibiotics, can cause loose, watery stools (**diarrhea**).
- Iron can make the stool black; in some residents iron can cause loose stools, whereas others experience **constipation** (difficult bowel movements).
- Dark stool may also indicate the presence of blood from the intestines; bright red blood in the stool may be from distended and bleeding blood vessels in the rectum (hemorrhoids).

Conditions resulting from lower digestive tract dysfunction include:

- Constipation
- Flatus (gas)
- Diarrhea
- Anal incontinence

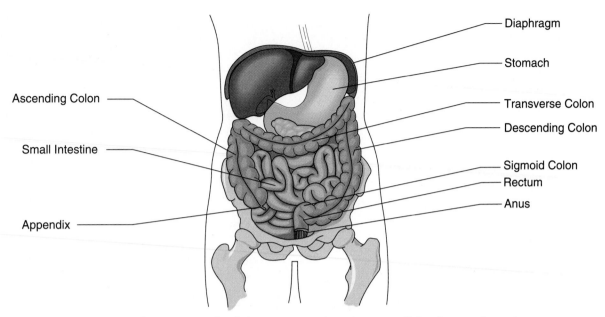

**FIGURE 18-7** Elimination of solid wastes involves organs of the lower digestive tract.

## THE RESIDENT WITH CONSTIPATION

Constipation (difficulty in emptying the bowels) is a problem for many residents in long-term care. This is due to food passing more slowly through the digestive tract. In addition, the residents do not:

- Take in adequate fluids
- Exercise sufficiently
- Take in enough bulk to stimulate peristalsis

Other causes include depression, disease, and certain drugs.

The resident with constipation may not have an appetite and may complain of abdominal discomfort. The abdomen may be **distended** (stretched). If **fecal impaction**—the most serious form of constipation—is present, there may be frequent instances of diarrhea.

Fecal impaction results when the fecal mass loses so much water that it becomes dehydrated (dry and hard) and impossible to eliminate. The dried waste acts as an irritant to the bowel. Mucus tends to dissolve the outer part of the mass, which then drains from the bowel as diarrhea. Whenever there are frequent, small amounts of diarrhea, report this to the nurse who will check the resident for fecal impaction.

### Checking for Fecal Impaction

In some facilities, nursing assistants are permitted to check for fecal impaction. If it is determined that a resident has a fecal impaction, an order is placed for a **suppository** or **enema** to provide relief. To check for fecal impaction, the resident must be in bed on the left side with the right leg flexed. *Be sure your facility permits nursing assistants to perform this procedure.*

Nursing assistant actions to help residents who are constipated include:

- Encouraging as much activity as possible
- Encouraging a high roughage diet
- Offering fluids frequently
- Assisting the resident to the bathroom and allowing adequate time for defecation
- Administering bowel aids as ordered

## BOWEL AIDS

Nursing assistants may give oil-retention enemas and soapsuds enemas. In some facilities, they may be permitted to insert lubricating suppositories. Each of these procedures requires a specific order.

## PROCEDURE 42

# Checking for Fecal Impaction

*Note:* Check the facility policy to be sure that this is a nursing assistant function.

1. Carry out each beginning procedure action.
2. Assemble equipment:
   - Disposable gloves
   - Lubricant
   - Protective pad
   - Bath blanket
   - Toilet tissue
   - Basin of warm water (105°F)
   - Washcloth and towel
3. Raise side rail on side opposite to you.
4. Raise bed to comfortable working height.
5. Put on disposable gloves.
6. Ask resident to raise hips.
7. Place bed protector under hips.
8. Turn resident to side, facing away from you.
9. Cover resident with bath blanket and fanfold top bedclothes to foot of bed.
10. Lubricate index finger of dominant hand.
11. Ask resident to take deep breath and bear down as you insert lubricated finger into rectum.
    *Note:* Rectum should feel soft and pliable. You may feel no feces or you may feel a soft stool, a large solid mass, or multiple hard formations.
12. Withdraw finger.
    *Note:* If a spontaneous bowel movement occurs, note amount and character.
13. Wash the resident's buttocks with warm water and dry.
14. Assist the resident onto back.
15. Ask resident to raise hips and withdraw bed protector.
16. If protector is soiled, fold inward so soiled portion is inside. Discard as biohazardous waste according to facility policy. Otherwise, discard in normal manner.
17. Remove gloves and discard according to facility policy. Wash hands.
18. Pull bedding up and remove bath blanket.
19. Fold bath blanket and store appropriately or place in laundry hamper (according to facility policy).
20. Make resident comfortable and lower bed.
21. Raise side rail, if required for safety.
22. Leave call bell within reach.
23. Empty basin, clean and dry. Return to bedside stand.
24. Remove gloves and discard according to facility policy.
25. Carry out each procedure completion action.

## Enemas

An enema is the introduction of fluid into the rectum, through the anal sphincter, to remove feces (stool) or flatus (gas). The fluid is expelled a short time after introduction, along with the waste products. The need to empty the bowel is signaled by a feeling of urgency. Sometimes a small amount of warm oil is given to soften the stool (oil-retention enema). This is followed by a cleansing soapsuds enema.

Prepackaged commercial enema solutions may be used. A specific order is required for an enema before it is given. Some facilities do not permit nursing assistants to give enemas of any kind. You are responsible for knowing the regulations of your facility.

**General Considerations.** Some general considerations to keep in mind when giving an enema are:

- If the resident is to use the bathroom after the enema, make sure the bathroom is not in use before giving the enema.
- When possible, the enema should be given before breakfast or morning care.
- Do not give an enema within an hour after a meal.

- Remember that you must have a physician's order for any enema and that you can give an enema only if it is a nursing assistant responsibility in your facility.

  Enemas commonly ordered are:
- Commercial preparations
  - Phosphosoda
  - Oil
- Soapsuds enema (SSE)
- Tap water enema (TWE)

---

## PROCEDURE 43

## Giving an Oil-Retention Enema

1. Carry out each beginning procedure action.
2. Assemble equipment:
   - Disposable gloves
   - Bedpan and cover
   - Toilet tissue
   - Towel, soap, basin
   - Prepackaged oil for retention enema
   - Bed protector
   - Bath blanket
3. Instruct the resident that it will be necessary to hold the solution at least 20 minutes.
4. Place chair at foot of bed and cover with towel. Place bedpan on it.
5. Cover resident with bath blanket and fanfold linen to foot of bed.
6. Place bed protector under buttocks.
7. Help resident turn to the left side and flex the right leg.
8. Open the prepackaged oil-retention enema.
9. Wash hands and put on gloves.
10. Expose the resident's anus. Remove cap from enema and insert the prelubricated tip into anus as the resident takes a deep breath.
11. Squeeze container until all the solution has entered the rectum.

12. Remove container and place in package box to be discarded (Figure 18-8).

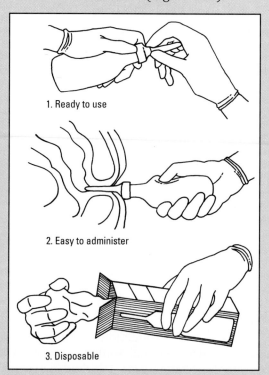

1. Ready to use

2. Easy to administer

3. Disposable

**FIGURE 18-8** Administering an oil-retention enema (Courtesy of C. B. Fleet Co., Inc.)

*(continues)*

**PROCEDURE** *43 (continued)*

13. Encourage resident to remain on the side.
14. Discard enema box. Remove and dispose of gloves according to facility policy. Wash hands.
15. Check resident every 5 minutes until fluid has been retained for 20 minutes.
16. Wash your hands and put on gloves.
17. Position resident on bedpan or assist to bathroom.
18. If resident is on the bedpan, raise head of bed to comfortable height.
19. Place toilet tissue and signal cord within easy reach of resident. If resident is in bathroom, stay nearby. Caution resident not to flush toilet.
20. Discard disposable materials in biohazardous waste according to facility policy.
21. Remove bedpan and cover or assist resident to return to bed.
    - Observe contents of bedpan or toilet.
    - Dispose of contents of bedpan or flush toilet.
22. Cleanse the anal area of the resident, if required.
23. Remove gloves and dispose of properly. Wash hands.
24. Give resident soap, water, and towel to wash and dry hands.
25. Replace top bedding and remove bath blanket and bed protector. Dispose of according to facility policy.
26. Carry out each procedure completion action.

**PROCEDURE 44**

# Giving a Soapsuds Enema

1. Carry out each beginning procedure action.
2. Assemble equipment:
   - Disposable gloves
   - Disposable enema equipment, consisting of a plastic container, tubing with rectal tube, clamp, and lubricant (equipment is commercially available as a kit)
   - Bedpan and cover
   - Bed protector
   - Toilet tissue
   - Bath blanket
   - Castile soap packet
   - Towel, soap, basin
3. In the utility room:
   a. Connect tubing to solution container (Figure 18-9A).

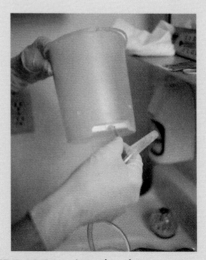

**FIGURE 18-9A** Attach tubing to container.

*(continues)*

**PROCEDURE 44** *(continued)*

b. Adjust clamp on tubing and snap shut (Figure 18-9B).
c. Fill container with warm water (105°F) to the 1,000-mL line (500 mL for children) (Figures 18-9C and D).
d. Open packet of liquid soap and put the soap in the water (Figure 18-9E).
e. Using the tip of the tubing, mix the solution (mix gently so that no suds form) or rotate the bag to mix. Do not shake.

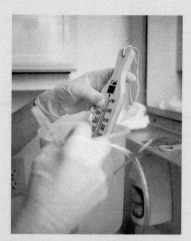

**FIGURE 18-9D** Use a bath thermometer to be sure water temperature is about 105°F.

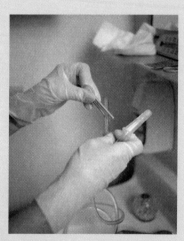

**FIGURE 18-9B** Slip clamp over tubing.

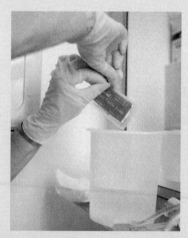

**FIGURE 18-9E** Add liquid soap from packet.

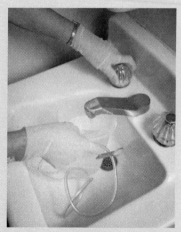

**FIGURE 18-9C** Fill container with warm water.

f. Run small amount of solution through tube to eliminate air and warm the tube (Figure 18-9F). Clamp the tubing (Figure 18-9G).
4. Place chair at foot of bed and cover with bed protector. Place the bedpan on it.
5. Elevate bed to comfortable working height. Be sure opposite side rail is up and secure for safety.

*(continues)*

**PROCEDURE 44** *(continued)*

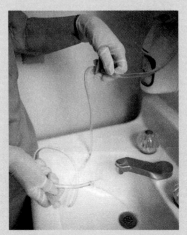

**FIGURE 18-9F**   Let a small amount of water flow through the tube to expel air.

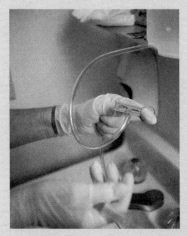

**FIGURE 18-9G**   Clamp tubing.

6. Cover the resident with a bath blanket and fanfold linen to foot of bed.
7. Wash hands and put on gloves.
8. Place bed protector under buttocks.
9. Help resident turn to left side and flex knees.
10. Place container of solution on chair so tubing will reach resident.
11. Adjust bath blanket to expose anal area.
12. Expose anus by raising upper buttock.

13. Lubricate tip of tube. Resident should breath deeply and bear down as tube is inserted to relax the anal sphincter. Insert tube 2 to 4 inches into the anus.
14. Never force the tube. If tube cannot be inserted easily, get help. There may be a tumor or a mass of feces blocking the bowel.
15. Open the clamp and raise the container 12 inches above the level of the anus so that the fluid flows in slowly (Figure 18-9H).
    - Ask the resident to take deep breaths to relax the abdomen.
    - If the resident complains of cramping, clamp tube and wait until cramping stops. Then open the tubing to continue fluid flow.
16. Clamp the tubing before container is completely empty.
17. Tell the resident to hold breath while upper buttock is raised and tube is gently withdrawn.
18. Wrap tubing in paper towel. Put it in the disposable container.
19. Place resident on bedpan or assist to bathroom.

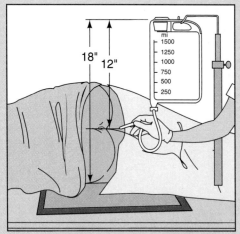

**FIGURE 18-9H**   Raise container above level of anus so fluid flow is unobstructed.

*(continues)*

## PROCEDURE 44 *(continued)*

20. Holding a paper towel in the hand so glove does not contaminate control or crank, raise head of bed to comfortable height if resident is on bedpan. Raise side rail for safety if bed is left in the higher horizontal position.
21. Place toilet tissue and signal cord within reach of resident. If resident is in bathroom, stay nearby. Caution resident not to flush toilet.
22. Discard disposable materials in biohazardous waste according to facility policy.
23. Remove gloves and discard according to facility policy. Wash hands.
24. Return to bedside. Wash hands and put on gloves.
25. Remove bedpan. Place it on a bed protector on chair and cover.
26. Cleanse the anal area.
27. Remove the bed protector and discard according to facility policy.
28. Remove gloves and wash hands.
29. Give resident soap, water, and towel to wash and dry hands.
30. Replace top bedding and remove bath blanket.
31. Put on gloves. Take bedpan to bathroom. Dispose of contents according to facility policy or, using a paper towel, flush toilet.
32. Remove gloves and dispose of according to facility policy.
33. Wash hands.
34. Air the room and leave room in order.
35. Unscreen unit.
36. Clean and replace all other equipment used according to facility policy.
37. Carry out each procedure completion action.

## Giving an Enema with a Commercially Prepared Chemical Enema Solution

Commercially prepared enemas are convenient to administer and more comfortable for the resident.

- The chemical solution is already measured and ready to use.
- A small amount of fluid will remain in the container after administration.
- The solution in a prepared enema draws fluid from the body to stimulate peristalsis.
- The amount of solution administered is about 4 ounces.
- The tip of the container is prelubricated.
- The enema solution is in an easy-to-handle plastic container.
- The solution is sometimes used at room temperature.
- You may be asked to warm the solution by placing the container in warm water before administration. Check with the nurse regarding your facility's policy.

## PROCEDURE 45 Giving a Commercially Prepared Enema

1. Carry out each beginning procedure action.
2. Assemble equipment:
   - Disposable gloves
   - Disposable prepackaged enema
   - Bedpan and cover
   - Bed protector
   - Pan of warm water (if enema solution is to be warmed)

*(continues)*

**PROCEDURE** *45* *(continued)*

3. Open package and remove plastic container with enema solution. Place solution container in warm water (if it is to be warmed).
4. Lower head of bed to horizontal position and elevate bed to comfortable working height. Raise side rail on opposite side of bed for safety.
5. Put on gloves.
6. Place bedpan and cover on the chair close at hand.
7. Assist resident to turn to the left side and flex the right leg.
8. Place bed protector under the resident.
9. Expose only the resident's buttocks by drawing the bedding upward in one hand.
10. Remove the cover from the enema tip (Figure 18-10). Gently squeeze to make sure tip is patent.

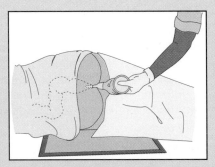

**FIGURE 18-11** Squeeze bottle from bottom until all the liquid has gone into the rectum.

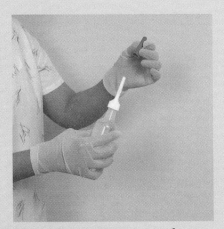

**FIGURE 18-10** Remove cover from prelubricated tip of container.

11. Separate buttocks, exposing anus, and ask resident to breathe deeply and bear down slightly.
12. Insert lubricated enema tip 2 inches into the rectum.
13. Squeeze the plastic container slowly from the bottom of the container until all fluid has entered the resident's body (Figure 18-11).

14. Remove the tip from the resident and place the container in the box. Encourage the resident to hold the solution as long as possible.
15. Remove gloves and dispose of properly and wash hands.
16. Discard the used enema in the biohazard waste.
17. Provide privacy. This enema should be retained for 20 minutes. Give the resident the call signal and leave.
18. When the resident feels the urge to defecate, lower bed and assist resident to the bathroom or commode or position on the bedpan.
19. Raise the head of the bed to a comfortable height if the resident is on the bedpan.
20. Place toilet tissue and signal cord within reach of the resident. Raise side rail for safety if bed is left in high position. If resident is in bathroom, stay nearby. Caution resident not to flush toilet.
21. Return to the resident when signaled. Wash hands. Lower nearest side rail if up. Put on gloves.
22. Remove bedpan and place on bed protector on chair. Observe contents of bedpan. Cover bedpan.
23. Clean anal area of resident if required.
24. If the resident has used commode or toilet:
    a. Clean anal area if required.
    b. Observe contents of commode or toilet.

*(continues)*

---

**PROCEDURE 45** *(continued)*

c. Flush toilet using paper towel or cover commode.

d. Remove gloves and discard according to facility policy. Assist resident into bed.

**25.** Put on gloves. Take bedpan or commode container and equipment to the bathroom. Dispose of contents according to facility policy.

**26.** Remove and dispose of gloves properly. Wash your hands.

**27.** Give the resident soap, water, and a towel to wash hands. Return equipment. Leave side rails down unless needed for safety and leave bed in low position.

**28.** Carry out each procedure completion action.

---

## Rectal Suppositories

Rectal suppositories are used to stimulate bowel evacuation or administer medication. Medicinal suppositories must be inserted by the nurse. You may be asked to insert the type of suppository that softens stool and promotes elimination.

Check your facility policy to be sure this is a nursing assistant function. The suppository must be placed beyond the rectal **sphincter** (circular muscle that controls the anal opening) and against the bowel wall so it can melt and lubricate the rectum.

---

**PROCEDURE 46** Inserting a Rectal Suppository

*Note:* Be sure this is a nursing assistant procedure at your facility.

**1.** Carry out each beginning procedure action.

**2.** Assemble equipment:

- Disposable gloves
- Suppository as ordered
- Toilet tissue
- Bedpan and cover, if needed
- Lubricant
- Bed protector

**3.** Wash hands and put on gloves.

**4.** Help resident turn on the left side and flex the right leg. Place bed protector under hips.

**5.** Adjust bed linen to expose buttocks only.

**6.** Unwrap suppository.

**7.** With left hand, separate the buttocks, exposing the anus.

**8.** Apply a small amount of lubricant to anus and to the suppository and insert the suppository. Suppository must be inserted deeply enough to enter the rectum beyond the sphincter (approximately 2 inches (Figure 18-12).

**9.** Encourage resident to take deep breaths and relax (until the need to defecate is felt in 5 to 20 minutes).

**10.** Remove gloves and dispose of properly. Wash hands.

*(continues)*

## PROCEDURE *46* (continued)

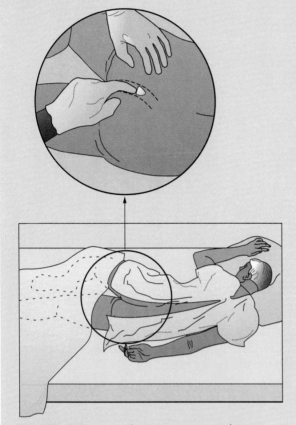

**FIGURE 18-12** Lubricate anus and insert suppository beyond the rectal sphincter muscle.

11. Adjust the bedding, helping resident to assume a comfortable position.
12. Place call bell near resident's hand, but check every 5 minutes.
13. Wash hands and put on gloves.
14. Assist resident to bathroom or commode or position on bedpan.
15. Provide privacy. Once the resident is finished, assist with hygiene if necessary.
16. Observe results and note any unusual characteristics of stool. If stool is unusual, save and report to nurse.
17. Dispose of stool and clean equipment according to facility policy. Store equipment as required.
18. Remove and dispose of gloves according to facility policy. Wash hands.
19. Carry out each procedure completion action.

## RECTAL TUBE AND FLATUS BAG ····

The rectal tube is used to reduce flatus (gas) in the bowel. Placing a rectal tube into the rectum provides a passageway for the gas to escape.

Flatus distends the intestines, causing pain and stress on incisions. Flatus is a problem for many residents in long-term care. If unexpelled, it can cause the resident to feel very uncomfortable.

You can assist the resident as follows:

- Encourage activity.
- Promote regularity.
- Accept the expulsion of gas as a natural body function. Do not contribute to the resident's embarrassment.
- Use flatus-reducing procedures when ordered.
- Insert a rectal tube with flatus bag if ordered. (Remember that your facility policies must state that nursing assistants can perform this procedure.)

The disposable tube is used once in a 24-hour period for no more than 20 minutes.

- Relief may occur as soon as the tube is inserted.
- Check the amount of abdominal distention (stretching).
- Question resident about amount of relief.

**PROCEDURE 47**

## Inserting a Rectal Tube and Flatus Bag

1. Carry out each beginning procedure action.
2. Assemble equipment:
   - Disposable gloves
   - Disposable rectal tube and flatus bag
   - Bed protector
   - Lubricant
   - Tissue
   - Tape
   - Paper towel
3. Lower the head of the bed to horizontal position.
4. Wash hands and put gloves on.
5. Assist the resident to turn to the left side and flex the right leg. Place bed protector under hips.
6. Adjust bed linen to expose only the resident's buttocks.
7. Lubricate tip of rectal tube.
8. Separate buttocks, exposing anus, and ask resident to breathe deeply and bear down gently.
9. Insert lubricated tip of rectal tube 2 to 4 inches.
10. Secure rectal tube in place with small piece of hypoallergenic adhesive (Figure 18-13).
11. Remove gloves and dispose of properly. Wash hands.
12. Adjust bedding and make resident comfortable. Leave unit neat and tidy. Place signal cord within reach of resident.
13. Return to unit in 20 minutes. Wash your hands.

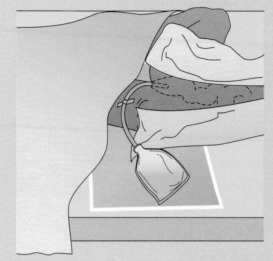

**FIGURE 18-13** Secure rectal tube with flatus bag in place using a small amount of hypoallergenic tape.

14. Identify resident and screen unit. Explain what you plan to do.
15. Put on gloves.
16. Gently remove rectal tube and place on paper towel.
17. Clean area around anus as needed.
18. Dispose of wrapped rectal tube and bag according to facility policy.
19. Remove and dispose of gloves according to facility policy. Wash hands.
20. Carry out each procedure completion action.

## OSTOMIES

The surgical removal of a section of diseased bowel requires the creation of an artificial opening (**ostomy**) in the abdominal wall for solid waste elimination. When the colon is brought through the abdominal wall, the opening is called a **colostomy**. The mouth of the opening is called a **stoma** (Figure 18-14). The ostomy may be temporary or permanent. The location of

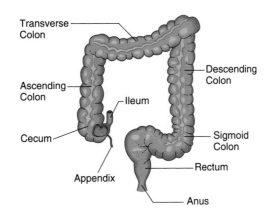

**FIGURE 18-14** Typical colostomy stoma

the ostomy (Figure 18-15) determines if the feces are formed, soft and mushy, semiliquid, or liquid.

The resident with a colostomy does not have normal sphincter control. This means the resident cannot voluntarily control emptying of the bowel in the same manner as emptying through the anus. If the colostomy is located in the bowel where stool is formed, regularity of elimination may be established. As elimination is controlled, the stoma may be covered with a simple dressing between evacuations. Liquid to mushy fecal drainage from a stoma is collected in a disposable drainage pouch, called an appliance, that is attached over the stoma.

## Stoma Care

Proper care is needed to keep the tissue around the stoma healthy. The waste eliminated from

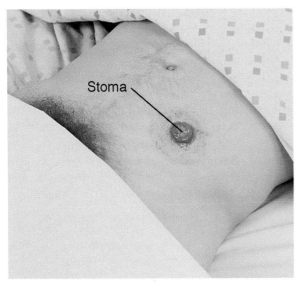

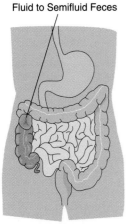
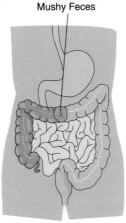
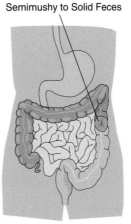
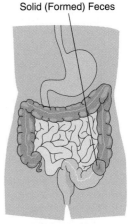

Ascending Colostomy — Transverse Colostomy — Descending Colostomy — Sigmoid Colostomy

**FIGURE 18-15** The site of the colostomy determines the character of the feces.

the stoma may be irritating to the tissue, especially the liquid or semiliquid feces. Other problems may include leakage and odor.

You can assist the resident with a colostomy by:

- Encouraging the resident to eat food helpful in controlling elimination. Restricting foods determined to cause flatus or loose feces (depending on location of ostomy) can make management of the ostomy easier.
- Performing routine stoma care
- Keeping the area around the opening clean and dry

- Protecting the skin around the stoma according to facility policy. Follow the care plan exactly.
- Adding deodorizer to ostomy bag, if instructed, to reduce odor
- Attaching the appliance securely over the stoma
- Reporting the nature of the colostomy output
- Reporting to the nurse if area around the stoma is red, irritated, or nonintact

If the colostomy appliance is reusable, it should be washed with soap and water and dried while a clean alternate is applied. If the pouch is not reusable, dispose of it according to facility policy.

---

**PROCEDURE**
## 48  Giving Routine Stoma Care (Colostomy)

1. Carry out each beginning procedure action.
2. Assemble equipment:
   - Disposable gloves
   - Washcloth and towel
   - Basin of warm water
   - Bed protector
   - Bath blanket
   - Disposable colostomy bag and belt
   - Bedpan
   - Skin lotion as directed
   - Prescribed solvent/dropper
   - Cleansing agent
   - Adhesive wafer
   - 4 × 4 gauze square
   - Toilet tissue
3. Place bath blanket over resident. Fanfold top bedding to foot of bed.
4. Wash hands and put on disposable gloves.
5. Place bed protector under the resident's hips.
6. Place bedpan and cover on bed protector on chair.
7. Remove the soiled disposable stoma bag (appliance) and place in bedpan—note amount and type of drainage.

8. Remove belt that holds stoma bag and save if clean.
9. Gently clean area around stoma with toilet tissue to remove feces and drainage (Figure 18-16A). Dispose of tissue in bedpan.
10. Wash area around stoma with soap and water. Rinse thoroughly and dry.
11. If ordered, apply barrier cream lightly around the stoma—too much lotion may interfere with proper seal of fresh ostomy bag.

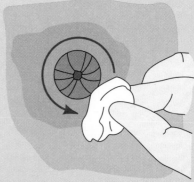

**FIGURE 18-16A** The area around the stoma is cleaned well but gently and dried before a new appliance is applied.

*(continues)*

**PROCEDURE** *48* *(continued)*

12. Position clean belt around resident— inspect skin under belt for irritation or breakdown.
13. It may be necessary to remove the adhesive wafer. To select the proper size of wafer, a commercial guide can be used to size the stoma (Figure 18-16B).
14. Replace adhesive wafer (Figure 18-16C). Place clean ostomy bag over stoma and secure belt.
15. Remove bed protector. Check to be sure bottom bedding is not wet. Change if necessary.

16. Remove gloves and discard according to facility policy. Wash hands.
17. Replace bath blanket with top bedding, making resident comfortable.
18. Using a paper towel to protect hands, gather and cover soiled materials and bedpan. Take to utility room. Dispose of materials according to facility policy.
19. Empty, wash, and dry bedpan. Store according to facility policy.
20. Carry out each procedure completion action.

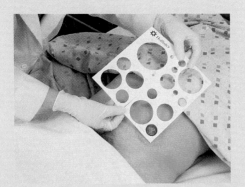

**FIGURE 18-16B**  Check the size of the stoma to be sure the proper size of barrier is used.

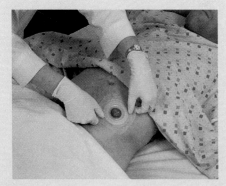

**FIGURE 18-16C**  A new barrier adhesive wafer is applied around the stoma.

## Care of the Resident with an Ileostomy

An **ileostomy** is a permanent artificial opening in the ileum (Figure 18-17) that drains through a stoma on the surface of the abdomen. The drainage from the ileum is in liquid form and contains digestive enzymes that are irritating to the skin.

Considerations for caring for a resident with an ileostomy include:

* The professional nurse cares for the resident with a fresh ileostomy.
* Routine care may be given by nursing assistants.
* The drainage from an ileostomy is very irritating to the skin, so care of the skin surrounding the stoma is crucial.

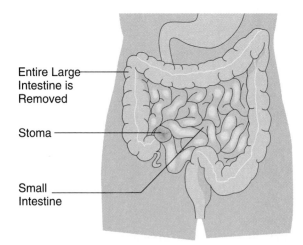

Entire Large Intestine is Removed

Stoma

Small Intestine

**FIGURE 18-17**  An ileostomy brings a section of the ileum through the abdominal wall.

• The fit of the ileostomy ring is critical to prevent leakage. This is true for both the disposable and reusable types of appliances.

# FECAL INCONTINENCE

Feces are highly irritating and contain many microbes that can be sources of infection. Fecal incontinence is distressing to residents. Residents must be cleaned immediately after involuntary defecation and every attempt must be made to establish continence through retraining and dietary management.

When there are frequent liquid stools, a drainable fecal incontinence collector may be needed (Figure 18-18).

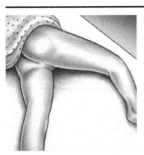

1. Position patient on side.

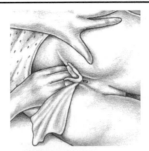

2. Clean and dry skin.

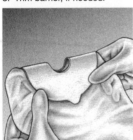

3. Trim barrier, if needed.

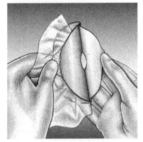

4. Remove release paper.

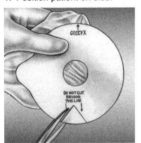

5. Fold barrier.

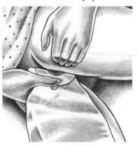

6. Separate buttocks.

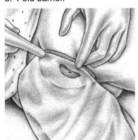

7. Position collector.

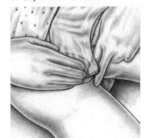

8. Press and seal barrier.

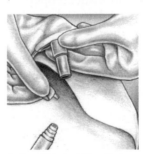

9. Connect to bedside collector.

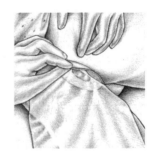

10. Remove.

## DRAINABLE FECAL INCONTINENCE COLLECTOR WITH FLEXTEND SKIN BARRIER

### Preparation and Application

1. Turn patient on one side, bending the upper knee up towards the chest.
2. Clean and dry the perineal area thoroughly.
3. If necessary, trim the skin barrier to fit perineal area.
   - For females with a narrow perineal bridge, the skin barrier should be cut to fit.
   - Follow the cutting guide, leaving as much of the skin barrier as possible. The barrier should not cover the labia or the vaginal opening.
4. Remove the release paper.
5. Fold the skin barrier in half.
6. Separate the buttocks.
7. Position the pre-cut hole over the anus. Do not enlarge pre-cut hole.
8. Apply and press firmly.
   - Apply barrier to perineal area first, pressing firmly after positioning correctly. Using your other hand, press the barrier firmly, holding for thirty seconds to allow it to adhere properly.
9. To empty, open drain cap and direct the stool into an appropriate receptacle. For best results, connect to a bedside drainage collector.
10. To remove, gently ease the barrier from the patient's skin, using fabric tab.

### Preparation and Application

- Remove oily substances or powders from the skin which interferes with skin barrier adhesion.
- Skin gel wipes on skin may decrease wear time.
- DO NOT cut the barrier opening.
- Trim excess hair with scissors. DO NOT use a razor.

**FIGURE 18-18** Fecal incontinence collection system (Permission to reproduce this copyrighted material has been granted by the owner, Hollister Incorporated, Libertyville, IL)

## COLLECTING A STOOL SPECIMEN ····

A stool specimen is usually required when infection, bleeding, or parasites in the colon are suspected. You may be asked to collect a stool specimen. When carrying out this task:

- Wear gloves.
- Collect the specimen in a bedpan, commode receptacle, toilet insert, or from a fecal collection bag or bed linens.

- Do not place toilet paper in the collection container.
- Do not allow the specimen to touch the outside of collection container.
- Use tongue depressors to handle the specimen.
- Make sure that the specimen is properly labeled and promptly transported.

**PROCEDURE**

**49**

# Collecting a Stool Specimen

1. Carry out each beginning procedure action.
2. Assemble equipment:
   - Disposable gloves
   - Bedpan and cover or collection container
   - Specimen container and cover
   - Biohazard specimen transport bag
   - Label including:
     - Resident's full name
     - Room number
     - Date and time of collection
     - Physician's name
     - Examination to be performed
     - Other information required
   - Toilet tissue
   - Tongue depressors
   - Basin
3. Wash hands and put on disposable gloves.
4. Uncover container used to collect bowel movement (bedpan or commode receptacle). (If toilet insert is used, specimen will be collected from insert.) If resident is incontinent of feces, use tongue depressors to obtain specimen from bed linens, diaper, or protective padding. A specimen may

also be obtained from a fecal incontinence collection bag when it is changed.
5. Following defecation, resident is to wash hands. Fill basin with water at 105°F. Assist resident if needed. If resident is incontinent, carefully clean and dry area around anus. Change bed linens as needed.
6. Take container with bowel movement to the bathroom. Use tongue blades to remove specimen and place in specimen container (Figure 18-19). Do not contaminate the outside of the specimen container or the cover. If possible, take a sample (about 1 teaspoon) from each part of the specimen.
7. Empty collection container into toilet. Clean or dispose of collection container according to facility policy. If the resident was incontinent, dispose of soiled brief or padding as biohazardous waste. Place soiled linen in proper hamper.
8. Remove and dispose of gloves according to facility policy.
9. Wash your hands.

*(continues)*

**PROCEDURE 49** *(continued)*

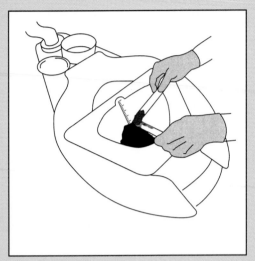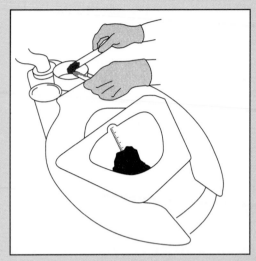

**FIGURE 18-19** Use tongue blades to transfer the stool specimen from the collection container (left) to the specimen container (right).

**10.** Cover container and attach completed label. Make sure cover is on container tightly. Place container in biohazard transport bag.

**11.** Take or send specimen to laboratory promptly. (Stool specimens are never refrigerated.)

**12.** Carry out each procedure completion action.

## URINARY SYSTEM

Most liquid wastes are eliminated from the body through the urinary system in the form of urine.

The urinary system consists of the kidneys (filter blood and form urine) and the ureters and urethra (tubes that carry the urine to the outside of the body) (Figure 18-20). The urinary system:

- Forms urine
- Stores urine
- Excretes urine
- Manages blood chemistry
- Manages fluid balance

### Kidneys

The kidneys are two bean-shaped organs about 6 inches long. They are located on either side of the spinal column in the lumbar area. They are made up of the:

- Cortex—the dark reddish brown outer part that contains the urine-producing unit called the **nephron** (Figure 18-21).
- Medulla—the lighter-colored middle part contains collecting tubules that receive the formed urine.
- Renal pelvis—the central basin-like area into which the urine passes. The renal pelvis directs the urine out of each kidney and into the ureters.

### Ureters

The **ureters** are tubes about 12 inches long that lead from each kidney to the urinary bladder.

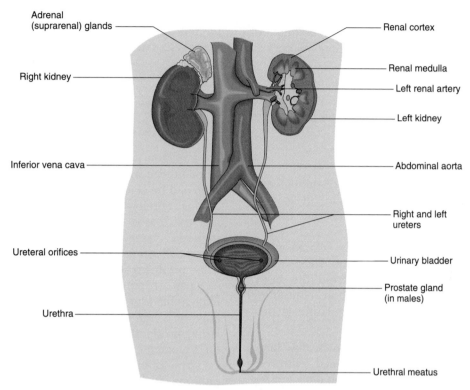

**FIGURE 18-20**   Structures of the urinary system

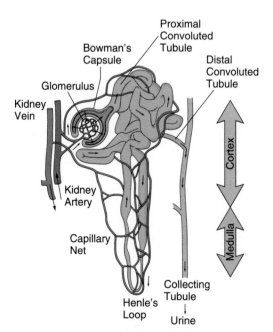

**FIGURE 18-21**   Nephron and related structures. Small arrows indicate the flow of blood through the nephron. The urine produced by the nephron flows through the collecting tubule.

## Urinary Bladder

The **bladder**, a hollow muscular organ in the pelvis, has the following functions:

- Receives the urine from the ureters
- Stores urine until it can be eliminated from the body (holds about 1 cup or 250 mL of urine before urge to void is felt)
- The exit from the bladder is guarded by a small, circular (sphincter) muscle that prevents urine from escaping involuntarily.

## Urethra

The **urethra** is a small tube that carries the urine from the bladder out of the body. The opening to the outside is called the **meatus**. The male and female urethra differ as follows.

The female urethra:

- Is about $1\frac{1}{2}$ inches long
- Transports urine only

The male urethra:

- Is 8 to 10 inches long.
- Is surrounded by a gland called the **prostate gland**, which is part of the reproductive system

- Transports urine
- Transports reproductive fluids to the outside. (Urine and reproductive fluids may not pass at the same time.)

Enlargement of the prostate gland can press on the urethra, making the passage of urine difficult. This often happens in men as they reach later middle age.

### Urine Formation

The nephron is a filtering system of tubules and blood vessels that produces urine. It is estimated that each kidney contains one million nephrons.

Blood arriving at the kidneys carries waste products such as acids and salts. These waste products must be eliminated from the body. Urine is a liquid waste solution containing water and dissolved substances. Urine is produced as follows:

- Waste products, helpful products, and large quantities of water are passed (filtered) through the capillary walls of the **glomerulus** (capillary bed) into **Bowman's capsule**, forming a liquid called filtrate. (See Figure 18-21.)
- The filtrate moves slowly along the convoluted tubules where some water and helpful substances like sugar are reabsorbed into the blood.
- The liquid remaining in the convoluted tubules is urine and contains wastes.
- The urine passes into the collecting tubules of the medulla, then out of the kidney to the ureter and into the urinary bladder.
- *Normal* urine is acid in reaction and pale to deep yellow in color.
- *Dilute* urine has more water and fewer dissolved substances, so it is white to pale yellow.
- *Concentrated* urine has less water and more dissolved substances, so it is darker in color and has a stronger odor.
- The amount of urine produced depends on the amount of intake and various physical conditions. Inadequate water intake leading to dehydration results in a small amount of concentrated urine.

The substances in the urine provide good information about the chemistry of the body and how well it is functioning. Tests are frequently performed on the urine (**urinalysis**).

During your care of the resident, note the amount, color, and odor of the urine, and the presence of any sediment.

## CHANGES IN THE URINARY SYSTEM CAUSED BY AGING

As a person ages, the kidneys decrease somewhat in size and some renal cells are lost and replaced by scar tissue. This means the kidneys are less efficient filters. The blood vessels carrying the blood to the kidneys for filtration undergo changes that reduce the amount of blood delivered. The lower blood flow decreases urine production.

Loss of pelvic muscle tone and strength makes bladder emptying less efficient. Urine may be retained in the bladder (**retention**). Urine production influences the acid-base and fluid balances of the body.

Urine is produced continuously. In younger persons, it is more concentrated during the night. An older person loses some concentrating ability and experiences more need to empty the bladder at night. This problem is called **nocturia**. Make sure the call bell is available and that lighting is adequate for safe ambulation at night. Figure 18-22 summarizes the urinary system changes caused by aging.

| **FIGURE 18-22** Changes in the urinary system as a result of aging |
| --- |
| • Kidneys decrease in size |
| • Scar tissue replaces some renal cells |
| • Reduced blood flow through the kidneys means lower urine production |
| • Reduced renal concentration, leading to nocturia |
| • Less efficient bladder emptying |
| • Reduced filtration ability |

# URINE ELIMINATION

The act of eliminating urine from the bladder is known by various terms:

- **Micturition**
- **Urination**
- **Voiding**

A common phrase is "passing water." Voiding or urinating are the terms most frequently used to describe emptying the bladder.

Voiding can occur involuntarily when the bladder fills to about 250 mL. Urine is released as the sphincter muscle relaxes and the bladder walls contract. With training, the signal that the bladder is filling is brought to the level of conscious thought so that voiding can be voluntarily controlled.

# URINARY RETENTION AND INCONTINENCE

Elderly residents face two major problems related to the urinary system. The problems are retention and incontinence.

Urinary retention is due to poor bladder tone or incomplete emptying because of an obstruction. Poor tone may be related to the aging process or prolonged catheter drainage. Obstruction may be due to tumor growth. In, men, obstruction is often due to the enlargement of the prostate gland. Urinary retention due to a tumor may require surgery to relieve the obstruction.

Urinary retention is due to one or more factors, including:

- Inability to reach toileting facilities in time
- Emotional withdrawal
- Lack of awareness of need
- Physical changes
- Infection of the urinary tract
- Fecal impaction
- Neurologic damage such as in a stroke
- Inability to communicate the need to toilet
- Mental confusion
- Ineffective muscle control

Urinary incontinence may be temporary or established. If attention is given to the underlying causes, the temporary use of incontinence pads may be all that is needed. When the incontinence is prolonged, tests to determine the cause may be ordered. If needed, a urinary retraining program will be started.

## Nursing Assistant Actions

Urinary incontinence is uncomfortable and embarrassing to the resident. In addition, prolonged exposure of the skin to urine is a major cause of skin breakdown. The warm, moist conditions also encourage bacterial growth. Pathogens on the skin grow quickly and move upward through the urinary tract to cause serious urinary infections. These can lead to life-threatening **septicemia** (**sepsis**). Wet linen that is not changed promptly has a disagreeable odor. Residents who are incontinent fear having "accidents" and tend to limit social interactions with others.

Every effort must be made to help the resident become continent. Little reference should be made to the temporary incontinence. Nursing assistants can do much to give emotional support and reassurance to residents who are incontinent. Nursing assistant responsibilities include:

- Assisting residents to toilet regularly
- Answering call lights promptly
- Always being courteous and patient when assisting residents with toileting
- Maintaining a positive attitude when changing soiled garments and bed linen and never being critical
- Performing good perineal care and being sure resident is clean and dry
- Checking the skin for signs of irritation whenever you toilet or bathe resident or perform perineal care
- Giving special attention to residents who are confused or forgetful because they may be unable to clearly state their need for assistance

# INTERNAL URINARY CATHETER DRAINAGE

At times, it may be necessary to assist urinary elimination by the use of an **indwelling catheter**. The **catheter** is a slender rubber or plastic tube that is inserted into the bladder using sterile technique. The urine drains out of the bladder through the catheter. A balloon around the neck of the catheter is inflated once the catheter is in place. The inflated balloon keeps the catheter in place so that it will not easily slip out. The other end of the catheter is connected to a drainage tube and collection bag (Figure 18-23). This is a closed system and is sterile as long as it is not opened. Opening the system greatly increases the risk of infection. The insertion of a sterile catheter is the responsibility of the nurse.

## Catheter Care

The nursing assistant provides daily care of the catheter when the resident has an indwelling catheter for urinary drainage. This care consists of the following actions:

- Applying the principles of standard precautions
- Keeping the urinary meatus clean
- Washing the area around the meatus daily with a solution approved by your facility
- Checking regularly for signs of irritation or urinary discomfort and reporting to the nurse
- Securing the tubing in such a way that there is no strain on the catheter or tubing (A catheter strap should be applied to the leg to secure the tubing.)
- Maintaining the drainage bag below the level of the bladder
- Clamping and unclamping the catheter tubing at specific times. The clamping allows the bladder to fill, stimulating muscle tone.
- Not opening the closed system
- Making sure the tubing is not kinked or obstructed
- Ensuring that the collection bag does not touch the floor
- Measuring the amount of drainage in the collection bag at the end of each shift, noting the character of the urine, and reporting and recording the information
- Checking the entire drainage setup each time care is given and at the beginning and end of your shift
- Reporting changes in the character or quantity of urine

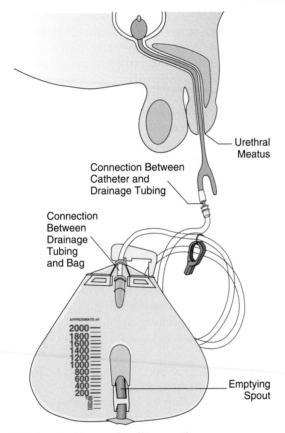

Urethral Meatus

Connection Between Catheter and Drainage Tubing

Connection Between Drainage Tubing and Bag

APPROXIMATE ml
2000
1800
1600
1400
1200
1000
800
600
400
200

Emptying Spout

**FIGURE 18-23** Indwelling catheter connected to a urine drainage bag

---

**PROCEDURE**

## *50* Routine Drainage Check

**1.** Carry out each beginning procedure action.

**2.** Wash hands. Put on gloves.

**3.** Raise bedding to observe tubing.

*(continues)*

**PROCEDURE *50* (continued)**

4. Check condition of catheter and meatus.
5. Keep drainage tubing coiled on bed so there is a direct drop to collection bag (Figure 18-24).
6. Collection bag height must be lower than resident's hips.
7. Keep end of drainage tube above urine level in bag.
8. Be sure drainage bag is attached to bed frame.
9. Note color and character and flow of urine.
10. Measure urine using proper technique.
11. Remove gloves and discard according to facility policy.
12. Carry out each procedure completion action.

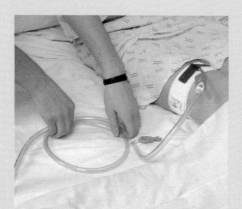

**FIGURE 18-24** Check the catheter tubing to be sure it is secured but not obstructed by the Velcro® leg band and that it is coiled on the bed.

**PROCEDURE *51*** Giving Indwelling Catheter Care

1. Carry out each beginning procedure action.
2. Assemble equipment:
   • Disposable gloves
   • Bed protector
   • Bath blanket
   • Plastic bag for disposables
   • Daily catheter care kit (if available)
   • Washcloth, towel, basin, and soap if kit is unavailable
   • Antiseptic solution
   • Sterile applicators
   • Tape
3. Elevate bed to comfortable working height. Be sure opposite side rail is up and secure. Position patient on back,

with legs separated and knees bent, if permitted.
4. Cover resident with bath blanket and fan-fold bedding to foot of bed.
5. Ask resident to raise hips. Place bed protector underneath resident.
6. Position bath blanket so that only genitals will be exposed.
7. Arrange catheter care kit and plastic bag on overbed table. Open kit.
8. Wash hands and put on gloves and draw drape back.
9. For the male resident:
   • Gently grasp penis and draw foreskin back, if not circumcised (Figure 18-25).

*(continues)*

**PROCEDURE *51*** *(continued)*

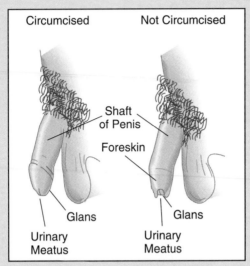

**FIGURE 18-25** Comparison of circumcised and uncircumcised penis

- Using a new applicator dipped in antiseptic solution for each stroke, cleanse the glans from meatus toward shaft for approximately 4 inches.
- After one stroke, dispose of each used applicator in plastic bag.
  **Alternate Action:** Going around the catheter first and then around meatus and glans. Wash with soap and water using a circular motion. Dry in the same manner. Make sure to return the foreskin (if not circumcised) to its proper position.

For the female resident:
- Separate the labia.
- Using a new applicator dipped in antiseptic for each stroke, cleanse from front to back.
- After one stroke, dispose of each used applicator in plastic bag.
  **Alternate Action:** Using a clean cloth, soap and water, clean labia majora from front to back. Repeat, cleaning labia minora and then wash

meatus. Clean catheter down about 4 inches. Dry carefully.
**10.** Remove gloves and discard in plastic bag. Wash hands.
**11.** Check catheter to be sure it is secured properly to the leg. (See Figure 18-24.) Readjust Velcro® strap for slack, if needed. If a Velcro® strap is not available, use tape (Figure 18-26).

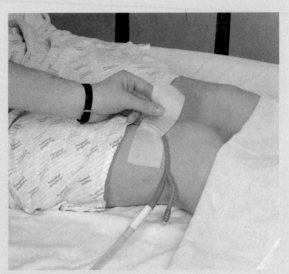

**FIGURE 18-26** The catheter tubing can also be taped to the thigh using hypoallergenic tape preferably.

**12.** Check to be sure tubing is coiled on bed (see Figure 18-24) and hangs straight down into drainage container. Empty bag and measure if necessary. Do not raise bag above level of resident's hips.
**13.** Replace bedding and remove bath blanket.
**14.** Fold bath blanket and store or put in linen hamper.
**15.** Lower bed. Adjust side rails for safety.
**16.** Carry out each procedure completion action.

## Ambulating with a Catheter

When residents are ambulatory or using a geri-chair or wheelchair, you must be careful about the placement of the urinary drainage bag. Remember that the drainage bag must always be lower than the bladder so the urine cannot flow back into the bladder. The bag may be secured to the resident's leg or clothing when the resident ambulates.

When the resident is seated in a wheelchair, the tubing should run below and under the wheelchair so the drainage bag can be secured to the wheelchair back. The drainage bag or tubing must never touch the floor.

At times, the catheter may be disconnected to make ambulation easier. However, there is always the danger of contamination.

## Infection Risk

You must follow the procedure for disconnecting the catheter carefully. The resident who has an indwelling catheter is at risk for infection. There are several sites where infection can enter the drainage system:

- Urinary meatus, where the catheter is inserted
- Connection between the catheter and drainage tube
- Connection between the drainage bag and drainage tubing
- Opening used to empty the drainage bag

## Disconnecting the Catheter

It is preferable never to disconnect the drainage setup, but at times, it is necessary. If sterile caps and plugs are available, they should be used. If not, the disconnected ends must be protected with sterile gauze sponges.

---

**PROCEDURE**
## 52 Disconnecting the Catheter

**1.** Carry out each beginning procedure action.
**2.** Assemble equipment:
   - Disposable gloves
   - Antiseptic wipes
   - Gauze sponges
   - Sterile caps/plugs
   - Clamps
**3.** Wash hands and put on gloves.
**4.** Clamp the catheter.
**5.** Disconnect the catheter and drainage tubing. Do not put the ends down or allow them to touch anything. If accidental contamination occurs, wipe the ends with antiseptic wipes before inserting plug or placing cap. Dispose of antiseptic wipes in plastic bag.

**6.** Insert a sterile plug in the end of the catheter. Place a sterile cap over the exposed end of the drainage tube (Figure 18-27).
**7.** Secure the drainage tube to the bed frame in such a way that it will not touch the floor.
**8.** Remove and dispose of gloves according to facility policy. Wash hands.
**9.** Carry out each procedure completion action.
   *Note:* Reverse the procedure to reconnect the catheter. If you find an unprotected, disconnected tube in the bed or on the floor, *do not reconnect it. Report it at once.*

*(continues)*

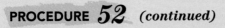

**PROCEDURE** *52* *(continued)*

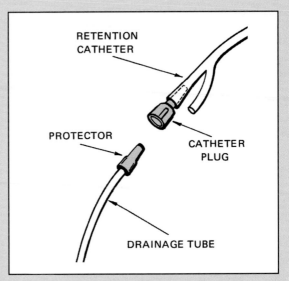

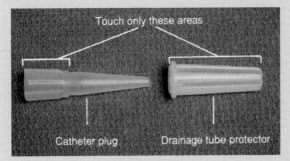

**FIGURE 18-27** Sterile catheter plug and protective cap (left). Plug and protective cap in place (right)

## INTAKE AND OUTPUT (I&O) ·········

### Intake

Intake includes everything taken in that is liquid at room temperature, such as:

- Water or tea
- Gelatin, junket, or pudding
- Fluids given directly into a vein (IV)

### Output

Normal fluid output includes all fluids that leave the body, including:

- Urine
- Perspiration
- Moisture from the lungs
- Moisture from the bowels

Excessive fluid loss results in dehydration (inadequate water content in body tissue). This loss can occur through:

- Diarrhea
- Vomiting
- Excessive urine output (diuresis)
- Excessive perspiration (diaphoresis)

Retention of fluids results in edema (swelling of body tissues). This may be caused by:

- Kidney dysfunction
- Cardiovascular disease

### Recording Output

An accurate recording of intake and output is basic to the care of many residents. Intake and output totals are usually kept on the same form. Records are kept when ordered by the physician and when residents:

- Are dehydrated
- Receive intravenous infusions
- Have a urinary catheter
- Are perspiring profusely or vomiting
- Have specific diagnoses such as congestive heart failure or renal disease that require accurate monitoring of I&O

If the resident is incontinent, indicate the number of times on the output record. Do not forget to check the resident often and to change the bed linen each time it is wet. After each incident, clean resident and give perineal care. Change soiled clothing.

PROCEDURE
*53*
# Measuring and Recording Fluid Output

1. Carry out each beginning procedure action.
2. Assemble equipment:
   * Disposable gloves
   * Graduate pitcher
   * Pen for recording
3. Wash hands and put on disposable gloves.
4. Save urine **specimen** (amount collected) and take to utility room or resident's bathroom.
   * Instruct the resident who is able to ambulate to the bathroom to use the hat-shaped specimen collection container (Figure 18-28).

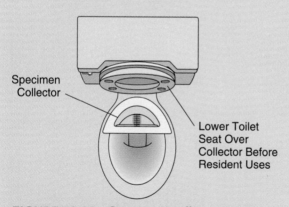

Specimen Collector

Lower Toilet Seat Over Collector Before Resident Uses

**FIGURE 18-28** Specimen collection container is placed on toilet under seat. Seat is lowered to hold container in place during use.

5. Pour urine from bedpan or urinal into graduate pitcher and measure (Figures 18-29A and B).
6. Empty urine.
   * If specimen is accidentally lost, estimate amount and make notation that it is an estimate.
   * In some cases, the physician will request that the incontinent resident's

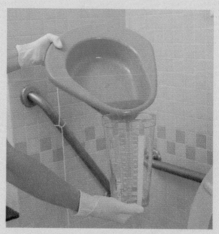

**FIGURE 18-29A**   Pour urine into graduate pitcher. Make sure there is no toilet paper in the bedpan.

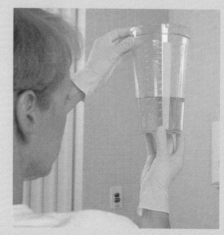

**FIGURE 18-29B**   Read the amount of urine in the graduate pitcher at eye level. The measuring scale is marked in cc or mL.

protective pads or briefs be weighed to determine output.

*Note:* Some health care facilities have guidelines for estimating the amount of urine or blood on pads or linen by the diameter of the wet area.

*(continues)*

**PROCEDURE *53* (continued)**

7. Rinse graduate pitcher with cold water. Clean according to facility policy.
8. Clean bedpan or urinal or specimen container and store properly, according to facility policy.
9. Remove and dispose of gloves according to facility policy. Wash hands.
10. Record amounts immediately under output column on bedside intake and output record (Figure 18-30). All liquid output should be recorded. Output includes:

- Urine
- Vomitus—also called **emesis**
- Drainage from a wound or the stomach
- Liquid stool—record an estimated amount
- Blood loss—record an estimated amount if on sheets or dressings, otherwise measure with a graduate
- Perspiration—record an estimated amount

*Note:* Fluids used to irrigate the bladder or for an enema are not included in calculating the output.

**FIGURE 18-30** Bedside intake and output sheet. In this example, the output amounts are highlighted.

| Date | Time | Method of Adm. | Solution | Intake Amounts Rec'd | Time | Output Urine Amount | Others | |
|---|---|---|---|---|---|---|---|---|
| | | | | | | | Kind | Amount |
| 7/16 | 0700 | PO | water | 120 mL | | 500 mL | | |
| | 0830 | PO | coffee | 240 mL | | | | |
| | | | or. ju. | 120 mL | | | | |
| | 1030 | PO | cran. ju. | 120 mL | | | | |
| | 1100 | | | | | 300 mL | | |
| | 1230 | PO | tea | 240 mL | | | | |
| | 1400 | PO | water | 150 mL | | | | |
| Shift Totals | 1500 | | | 990 mL | | 800 mL | | |
| | 1530 | PO | gelatin | 120 mL | | | | |
| | 1700 | PO | tea | 120 mL | | | | |
| | | | soup | 180 mL | | | | |
| | 2000 | | | | | 512 mL | | |
| | 2045 | | | | | | vomitus | 500 mL |
| | 2205 | | | | | | vomitus | 90 mL |
| Shift Totals | 2300 | | | 420 mL | | 512 mL | | 590 mL |
| | 2345 | | | | | | vomitus | 80 mL |
| | 0130 | IV | D/W | 500 mL | | | | |
| | 0315 | | | | | 400 mL | | |
| Shift Totals | 0700 | | | 500 mL | | 400 mL | | 80 mL |
| 24 Hour Totals | | | | 1910 mL | | 1712 mL | | 670 mL vomitus |

*(continues)*

**PROCEDURE 53** *(continued)*

11. Carry out each procedure completion action.
12. Copy information on resident's record from intake and output sheet according to facility policy.
    - Perspiration and blood loss may be described as *little, moderate,* or *excessive.*

- Also record the number of times linens or dressings have been changed or reinforced because of such fluid losses.
- Blood loss is determined by the size of the wet area on dressings and by measuring amounts in Hemovac containers.

**PROCEDURE 54** Emptying a Urinary Drainage Unit

1. Carry out each beginning procedure action.
2. Assemble equipment:
   - Disposable gloves
   - Graduated container
   - Sterile cap or sterile 4 × 4 (needed if container has no bottom drain tube)
   - Antiseptic wipes
3. Wash hands and put on gloves.
4. Place paper towel on the floor under the drainage bag. Place a graduate on paper towel under drain of collection bag.
5. Remove drain from holder (Figure 18-31) and open. Allow the urine to drain into the graduate using aseptic technique. Do not allow the tip of the tubing to touch the sides of the graduate.
6. Close the drain and replace it in the holder (Figure 18-32). If accidental contanimation occurs, wipe the drain tip with antiseptic wipe before returning it to the holder. Dispose of antiseptic wipe in plastic bag.

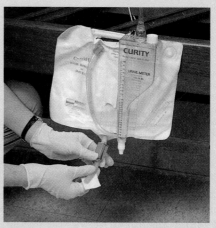

**FIGURE 18-31** Remove drain from holder and wipe with an antiseptic wipe.

7. Pick up paper towel, touching top surface only, and discard.
8. Check position of drainage tube.
9. Take graduate to bathroom and empty it.
10. Wash and dry graduate and store it according to facility policy.

*(continues)*

**PROCEDURE 54** *(continued)*

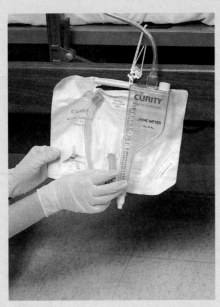

**FIGURE 18-32** Wipe the drain with an antiseptic wipe and return it to the holder.

**11.** Remove gloves and discard according to facility policy.
**12.** Record amount of urine and note character.
**13.** Carry out each procedure completion action.

## LEG BAG DRAINAGE

Some residents find it easier to ambulate when urine drainage is collected in a leg bag instead of the larger urinary drainage bag. The leg bag is held to the resident's leg by Velcro® straps around either the thigh or the lower leg (Figure 18-33). Points to keep in mind when residents use a leg bag are:

• The leg bag is smaller and must be emptied more often.
• The bag must be placed so there is a straight drop down from the catheter.
• Tension on the catheter tubing must be minimal.
• Care must be taken not to introduce germs when connecting and disconnecting the bag and catheter.

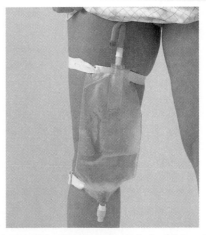

**FIGURE 18-33** The leg bag is held in place by adjustable straps. Because it is smaller than the standard drainage bag, it must be emptied more often.

## PROCEDURE 55
# Emptying a Leg Bag

1. Carry out beginning procedure actions.
2. Assemble equipment:
   - Disposable gloves
   - Antiseptic wipes
   - Emesis basin
   - Graduate pitcher
   - Paper towels
3. Position resident safely.
4. Wash hands and put on gloves.
5. Release Velcro® straps holding leg bag so it can be moved away from leg.
6. Place paper towel on floor under drainage outlet of leg bag.
7. Place graduate on paper towel under drainage outlet.
8. Remove cap, being careful not to touch tip. Drain urine into the graduate. Do not put cap down and do not touch inside of cap. If accidental contamination occurs, wipe the area with antiseptic wipes before replacing cap. Dispose of antiseptic wipes in a plastic bag.
9. Wipe drainage outlet with an antiseptic wipe and replace cap.
10. Refasten Velcro® straps to secure drainage bag to leg.
11. Make sure resident is comfortable and safe.
12. Discard paper towel.
13. Measure urine and note amount if required.
14. Discard urine. Clean graduate and store.
15. Remove gloves and discard according to facility policy.
16. Carry out each procedure completion action.

## PROCEDURE 56
# Connecting Catheter to Leg Bag

*Note:* Always check with the nurse before using a leg bag.

1. Carry out beginning procedure actions.
2. Assemble equipment:
   - Disposable gloves
   - Antiseptic wipes
   - Leg bag and tubing
   - Emesis basin
   - Bed protector
   - Sterile cap/plug
   - Clamp
3. Wash hands and put on gloves.
4. Place bed protector under the connection between catheter and drainage tube.
5. Clamp the catheter.
6. Disconnect the catheter and drainage tubing. Do not put them down or allow them to touch anything.

*(continues)*

**PROCEDURE 56** *(continued)*

7. Insert a sterile plug in the end of the catheter. Place a sterile cap over the exposed end of the drainage tube. *Note:* If accidental contamination occurs, wipe the area with antiseptic wipes before inserting sterile plug or replacing sterile cap over exposed end of drainage tubing. Dispose of antiseptic wipes in plastic bag.
8. Secure the drainage tube to the bed frame. The drainage tube must not touch the floor.
9. Remove catheter plug.
10. Insert the end of the leg bag tubing into the catheter (Figure 18-34).
11. Release the catheter clamp.
12. Secure the leg bag with Velcro® straps to the resident's leg so there is no tension on the tubing. Be sure there is a straight drop down from the catheter to the bag for urine flow. Check for leakage.
13. Remove bed protector and discard.
14. Remove gloves and discard according to facility policy. Wash hands.
15. Assist resident to get out of bed. The single-use leg bag should be discarded in biohazardous waste container.

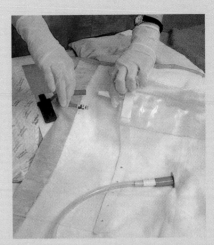

**FIGURE 18-34** Connecting leg bag to catheter tubing. Do not let the catheter tubing touch anything that could contaminate it. Note that the tubing to the drainage bag is covered with a sterile cap to protect it until it is reconnected to the catheter.

16. Carry out procedure completion actions. *Note:* To reconnect the regular drainage bag, reverse the procedure.

**PROCEDURE 57**   Collecting a Routine Urine Specimen

1. Carry out each beginning procedure action.
2. Assemble equipment:
   - Disposable gloves
   - Bedpan/urinal

- Sterile specimen container and cover
- Label including:
  - Resident's full name
  - Room number
  - Facility identification

*(continues)*

**PROCEDURE 57** *(continued)*

- • Date and time of collection
- • Physician's name
- • Examination to be done
  - • Other information requested
- • Graduate pitcher
- • Laboratory requisition slip, properly filled out
- • Biohazard specimen transport bag

3. Completely fill out the label of the specimen container.
4. Wash hands and put on disposable gloves.
5. Offer bedpan or urinal.
6. Instruct the resident not to discard toilet tissue in the pan with the urine. Provide a small plastic bag in which to place the soiled tissue.
7. After resident has voided, cover pan and place on bed protector on chair. Offer wash water to resident.
8. If resident can ambulate to bathroom, place specimen collector in toilet.
9. Assist resident to bathroom. Ask resident to void into specimen collector. Instruct resident to discard soiled toilet tissue in plastic bag provided. Tissue must not be placed in collector.
10. Provide privacy.
11. Put on gloves. Remove specimen collector from toilet. If resident is on I&O, note amount of urine (Figure 18-35). If resident used bedpan, pour urine into graduate to measure. Note amount. Remove gloves and discard according to facility policy. Wash hands.
12. Remove cap from specimen container, and place it (inside up) on shelf or other flat surface in bathroom or utility room. Do not touch inside of cap or container.
13. Put on gloves. Carefully pour about 120 mL urine into specimen container from collector (Figure 18-36).
14. Remove and discard gloves according to facility policy.

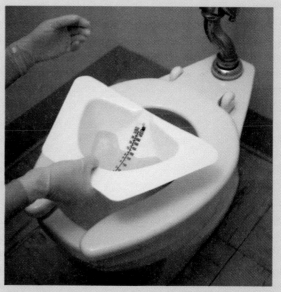

**FIGURE 18-35** Remove specimen collector from toilet. Note amount of urine if resident is on I&O.

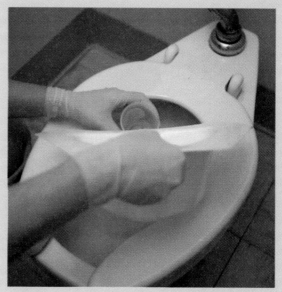

**FIGURE 18-36** Carefully pour about 120 mL of urine from collector into specimen container.

*(continues)*

**PROCEDURE 57** *(continued)*

15. Wash your hands.
16. Place cap on specimen container. Do not contaminate outside of container. Attach completed label to container (Figure 18-37). Place specimen container in biohazard specimen transport bag and attach laboratory requisition slip (Figure 18-38).
17. Carry out each procedure completion action.
18. Follow facility policy for transporting specimen to laboratory.

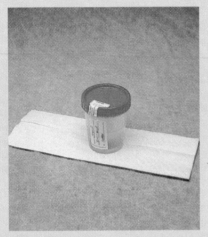

**FIGURE 18-37** After specimen is placed in container and cap is put on, place label on container.

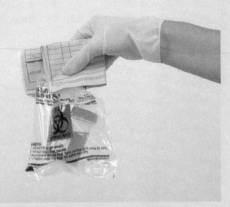

**FIGURE 18-38** Properly labeled specimen container is placed in biohazard specimen transport bag and laboratory requisition is attached.

**PROCEDURE 58** Collecting a Clean-Catch Urine Specimen

1. Carry out each beginning procedure action.
2. Assemble equipment:
   - Disposable gloves
   - Sterile specimen container and cover
   - Label for container with:
     - Resident's full name
     - Room number
   - Facility identification
   - Date and time of collection
   - Physician's name
   - Type of specimen test to be performed
   - Any other information requested
   - Gauze squares or cotton
   - Antiseptic solution

*(continues)*

**PROCEDURE** *58* *(continued)*

- Laboratory requisition slip, properly filled out
- Biohazard specimen transport bag

**3.** Wash hands and put on disposable gloves.

**4.** Wash the resident's genital area properly or instruct the resident to do so. If soiled due to incontinence, perform perineal care.

a.  For female residents:

1.  Using the gauze or cotton and the antiseptic solution, cleanse the outer folds of the vulva (folds are also called labia or lips) from front to back. Use separate cotton/gauze for each size. Discard the gauze/cotton in plastic bag.

2.  Cleanse the inner folds of the vulva with two pieces of gauze and antiseptic solution, again from front to back. Discard gauze/cotton in plastic bag.

3.  Cleanse the middle, innermost area (meatus or urinary opening) in the same manner. Discard the gauze/cotton in plastic bag.

4.  Keep the labia separated so that the folds do not fall back and cover the meatus.

b.  For male residents:

1.  Using the gauze/cotton and the antiseptic solution, cleanse the tip of the penis from the urinary meatus down, using a circular motion.

2.  Discard gauze/cotton in plastic bag.

**5.** Instruct the resident to void, allowing the first part of the urine to escape. Then:

a.  Catch the urine stream that follows in the sterile specimen container.

b.  Allow the last portion of the urine stream to escape.

*Note:* If the resident's I&O is being monitored, or if the amount of urine passed must be measured, catch the first and last part of the urine in a bedpan, urinal, or specimen collection container.

**6.** Place the sterile cap on the urine container immediately to prevent contamination of the urine specimen.

**7.** Allow the resident to wash hands.

**8.** With the cap securely tightened, wash the outside of the specimen container. Dry the container.

**9.** Remove and dispose of gloves according to facility policy.

**10.** Wash your hands.

**11.** Attach completed label to the container and place specimen in the transport bag.

**12.** Carry out procedure completion actions.

**13.** Follow facility policy for transporting specimen to laboratory.

# EXTERNAL URINARY DRAINAGE (MALE)

External urinary drainage is preferred for male residents who require drainage for long periods of time. In this form of drainage, an internal catheter is not inserted in the urethra. Thus, there is a less danger of infection.

A **condom** (sheath) or some other type of appliance is placed on the penis. The condom is attached to drainage tubing and a collection bag. The condom is removed every 24 hours and the penis is washed and dried.

## PROCEDURE
### 59

## Applying a Condom for Urinary Drainage

1. Carry out each beginning procedure action.
2. Assemble equipment:
   - Disposable gloves
   - Basin of warm water
   - Condom with drainage tip
   - Bed protector
   - Bath blanket
   - Towel
3. Arrange equipment on overbed table.
4. Raise bed to comfortable working height. Be sure opposite side rail is up and secure for safety.
5. Lower side rail on the side where you will be working.
6. Cover resident with bath blanket and fan-fold bedding to foot of bed.
7. Wash hands and put on gloves.
8. Place bed protector under resident's hips.
9. Adjust bath blanket to expose genitals only.
10. Carefully wash and dry penis. Observe for signs of irritation. Check to be sure condom has "ready stick" surface.
11. Apply condom and drainage tip to penis by placing condom at top of penis and rolling toward base of penis. Leave space between drainage tip and glans of penis to prevent irritation (Figure 18-39). If the resident is not circumcised, be sure that foreskin is in normal position.
12. Apply tape provided with condom to secure it to the penis (Figure 18-40).
13. Condom is now ready to be connected to drainage tubing leading to collection bag.
14. Remove gloves and discard according to facility policy.
15. Wash hands.
16. Adjust bedding and remove bath blanket. Fold bath blanket and store in room or place in laundry hamper.
17. Lower bed. Adjust side rails for safety.
18. Carry out procedure completion actions.

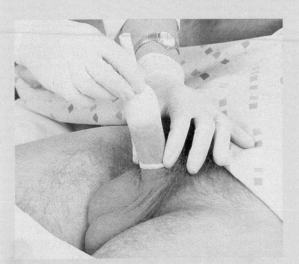

**FIGURE 18-39** When condom is placed on penis, leave room between the drainage tip and the glans of the penis to prevent irritation. Roll condom to base of penis.

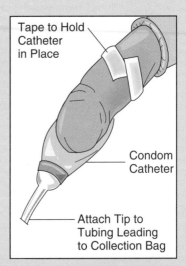

**FIGURE 18-40** Correctly applied and secured condom ready to be attached to tubing leading to drainage bag

## COMMON CONDITIONS ·················

### Rectocele and Cystocele

The urinary bladder, ureters, and the urethra are found in the pelvic cavity. Some of the female reproductive organs are also in the pelvis. Each group of organs can be affected by disease or stress in the other group.

Frequent pregnancies and general loss of muscle tone due to the aging process may cause the bladder to protrude into the vagina (**cystocele**) and the rectum into the vagina (**rectocele**).

The weakness of the bladder wall can cause urinary incontinence, especially with extra stress such as laughing or coughing. The weakened rectal wall can lead to constipation and hemorrhoids. Surgery can be helpful in repairing the cystocele and rectocele.

### Renal Calculi

**Renal calculi**, or kidney stones, form as various salts and compounds settle out of the forming urine. Starting as tiny grains of sediment, they become larger and larger until they block part of the drainage system, often a ureter. When blockage occurs the resident experiences extreme pain. Pain associated with urine elimination is known as **dysuria**. Most kidney stones are passed when fluids are forced, but surgery may be required to relieve the obstruction.

The urine may be strained through gauze or filter paper before being measured and discarded to determine when the stone is passed. Blood may cause the urine to become pink to deep red in color. Blood in the urine is called **hematuria**.

### Renal Failure

Renal failure (**uremia**) may occur suddenly but it is usually a chronic situation that develops gradually over a period of years. Causes include changes in the blood vessels that serve the kidneys, hypertension, and the aging process.

The resident in chronic renal failure does not eliminate effectively, so water and wastes build up in the body. Urine output is reduced (**oliguria**). In the terminal stage of renal failure, urine output ceases altogether (**anuria**). Blood pressure increases and edema and chemical imbalance develop throughout the body. The resident may complain of headache, nausea, and a bad taste in the mouth. Uric acid is eliminated in the

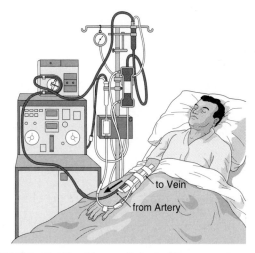

**FIGURE 18-41**   Hemodialysis filters wastes from the resident's blood. Blood leaves the body from an artery, is filtered by the machine, and is returned to the body through a vein.

perspiration. The uric acid accumulates as white crystals on the skin and is called **uremic frost**. The perspiration has an unpleasant odor. Careful attention is needed to keep the skin clean and free from breakdown.

Renal failure is treated by:

- Surgery to implant a healthy kidney
- Hemodialysis, a procedure that uses a machine to filter wastes and impurities from the blood (Figure 18-41).

Residents receiving hemodialysis may leave the facility for the treatment, which normally requires several hours. When residents return to the facility after hemodialysis, they are observed closely for dizziness and fainting. They are often placed on fluid restriction, I&O, and a specialized diet. Hemodialysis is often performed more than once a week. Two connectors (cannulas) are implanted in the resident's body, usually in an arm. One cannula is placed in an artery and the other is placed in a vein.

When caring for the resident with implanted hemodialysis cannulas:

- Be careful not to dislodge the cannulas.
- Notify the nurse if there is pain, swelling, redness, or drainage in the arm.
- Do not use the arm for blood pressure measurements.
- Do not apply tight clothing to the arm.
- Encourage resident to follow any special exercises that may have been ordered.

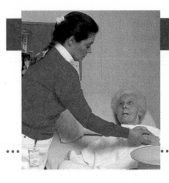

## LESSON SYNTHESIS: Putting It All Together

*Y*ou have just completed this lesson. Now go back and review the Clinical Focus. Try to see how the Clinical Focus relates to the concepts presented in the lesson. Then answer the following questions.

1. What do you think Ms. Beebe's problem is?

2. What made the nursing assistant think to ask Ms. Beebe when she had her last bowel movement?

3. What actions could the nursing staff take that might help the resident avoid a similar situation in the future?

4. Why is the attitude of the staff an important factor in the success or failure of managing elimination problems?

## REVIEW

**A. Match each term (items a.–e.) with the proper definition.**

a. constipation     d. micturition
b. diarrhea     e. retention
c. feces

1. _____ loose, liquid stools

2. _____ inability to urinate

3. _____ hard and difficult to evacuate stool

4. _____ solid waste

5. _____ another term for urination

**B. Complete the sentence by providing the proper term.**

6. Elimination of feces is called _____.

7. Blood in the urine is called _____.

8. Painful urination is _____.

9. Inability to control elimination is _____.

10. An artificial opening in the wall of the abdomen for the elimination of feces is called a(an) _____.

**C. Fill in the blanks by selecting the correct word or phrase from the list.**

| | |
|---|---|
| liquid | sit upright |
| left side | I&O sheet |
| floor | incontinent |
| coiled | dehydration |
| oil-retention enema | tongue depressors |
| voiding | stoma |

11. The best position for the resident receiving an enema is on the _____ with the knees flexed.

12. One type of enema that should be retained for 20 minutes is the _____.

13. When collecting a stool specimen, use _____ to transfer the sample from the bedpan to the specimen container.

14. The best position to encourage voiding in a female resident is to have her _____.

15. A person who is unable to control urine output voluntarily is said to be _____.

16. Intake includes everything taken in that is _____ at room temperature.

17. Intake and output are recorded on the _____.

18. When a resident has a colostomy, the opening is called the _____.

19. During a routine urinary drainage check, the tubing should be _____ on the bed.

20. A urine collection bag must never touch the _____.

21. A common term for eliminating urine from the bladder is _____.

22. Excessive fluid loss from the body results in _____.

D. **Select the one best answer for each of the following.**

23. The proper temperature for a soapsuds enema is
    a. 80°F
    b. 95°F
    c. 105°F
    d. 120°F

24. A rectal tube should be inserted into the rectum
    a. ½ inch
    b. 1 to 1½ inches
    c. 2 to 4 inches
    d. 6 inches

25. Gloves should be worn when
    a. inserting a flatus tube
    b. giving perineal care

c. applying a leg drainage bag
d. all of these

26. A resident with a colostomy evacuates feces through the
    a. anus
    b. ileum
    c. jejunum
    d. colon

27. Normal urine color is
    a. red
    b. yellow
    c. colorless
    d. brown

E. **Clinical Experience**

Mrs. Duff has an indwelling catheter and is in a wheelchair. You are assigned to her care. Answer the following questions.

28. May the collection bag touch the floor at any time?

29. Should the collection bag or tubing be higher or lower than the resident's bladder?

30. Is perineal care necessary?

31. How often should the drainage be emptied?

32. When Mrs. Duff is in her wheelchair, how should the urinary drainage tubing be positioned?

# SECTION

# 6

# Special Nursing Assistant Activities

## LESSONS

**19** Measuring and Recording Residents' Data

**20** Admission, Transfer, and Discharge

**21** Warm and Cold Applications

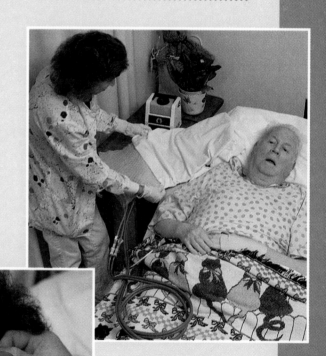

# Measuring and Recording Residents' Data

## CLINICAL FOCUS

Think about situations in which the measuring and recording of data are an important part of your duties as you study this lesson and meet:

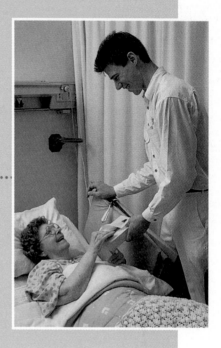

*G*eraldine Hoden, 72 years old, who is a resident in your facility. Mrs. Hoden has heart problems that cause her to retain fluid (edema). She becomes short of breath with any physical exertion. Mrs. Hoden is taking medication to strengthen and regulate her heart activity. She also has a history of hypertension. Mrs. Hoden is alert and cooperative.

## OBJECTIVES

*After studying this lesson, you should be able to:*

- Define and spell vocabulary words and terms.
- Properly select and use equipment to measure vital signs.
- Identify the range of normal values.
- State the reasons for measuring weight and height.
- Demonstrate the following:
  Procedure 60 Measuring an Oral Temperature (Glass Thermometer)
  Procedure 61 Measuring a Rectal Temperature (Glass Thermometer)
  Procedure 62 Measuring an Axillary Temperature (Glass Thermometer)
  Procedure 63 Measuring an Oral Temperature (Electronic Thermometer)
  Procedure 64 Measuring a Rectal Temperature (Electronic Thermometer)
  Procedure 65 Measuring an Axillary Temperature (Electronic Thermometer)
  Procedure 66 Measuring a Tympanic Temperature
  Procedure 67 Counting the Radial Pulse Rate
  Procedure 68 Counting the Apical-Radial Pulse
  Procedure 69 Counting Respirations
  Procedure 70 Taking Blood Pressure
  Procedure 71 Weighing and Measuring the Resident Using an Upright Scale

# OBJECTIVES

· · · · · · · · · · · · · · · · · · · · ·

**Procedure 72** Measuring Weight with an Electronic Wheelchair Scale

**Procedure 73** Weighing the Resident in a Chair Scale

**Procedure 74** Measuring and Weighing the Resident in Bed

# VOCABULARY

· · · · · · · · · · · · · · · · · · · · ·

**accelerated**   *(ack-**SELL**-er-**ay**-ted)*

**antihypertensive**   *(**an**-tee-**high**-per-**TEN**-siv)*

**apex**   *(**AY**-pecks)*

**apical pulse**   *(**AP**-ih-kal puls)*

**bradycardia**   *(**brad**-ee-**KAR**-dee-ah)*

**Celsius**   *(**SELL**-see-us)*

**centimeter**   *(**SEN**-tih-**mee**-ter)*

**cyanotic**   *(**sigh**-ah-**NOT**-ick)*

**depressant**   *(dee-**PRESS**-ant)*

**diastolic**   *(**die**-ah-**STOL**-ick)*

**expiration**   *(**ecks**-pih-**RAY**-shun)*

**Fahrenheit**   *(**FAIR**-en-hight)*

**fasting**   *(**FAST**-ing)*

**hypertension**   *(**high**-per-**TEN**-shun)*

**hypotension**   *(**high**-poh-**TEN**-shun)*

**inspiration**   *(**in**-spih-**RAY**-shun)*

**kilogram**   *(**KILL**-oh-gram)*

**mercury**   *(**MER**-kyou-ree)*

**oral**   *(**OR**-al)*

**pulse**   *(puls)*

**pulse deficit**   *(puls **DEF**-ih-sit)*

**pulse rate**   *(puls rayt)*

**radial artery**   *(**RAY**-dee-al **ARE**-ter-ee)*

**rales**   *(rahls)*

**respiration**   *(**res**-pih-**RAY**-shun)*

**rhythm**   *(**RITH**-um)*

**sheath**   *(sheeth)*

**sphygmomanometer**   *(**sfig**-moh-mah-**NOM**-eh-ter)*

**stethoscope**   *(**STETH**-oh-skohp)*

**systolic**   *(sis-**TOL**-ick)*

**tachycardia**   *(**tack**-ee-**KAR**-dee-ah)*

**thermometer**   *(ther-**MOM**-eh-ter)*

**tympanic**   *(tim-**PAN**-ick)*

**vital signs**   *(**VIGH**-tal signs)*

**volume**   *(**VOL**-youm)*

· · · · · · · · · · · · · · · · · · · · · · · · · · · · · · · · · · · · · · · · · · · · · · · · · · · · · · · · · · · · · · · ·

## MEASURING VITAL SIGNS · · · · · · · · · · · · ·

Each resident must have **vital signs** *(vital means living)* measured and recorded on admission. Vital signs are also frequently measured throughout the resident's stay. The vital signs are:

- Temperature
- Pulse rate
- Respiratory rate
- Blood pressure

The vital signs give information about the general health of the individual and changes in the health status. It is essential that these measurements be accurate and you record them properly.

To do this accurately you must know how to:

- Read a clinical thermometer using the **Celsius** and **Fahrenheit** scales
- Read a **sphygmomanometer** (blood pressure cuff)

In addition to vital signs, you will also measure residents' weight and height on a regular basis. To do this accurately you must know how to:

- Read a scale for weight in pounds and **kilograms**.

| FIGURE 19-1 | Temperature variations related to method of measurement | | |
|---|---|---|---|
| | **Oral** | **Axillary** | **Rectal** |
| Average Temperature | 98.6°F | 97.6°F | 99.6°F |
| Acceptable Range | 97.6–99.6°F (36.5–37.5°C) | 96.6–98.6°F (36–37°C) | 98.6–100.6°F (37–38.1°C) |

- Read a scale for height in feet and inches and in **centimeters**.

Procedures for measuring weight and height are described later in this lesson.

Celsius, kilograms, and centimeters are metric measurements. Facilities that use the metric system for these temperature, weight, and height measurements will have thermometers and scales with the metric values. You do not have to convert measurements from one system to the other.

### Equipment Needed

Clinical **thermometers** are used to determine temperature. A watch with a second hand is needed to count the pulse and respiratory rate. A **stethoscope** and sphygmomanometer are needed to measure the blood pressure. Each vital sign will be discussed separately, although actual measurements are usually done as a combined activity.

## TEMPERATURE

Temperature is the measurement of body heat. One of two temperature scales may be used: Fahrenheit or Celsius. Normal body temperature is about 98.6° Fahrenheit (37° Celsius).

Temperatures taken with glass or electronic thermometers are usually measured orally. The temperature can also be taken with a thermometer placed and held in the rectum (rectal temperature). Alternatively, the thermometer can be placed in the armpit (axillary temperature) if the resident:

- Is unable to keep the mouth closed
- Has respiratory difficulty

- Is receiving oxygen
- Is receiving oral tube feeding

The rectal temperature registers 1° higher and the axillary temperature registers 1° lower than an **oral** temperature in the same person (Figure 19-1).

The temperature of the blood in the vessels of the eardrum may also be measured. This is known as **tympanic** temperature. It is the most accurate temperature reading. The temperature taken in the axilla is the least accurate reading.

Temperature can be increased by:

- Infection
- Dehydration
- Physical exercise
- Hot water
- Brain damage

It can be decreased by:

- Shock
- Cold weather
- Sponge bath
- Medications
- Approaching death

### Clinical Thermometers

Three types of glass clinical thermometers (Figure 19-2) are in general use:

- Oral
- Security
- Rectal

These thermometers differ mainly in the size and shape of the bulb (the end that is inserted into the resident). When only security or stubby-type thermometers are in use, the rectal thermometers are marked with a red dot at the end of the stem. Figure 19-3 shows rectal thermome-

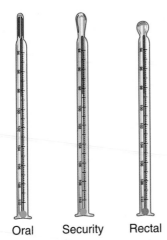

**FIGURE 19-2** Clinical thermometers: from left to right—oral, security, rectal

ters: A has a Fahrenheit scale and B has a Celsius scale.

**Reading the Glass Thermometer.** **Mercury** is a heat-sensitive liquid metal that appears as a solid color line in the bulb of the thermometer. The mercury rises in the hollow center of the stem. To read the thermometer:

- Hold it at eye level.
- Find the solid column of mercury (Figure 19-4).
- Look along the sharper edge between the numbers and lines.
- Determine the point where the mercury ends.

Starting with 94°F (34°C), each long line indicates a 1° elevation in temperature. Only every other degree is marked with a number. In between each long line are four shorter lines. Each shorter line equals two tenths ($^2/_{10}$ or 0.2) of a degree. The thermometer is "read" at the point at which the mercury ends (stops rising). If it stops between two lines, read it to the closer line.

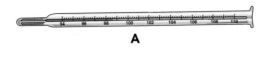

**A**

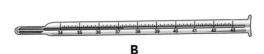

**B**

**FIGURE 19-3** A. Fahrenheit and B. Celsius thermometers

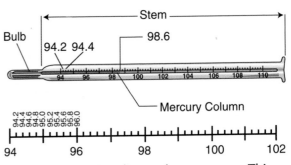

**FIGURE 19-4** Reading a thermometer. This thermometer reads 98.6°F.

*Note:* On a Celsius thermometer, the lines have different values. Each degree is marked (34, 35, 36, etc.). There are 10 small lines in between each number. Each of these small lines equals one tenth ($^1/_{10}$ or 0.1) of a degree.

## General Thermometer Safety Precautions

- Check glass thermometers for chips.
- Shake mercury down before use, *away* from resident or hard objects.
- Do not leave resident alone with thermometer in place.
- Allow glass thermometer to register for at least 3 minutes orally, 2 minutes rectally, or 10 minutes axillary.
- Hold rectal and axillary thermometers in place.
- When measuring a rectal temperature, lubricate bulb end of thermometer before inserting in rectum.
- Use an alcohol wipe or cotton ball to wipe thermometer from end to bulb before reading.

**Contraindications**—Oral Temperatures: An oral temperature is not taken if resident is

- Confused, disoriented
- Restless
- Unconscious
- Chilled
- Coughing
- Unable to breathe through the nose
- Very weak
- On seizure precautions

**Contraindications**—Rectal Temperatures: A rectal temperature is not taken if resident has

- Diarrhea
- Fecal impaction
- Combative behavior

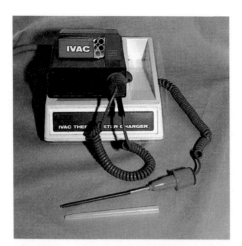

**FIGURE 19-5** An electronic thermometer. The temperature is registered in large, easy-to-read numerals. The disposable protective sheath is placed over the probe tip. (The blue probe is for oral temperatures and the red probe is for rectal temperatures.) The blue probe is then inserted into the resident's mouth in the usual manner.

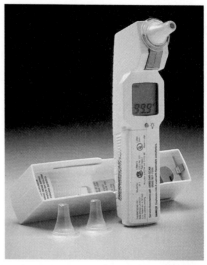

**FIGURE 19-6** The cordless, hand-held tympanic thermometer. The lens on the handset indicates the digital temperature reading. (Courtesy of Thermoscan® Inc., San Diego, CA)

- Rectal bleeding
- Hemorrhoids
- Colostomy

Some facilities use other types of thermometers to take temperatures, including

- Electronic thermometer
- Tympanic thermometer

### The Electronic Thermometer

The electronic thermometer is battery operated. The temperature is registered in large numbers on the screen. The probe is the portion that is placed into the resident. The probes or probe stems are colored blue for oral or axillary use and red for rectal use. The probe is covered with a disposable **sheath** that stays on during use and is then discarded (Figure 19-5).

The tympanic (ear) thermometer (Figure 19-6) measures the temperature from blood vessels in the tympanic membrane in the ear. This provides a reading close to the core body temperature. The instrument has a built-in converter that provides the equivalent temperature in rectal or oral values (in both Fahrenheit or Celsius systems). The type of thermometer reading (mode) is selected by the user.

---

**PROCEDURE**
**60**

# Measuring an Oral Temperature (Glass Thermometer)

**1.** Carry out each beginning procedure action.

**2.** Assemble equipment:
   - Disposable gloves
   - Container with clean thermometer

*(continues)*

## PROCEDURE *60*   *(continued)*

- Container for used thermometers
- Cotton balls
- Container for soiled tissues
- Container with tissues
- Pad and pencil
- Watch with second hand
- Disposable sheath for thermometer (if used in facility)

**3.** Put on gloves.

**4.** Have resident rest in a comfortable position in bed or chair.

**5.** Ask resident if he or she has had hot or cold liquids to drink or smoked within the last 15 minutes. If the answer is "yes," wait 15 minutes before taking oral temperature. Holding stem end remove thermometer from container. Wipe with tissue. Check to be sure the thermometer is intact with no chips or cracks. Read the mercury column. It should register below 96°F. If necessary, shake down. To shake down (Figure 19-7), move away from table or other hard objects. Grasp the stem tightly between your thumb and fingers. Shake down with downward motion.

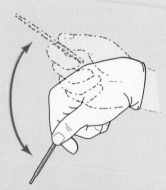

**FIGURE 19-7**   Shake mercury down in column by holding the thermometer by the stem and snapping the wrist. Check the reading. Repeat until the reading is below 96°F.

**6.** Insert thermometer in sheath, if used. Insert bulb end of thermometer under resident's tongue, toward base of tongue (Figure 19-8). Tell resident to hold thermometer gently with lips closed for 3 minutes.

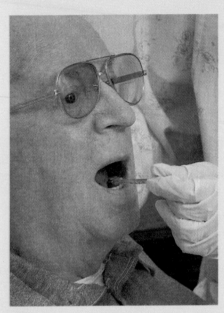

**FIGURE 19-8**   The bulb end of the thermometer is inserted under the tongue, left 3 minutes, then removed.

**7.** Remove thermometer, holding by stem. Remove sheath, if used, and place in proper container. Wipe from stem end toward bulb end.

**8.** Discard tissue in proper container.

**9.** Read thermometer (Figure 19-9) and record on pad.

**10.** Place thermometer in container for used thermometers. If thermometer is to be reused for this resident:

- Wash it twice in cold water and soap with two separate cotton balls, wiping from stem to bulb.
- Rinse and dry it.

*(continues)*

**PROCEDURE 60** *(continued)*

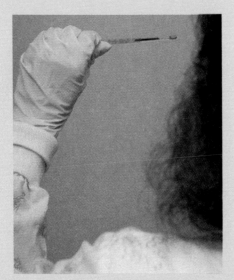

**FIGURE 19-9** Hold thermometer at eye level. Locate the column of mercury and read to the closest line.

- Return it to the individual disinfectant-filled holder.
11. Remove gloves and discard according to facility policy.
12. Carry out each procedure completion action.
13. Report any unusual variations to the nurse at once.

**PROCEDURE 61** Measuring a Rectal Temperature (Glass Thermometer)

1. Carry out each beginning procedure action.
2. Assemble equipment:
   - Disposable gloves
   - Container with clean rectal thermometer
   - Container for used thermometers
   - Container for soiled tissues
   - Lubricant
   - Container with tissues
   - Sheath for thermometer, if used
   - Pad and pencil
   - Watch with second hand

3. Put up opposite side rail if not already up. Lower backrest of bed. Ask resident to turn on her side. Assist resident, if necessary.
4. Place small amount of lubricant on tissue.
5. Put gloves on. Remove thermometer from container by holding stem end. Read mercury column. Be sure it registers below 96°F. Check thermometer for cracks and chips. Insert thermometer in sheath if used.

*(continues)*

**PROCEDURE 61** *(continued)*

6. Using tissue apply small amount of lubricant to bulb.
7. Fold the top bedclothes back to expose anal area.
8. Refer to Figure 19-10. Separate buttocks with one hand. Insert the thermometer gently into rectum 1½ inches. Hold in

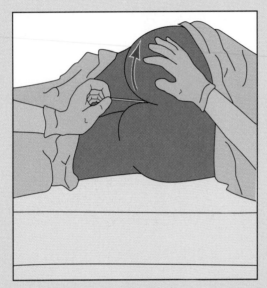

**FIGURE 19-10** The rectal thermometer is lubricated and then inserted 1½ inches into the rectum and held in place.

place. Replace bedclothes as soon as thermometer is inserted.
9. Thermometer should remain inserted for 3 minutes.
10. Remove thermometer, holding by stem. Remove sheath, if used, and dispose of in proper container. Wipe from stem toward bulb end.
11. Discard tissue in proper container.
12. Read thermometer. Record reading on pad.
13. Wipe lubricant from resident. Discard tissue.
14. Place thermometer in container for used thermometers. If thermometer is to be reused for this resident:

- Wash it in cold water and soap.
- Rinse and dry it.
- Return it to the individual disinfectant-filled holder.

15. Remove gloves and discard according to facility policy.
16. Lower opposite side rail if indicated.
17. Carry out each procedure completion action.
*Note:* Remember that when a rectal temperature is recorded, add (R) after the reading.

---

**PROCEDURE 62** Measuring an Axillary Temperature (Glass Thermometer)

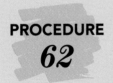  

1. Carry out each beginning procedure action.
*Note:* Use disposable gloves if there may be contact with open lesions, wet linens, or body fluids.

2. Assemble equipment:
- Container with clean oral thermometers
- Container for used thermometers
- Container for soiled tissues

*(continues)*

**PROCEDURE 62** *(continued)*

- Container with tissues
- Pad and pencil
- Watch with a second hand
- Sheath for thermometer, if used

3. Wipe the area dry and place sheath on the thermometer, if used. Place thermometer in armpit.
   a. The resident's arm is kept close to his body if axillary site is used (Figure 19-11).
   b. Leave the thermometer in place 10 minutes.
   c. Remove sheath, if used, and dispose of in proper container. Wipe and read thermometer. Note reading on pad.
   d. Clean and replace as with oral thermometer if it is to be reused.

4. Carry out each procedure completion action.
   *Note:* Remember that when an axillary temperature is recorded, add (AX) after the reading.

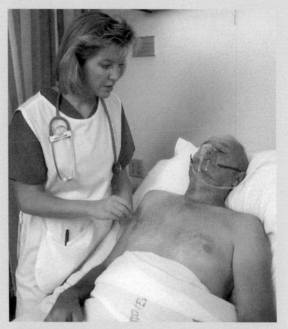

**FIGURE 19-11**   When the thermometer is placed in the axilla, it must be held in place.

---

**PROCEDURE 63**

# Measuring an Oral Temperature (Electronic Thermometer)

1. Carry out each beginning procedure action.
2. Obtain electronic thermometer, disposable sheaths, and gloves (if this is your facility policy). (Gloves are not necessary with an oral temperature using this type of thermometer. Know and follow your facility policy.)
3. Ask resident if he or she has had hot or cold liquids to drink or smoked within the last 15 minutes. If the answer is "yes," wait 15 minutes before taking oral temperature.
4. Cover probe (blue) with protective sheath.
5. Insert covered probe under resident's tongue, toward side of mouth (Figure 19-12).
6. Hold probe in position.
7. When buzzer signals temperature has been determined, take reading and record on pad.

*(continues)*

**PROCEDURE 63** *(continued)*

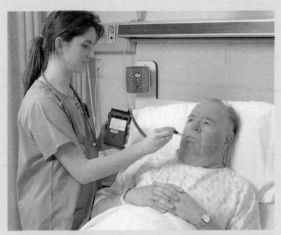

**FIGURE 19-12** Inserting the blue probe of the electronic thermometer in the resident's mouth

8. Discard sheath in wastebasket. Do not touch sheath. Remove gloves and discard according to facility policy.
9. Return probe to proper position and entire unit to charging.
10. Carry out each procedure completion action.

**PROCEDURE 64**

# Measuring a Rectal Temperature (Electronic Thermometer)

1. Carry out each beginning procedure action.
2. Assemble equipment:
   - Disposable gloves
   - Electronic thermometer with red probe
   - Sheaths
   - Lubricant
3. Lower backrest of bed. Ask resident to turn on his side. Assist resident, if necessary.
4. Put on disposable gloves.
5. Place a small amount of lubricant on the tip of the sheath (Figure 19-13).
6. Fold the top bedclothes back to expose anal area.

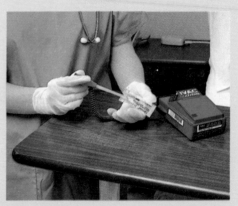

**FIGURE 19-13** Lubricating the tip of the sheath-covered probe

*(continues)*

**PROCEDURE 64** *(continued)*

7. Separate buttocks with one hand. Insert sheath-covered probe about 1½ inches into rectum or as recommended by manufacturer. Hold in place. Replace bedclothes as soon as thermometer is inserted.
8. Read temperature when registered on digital display. Note reading on pad.

9. Remove probe and discard sheath. Wipe lubricant from resident. Discard tissue.
10. Remove gloves and discard according to facility policy.
11. Carry out each procedure completion action.

**PROCEDURE 65**

# Measuring an Axillary Temperature (Electronic Thermometer)

1. Carry out each beginning procedure action.
   *Note:* Use disposable gloves if there may be contact with open lesions, wet linens, or body fluids.
2. Equipment needed: same as for oral temperature measurement using an electronic thermometer.

3. Wipe axillary area dry and place covered probe in place. Keep resident's arm close to the body. Hold probe in place until temperature records on digital display and buzzer signals.
4. Remove thermometer probe. Dispose of sheath.
5. Carry out each procedure completion action.

Many facilities use tympanic (aural) thermometers. The temperature is taken by measuring the heat that is given off by the tympanic membrane (in the ear). This method has several advantages:

- Tympanic thermometers are accurate and easy to use.
- The temperature registers in a few seconds. Because of this, taking the temperature of an agitated resident is safer and faster.
- Temperatures that cannot be taken orally can be taken by the tympanic method, eliminat-

ing the need to take rectal or axillary temperatures.
- The tympanic thermometer allows you to select a core, oral, or rectal mode. This means the reading will correlate with the mode selected. Choose the mode according to your facility's policy.
- Wait for 15 minutes to take the temperature if the resident has been outdoors or if the resident has been lying on the ear you will use.

**PROCEDURE**

**66**

# Measuring a Tympanic Temperature

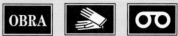

1. Carry out each beginning procedure action.
2. Assemble equipment:
   - Disposable gloves if there may be contact with blood or body fluids, open lesions, or wet linens
   - Tympanic thermometer
   - Probe covers
3. Place a clean probe cover on the probe.
4. Select the appropriate mode on the thermometer.
5. Check the lens to make sure it is clean and intact (Figure 19-14).

6. Put on disposable gloves if you may have contact with blood or body fluids, open lesions, or wet linens.
7. Position the resident so you have access to the ear you will be using.
8. Gently pull the ear pinna back and up (Figure 19-15). This straightens the ear canal so the thermometer can be placed for an accurate reading.
9. Place the probe in the resident's ear, aiming it toward the tympanic membrane. Insert the probe until it seals the ear canal (Figure 19-16). Do not apply pressure.

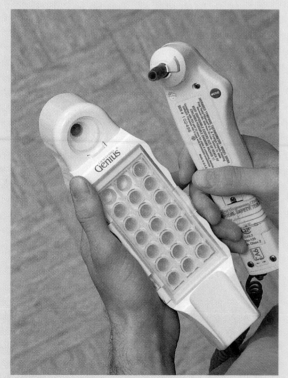

**FIGURE 19-14** Check the lens of the tympanic thermometer to make sure it is clean and intact.

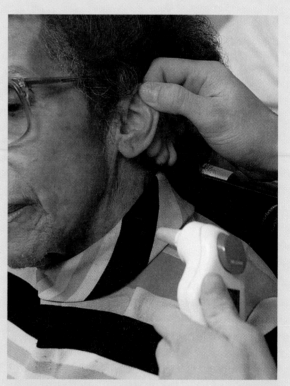

**FIGURE 19-15** Gently pull the ear pinna back and up.

*(continues)*

**PROCEDURE** *66* *(continued)*

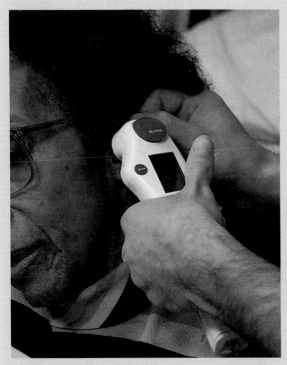

**FIGURE 19-16**  Place the probe in the resident's ear, aiming it toward the tympanic membrane. Insert the probe until it seals the ear canal.

10. Press the activation button (Figure 19-17). Leave the thermometer in the ear for the time recommended by the manufacturer.

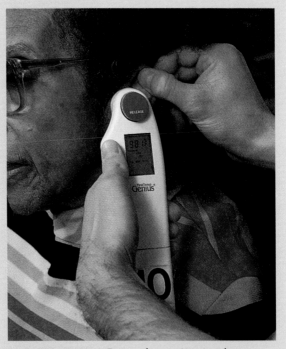

**FIGURE 19-17**  Press the activation button and leave the thermometer in the ear for the time recommended by the manufacturer.

11. When you have a reading, remove the probe from the resident's ear and dispose of the cover.
12. Carry out each procedure completion action.

## PULSE AND RESPIRATION

The **pulse** and **respiration** of the resident are usually counted during the same procedure.

Pulse is the pressure of the blood felt against the wall of an artery as the heart alternately beats (contracts) and rests (relaxes). The pulse is more easily felt in arteries that are fairly close to the skin surface and can be gently pressed against a bone by the fingers. The pulse rate and its character provide a good indication of how the cardiovascular system is able to meet the body's needs.

### Radial Pulse

The pulse is usually measured over the **radial artery** (at the base of the wrist on the thumb side) (Figure 19-18). The age, sex, size, and condition of the resident affect the character of the pulse. Pulse character means:

- Rate (speed)
- **Volume** (fullness)
- **Rhythm** (regularity)

Pulse character should always be noted when counting the pulse.

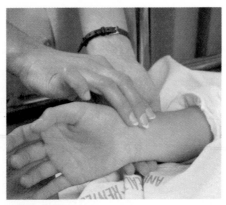

**FIGURE 19-18**   Locate the pulse on the thumb side of the wrist with the tips of your fingers.

## Apical Pulse

The heart rate is usually the same as the **pulse rate**. At times, however, some of the heartbeats are not strong enough to be transmitted and felt along the radial artery. This results in a difference between the heart rate and the pulse rate. This difference is called a **pulse deficit**. Pulse deficits are found in some forms of heart disease. If a pulse deficit is suspected, it may be necessary to count the heart rate and the pulse rate at the same time. One person determines the heart rate by placing a stethoscope on the chest over the **apex** or point of the heart. The apex is the lowest point of the heart and can eas-

---

**PROCEDURE**
**67**

# Counting the Radial Pulse Rate

1. Carry out each beginning procedure action.
   *Note:* Use disposable gloves if there may be contact with open lesions, wet linens, or body fluids.
2. Place resident in a comfortable position. The palm of the hand should be down and the arm should rest across the resident's chest.
3. Locate the pulse on the thumb side of the wrist with the tips of your first three fingers. Do not use your thumb because it contains a pulse that may be confused with the resident's pulse. Refer to Figure 19-19 for the location of other sites on the body where the pulse rate can be counted.

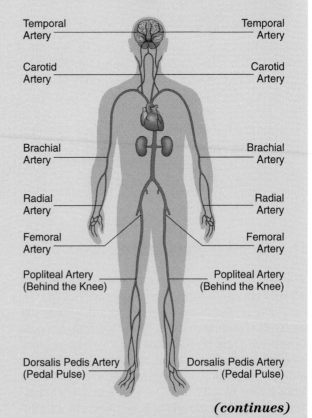

Temporal Artery — Temporal Artery

Carotid Artery — Carotid Artery

Brachial Artery — Brachial Artery

Radial Artery — Radial Artery

Femoral Artery — Femoral Artery

Popliteal Artery (Behind the Knee) — Popliteal Artery (Behind the Knee)

Dorsalis Pedis Artery (Pedal Pulse) — Dorsalis Pedis Artery (Pedal Pulse)

**FIGURE 19-19**   Pulses may be felt in areas other than the wrist. These are called pulse sites.

*(continues)*

**PROCEDURE** *67* *(continued)*

4. When the pulse is felt, exert slight pressure. Use second hand of watch and count for 1 minute. It is the practice in some facilities to count for 30 seconds, multiply the value by two, and then record the rate for 1 minute. For accuracy, a 1-minute count is preferred and must be done if the pulse is irregular. Figure 19-20 lists average pulse rates.
5. Carry out each procedure completion action.

| **FIGURE 19-20** Average pulse rates | | |
|---|---|---|
| Adult men | 60–70 | beats per minute |
| Adult women | 65–80 | beats per minute |
| Children over 7 years | 75–100 | beats per minute |
| Preschoolers | 80–110 | beats per minute |
| Infants | 120–160 | beats per minute |

ily be located near the left nipple or under a woman's left breast. The second person counts the radial pulse at the same time and the rates are compared. This is called taking an **apical pulse**. The average pulse rate is about 72 beats per minute (bpm). Pulse rates under 60 or over 90 should be reported.

- **Tachycardia**—unusually fast pulse rate (over 90 bpm)
- **Bradycardia**—unusually slow pulse rate (under 60 bpm)

Any irregularities in the rate, rhythm, or volume of the resident's pulse should be reported immediately.

**PROCEDURE 68** Counting the Apical-Radial Pulse

1. Carry out each beginning procedure action.
   *Note:* Use disposable gloves if there may be contact with open lesions, wet linens, or body fluids.
2. Clean stethoscope earpieces and bell with disinfectant.
3. Two people measure the heart rate and the radial pulse at the same time. The nurse places the stethoscope earpieces in the ears and the stethoscope diaphragm over the apex of the resident's heart. (The diaphragm may be warmed in the hands before placing it on the resident's chest.) The heartbeats are counted for 1 minute.
4. At the same time, the nursing assistant counts the radial pulse for 1 minute (Figure 19-21).

*(continues)*

**PROCEDURE 68** *(continued)*

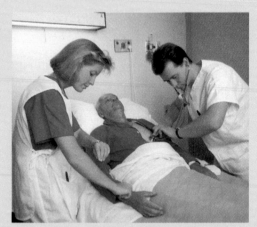

**FIGURE 19-21** Taking the apical and radial pulses

5. Compare the results and note them on the pad.
6. Clean earpieces and bell of stethoscope with disinfectant.
7. Carry out each procedure completion action. Record date, time, pulse values as in example, and character, such as weak and irregular.

*Example:*

| | |
|---|---|
| Apical pulse | A 108 |
| Radial pulse | R 82 |

Pulse deficit is 26
(108 − 82 = 26)

## Respiration

Respiration supplies the cells in the body with oxygen and rids the body of excess carbon dioxide. When respirations are inefficient, carbon dioxide gas builds up in the bloodstream, making the skin dusky, bluish, or **cyanotic**.

There are two parts to each respiration:

- One **inspiration** (inhalation)
- One **expiration** (exhalation)

The character (rhythm and volume) and the rate of respirations must be noted. Respirations are described as:

- Normal
- Shallow
- Deep
- Labored
- Difficult

The normal respiration rate for adults is 16 to 20 per minute. If the rate is more than 25 per minute, it is **accelerated** and is reported. If the rate is less than 12 per minute, it is too low and is reported. Special terms are used to describe different types of breathing (Figure 19-22).

The rate is determined by counting the rise and fall of the chest for 1 minute while using a watch equipped with a second hand.

**FIGURE 19-22** Special terms describe different breathing patterns.

- Tachypnea—rapid, shallow breathing

- Dyspnea—difficult or labored breathing

- Shallow—breaths that partially fill the lungs

- Apnea—a period of no respirations

- Cheyne-Stokes respirations—a period of dyspnea followed by periods of apnea

- Stertorous—Snoring-like respirations

- **Rales** (gurgles)—moist respirations. At times, fluid (mucus) will collect in the air passages. This causes a bubbling type of respiration. Rales are common in the dying resident.

- Wheezing—difficult breathing accompanied by a whistling or sighing sound due to narrowing of bronchioles (as in asthma) or an increase of mucus in bronchi

| **FIGURE 19-23**  Factors affecting respiratory rates | |
|---|---|
| • Illness | • Exercise |
| • Emotions | • Position |
| • Elevated temperature | • Drugs |
| • Age | |

| **FIGURE 19-24**  Factors influencing blood pressure readings |
|---|
| • Amount of blood in circulatory system |
| • Force of the heartbeat |
| • Age |
| • Sleep |
| • Weight |
| • Emotion |
| • Heredity |
| • Viscosity of blood |
| • Condition of blood vessels |

Breathing is partially under voluntary control; that is, a person is able to stop breathing for a short period of time. This frequently happens when a resident realizes that breathing is being watched and counted. The breathing pattern is altered unintentionally. To avoid this, the respirations are counted immediately following the pulse count. The resident's hand is kept in the same position on the chest and your fingers remain on the pulse.

Factors affecting respiratory rates are listed in Figure 19-23.

## BLOOD PRESSURE

The factors that influence blood pressure are listed in Figure 19-24.

There is greater resistance to blood flow in arteries that have lost their elasticity or ability to stretch due to disease. This causes higher blood pressure. Blood pressure is also increased by:

- Exercise
- Eating
- Stimulants
- Emotional anxiety
- Some drugs

Blood pressure is decreased by:

- **Fasting** (not eating)
- Rest
- **Depressants** (drugs that slow down body functions)
- Excessive loss of blood

## PROCEDURE
## *69*   Counting Respirations

**1.** After counting the pulse rate, leave your fingers on the radial pulse.
**2.** Start counting the number of times the chest rises and falls during a period of 1 minute.

**3.** Note depth and regularity of respirations.
**4.** Record the time, rate, depth, and regularity of respirations.

- **Antihypertensives** (drugs that lower blood pressure in persons who have hypertension)

If the resident is resting, any reading between 60 and 90 diastolic (lower reading) is considered normal. Blood pressure rises slightly with age.

**Hypertension** is high blood pressure (greater than 140/90). Uncontrolled hypertension can lead to stroke, kidney disease, or heart damage.

**Hypotension** is low blood pressure (below 100/70). Excessive hypotension can lead to shock.

In either case, unusual or changed findings must be recorded and reported.

## Blood Pressure Equipment

Blood pressure equipment includes the sphygmomanometer (Figure 19-25) and the stethoscope (Figure 19-26). The commonly used sphygmomanometer consists of a cuff with a rubber bladder inside with two tubes—one connected to the pressure control bulb and the other to the pressure gauge (Figure 19-25B). The gauge may be a round dial or a column of mercury. Both are marked in numbers. Be sure to use a cuff of the proper size. Cuffs that are too wide or too narrow for the arm will give inaccurate readings.

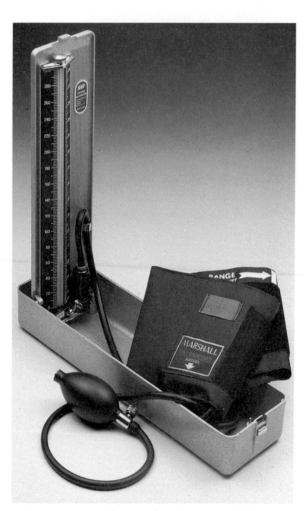

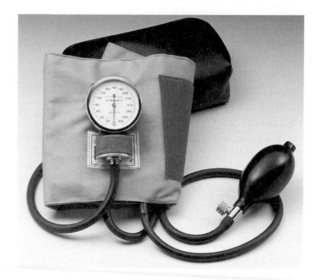

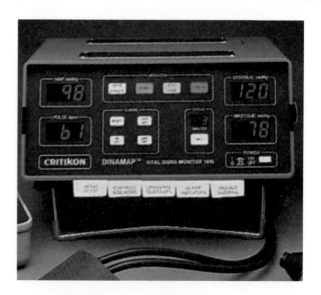

**FIGURE 19-25** Types of sphygmomanometers (Left) Mercury gravity sphygmomanometer (Top, right) Dial (aneroid) sphygmomanometer (Bottom, right) Electronic sphygmomanometer

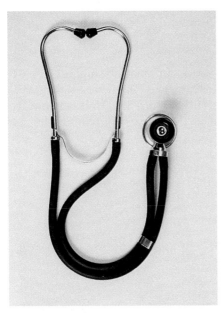

**FIGURE 19-26**   A stethoscope

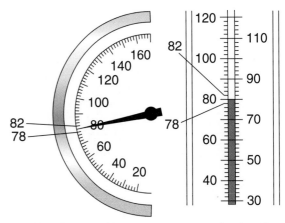

**FIGURE 19-27**   The gauges are marked with a series of large lines at 10-mm (millimeter) intervals.

The length of the bladder portion of the cuff should be about 80% of the circumference of the resident's arm.

**How to Read the Gauge.** The gauges are marked with a series of large lines at 10-mm (millimeter) intervals (Figure 19-27). In between the large lines are shorter lines, each of which indicates 2 mm. For example, the small line above 80 mm is 82 mm, and the small line below 80 mm is 78 mm. For accuracy, the gauge should be at eye level when reading. The mercury col-

umn gauge must not be tilted. The level of the top of the column of mercury or the pointer of the dial is taken for the reading. Two readings are recorded:

- **Systolic**—first sound heard. It represents the highest pressure in the arteries.
- **Diastolic**—the level at which sound stops. The smaller number indicates when this change in sound is heard.

The blood pressure is recorded as a fraction with the larger number on top. For example, 112/68 means:

- 112 is the systolic pressure
- 68 is the diastolic pressure

---

*G*uidelines for

## Preparing to Measure Blood Pressure

**Before using the stethoscope:**
1. Clean the earpieces with an alcohol wipe and clean the bell with a different alcohol wipe.
2. Point the earpieces forward when inserting them in your ears.
3. Use the bell portion of the stethoscope (Figure 19-28).

4. Be sure the bell portion is open so you will hear the beats.

**Before using a sphygmomanometer:**
1. If using a mercury manometer—if the mercury moves up the column very slowly (Figure 19-29), it may have oxidized. Report this to the nurse and use another sphygmomanometer.

*(continues)*

## $\mathcal{G}$uidelines *(continued)*

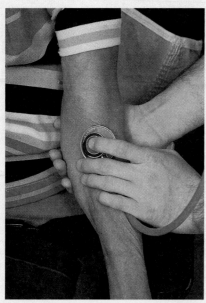

**FIGURE 19-28** Use the bell portion of the stethoscope when taking a blood pressure.

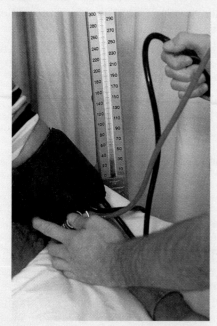

**FIGURE 19-29** Do not use the sphygmomanometer if the mercury moves up the column very slowly.

2. If using an aneroid manometer—make sure the needle is on zero before inflating the cuff (Figure 19-30). If it is not, report this to the nurse and use another sphygmomanometer.

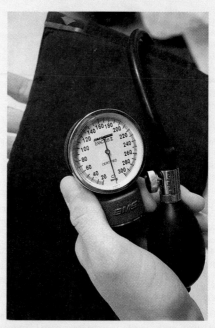

**FIGURE 19-30** Make sure the needle is on zero before inflating the cuff of the aneroid manometer.

Turn off radio and television when taking blood pressure. Ask the resident not to talk. Do not take blood pressure on an arm that:

- Has an intravenous feeding or other device inserted
- Is being treated for burns, fractures, or other injuries

## PROCEDURE
### *70*
## Taking Blood Pressure

1. Carry out each beginning procedure action.
2. Assemble equipment:
   - Sphygmomanometer with appropriate size cuff
   - Stethoscope
   - Alcohol wipes
3. Remove resident's arm from sleeve or roll sleeve 5 inches above elbow; it should not be tight or binding.
4. Locate the brachial artery with your fingers (Figure 19-31).
5. Place resident's arm palm upward, supported on bed or table.
6. Wrap the cuff smoothly and snugly around resident's arm. Center the bladder over the brachial artery. The bottom of the cuff should be 1 inch above the antecubital space (inner elbow) (Figure 19-32).

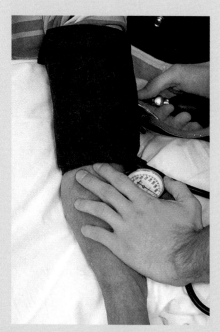

**FIGURE 19-32**  The bottom of the cuff should be 1 inch above the antecubital space (inner elbow).

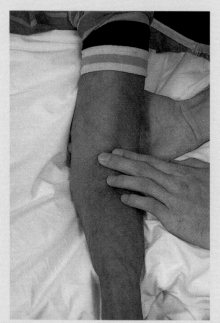

**FIGURE 19-31**  Locate the brachial artery with your fingers.

7. Place the bulb in your dominant hand and feel for the radial pulse with the fingers of your other hand (Figure 19-33). To find out how high to pump the cuff:
   - Rapidly inflate the cuff until you no longer feel the radial pulse.
   - Add 30 mm to that reading. (If you no longer feel the pulse when the mercury or needle reaches 130, add 30 mm for a reading of 160).

*(continues)*

**PROCEDURE** *70* *(continued)*

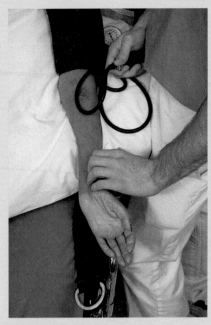

**FIGURE 19-33** Place the bulb in your dominant hand and feel for the radial pulse with the fingers of your other hand.

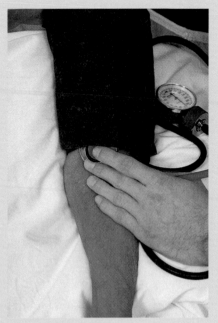

**FIGURE 19-34** Place the stethoscope over the brachial artery.

8. Quickly and steadily deflate the cuff. Wait 15 to 30 seconds.
9. Place the stethoscope over the brachial artery (Figure 19-34).
10. Reinflate the cuff quickly and steadily to the level you calculated (in example in Step 7, to 160) (Figure 19-35).
11. Release the air at an even pace, about 2 to 3 mm per second. Keep your eyes on the needle or the mercury.
12. Listen for the onset of at least two consecutive beats. Note where the needle is on the sphygmomanometer when you hear the sound. (Do not stop deflating the cuff). This is your systolic reading.
13. Continue deflating the cuff. The last sound you hear is the diastolic reading. Continue to deflate and to listen for 10 to 20 mm more to make sure you have the correct diastolic reading.

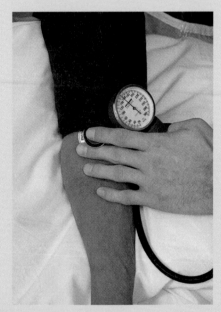

**FIGURE 19-35** Reinflate the cuff quickly and steadily to the level you calculated.

*(continues)*

**PROCEDURE** *70* *(continued)*

14. Record the reading (blood pressure is always recorded in even numbers with the systolic on top and the diastolic on the bottom, e.g., 128/82). Indicate the arm used and the position of the resident—sitting, lying down, or standing.
15. If you are not sure of the reading and need to retake the blood pressure, wait

1 to 2 minutes before repeating the procedure.
16. Clean the earpieces of the stethoscope with alcohol wipes.
17. Return equipment to appropriate area.
18. Carry out each procedure completion action.

## WEIGHING AND MEASURING THE RESIDENT

Maintaining a record of the height and weight of all residents is important for several reasons:

- Medication dosages may be calculated based on height and weight.
- Weight is monitored to determine if the resident is retaining fluid (edema).
- Weight indicates if the resident's nutritional intake is adequate.

Baseline (original) measurements are obtained on admission. Residents are weighed at least monthly thereafter. Some residents may need to be weighed more often.

### Methods of Measurement

Height and weight may be measured using the metric system: centimeters for height and kilograms for weight. If your facility uses this method, the scales will be calibrated for the metric system. There is no need to convert from the inch and pound system to the metric system. There are several types of scales:

- An upright scale is used only for residents who can stand unattended on the platform (Figure 19-36).
- Chair scales are used for residents in wheelchairs who cannot stand on an upright scale (Figure 19-37).
- A mechanical lift with scale is used to weigh residents in bed who cannot stand on an

upright scale and who cannot sit in a wheelchair (Figure 19-38).

Height is measured with the ruler attached to an upright scale or with a tape measure when the resident is in bed.

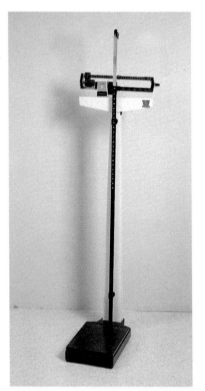

**FIGURE 19-36**   An upright scale is used only for residents who can stand unattended on the platform.

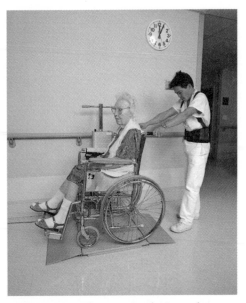

**FIGURE 19-37** Electronic chair scales are used for residents in wheelchairs who cannot stand on an upright scale.

## Obtaining Accurate Weights

To obtain an accurate measurement of weight, you must:

- Weigh the resident at the same time of day each time.
- Have the resident wear the same type of clothing each time.
- Use the same method and the same scale each time, if possible.

You must learn to read the scale correctly. There are two bars on the upright scale shown in Figure 19-36. The balance bar should hang free to start.

- The lower bar indicates weights in large 50-pound increments.
- The upper bar indicates smaller pound weights (Figure 19-39). The even-numbered pounds are marked with numbers.
- The long line between each number indicates the odd-numbered pounds.

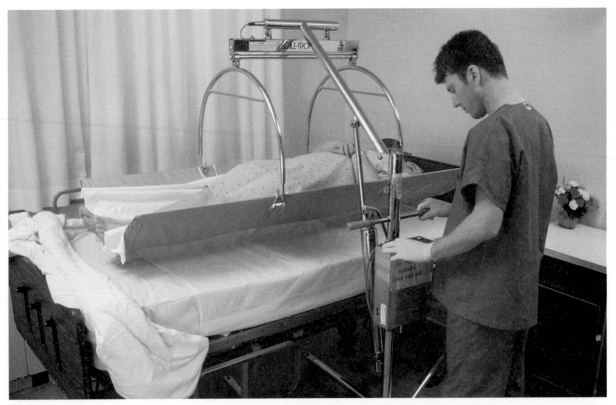

**FIGURE 19-38** A mechanical lift with scale is used to weigh residents in bed who cannot stand on the upright scale and cannot sit up in a wheelchair.

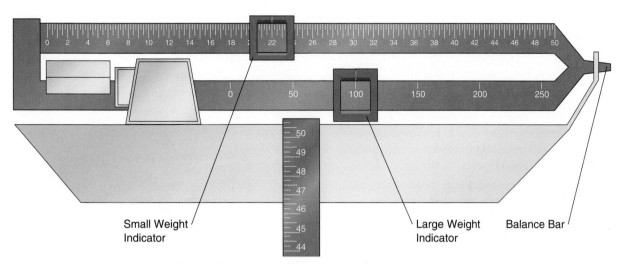

Small Weight Indicator

Large Weight Indicator    Balance Bar

**FIGURE 19-39**   The upper bar indicates smaller pound weights. The weight shown on the lower bar is added to the weight shown on the upper bar.

• Each small line indicates one quarter of a pound, or 4 ounces.

The two figures are added and recorded as the person's total weight. The sum is recorded according to facility policy in either pounds or kilograms.

Large weight = 100 pounds
Small weight = +22 pounds
          Total = 122 pounds

Measuring the resident may be done during the weighing procedure with an upright scale. The information is recorded in feet and inches or in centimeters, according to facility policy.

*Example:*

A height measurement of 62 inches may be recorded as 62 inches, or 5 feet 2 inches or 155 cm.

**PROCEDURE 71**   Weighing and Measuring the Resident Using an Upright Scale

**1.** Carry out each beginning procedure action.
*Note:* Use disposable gloves if there may be contact with open lesions, wet linens, or body fluids.

**2.** Check previous weight as documented. Then escort the resident to the scales.

**3.** Place a paper towel on the platform of the scale.

**4.** Be sure the weights are to the extreme left and the balance bar (bar with weight markings) hangs free.

• The lower bar (large indicator) is calibrated (marked) in increments (amounts) of 50 pounds.

• The upper bar (small indicator) is calibrated in increments of single pounds.

*(continues)*

**PROCEDURE** *71* *(continued)*

- The even-numbered pounds are marked with numbers.
- The long line between even numbers indicates the odd-numbered pounds.
- Each small line indicates one quarter of a pound.

5. Assist the resident to remove shoes and step up onto the scale platform, facing the balance bar. The balance bar will rise to the top of the bar guide. The resident should not hold the bar or other parts of the scale.

6. Move the large weight to the right to the closest estimated resident weight.

7. Move the small weight to the right until the balance bar hangs freely halfway between the upper and lower bar guides.

8. Add the two figures and record the total as the resident's weight in pounds or kilograms, according to the type of scale used.

9. Assist the resident to turn on the platform until facing away from the balance bar. Raise the height bar until it is level with the top of the resident's head.

10. The reading is made at the movable point of the ruler (Figure 19-40).

11. Note the number of inches indicated. Record this information in inches ("), feet (') and inches ("), or centimeters (cm)

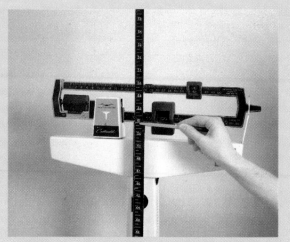

**FIGURE 19-40** The resident's height is read at the movable point of the ruler.

according to the type of scale. The height shown in Figure 19-40 is 62 inches. This may be recorded as 62 inches or 5 feet 2 inches (62 ÷ 12 = 5 feet 2 inches). Record value on your note pad.

12. Assist the resident off the platform. Help resident to put on shoes, if necessary, and return to the room.

13. Carry out each procedure completion action.

---

**PROCEDURE** *72*

## Measuring Weight with an Electronic Wheelchair Scale

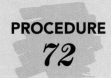  

1. Carry out each beginning procedure action.
2. Assemble equipment:
   - Wheelchair scale (Figure 19-41A)
3. Determine empty weight of wheelchair by weighing it on the scale.

4. Take wheelchair to resident's room. Help the resident into the wheelchair and take the resident to the electronic wheelchair scale.
5. Open metal ramp sides on scale to rest on floor. This allows wheelchair access to scale.

*(continues)*

**PROCEDURE *72* (continued)**

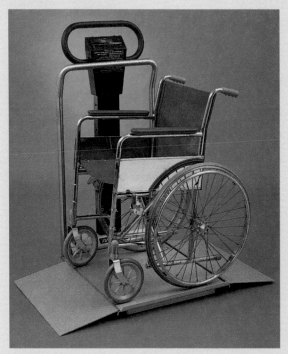

**FIGURE 19-41A**  Wheelchair scale

6. Press "on" button; scale zeros automatically (Figure 19-41B).
7. Roll wheelchair with resident onto platform of scale. Lock wheels of wheelchair.

8. Digital readout will show weight.
9. Record weight of resident and wheelchair. Subtract wheelchair weight to obtain resident weight.
10. Unlock wheels of wheelchair. Roll wheelchair with resident off scale.
11. Fold scale ramps back in place.
12. Carry out each procedure completion action.

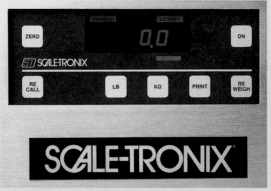

**FIGURE 19-41B**  Press "on" button to zero scale automatically. (Courtesy of Scale-Tronix, White Plains, NY)

**PROCEDURE *73*  Weighing the Resident in a Chair Scale**

1. Carry out each beginning procedure action.
2. Assemble equipment:
   • Chair scale
3. Take resident in wheelchair to chair scale.
4. Apply transfer belt to resident and assist in a pivot transfer to chair on scale. Instruct resident to sit down when the chair is felt against the back of the legs. Be sure resident's feet are on footrest of scale.
5. Walk behind the scale to obtain the reading.
6. Transfer resident back to wheelchair.
7. Carry out each procedure completion action.

**PROCEDURE 74** Measuring and Weighing the Resident in Bed

1. Carry out each beginning procedure action.
2. Obtain assistance from coworker.
3. Assemble equipment:
   - Overbed scale
   - Tape measure
   - Pencil
4. Check scale sling and straps for frayed areas or poorly closing straps.
5. Lower side rail on your side. Make sure side rail is up on other side.
6. Fanfold top linen to foot of bed.
7. Position resident flat on back with arms and legs straight and body in good alignment.
8. Make a small pencil mark at the top of the resident's head on the sheet.
9. Make a second pencil mark even with the feet.
10. Using the tape measure, measure the distance between the two pencil marks.
11. Note this on a pad with resident's height in feet and inches.
12. Remove the scale sling from suspension straps and position half under the resident.
    - Turn the resident away from you.
    - Place the sling folded lengthwise under the resident.

- Return resident to recumbent position and place sling so that the resident rests securely within it.
- Attach sling to suspension straps. Check to be sure attachments are secure.

13. Position lift frame over bed with base legs in maximum open position and lock.
14. Elevate head of bed and bring resident to sitting position.
15. Attach suspension straps to frame. Position resident's arms inside straps.
16. Slowly raise sling so resident's body is free from bed. Be reassuring.
17. Guide the lift away from the bed so that no part of the resident touches the bed.
18. Balance scale according to manufacturer's instructions.
19. Take and note reading.
20. Reposition sling over center of bed.
21. Release knob slowly, lowering resident to bed.
22. Remove sling by reversing the process in Step 12.
23. Assist resident to comfortable position.
24. Move overbed scale out of the way.
25. Replace top bed linen over resident. Raise side rail and lower bed to lowest horizontal height.
26. Carry out each procedure completion action.

## RECORDING VITAL SIGNS

Temperature, pulse, and respiration (TPR), and height and weight values are recorded in a notebook and then transferred to the resident's chart (Figure 19-42) by a secretary or a nurse.

**Bay Shore Convalescent Home**
**4782 Bay Shore Drive**
**Watertown, Mich.**

Vital signs are to be checked on all residents once each
day unless ordered otherwise.

Date 4/10/XX

| Resident | Room | Temp. | Pulse | Resp. | B/P | Comments |
|---|---|---|---|---|---|---|
| Estrada, Luisa 101A | | | | | | |
| Hartong, Mary 101B | | | | | | |
| Diette, Marie | 102A | | | | | |
| Aquino, Lucy | 102B | | | | | |
| Ihli, Fred | 103A | | | | | |
| Dyment, Frank 103B | | | | | | |
| Lightfoot, Wm. 104A | | | | | | |
| Lee, Sayo | 104B | | | | | |
| Salcido, Rose | 105A | | | | | |
| Tham, Peou | 105B | | | | | |
| Wilde, Rose Marie | 106A | | | | | |
| Hubbard, Marta | 106B | | | | | |
| Lam, Lotruc | 107A | | | | | |
| Uy, Aime | 107B | | | | | |
| Valasco, Mary 108A | | | | | | |
| Lobliner, Esther | 108B | | | | | |
| | 109A | | | | | |
| Moak, Loreta | 109B | | | | | |
| Ocha, Vario | 110A | | | | | |
| | 110B | | | | | |
| | | | | | | |
| | | | | | | |

**FIGURE 19-42** Vital signs may be taken and recorded on the unit sheet and later transferred to
the resident's record.

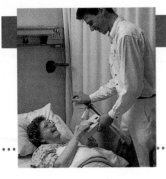

## LESSON SYNTHESIS: Putting It All Together

*Y*ou have just completed this lesson. Now go back and review the Clinical Focus. Try to see how the Clinical Focus relates to the concepts presented in the lesson. Then answer the following questions.

1. The physician has ordered that Mrs. Hoden be weighed daily. Why do you think this is important?

2. Which method would be the most appropriate for weighing Mrs. Hoden?

3. An apical/radial pulse is taken on Mrs. Hoden because she has a pulse deficit. What does this mean?

4. What type of respirations would you expect to note on Mrs. Hoden?

## REVIEW

**A. Select the one best answer for each of the following.**

1. The term vital signs includes
   a. height and weight
   b. temperature, pulse, respirations, and blood pressure
   c. temperature, pulse, and respirations
   d. all of these

2. Temperature can be increased by
   a. medications
   b. shock
   c. dehydration
   d. cold weather

3. Oral temperatures should not be taken on residents who are
   a. confused and disoriented
   b. on seizure precautions
   c. unconscious
   d. all of these

4. A temperature taken in the ear is called
   a. oral
   b. axillary
   c. rectal
   d. tympanic

5. The most accurate method of taking temperature is
   a. oral
   b. axillary

   c. rectal
   d. tympanic

6. The pulse is usually taken at which artery?
   a. brachial
   b. radial
   c. femoral
   d. carotid

7. The average pulse rate per minute for adult women is
   a. 80–110
   b. 60–70
   c. 65–80
   d. 75–100

8. Blood pressure can be increased by
   a. exercise
   b. eating
   c. emotional anxiety
   d. all of these

9. Medications prescribed to lower blood pressure are called
   a. antihypertensives
   b. stimulants
   c. depressants
   d. antibiotics

10. The first sound heard when taking blood pressure is called
    a. diastolic
    b. systolic

c.  pulse pressure

d.  apical

**B.  Match each term (items a.–j.) with the proper definition.**

a.  sphygmomano-  f.  hypotension
    meter            g.  bradycardia
b.  tachycardia     h.  hypertension
c.  thermometer     i.  pulse deficit
d.  volume          j.  rales
e.  fasting

11.  _____  low blood pressure

12.  _____  fullness (amount)

13.  _____  moist respirations

14.  _____  not eating

15.  _____  rapid heart rate

16.  _____  slow heart rate

17.  _____  used to determine blood pressure

18.  _____  used to determine temperature

19.  _____  high blood pressure

20.  _____  difference between radial and apical pulse rates

**C.  Identification**

21.  Read the temperature indicated on each thermometer
     oral:
     security:
     rectal:

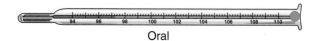

Oral

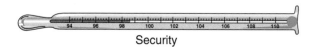

Security

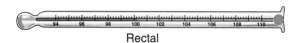

Rectal

**D.  Fill in the blanks by selecting the correct word or phrase from the list.**

axillary              rate
bradycardia           rectal
centimeters           rhythm
cyanotic              sphygmomanometer
dyspnea               stethoscope
expiration            tachycardia
inspiration           vital signs
kilograms             volume
rales

22.  Temperature, pulse, respiration, and blood pressure are: _____.

23.  The instrument used to listen to the heart is a (an): _____.

24.  The instrument used to measure blood pressure is a (an): _____.

25.  A _____ temperature is usually 1° higher than an oral temperature.

26.  An _____ temperature is usually 1° lower than an oral temperature.

27.  In the metric system, height is measured in _____.

28.  In the metric system, weight is measured in _____.

29.  When taking a pulse, you should note _____, _____, _____.

30.  A rapid pulse rate is called _____.

31.  A slow pulse rate is called _____.

32.  The two parts to each respiration are called _____ and _____.

33.  The term _____ means a dusky, bluish color to the skin.

34.  Moist respirations are called _____.

35.  Labored breathing is called _____.

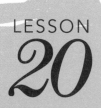
# *20* Admission, Transfer, and Discharge

## CLINICAL FOCUS

Think about situations that require admission to, or transfer and discharge from, the long-term care facility as you study this lesson and meet:

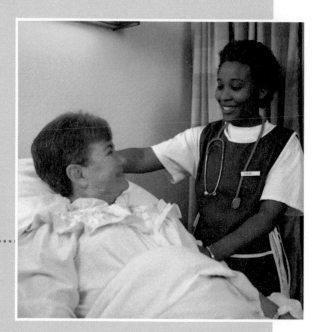

*F*iona Lyon-Ravens, age 61, who has just been transferred by ambulance to your facility from the local acute care hospital. She fractured her hip at home. The fracture was repaired with surgery. She will be receiving rehabilitation at your facility and then will be discharged to go home. She is alert and able to follow instructions.

## OBJECTIVES

*After studying this lesson, you should be able to:*

- Define and spell vocabulary words and terms.
- List reasons why residents are admitted to long-term care facilities.
- Describe the emotional reactions of the resident and the family to admission.
- Identify the responsibilities of the nursing assistant related to admission procedures.
- List reasons why residents may be transferred out of the facility.
- Identify the responsibilities of the nursing assistant related to transfer procedures.

- List reasons why residents are discharged from long-term care facilities.
- Describe the actions involved in the discharge of a resident.
- Identify the responsibilities of the nursing assistant related to discharge procedures.
- Demonstrate the following:
  Procedure 75 Admitting the Resident
  Procedure 76 Transferring the Resident
  Procedure 77 Discharging the Resident

# VOCABULARY

**community services**   *(kom-**MYOUN**-ih-tee*
   ***SIR**-vih-sez)*

**diagnosis-related group (DRG)**   *(**die**-ag-*
   ***NOS**-is ree-**LAY**-ted groop)*

**discharge planner**   *(**DIS**-charj **PLAN**-er)*

**discharge planning**   *(**DIS**-charj **PLAN**-ing)*

**kidney dialysis**   *(**KID**-nee die-**AL**-ih-sis)*

**personal inventory**   *(**PER**-son-al **IN**-ven-*
   ***tor**-ee)*

## ADMITTING THE RESIDENT

### Reasons for Admission

A resident may be admitted to a long-term care facility because the individual:

- Requires 24-hour-a-day supervision and nursing care
- Requires specialized treatments
- Requires rehabilitation services before returning home
- Has a progressive, chronic disease that requires more care
- Has Alzheimer's disease or another dementia and can no longer be cared for at home

   The resident may be admitted from

- An acute care hospital
- Home
- Another extended care facility

There may be varying circumstances surrounding the admission. Some residents are admitted to the hospital as emergencies requiring immediate care. An example of this would be a person who fell and broke a hip or the person who had a stroke. The individual can stay in the hospital for a limited number of days according to the **diagnosis-related group (DRG)** that covers the person's diagnosis. At the end of this time most people are not yet ready to care for themselves. The **discharge planner** (the person who arranges care after discharge from the hospital) may arrange for home care or for the person to be admitted to a long-term care facility until the person is more independent. In these situations the family and resident may need to make a quick decision about placement (Figure 20-1).

   Some residents are admitted because they have Alzheimer's disease or another dementia.

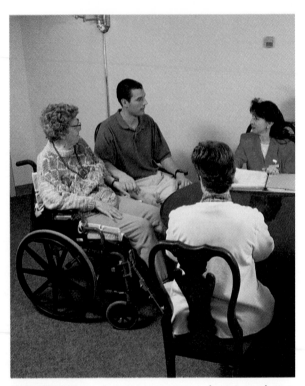

**FIGURE 20-1**   In some cases a decision about a long-term care facility may need to be made in a hurry.

These diseases are progressive and eventually require 24-hour-a-day supervision. Most families do not have the energy resources to cope with the situation. Other chronic diseases such as Parkinson's disease or multiple sclerosis may progress to the point that the individual is unable to perform the activities of daily living without maximal assistance.

   In some situations, residents require specialized care because they need:

- Artificial ventilation to breathe
- **Kidney dialysis** (treatment when kidneys fail)
- Complicated wound care
- Rehabilitation services

## Anxiety About Admission

Some admissions are considered permanent, which means the resident will live in the facility for the rest of his life. Other admissions are temporary and the resident will eventually be discharged.

The new resident who is considered a permanent admission probably has experienced many losses. Admission means a further loss of independence. He or she may have lost a spouse and now, along with failing strength and health, the comfort and security of familiar surroundings is about to be lost. Families often feel guilty because the family member cannot be provided for at home. They may also be physically and emotionally exhausted from giving care for several years before this admission. Burdens also may be intensified by the financial costs of admission. Residents who need to apply for Medicaid usually feel embarrassed because they cannot pay their own way.

Both the family and the new resident will feel uncertain about and somewhat fearful of the new environment. They will need support and encouragement. Their anxiety may make it difficult for them to remember things that you explain to them. Be prepared to repeat statements. Reassure them that their feelings are natural and help them express these feelings. Make their first impression of you and the facility a positive one.

## Preadmission Activities

Arranging for admission to a long-term care facility involves many activities that occur before the resident arrives. The family is often responsible for participating in these procedures, especially if the resident is in the hospital. The family will need to:

- Choose (with the resident's input if possible) a facility
- Meet with someone from the Social Services Department to arrange for the admission
- Apply for Medicaid, if necessary, to pay for the cost of services

If the resident is coming from a hospital, the discharge planner at the hospital will need to:

- Confirm admission with the Social Services Department of the facility to be sure a bed is available and that the facility can provide the care and treatment the person needs
- Complete transfer forms to ensure continuity of care
- Arrange for the resident's transfer (usually by ambulance) from hospital to facility

The Social Services Department staff of the receiving facility will need to:

- Meet with the discharge planner to determine services needed. The social worker may visit the resident to make an initial assessment.
- Meet with the nursing staff of the receiving facility to determine if special equipment, such as traction, will be needed
- Meet with the family (and resident if possible) to explain the facility's services and the responsibilities of the family and resident
- Explain and provide a copy of the Residents' Rights to family and resident
- Determine the method of payment for services
- Inform appropriate departments of the resident's pending admission and the services that will be needed
- Inform any residents who may be sharing the room of the new resident's arrival

In-service meetings or training for the staff may be needed if the resident has an unusual diagnosis, requires special treatment, or needs special equipment.

## Day of Admission

On the day of admission, you may be expected to check the room to be sure it is ready for the new resident's arrival.

- Check the room lights to be sure they are working.
- Check the call light to be sure it is working. Attach it to the bed.
- Check bed controls and attach to bed.
- Check the bed for clean sheets, a pillow, and a spread. Lock the wheels of the bed. Place bed in lowest position.
- Check the telephone for a dial tone.
- Move overbed table, if necessary, so it is not in the way.

- Place a pitcher and glass on the bedside table. Wait to fill the pitcher with fresh water until the resident's arrival.
- Place personal care items in the bedside table. In the top drawer place:
  - Emesis basin
  - Toothbrush and toothpaste
  - Mouthwash
  - Lotion
  In the middle drawer place:
  - Wash basin
  - Soap in soap dish
  In the bottom drawer place:
  - Bedpan
  - Toilet tissue
  - Urinal if resident is male

*Note:* The arrangement of items may be different for each facility. Remember that "dirty" items such as bedpans and urinals should not be placed with clean items like the wash basin and toothbrush.

- Check the resident's bathroom for:
  - Cleanliness
  - Soap in soap dispenser
  - Paper towels in dispenser
  - Towels and washcloths for the resident
  - Toilet tissue
- Check dresser drawers for cleanliness.
- Check the closet for hangers.

The bed may be opened (top covers folded to end of bed) or left closed depending on the condition of the resident. The nurse or the unit secretary will set up a chart, care plan, and other forms to be used on admission.

## Admission Assessments

The members of the interdisciplinary health care team will each make an assessment of the new resident (Figure 20-2). This includes the Minimum Data Set (MDS) 2.0 form required by OBRA and other assessments required by the facility. This information will be used to start the plan of care.

## Meeting the New Resident

First impressions are important. Remember that this is a new and strange experience for the resident and family. Someone from the facility is

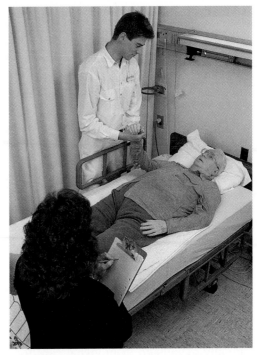

**FIGURE 20-2** Each member of the interdisciplinary team will make an assessment of the new resident.

designated to meet the resident and family and to accompany them to the assigned room. The social worker or nurse may be responsible for this procedure.

## Responsibilities of the Nursing Assistant

The nurse and social worker need to complete a number of procedures once the resident is in the room. At the appropriate time you will need to complete the nursing assistant's part of the admission procedure.

In most facilities the social worker or nurse will inform the resident and family about:
- Facility rules such as limitations on smoking
- Visiting periods
- Availability of services and activities

The resident (if possible) and the family will be taken on a tour of the building so they know the location of:
- Stairs, elevators
- Dining room

## PROCEDURE 75

# Admitting the Resident

**1.** Wash hands and assemble equipment:
- Urine specimen container
- Equipment for taking temperature
- Worksheet for recording information
- Stethoscope
- Sphygmomanometer
- Watch with second hand
- Appropriate scales

**2.** Prepare unit as described above if that has not yet been done.

**3.** Identify the resident both by asking the name and checking the identification bracelet.

**4.** Introduce yourself.

**5.** Help the resident undress if instructed by the nurse to do so. If resident will remain dressed, have resident sit in chair.

**6.** Show the resident how to use the call light.

**7.** Help the resident unpack. Hang up clothing or place it in the dresser drawers.

**8.** Set up personal items such as photographs, plants, religious articles (Figure 20-3).

**9.** Fill the pitcher with fresh water and ice (if appropriate).

**10.** Take the resident's vital signs.

**11.** Obtain the resident's height and weight.

**12.** Collect urine specimen if instructed to do so.

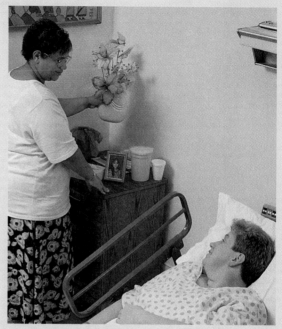

**FIGURE 20-3** The nursing assistant can help the new resident set up personal items.

**13.** Show the resident and family how to operate equipment such as electric bed, telephone, and television.

**14.** Carry out each procedure completion action.

---

- Activity areas
- Visiting areas outside the resident's room
- Offices of administrative staff
- Public telephones
- Public restrooms
- Rehabilitation services areas

You should be familiar with this information so you can accurately answer any questions the resident may have later.

## Completing a Personal Inventory

A **personal inventory** is completed for every resident who is admitted. This is a special form that lists and describes all items the resident brings to the facility (Figure 20-4). All items must be labeled with the resident's name. Follow the facility policy for this procedure. This task may be completed by the nurse, the unit secretary, the nursing assistant, or housekeeping staff.

Form 883/2   BRIGGS, Des Moines, Iowa 50306
PRINTED IN U.S.A.

## INVENTORY LIST

| QTY. | ARTICLES | QTY. | APPLIANCES | QTY. | PROSTHETIC DEVICES | | ACQUIRED AFTER ADMISSION |
|---|---|---|---|---|---|---|---|
| | Belts | | T.V. - Ser. #: | | Dentures: ☐ Upper | | |
| | Blouses | | Radio - Ser. #: | | ☐ Lower ☐ Partial | Date | Item |
| | Coats | | Hair Dryer | | Eye Wear | | |
| | Dresses | | Electric Razor | | Cane | | |
| | Gloves | | | | Walker - Ser. #: | | |
| | Hats | | | | W/chair - Ser. #: | | |
| | Housecoats - Robes | | JEWELRY | | Brace | | |
| | Jackets | | Ring (Describe) | | | | |
| | Nightgowns - Pajamas | | | | | | |
| | Purses | | Watch (Describe) | | OTHER | | |
| | Shaving Kit | | | | | | |
| | Shoes | | Other | | | | |
| | Shorts | | | | | | |
| | Slacks | | | | | | |
| | Slippers | | | | | | |
| | Slips | | FURNITURE | | | | |
| | Socks/Hose | | | | | | |
| | Suitcases | | | | | | |
| | Suits | | | | VALUABLES RELEASED FROM SAFE | | |
| | Sweaters | | | | | | |
| | Ties | | | | | | |
| | Undershirts | | | | | | |
| | Underwear | | | | | | |

I received on discharge in satisfactory condition the above articles and a copy of this list.
Disposition of belongings: _____

▶ _____   _____   ▶ _____   _____
Signature of Patient/Resp. Party      Date        Signature of Facility Representative      Date

**NOTE** ▶ Patient/Responsible Party is responsible for assuring that all personal belongings are properly marked. All items brought in after admission are added to this inventory at the request of Patient/Responsible Party.

| QTY. | ARTICLES | QTY. | APPLIANCES | QTY. | PROSTHETIC DEVICES | | ACQUIRED AFTER ADMISSION |
|---|---|---|---|---|---|---|---|
| 1 | Belts (black) | | T.V. - Ser. #: | | Dentures: ☐ Upper | | |
| 2 | ~~Blouses~~ Shirts (polo) | | Radio - Ser. #: | | ☐ Lower ☐ Partial | Date | Item |
| | Coats | | Hair Dryer | | Eye Wear | | |
| | Dresses | 1 | Electric Razor | | Cane | | |
| | Gloves | | | | Walker - Ser. #: | | |
| | Hats | | | | W/chair - Ser. #: | | |
| 1 | ~~Housecoats~~ - Robes (red) | | JEWELRY | | Brace | | |
| | Jackets | 1 | Ring (Describe) | | | | |
| | Nightgowns - Pajamas | | yellow metal wedding band | | | | |
| | Purses | 1 | Watch (Describe) | | OTHER | | |
| | Shaving Kit | | Timex silver metal | 1 | Bible | | |
| 1 pr | Shoes (black laced) | | Other | 8 | handkerchiefs, white | | |
| | Shorts | | | | | | |
| 2 | Slacks (knit, black, grey) | | | | | | |
| 1 pr | Slippers (brown felt) | | | | | | |
| | Slips | | FURNITURE | | | | |
| 6 pr | Socks/~~Hose~~ (black) | | | | | | |
| | Suitcases | | | | | | |
| | Suits | | | | VALUABLES LOCKED IN SAFE | | |
| | Sweaters | | | | | | |
| | Ties | | | | | | |
| 6 | Undershirts (white T) | | | | | | |
| 6 | Underwear (white jockey) | | | | | | |

I certify that this is a correct list of my clothes and belongings which I wish to retain in my possession and for which I take ENTIRE RESPONSIBILITY. I have received a copy of this list.

▶ *Joseph Cervanti*   7-26-97   ▶ *Della Sheeling*   7-26-97
Signature of Patient/Resp. Party      Date        Signature of Facility Representative      Date

If the patient is unable to sign, state reason: _____

▶ Signature of Witness: _____

| PATIENT NAME—LAST | FIRST | MIDDLE | HOSP. NO. | ROOM NO. |
|---|---|---|---|---|
| Cervanti | Joseph | — | | 203B |

## INVENTORY LIST

Form 883/2   BRIGGS, Des Moines, Iowa 50306
PRINTED IN U.S.A.

**FIGURE 20-4** The personal inventory lists and describes all items that the resident brings into the facility. (Reprinted with permission of Briggs Corporation, Des Moines, IA 50306 [800]247-2343)

The personal inventory includes:

- All items of clothing
- Jewelry including wedding rings and watches
- Personal equipment such as razors, combs, brushes
- Religious items such as bibles, rosaries
- Books, magazines, plants, photographs, afghan, quilt
- Furniture such as a chair, dresser, television
- Assistive devices: glasses, dentures, hearing aid(s), cane, walker

The items listed are also described. Be careful in your descriptions. For example, do not describe a ring as a "diamond in a gold setting." The correct description is "clear stone in a yellow metal setting." This is done because the staff is not qualified to determine whether the stone is a diamond or whether it is glass. After the inventory is completed sign the form. The resident or a family member also signs the form. Residents are discouraged from keeping large sums of money or valuable items in their rooms. Facilities are required to provide accounts for residents so they can deposit and withdraw money as it is needed. Other valuable items can be placed in the facility safe.

## Helping the Resident Adapt to the Facility

Remember that living in the long-term care facility is a very different experience for the resident. It will take the resident time to adapt to the environment, the routine, and the caregivers. Some residents may have a temporary period of confusion and disorientation until they become familiar with the facility. Residents may feel overwhelmed by the amount of information they are expected to remember. Be patient in repeating and reinforcing the information.

Introduce the resident to other residents and caregivers. Take time to talk with new residents so they feel safe and secure in their new home. Fire drills and other routine procedures may be frightening. Explain what is happening and guide the resident through the process.

Welcome the family and consider them members of the care team. Follow your facility policies regarding such issues as:

- Family members taking residents outside the facility
- Family members feeding residents or providing other types of care

## TRANSFERRING THE RESIDENT

There are two types of resident transfers:

- Within the facility, transferring the resident from one room or nursing unit to another
- Outside the facility to another health care agency

There are several reasons why a resident may be transferred within the facility:

- The resident's condition changes, requiring a different level of care
- Residents in the same room do not get along
- Resident requests a different room

When a transfer within the facility occurs, all items go with the resident to the new room or unit (Figure 20-5).

- Clothing and all personal items belonging to the resident
- Items in the bedside stand
- Chart, care plan, other medical records, and medications if resident is moving to another unit
- Medications

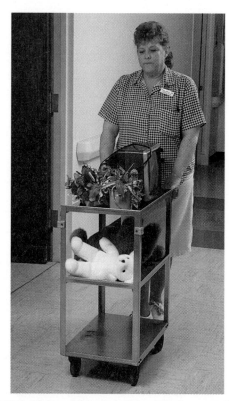

**FIGURE 20-5** All items go with the resident when she is transferred to another room in the same facility.

A resident may be transferred out of the facility to another health care agency because the resident needs:

- The services of an acute care hospital
- Evaluation and treatment for psychiatric problems

If the resident is transferred outside the facility, personal possessions, medical records, and personal care items remain in the facility. The only item going with the resident is a transfer record. The transfer record contains information for the receiving facility (Figure 20-6).

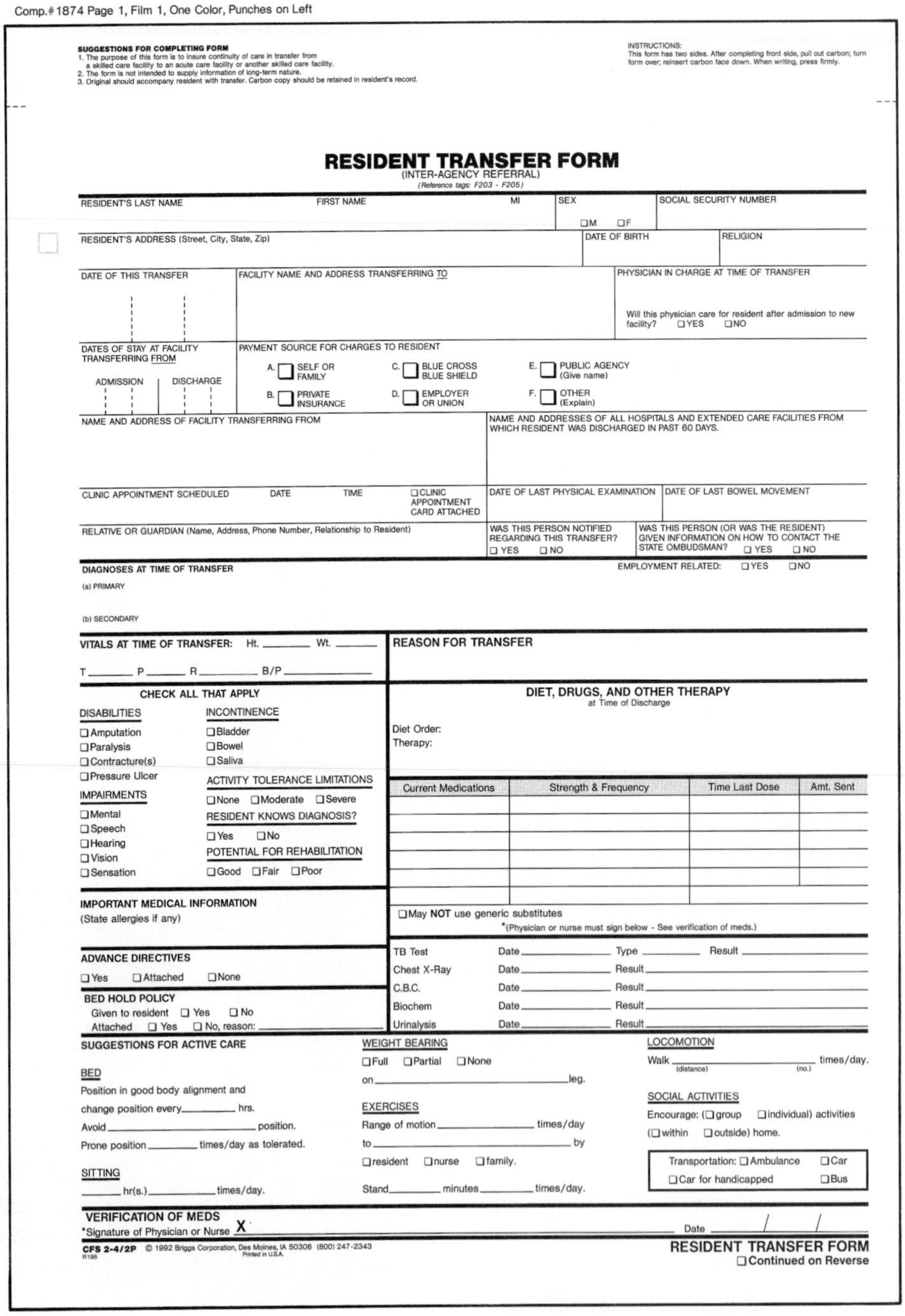
Comp.#1874 Page 1, Film 1, One Color, Punches on Left

SUGGESTIONS FOR COMPLETING FORM
1. The purpose of this form is to insure continuity of care in transfer from a skilled care facility to an acute care facility or another skilled care facility.
2. The form is not intended to supply information of long-term nature.
3. Original should accompany resident with transfer. Carbon copy should be retained in resident's record.

INSTRUCTIONS:
This form has two sides. After completing front side, pull out carbon; turn form over; reinsert carbon face down. When writing, press firmly.

RESIDENT TRANSFER FORM
(INTER-AGENCY REFERRAL)
(Reference tags: F203 - F205)

RESIDENT'S LAST NAME | FIRST NAME | MI | SEX ☐M ☐F | SOCIAL SECURITY NUMBER
RESIDENT'S ADDRESS (Street, City, State, Zip) | DATE OF BIRTH | RELIGION
DATE OF THIS TRANSFER | FACILITY NAME AND ADDRESS TRANSFERRING TO | PHYSICIAN IN CHARGE AT TIME OF TRANSFER
Will this physician care for resident after admission to new facility? ☐YES ☐NO
DATES OF STAY AT FACILITY TRANSFERRING FROM: ADMISSION | DISCHARGE
PAYMENT SOURCE FOR CHARGES TO RESIDENT: A. ☐ SELF OR FAMILY; B. ☐ PRIVATE INSURANCE; C. ☐ BLUE CROSS BLUE SHIELD; D. ☐ EMPLOYER OR UNION; E. ☐ PUBLIC AGENCY (Give name); F. ☐ OTHER (Explain)
NAME AND ADDRESS OF FACILITY TRANSFERRING FROM | NAME AND ADDRESSES OF ALL HOSPITALS AND EXTENDED CARE FACILITIES FROM WHICH RESIDENT WAS DISCHARGED IN PAST 60 DAYS.
CLINIC APPOINTMENT SCHEDULED | DATE | TIME | ☐CLINIC APPOINTMENT CARD ATTACHED | DATE OF LAST PHYSICAL EXAMINATION | DATE OF LAST BOWEL MOVEMENT
RELATIVE OR GUARDIAN (Name, Address, Phone Number, Relationship to Resident) | WAS THIS PERSON NOTIFIED REGARDING THIS TRANSFER? ☐ YES ☐ NO | WAS THIS PERSON (OR WAS THE RESIDENT) GIVEN INFORMATION ON HOW TO CONTACT THE STATE OMBUDSMAN? ☐ YES ☐ NO
DIAGNOSES AT TIME OF TRANSFER | EMPLOYMENT RELATED: ☐YES ☐NO
(a) PRIMARY
(b) SECONDARY

VITALS AT TIME OF TRANSFER: Ht. ______ Wt. ______
T______ P______ R______ B/P ______
REASON FOR TRANSFER

CHECK ALL THAT APPLY
DISABILITIES: ☐Amputation ☐Paralysis ☐Contracture(s) ☐Pressure Ulcer
IMPAIRMENTS: ☐Mental ☐Speech ☐Hearing ☐Vision ☐Sensation
INCONTINENCE: ☐Bladder ☐Bowel ☐Saliva
ACTIVITY TOLERANCE LIMITATIONS: ☐None ☐Moderate ☐Severe
RESIDENT KNOWS DIAGNOSIS? ☐Yes ☐No
POTENTIAL FOR REHABILITATION: ☐Good ☐Fair ☐Poor

DIET, DRUGS, AND OTHER THERAPY
at Time of Discharge
Diet Order:
Therapy:

| Current Medications | Strength & Frequency | Time Last Dose | Amt. Sent |
|---|---|---|---|
| | | | |
| | | | |
| | | | |
| | | | |
| | | | |
| | | | |

☐May NOT use generic substitutes
*(Physician or nurse must sign below - See verification of meds.)

IMPORTANT MEDICAL INFORMATION
(State allergies if any)

ADVANCE DIRECTIVES: ☐Yes ☐Attached ☐None
BED HOLD POLICY
Given to resident ☐ Yes ☐ No
Attached ☐ Yes ☐ No, reason: ______

TB Test Date ______ Type ______ Result ______
Chest X-Ray Date ______ Result ______
C.B.C. Date ______ Result ______
Biochem Date ______ Result ______
Urinalysis Date ______ Result ______

SUGGESTIONS FOR ACTIVE CARE
BED
Position in good body alignment and change position every______ hrs.
Avoid ______ position.
Prone position______ times/day as tolerated.
SITTING
______ hr(s.)______ times/day.

WEIGHT BEARING
☐Full ☐Partial ☐None
on ______ leg.
EXERCISES
Range of motion ______ times/day to ______ by ☐resident ☐nurse ☐family.
Stand______ minutes______ times/day.

LOCOMOTION
Walk ______ (distance) ______ (no.) times/day.
SOCIAL ACTIVITIES
Encourage: (☐group ☐individual) activities (☐within ☐outside) home.
Transportation: ☐Ambulance ☐Car ☐Car for handicapped ☐Bus

VERIFICATION OF MEDS
*Signature of Physician or Nurse X ______ Date __/__/__

CFS 2-4/2P © 1992 Briggs Corporation, Des Moines, IA 50306 (800) 247-2343 R195 Printed in U.S.A.
RESIDENT TRANSFER FORM
☐Continued on Reverse

**FIGURE 20-6** The transfer record goes with the resident from one facility to the next. (Reprinted with permission of Briggs Corporation, Des Moines, IA 50306 [800]247-2343)

Comp.# 1874 Page 2, Film 1, One Color, Backer

**RESIDENT TRANSFER FORM (continued)**

SELF CARE STATUS
(Check level of ability. Write S in space if needs supervision only. Draw line across if inapplicable.)

| | | Independent | Needs Assistance | Unable To Do |
|---|---|---|---|---|
| **Bed Activity** | Turns | | | |
| | Sits | | | |
| **Personal Hygiene** | Face, Hair, Arms | | | |
| | Trunk & Perineum | | | |
| | Lower Extremities | | | |
| | Bladder Program | | | |
| | Bowel Program | | | |
| **Dressing** | Upper Extremities | | | |
| | Trunk | | | |
| | Lower Extremities | | | |
| | Appliance, Splint | | | |
| **Feeding** | | | | |
| **Transfer** | Sitting | | | |
| | Standing | | | |
| | Tub | | | |
| | Toilet | | | |
| **Loco-motion** | Wheelchair | | | |
| | Walking | | | |
| | Stairs | | | |

BED ☐Low Mattress: ☐Firm ☐Reg.
Other ______
Side Rails: ☐Yes ☐No

BEHAVIOR ☐Cooperative ☐Oriented X______
☐Disruptive ☐Belligerent ☐Combative
☐Senile ☐Suspicious ☐Withdrawn

MENTAL STATUS
☐Alert ☐Forgetful ☐Confused

| COMMUNICATION ABILITY | Yes | No |
|---|---|---|
| Able to make needs known | | |
| Can speak | | |
| Can hear | | |
| Can write | | |
| Understands speaking | | |
| Understands writing | | |
| Understands gestures | | |
| Understands English | | |

If no, state language spoken or understood: ______

DIET
☐Regular ☐Low Salt ☐Diabetic ☐Bland
☐Low Residue ☐Other ______
☐Feeds Self ☐Needs Help
☐Partial Assist ☐Total Assist

RESIDENT USES
☐Appliance
☐Catheter (date of last change___/___/___
☐Colostomy ☐Cane ☐Crutches ☐Prosthesis
☐Walker ☐Chair ☐Hearing Aid
☐Dentures (Specify ______ )

OTHER EQUIPMENT

ADDITIONAL PERTINENT INFORMATION
(Explain necessary details of care, diagnosis, medications, treatments, prognosis, teaching, habits, preferences, etc. Therapists and social workers add signature and title to notes.)

SOCIAL INFORMATION
(Adjustment to disability, emotional support from family, motivation for self-care, socializing ability, financial plan, family health problem, etc.)

PERSON COMPLETING THIS FORM: Signature/Title ______ Date ___/___/___
RESIDENT TRANSFER FORM

**FIGURE 20-6** *(continued)*

## Discharging the Resident

Discharging of residents from the long-term care facility has become a common occurrence. Residents are discharged because they:

- Have improved enough to go home
- Do not need the high level services of the facility but can function in a less restrictive environment such as an assisted living facility
- Require care that can be provided by another long-term care facility

## PROCEDURE
# 76  Transferring the Resident

1. Find out if the resident is to be transferred within the facility or out of the facility.
2. If within the facility, find out if the resident will be moved by wheelchair or in the bed.
3. If out of the facility, find out if the resident will be taken to the exit by wheelchair to a car or if the resident will be transferred by ambulance.
4. Carry out each beginning procedure action.
5. For transfer within the facility, the following items will be moved with the resident:
   - Resident's belongings
   - Personal care items from bedside table
   - Supplies or equipment used for resident's care
   - Medical records, care plan, and medications (if moving to another unit)
6. Help resident dress if necessary.
7. Move resident to new unit as indicated.
8. Help resident get settled in new room.
9. Introduce resident to staff and other residents.
10. Tell the resident good-bye and wish him well.
11. Carry out each procedure completion action.

If resident is being transferred out of facility:

1. If resident is going by car, make sure the resident is well groomed and dressed appropriately for the weather, then assist into wheelchair and take to exit. Assist in transferring into car.
2. If resident is going by ambulance, follow nurse's instructions.
3. The nurse will give appropriate records and transfer form to family or ambulance drivers.
4. Tell the resident good-bye.
5. Carry out each procedure completion action.

---

The discharge procedure is usually simple if the resident is going to another facility. The social worker and nurse relay information to the receiving facility. The resident's belongings are sent to the new facility.

Discharge to the resident's home is more complicated and requires a number of actions called **discharge planning**. Discharge planning is a cooperative procedure that involves all members of the interdisciplinary health care team. The social worker is the coordinator for discharge planning and is responsible for arranging for **community services**. Community services may include intermittent services of a:

1. Registered nurse for ongoing assessment, monitoring, supervision of other caregivers, planning of care, teaching, and implementation of treatments
2. Home health aide for personal care including bathing, positioning, passive range of motion exercises, taking vital signs, and doing simple treatments
3. Rehabilitation staff for physical therapy, occupational therapy, and speech therapy
4. Homemaker for completing routine household chores such as light cleaning, laundry, cooking, and grocery shopping
5. Home-delivered meals. These are delivered for the noon meal and meet the nutritional

---

## 77  Discharging the Resident

**1.** Check with the nurse to be sure the resident has an order to be discharged.

**2.** Carry out each beginning procedure action.

**3.** Collect equipment:

- Wheelchair
- Cart to transport items to exit

**4.** Help the resident to dress if necessary.

**5.** Collect the resident's personal belongings.

- Check them against the admission inventory list.
- Help resident pack.
- Check bathroom, closets, dressers, and bedside table for overlooked items.

**6.** Check with nurse to see if there are other items such as records, unused supplies, or medications that will go home with the resident.

**7.** Help resident into wheelchair and take resident to exit.

- Help resident transfer into car.
- Be sure all items go with resident.
- Be gracious as you say good-bye.

**8.** Return wheelchair.

**9.** Return to resident's room.

- Strip bed. Dispose of soiled linens.
- Discard disposable items.

**10.** Notify housekeeping so room can be cleaned.

**11.** Record discharge according to facility policy.

- Time
- Method of transport
- Person(s) accompanying resident
- Resident's reaction
- Signature

**12.** Report completion of procedure to nurse.

---

requirements of the resident. Meals for persons on diabetic, low salt, low fat, and low cholesterol diets can usually be arranged.

### Factors to Consider Before Discharge

Before discharge planning proceeds, the interdisciplinary team must consider several factors:

1. Does the resident have the potential to regain enough independence to go home?
2. Is there a person (spouse, family member, or friend) willing to serve as a liaison (go-between) for the resident when he or she goes home? The person living alone will usually need someone to call or check on him, run errands, help with money management, and oversee the household management.

3. Are adequate community services available? If the resident needs continuing physical therapy, for example, there may not be an agency that provides this service. In some areas of the country there are not enough therapists to meet the demand.
4. Does the resident need 24-hour-a-day supervision or care? Medicare and private insurance will not pay for this type of care. Most people could not afford to pay for it themselves. (Continuous care may cost several hundreds of dollars per day.)
5. Will the structure of the resident's home allow the resident to function adequately and safely? For example, is there a bedroom and bathroom on the same floor?

These factors are especially critical if the resident will be living alone. If the resident, the family, and the care team determine that discharge is a reasonable expectation then planning proceeds.

1. The interdisciplinary team will prepare a discharge plan of care. This plan provides information to the resident and caregivers (family, friends, or community service providers) on how to help the resident maintain health (Figure 20-7).

2. The social worker arranges for the community services.

Comp.# 1872 Page 1, Film 1, One Color, Punches on Left

## POST-DISCHARGE PLAN OF CARE
(Reference tags: F203, F204; Cross reference tags: F157, F284)

The following discharge information is to help you maintain your health and independence.

You are being discharged : ☐ home    ☐ to a residential care facility (see facility name and address below).

Facility _____ Phone_____

Address _____ City/State/Zip_____

**THE FOLLOWING COMMUNITY RESOURCES ARE AVAILABLE TO MEET YOUR INDIVIDUAL NEEDS ▶**

State Ombudsman_____ Phone _____
Address _____ City/State/Zip_____

Visiting Nurse _____ Phone _____
Address _____ City/State/Zip_____

Other Agency_____ Phone _____
Address _____ City/State/Zip_____

**COMMUNITY RESOURCES AND SERVICES PLANNING ▶**

Nursing needs: _____

Personal care: _____

Transportation:_____
Meals: _____
Housekeeping: _____
Social support/Family system/Special requests: _____

Financial status/needs:_____
Financial access/Payment for services: _____
Therapy services: _____

Other:_____

Person completing this section: _____ ___/___/___
Signature and title                                    Date

**SCHEDULED APPOINTMENTS ▶**

| Appointment With | Date | Purpose | Telephone |
|---|---|---|---|
| | | | |
| | | | |
| | | | |
| | | | |

NAME—Last            First            Middle    Attending Physician            Chart No.

CFS 2-2/2P © 1992 Briggs Corporation, Des Moines, IA 50306 (800) 247-2343    **POST-DISCHARGE PLAN OF CARE**
Printed in U.S.A.                                                        ☐ Continued on Reverse

**FIGURE 20-7** Care plan for the resident who is to be discharged home (Reprinted with permission of Briggs Corporation, Des Moines, IA 50306 [800]247-2343)

Comp.#1872 Page 2, Film 1, One Color

## POST-DISCHARGE PLAN OF CARE (continued)

**DIETARY AND NUTRITIONAL NEEDS ▶**

Suggested food/fluids: _____

Special instructions: _____

Avoid: _____

☐ Copy of diet given   ☐ Diet explained to resident/caregiver   ☐ Restrictions explained (if applicable)

Person completing this section _____ ___/___/___
                                    *Signature and title*                              *Date*

**ACTIVITIES AND LEISURE PURSUITS ▶**

Suggested activities:   ☐ T.V./Movies   ☐ Radio   ☐ Reading   ☐ Senior Center   ☐ Talking books

   ☐ Volunteer Work   ☐ Other_____

Special instructions: _____

Activities to avoid: _____

Person completing this section _____ ___/___/___
                                    *Signature and title*                              *Date*

**MEDICATIONS ▶**

| Medication | Dose and Frequency | Purpose and Special Instructions | Amount Sent With Resident | Prescription Sent With Resident | Prescription Called To Pharmacy |
|---|---|---|---|---|---|
|  |  |  |  |  |  |
|  |  |  |  |  |  |
|  |  |  |  |  |  |
|  |  |  |  |  |  |
|  |  |  |  |  |  |

Person completing this section _____ ___/___/___
                                    *Signature and title*                              *Date*

**WOUND CARE, TREATMENTS, THERAPY ▶ Procedures you should do**

| Procedure | Purpose | Frequency |
|---|---|---|
|  |  |  |
|  |  |  |
|  |  |  |
|  |  |  |

Person completing this section _____ ___/___/___
                                    *Signature and title*                              *Date*

**IMPORTANT NAMES AND PHONE NUMBERS ▶**

Physician _____ Phone _____
              *Name and address*

Pharmacy _____ Phone _____
              *Name and address*

These discharge instructions have been reviewed with me in a language I understand. All questions have been answered to my satisfaction. I have received the medications or written prescriptions as indicated above.

Signature **X**_____ ___/___/___
              *Resident / Caregiver*                              *Date*

Please contact us if you have further questions.

Facility_____ Telephone _____

| NAME—Last | First | Middle | Attending Physician | Chart No. |
|---|---|---|---|---|

POST-DISCHARGE PLAN OF CARE

**FIGURE 20-7** *(continued)*

3. The physical therapist or a rehabilitation nurse may take the resident home for a short visit to evaluate the resident's ability to function in the home setting. The therapist will make recommendations, if necessary, that may include:

- Rearranging rooms, for example, turning the living room into the bedroom
- Building a ramp from the outside entrance
- Installing a telephone that is accessible to the resident

- Renting equipment such as a seat for the shower or tub
- Suggesting safety measures, such as the removal of throw rugs and electrical cords on the floor

4. The interdisciplinary health care team will determine what the resident and family need to learn before discharge and who will be responsible for teaching. Some examples follow. Not all residents need all of these, and some residents will need teaching not included here.

   - The physical therapist will teach the resident how to transfer in and out of bed, how to ambulate with an artificial leg (prosthesis), how to walk up and down stairs (Figure 20-8).

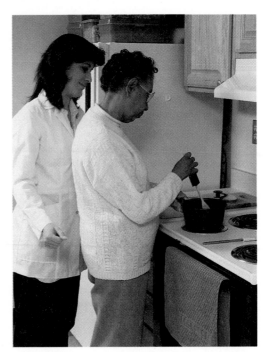

**FIGURE 20-9** The occupational therapist teaches the resident how to manage the activities of daily living before she goes home.

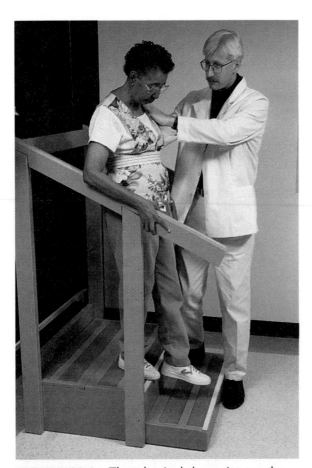

**FIGURE 20-8** The physical therapist teaches the resident how to go up and down stairs in preparation for going home.

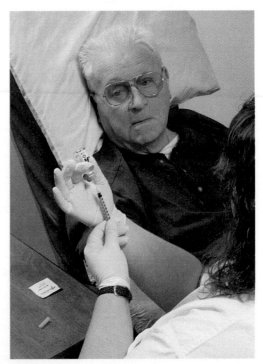

**FIGURE 20-10** The nurse teaches the resident how to inject his insulin.

- The occupational therapist will teach the resident how to dress and undress, how to use the telephone, or how to cook (Figure 20-9).

5. The dietitian will teach the resident and family the basics of planning and preparing diabetic meals.

6. The nursing staff will teach the resident how to give his own insulin (Figure 20-10), how to check his blood sugar, how to recognize signs and symptoms of complications, or how to change a colostomy or wound dressings.

A discharge date will be arranged and all members of the team including the resident and family will strive to meet the goals that will enable the resident to return home.

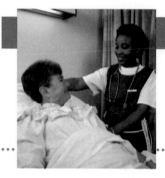

## LESSON SYNTHESIS: Putting It All Together

*Y*ou have just completed this lesson. Now go back and review the Clinical Focus. Try to see how the Clinical Focus relates to the concepts presented in the lesson. Then answer the following questions.

1. Would you expect Mrs. Lyon-Ravens to feel anxiety on admission to the long-term care facility? What is a likely reason for this anxiety? How may the interdisciplinary team help Mrs. Lyon-Ravens to overcome this anxiety?

2. How can you make her feel more comfortable and secure in her new environment?

3. What information would you want to learn about Mrs. Lyon-Ravens' present condition? How will you do this?

4. How will the nursing staff use the information that you obtain in formulating a care plan that is appropriate for this resident?

## REVIEW

**A. Select the one best answer for each of the following.**

1. Most residents are admitted to long-term care facilities because
   a. their families no longer want to deal with them
   b. the resident no longer wants the responsibility of keeping up a home
   c. the resident is tired and needs rest
   d. the resident requires health care services

2. Residents admitted to long-term care facilities may need
   a. specialized treatments
   b. 24-hour-a-day care and supervision
   c. rehabilitation services
   d. all of these

3. The length of hospital stays for acute illness is limited because
   a. of staff shortages
   b. of the inconvenience to the family
   c. of diagnosis-related groups
   d. all of these

4. Before admission, the family will need to
   a. choose a facility if the resident is unable to do so
   b. draw the resident's money out of the bank
   c. sell the resident's home
   d. try to care for the resident at home

5. The members of the interdisciplinary health care team will obtain assessments of new residents for the purpose of
   a. starting the plan of care
   b. keeping the resident busy
   c. making the family think the staff is attentive
   d. all of these

6. When a new resident is admitted, the nursing assistant will
   a. take the resident's vital signs
   b. weigh and measure the resident
   c. help the resident put away personal possessions
   d. all of these

7. When a resident is transferred from one nursing unit to another within the facility, the nursing assistant will
   a. move the resident's belongings to the new room
   b. give the resident any medication that is due before moving
   c. call the resident's family for permission before moving the resident
   d. move all the furniture in the room to the new room

8. Residents may be discharged because they
   a. have improved enough to go home
   b. do not need the high level of care offered by the facility
   c. cannot obtain the services they need in the present facility
   d. all of these

9. Community services include
   a. services of a registered nurse
   b. home-delivered meals
   c. services of a home health aide
   d. all of these

10. Community services are usually coordinated and arranged for by the
    a. administrator
    b. family
    c. director of nursing
    d. social worker

**B. Answer each statement true (T) or false (F).**

11. T  F  The discharge planner selects the long-term care facility for patients who need that service.

12. T  F  The family may need to apply for Medicaid if the resident has exhausted his funds.

13. T  F  Copies of the Residents' Rights are only given to residents who are able to read and understand them.

14. T  F  The physician makes out the personal inventory after the resident is admitted.

15. T  F  Residents are advised not to bring any personal possessions with them to the long-term care facility.

16. T  F  A resident may be transferred to another room because of friction between roommates.

17. T  F  Some admissions to long-term care facilities are considered permanent.

18. T  F  Families are discouraged from visiting residents.

19. T  F  Most families have concerns about admitting a family member to a long-term care facility.

20. T  F  First impressions on the family and resident are extremely important.

# Warm and Cold Applications

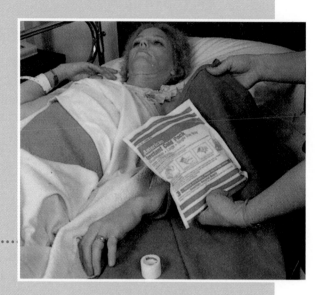

## CLINICAL FOCUS

Think about the reasons for warm and cold applications and the safety precautions to observe when they are carried out as you study this lesson and meet:

Mrs. Lipskin, who is assigned to your care. She tires easily and is returned to her bed for rest in the afternoon. As she was getting into bed, she slipped and hit her forearm against the side of the bed. To counteract pain and swelling from the injury, a disposable cold pack is ordered and applied to her arm.

## OBJECTIVES

*After studying this lesson, you should be able to:*

- Define and spell vocabulary words and terms.
- State the effects of warm and cold applications.
- Give reasons why warm and cold applications may be ordered.
- Describe precautions in carrying out warm and cold application procedures.

- Demonstrate the following:
  Procedure 78 Applying an Aquamatic K-Pad®
  Procedure 79 Applying a Disposable Cold Pack
  Procedure 80 Applying an Ice Bag
  Procedure 81 Assisting with the Application of a Hypothermia Blanket

## VOCABULARY

Aquamatic K-Pad® (*ack*-kwah-*MAT*-ick *KAY*-pad)
asepto syringe (*ay*-*SEP*-toh sih-*RINJ*)

diathermy (*DIE*-ah-*ther*-mee)
hypothermia (*high*-poh-*THER*-mee-ah)
ice bag (*ise bag*)

# VOCABULARY

thermal blanket *(THER-mal BLAN-kit)*

vasoconstriction *(vas-oh-kon-STRICK-shun)*

vasodilation *(vas-oh-die-LAY-shun)*

warm soak *(warm sohk)*

wet compress *(wet KOM-press)*

Warm and cold applications require a physician's order. Some facilities permit only licensed care providers to perform warm and cold applications. In other facilities, nursing assistants are permitted to carry out these procedures under the supervision of the nurse. All warm and cold applications must be performed carefully to prevent injury to the resident. *Be sure you know and follow the policy of your facility and are adequately prepared and supervised.*

Older people have less sensitivity to changes in temperature. They may not realize when an application is too hot or cold. If the temperature is too high, burns may result. Other types of tissue damage may occur if the temperature is too cold. Warm and cold applications that are left on too long can also cause damage.

## SAFETY

The older resident has less sensitivity to pain and is at greater risk for injury. *Note: Heat is especially dangerous.* When using warm or cold applications on older residents, it is very important that you:

- Frequently check the area that is being treated.
- Report unusual changes. You should check for excessive redness, blanching (whitening), or other discoloration. Report any complaints of discomfort or pain.
- Do not rely on the resident's ability to inform you of any problems; check carefully yourself. The resident may not be aware that a problem exists.
- Follow facility policy for discontinuing the treatment.

Applications of warm and cold may be either moist or dry (Figure 21-1). Moisture makes both heat and cold more penetrating. Therefore, moist

| **FIGURE 21-1** Warm and cold applications |
| --- |
| **Dry Warm Applications**<br>Aquamatic K-Pad®<br>Disposable warm pack |
| **Moist Warm Applications**<br>Warm soaks<br>Compresses<br>Tub bath<br>Sitz bath |
| **Dry Cold Applications**<br>Ice cap<br>Ice bag<br>Disposable cold pack<br>Aquamatic K-Pad®<br>Hypothermia blanket |
| **Moist Cold Applications**<br>Compresses<br>Soaks |

heat or moist cold is more likely to cause injury. Extra care must be taken to protect the resident when moist treatments are used. Be sure you know:

- Exact method to be used
- Correct temperature and placement
- Proper length of time the warm or cold application is to be performed
- How often to check the area being treated

## COMMERCIAL PREPARATIONS

Easy to use commercial warm and cold packs are available for dry applications. For one type of pack, a single blow to the pack before application activates the heat or cold. The pack is discarded after one use.

Reusable packs are also available, but infection control issues make them less desirable.

## USE OF WARM APPLICATIONS

Warm applications are ordered to:
- Relieve muscle spasms
- Reduce pain
- Promote healing
- Combat local infection
- Improve mobility before exercise periods
- Soothe the resident

The value of heat treatments (**diathermy**) lies in the fact that heat dilates or increases the size of blood vessels (**vasodilation**). This brings more blood to the area to promote healing. Warmth is very soothing when there is pain.

There must be a specific order for a warm application. Some groups of people require extra care when they receive warm applications (Figure 21-2).

### Cautions

Follow these cautions when working with residents.
- Constant warmth must be carefully monitored.
- Moisture intensifies the effect of warmth. Use extra caution.

---

**FIGURE 21-2** Use caution when applying warm and cold treatments.

Caution: Consider the age and condition of the resident when using warm or cold treatments.

Proceed with caution with:
- Elderly residents
- Uncooperative residents
- Unconscious residents
- Paralyzed residents
- Residents with tissue damage
- Residents with poor circulation

---

- Never allow a resident to lie on a constant heat unit because heat may be trapped and build up to dangerous levels.
- Temperature of a constant heat unit should be between 95° and 100°F.
- Always use a bath thermometer to check solution temperatures.
- Always remove the body part being soaked before adding warm solution.
- Always stay with the resident during the treatment.
- Protect areas not being treated from excessive exposure.
- Warmth is not applied to the head because it could cause blood vessels in the area to dilate, resulting in headaches.
- Rubber or plastic should never touch the resident's skin. Be sure all appliances are covered with cloth.

### Dry Warm Applications

The **Aquamatic K-Pad®** is commonly used to provide dry warmth. It consists of a plastic pad with fluid-filled coils and a control unit that maintains a constant temperature of the fluid.

The fluid in the pad is distilled water that is supplied from a reservoir in the control unit. The control unit is placed on the bedside stand and is plugged into an electrical outlet. In most facilities, the temperature is preset by the central supply department. The temperature is usually set at 95° to 100°F.

### Moist Warm Applications

*Remember:* Moisture intensifies heat and you must use extra care. For each of the warm treatments, follow the facility policy for:
- Method of applying the treatment
- Length of time treatment is to be applied
- How often resident is to be checked for condition of skin in the treatment area and general response to the treatment
- Signs that treatment should be discontinued

Moist warm treatments include:
- **Warm soaks**—The resident, or the part of the resident's body that is being treated, is immersed in a tub filled with water at a specific temperature, usually 105°.

### PROCEDURE 78
# Applying an Aquamatic K-Pad®

1. Carry out each beginning procedure action.
2. Assemble equipment:
   * K-Pad® and control unit
   * Distilled water
   * Covering for pad
3. Check the cord for frayed or damaged insulation. Also check that the tubing between the control unit and the pad is intact.
4. Place the control unit on the bedside stand (Figure 21-3).
5. Remove the cover of the control unit and check the level of the distilled water. If it is low, fill the unit two-thirds full or to the fill line using distilled water. Tilt the unit back and forth gently to clear the tubing of air.
6. Screw the cover in place and loosen it one-quarter turn.
7. If the temperature was not preset, check with the nurse for the proper setting before turning on the unit. Remove the key after setting the temperature.
8. Plug in the unit.
9. Cover pad with an appropriate cover, according to facility policy or as specified by the manufacturer of the unit. Do not use pins to hold the cover in place.
10. Expose the area of the resident to be treated. Place the covered pad on the resident and note the time.
    * Be sure the tubing between the control unit and the pad does not hang over the side of the bed. It should be coiled on the bed to promote the flow of liquid.

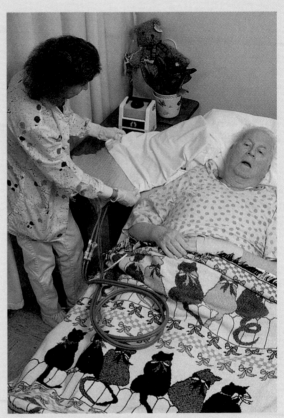

**FIGURE 21-3**   The disposable Aquamatic K-Pad® and control unit (reusable) maintain an even temperature.

11. Following facility policy, periodically check the skin under the pad.
12. Check the level of the water in the control unit. Refill if necessary to the fill line.
13. Remove the pad after the prescribed amount of time.
14. Carry out each procedure completion action.

- **Wet compresses**—Wet compresses are moistened with a solution and placed on the affected area.
  - An **asepto syringe** may be used to add water to the compresses to keep them moist.
  - The compresses can be kept warm by covering them with an Aquamatic K-Pad®.
  - Each time the pad is removed and replaced, be careful to reposition the protective covering.

# USE OF COLD APPLICATIONS ·········

Applications of cold are given only with a physician's order. The application of cold:

- Constricts or decreases the size of blood vessels (**vasoconstriction**) and reduces swelling
- Decreases sensitivity to pain
- Reduces temperature
- Slows inflammation
- Reduces itching

## Cautions

Remember, moisture intensifies the effect of cold just as it does heat. Caution must be used in the application of moist cold.

- Excessive cold can damage body tissues.
- Report color changes such as blanching (turning white) or cyanosis (becoming bluish).
- Report feelings of numbness or discomfort experienced by resident.

- Stop the cold treatment if shivering develops. Cover resident with blanket and report immediately to the nurse. Cold applications may be dry or moist.

## Dry Cold Applications

Several methods exist for applying therapeutic cold. For the elderly, careful attention to the application is required to prevent injury.

- **Disposable cold pack**—This single-use commercial pack can be stored until needed. Reusable commercial packs are also available (for both warm and cold applications). The pack remains effective for approximately 15 to 30 minutes. If the cold pack must be activated, follow the manufacturer's instructions exactly. When activating the pack, do not hold it in front of your face. If a leak occurs, the chemicals inside the pack may splash. Check the area being treated every 10 minutes.
- **Ice bag**—This reusable waterproof canvas container can be filled with ice to provide temporary local cold. An ice bag is never placed directly on the affected area because the weight of the bag will cause the resident discomfort.
- **Thermal blanket**—This is a large, fluid-filled blanket that is placed over or around the resident. The temperature of the fluid in the blanket may be raised or lowered. The blanket is used to lower or raise the resident's body temperature. However, it is most often used in care facilities to lower the body temperature. This process is called **hypothermia**. A licensed professional usually monitors the use of this type of blanket.

---

**PROCEDURE**
**79**

# Applying a Disposable Cold Pack

1. Carry out each beginning procedure action.
2. Assemble equipment:
   - Disposable commercial cold pack

- Cloth covering (towel, warm water bag cover, or other cover specified by the facility)
- Tape or rolls of gauze

*(continues)*

**PROCEDURE 79** *(continued)*

3. Expose area to be treated. Note condition of area.
4. Place cold pack in cloth covering.
5. Strike or squeeze cold pack to activate chemicals. (Follow manufacturer's instructions.)
6. Place covered cold pack on proper area and cover with a towel (Figure 21-4). Note time of application.
7. Secure cover with tape or gauze, if necessary, to hold in place.
8. Leave resident in comfortable position with signal cord within easy reach.
9. Return to bedside every 10 minutes. Check area being treated for discoloration or numbness. If these signs and symptoms occur, discontinue treatment and report them to your supervisor.
10. If no adverse symptoms occur, remove pack in 30 minutes, or after amount of time given in your instructions. Note condition of area. Continuous treatment requires application of a fresh pack.

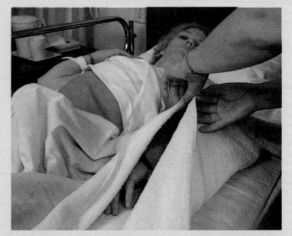

**FIGURE 21-4** Once the cold pack is in place, cover the entire application with a towel.

11. Remove pack from cover and discard according to facility policy. Return unused gauze and tape.
12. Put cover in laundry hamper.
13. Carry out each procedure completion action.

---

**PROCEDURE**
# 80
## Applying an Ice Bag

1. Carry out each beginning procedure action.
2. Assemble equipment:
   - Ice bag
   - Cover (usually cotton, such as a towel, or cover specified by your facility)
   - Paper towels
   - Spoon or similar utensil
   - Ice cubes or crushed ice
3. Prepare ice bag as follows:
   a. Fill ice bag with cold water and check for leaks.
   b. Empty the bag.
   c. If ice cubes are used, rinse them in water to remove sharp edges. The use of crushed ice gives more flexibility to the bag and is more comfortable for the resident.

*(continues)*

**PROCEDURE** *80* *(continued)*

d. Fill ice bag half full, using ice scooper, paper cup, or large spoon (Figure 21-5). Avoid making ice bags too heavy. Do not allow scoop to touch ice bag.

e. To remove air from ice bag:
- Rest ice bag flat on a paper towel on a flat surface.
- Put top in place, but do not screw on.
- Press bag until air is removed.

f. Fasten top securely.

g. Test for leakage.

h. Wipe dry with paper towels. Place in cloth cover.

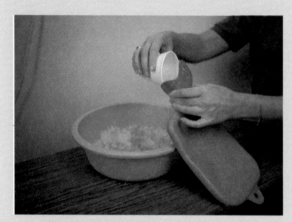

**FIGURE 21-5**   Fill ice bag half full.

*Note:* As an alternative, a gel pack stored in the freezer can be used for cold applications. These packs can be refrozen and reused if this is the facility policy.

4. Apply ice bag to the affected part.

5. Refill ice bag before all ice is melted.

6. Check skin area under the ice bag every 10 minutes. Report to supervising nurse immediately if skin is discolored or white or if resident reports skin is numb.

7. Continue the cold application for the amount of time specified by your supervisor. If the resident feels cold, cover with a blanket, but do not cover the area being treated.

8. Carry out each procedure completion action.

9. When the treatment is complete wash the bag with soap and water, rinse, dry completely, and then screw top on. Wipe with a disinfectant if this is your facility policy. Leave air in ice bag to prevent sides from sticking together.

10. If a reusable cold pack is used, wash it thoroughly with soap and water or wipe with a disinfectant, according to facility policy. Return pack to the refrigerator. Discard a disposable pack.

**PROCEDURE** *81*
# Assisting with the Application of a Hypothermia Blanket

*Note:* Applying a hypothermia blanket and monitoring a resident receiving a hypothermia treatment is a professional nursing responsibility. The nurse will supervise the procedure and monitor the resident throughout the treatment. The nurse will check the specific gravity of the resident's urine, vital signs, and nervous system response. The

*(continues)*

**PROCEDURE 81** *(continued)*

nursing assistant may be asked to assist in setting up equipment, positioning the resident and the thermal blanket, observing the resident during the treatment, and keeping the resident comfortable. In addition, the nursing assistant may be asked to transport equipment to and from the central supply service.

1. Wash hands, collect equipment, and take equipment to bedside.
2. Assemble equipment:
   - Disposable gloves
   - Hyperthermia/hypothermia control unit
   - Fluid for control unit
   - Thermometer probes (rectal or skin)
   - Adhesive tape
   - Sphygmomanometer
   - Stethoscope
   - Hyperthermia/hypothermia blanket (disposable or reusable), one or two as ordered
   - Bath blanket or sheet, one or two as ordered
   - Lanolin-based skin cream
3. Follow manufacturer's directions for setting up the equipment. Check equipment for safety. Be sure the control unit is grounded.
4. Connect blanket(s) to control unit and set control.
5. Turn on control unit and add liquid.
6. Allow blanket(s) to precool as you prepare resident.
7. Carry out each beginning procedure action.
8. Place resident in hospital-type gown with ties.
9. Measure vital signs and record.
10. Place hyperthermia/hypothermia blanket on bed and cover with sheet. Position resident on the sheet-covered thermal blanket in the recumbent position, with head on pillow that does not touch blanket.
11. Wash hands. Put on gloves.
12. Insert rectal thermometer probe into rectum (unless contraindicated) and tape in place. (Alternatively, place skin probe into axilla and secure in place with tape.)
13. Plug end of probe into proper jack on control panel.
14. Place second sheet over resident and place second thermal blanket over sheet, if ordered.
15. Apply lanolin-based cream to resident's skin where it contacts the blanket.
16. Remove gloves. Discard according to facility policy. Wash hands.
17. Monitor vital signs, neurologic response, and intake and output every 5 minutes until desired body temperature is reached, and then every 15 minutes as ordered.
18. Report color changes in skin or excessive shivering.
19. Resident should be repositioned every 30 minutes to 1 hour. Reapply skin cream as necessary. Covering sheets should be changed if they become moist. Put on gloves each time you care for resident. At the end of care, remove gloves, discard according to facility policy, and wash hands.
20. At completion of treatment, follow manufacturer's instructions for turning off unit, disconnecting blanket(s), and returning to storage.
21. Put on gloves. Continue to monitor resident as you remove the equipment.
22. Replace any damp bedding or garments and cover resident. Continue to monitor resident every 30 minutes until stable for 2 hours.
23. Clean thermometer probe and store according to facility policy.
24. Remove gloves and discard according to facility policy.
25. Carry out each procedure completion action.

## Moist Cold Application

- **Wet compresses**—The same cautions apply to cold as to warm compresses. They may be kept wet with an asepto syringe and cold by placing a covered ice cap against the area that is affected.

Follow facility policy for:
- Method of applying the treatment
- Length of time treatment is to be applied
- How often resident is to be checked for condition of skin in the treatment area and general response to the treatment
- Signs that treatment should be discontinued

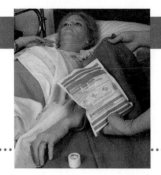

## LESSON SYNTHESIS: Putting It All Together

*Y*ou have just completed this lesson. Now go back and review the Clinical Focus. Try to see how the Clinical Focus relates to the concepts presented in the lesson. Then answer the following questions.

1. How was the disposable cold pack activated?

2. How might it have been secured in place?

3. Is the pack placed directly on the area of the body to be treated?

4. How often should you check the area in contact with the pack?

5. What signs or symptoms should be reported to the nurse during the treatment?

## REVIEW

**A. Write the definition for each of the following terms.**

1. diathermy
2. hypothermia
3. vasoconstriction
4. vasodilation
5. ice bag

**B. Answer each statement true (T) or false (F).**

6. T   F   Warm and cold treatments are part of the job description for all nursing assistants.

7. T   F   The elderly are usually more sensitive to warm and cold treatments.

8. T   F   A physician's order is required for all warm and cold applications.

9. T   F   Moisture increases the effect of both warm and cold treatments.

10. T   F   Heat may be applied to the head because it causes vasoconstriction and relieves headache.

11. T   F   All heat or cold appliances must be covered with cloth so that rubber or plastic never touches the skin.

12. T   F   Residents should not be left alone when receiving a heat treatment.

13. T   F   Always place a filled ice bag on top of the area being treated.

## C. Select the one best answer for each of the following.

14. Which resident is at greatest risk for injury during a heat treatment?
    a. resident who is conscious
    b. resident who is cooperative
    c. resident who is paralyzed
    d. resident who has warm pink skin

15. The control unit of the Aquamatic K-Pad® is filled
    a. to the top
    b. ⅓ full
    c. ½ full
    d. ¾ full

16. The tubes of the Aquamatic K-Pad® should be
    a. allowed to hang below bed level
    b. coiled on the bedside stand
    c. pinned to the headboard of the bed
    d. coiled on the bed

17. The temperature of the Aquamatic K-pad® is usually set at
    a. 95°F
    b. 98°F
    c. 100°F
    d. 110°F

18. Ice bags are
    a. filled to the top
    b. partially filled with air before adding ice
    c. filled with the largest ice cubes
    d. tested for leaks before filling

## D. Clinical Situations

19. Mrs. Maupin has an order for an Aquamatic K-Pad® to be applied for back pain. Shauna, the nursing assistant, notes that her lower back has become discolored and is more painful. What action should Shauna take?

20. Shauna's supervisor tells her to apply cold to Mrs. Bronson's injured ankle. Shauna replies that she needs more information to give proper care to Mrs. Bronson. What information does Shauna need?

# Introduction to Restorative Care

## LESSONS

**22** Restorative Care of the Resident

**23** Restoring Residents' Mobility

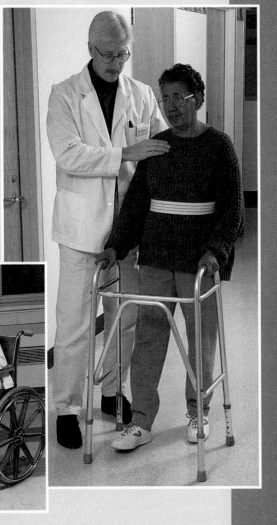

# 22

# Restorative Care of the Resident

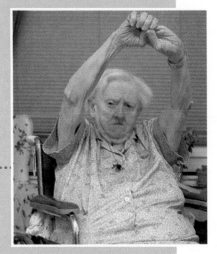

**CLINICAL FOCUS**

Think about the care you would give to residents with disorders for which restorative care is appropriate as you study this lesson and meet:

*M*rs. Murphy, who was admitted to the facility while you were on your day off. She is 5 feet, 9 inches tall, with a heavy frame. She is 78 years old and had a stroke 2 months ago. She is unable to use her left arm or leg. Mrs. Murphy is relearning mobility skills and how to perform the activities of daily living. You are assigned to care for her and must assist her in these tasks.

## OBJECTIVES

*After studying this lesson, you should be able to:*

- Define and spell vocabulary words and terms.
- List the complications associated with inactivity.
- Describe the reasons why some residents have self-care deficits.
- Describe the principles of restorative care.
- Explain the benefits of restorative care.
- Describe the responsibilities of the nursing assistant for implementing restorative care.
- State the guidelines for doing passive range of motion exercises.
- State the guidelines for positioning residents in bed and chair.
- Describe the purpose of an orthosis.
- List the reasons for implementing bowel and bladder programs.
- Describe the responsibilities of the nursing assistant for implementing bowel and bladder programs.

- Use correct body mechanics in carrying out all procedures in this lesson.
- Demonstrate the following:

  Procedure 82 Passive Range of Motion Exercises

  Procedure 83 Moving the Resident Toward the Head of the Bed

  Procedure 84 Moving the Resident Toward the Foot of the Bed

  Procedure 85 Moving the Resident Toward the Side of the Bed

  Procedure 86 Turning the Resident to the Side

  Procedure 87 Log Rolling the Resident onto the Side

  Procedure 88 Supine Position

  Procedure 89 Semisupine or Tilt Position

  Procedure 90 Lateral (Side-Lying) Position

# OBJECTIVES

Procedure 91 Lateral Position on the Affected Side

Procedure 92 Semiprone Position

Procedure 93 Fowler's Position

Procedure 94 Chair Positioning

Procedure 95 Repositioning a Resident in a Wheelchair

Procedure 96 Wheelchair Activities to Relieve Pressure

Procedure 97 Assisting with Independent Bed Movement

# VOCABULARY

**active assistive range of motion** *(**ACK**-tiv ah-**SIS**-tiv rainj of **MOH**-shun)*

**active range of motion** *(**ACK**-tiv rainj of **MOH**-shun)*

**activities of daily living (ADL)** *(ack-**TIV**-ih-tees of **DAY**-lee **LIV**-ing)*

**adaptive devices** *(ah-**DAP**-tiv dih-**VICE**-es)*

**amputation** *(**am**-pyou-**TAY**-shun)*

**arthritis** *(are-**THRIGH**-tis)*

**atrophy** *(**AT**-roh-fee)*

**body alignment** *(**BAH**-dee ah-**LINE**-ment)*

**chronic disease** *(**KRON**-ick dih-**ZEEZ**)*

**contracture** *(kon-**TRACK**-shur)*

**deconditioned** *(**dee**-kon-**DISH**-und)*

**disability** *(**dis**-ah-**BILL**-ih-tee)*

**dislocation** *(**dis**-loh-**KAY**-shun)*

**disorientation** *(dis-**oh**-ree-en-**TAY**-shun)*

**embolus** *(**EM**-boh-lus)*

**flaccid** *(**FLACK**-sid)*

**footboard** *(**FOOT**-bord)*

**functional ability** *(**FUNK**-shun-al ah-**BILL**-ih tee)*

**hemiplegia** *(**hem**-ee-**PLEE**-jee-ah)*

**incontinence** *(in-**KON**-tin-ens)*

**instrumental activities of daily living (IADL)** *(**in**-strew-**MEN**-tal ack-**TIV**-ih-tees of **DAY**-lee **LIV**-ing)*

**interdisciplinary health care team** *(**in**-ter-**DISS**-ih-plin-**air**-ee helth kair teem)*

**lateral** *(**LAT**-er-al)*

**mobility skills** *(moh-**BILL**-ih-tee skills)*

**orthosis** *(or-**THOH**-sis)*

**osteoporosis** *(**oss**-tee-oh-poh-**ROH**-sis)*

**paralysis** *(pah-**RAL**-ih-sis)*

**paraplegia** *(**pair**-ah-**PLEE**-jee-ah)*

**passive range of motion** *(**PASS**-iv rainj of **MOH**-shun)*

**perceptual deficit** *(per-**SEP**-tyou-al **DEF**-ih-sit)*

**pneumonia** *(new-**MOH**-nee-ah)*

**postural support** *(**POS**-chur-al sup-**PORT**)*

**pressure ulcer** *(**PRESH**-ur **UL**-sir)*

**progressive mobilization** *(proh-**GRESS**-iv moh-bill-ih-**ZAY**-shun)*

**prone** *(prohn)*

**protraction** *(proh-**TRACK**-shun)*

**quadriplegia** *(**kwahd**-rih-**PLEE**-jee-ah)*

**rehabilitation** *(**ree**-hah-**bill**-ih-**TAY**-shun)*

**residual limb** *(rih-**ZID**-you-al lim)*

**restorative care** *(ree-**STOR**-ah-tiv kair)*

**retraction** *(ree-**TRACK**-shun)*

**self range of motion** *(self rainj of **MOH**-shun)*

**sensory deprivation** *(**SEN**-soh-ree **deh**-prih-**VAY**-shun)*

**sensory stimulation** *(**SEN**-soh-ree stim-you-**LAY**-shun)*

**shearing** *(**SHEER**-ing)*

**sling** *(sling)*

**spasticity** *(spas-**TIS**-ih-tee)*

**splint** *(splint)*

**strengths** *(strenths)*

**subluxation** *(**sub**-luck-**SAY**-shun)*

**supine** *(**SOO**-pine)*

## VOCABULARY

**task segmentation** *(task seg-men-TAY-shun)*

**thrombus** *(THROM-bus)*

**turning sheet** *(TURN-ing sheet)*

# RESTORATIVE CARE AND THE INTERDISCIPLINARY HEALTH CARE TEAM

**Restorative care** is a process in which the **interdisciplinary health care team** assists the resident to reach an optimal level of ability.

Several sections of OBRA refer to restorative care. The Residents' Rights state that the residents' independence must be promoted. The section on nursing assistant training requires that all nursing assistant courses include basic restorative skills. These include:

- Training of the resident in self-care according to the resident's abilities
- Assisting residents in transferring, ambulating, eating, and dressing

**SECTION G. PHYSICAL FUNCTIONING AND STRUCTURAL PROBLEMS**

1. (A) ADL SELF-PERFORMANCE—*(Code for resident's **PERFORMANCE OVER ALL SHIFTS during last 7 days**—Not including setup)*

0. *INDEPENDENT*—No help or oversight—OR—Help/oversight provided only 1 or 2 times during last 7 days
1. *SUPERVISION*—Oversight, encouragement or cueing provided 3 or more times during last 7 days—OR—Supervision (3 or more times) plus physical assistance provided only 1 or 2 times during last 7 days
2. *LIMITED ASSISTANCE*—Resident highly involved in activity; received physical help in guided maneuvering of limbs or other nonweight bearing assistance 3 or more times—OR—More help provided only 1 or 2 times during last 7 days
3. *EXTENSIVE ASSISTANCE*—While resident performed part of activity, over last 7-day period, help of following type(s) provided 3 or more times:
   —Weight-bearing support
   —Full staff performance during part (but not all) of last 7 days
4. *TOTAL DEPENDENCE*—Full staff performance of activity during entire 7 days
8. *ACTIVITY DID NOT OCCUR* during entire 7 days

(B) ADL SUPPORT PROVIDED—*(Code for **MOST SUPPORT PROVIDED OVER ALL SHIFTS during last 7 days; code regardless** of resident's self-performance classification)*

0. No setup or physical help from staff
1. Setup help only
2. One person physical assist
3. Two+ persons physical assist
8. ADL activity itself did not occur during entire 7 days

| | | | (A) SELF-PERF | (B) SUPPORT |
|---|---|---|---|---|
| a. | BED MOBILITY | How resident moves to and from lying position, turns side to side, and positions body while in bed A = 1 = 5A; A = 2, 3, or 4 = 5A, 16; A = 8 = 16 | | |
| b. | TRANSFER | How resident moves between surfaces—to/from: bed, chair, wheelchair, standing position (EXCLUDE to/from bath/toilet) A = 1, 2, 3, or 4 = 5A | | |
| c. | WALK IN ROOM | How resident walks between locations in his/her room A = 1, 2, 3, or 4 = 5A | | |
| d. | WALK IN CORRIDOR | How resident walks in corridor on unit A = 1, 2, 3, or 4 = 5A | | |
| e. | LOCOMOTION ON UNIT | How resident moves between locations in his/her room and adjacent corridor on same floor. If in wheelchair, self-sufficiency once in chair A = 1, 2, 3, or 4 = 5A | | |
| f. | LOCOMOTION OFF UNIT | How resident moves to and returns from off unit locations (e.g., areas set aside for dining, activities, or treatments). If facility has only one floor, how resident moves to and from distant areas on the floor. If in wheelchair, self-sufficiency once in chair A = 1, 2, 3, or 4 = 5A | | |
| g. | DRESSING | How resident puts on, fastens, and takes off all items of street clothing, including donning/removing prosthesis A = 1, 2, 3, or 4 = 5A | | |
| h. | EATING | How resident eats and drinks (regardless of skill). Includes intake of nourishment by other means (e.g., tube feeding, total parenteral nutrition)A = 1, 2, 3, or 4 = 5A | | |
| i. | TOILET USE | How resident uses the toilet room (or commode, bedpan, urinal); transfers on/off toilet, cleanses, changes pad, manages ostomy or catheter, adjusts clothes A = 1, 2, 3, or 4 = 5A | | |
| j. | PERSONAL HYGIENE | How resident maintains personal hygiene, including combing hair, brushing teeth, shaving, applying makeup, washing/drying face, hands, and perineum (EXCLUDE baths and showers)A = 1, 2, 3, or 4 = 5A | | |

| | | |
|---|---|---|
| 2. | BATHING | How resident takes full-body bath/shower, sponge bath, and transfers in/out of tub/shower (EXCLUDE washing of back and hair). ***Code for most dependent** in self-performance and support.* A = 1, 2, 3 or 4 =5A<br>(A) BATHING SELF-PERFORMANCE codes appear below. (A) (B)<br>0. Independent—No help provided<br>1. Supervision—Oversight help only<br>2. Physical help limited to transfer only<br>3. Physical help in part of bathing activity<br>4. Total dependence<br>8. Activity itself did not occur during entire 7 days<br>*(Bathing support codes are as defined in **Item 1, code B above**)* |
| 3. | TEST FOR BALANCE (See training manual) | *(Code for ability during test in the **last 7 days**)*<br>0. Maintained position as required in test<br>1. Unsteady, but able to rebalance self without physical support<br>2. Partial physical support during test; or stands (sits) but does not follow directions for test<br>3. Not able to attempt test without physical help<br>a. Balance while standing<br>b. Balance while sitting—position, trunk control 1, 2, or 3 = 17* |
| 4. | FUNCTIONAL LIMITATION IN RANGE OF MOTION (see training manual) | *(Code for limitations during **last 7 days** that interfered with daily functions or placed resident at risk of injury)*<br>(A) ***RANGE OF MOTION*** — 0. No limitation; 1. Limitation on one side; 2. Limitation on both sides<br>(B) ***VOLUNTARY MOVEMENT*** — 0. No loss; 1. Partial loss; 2. Full loss<br>(A) (B)<br>a. Neck<br>b. Arm—Including shoulder or elbow<br>c. Hand—Including wrist or fingers<br>d. Leg—Including hip or knee<br>e. Foot—Including ankle or toes<br>f. Other limitation or loss |
| 5. | MODES OF LOCOMOTION | ***(Check all that apply** during **last 7 days**)*<br>Cane/walker/crutch a.<br>Wheeled self b.<br>Other person wheeled c.<br>Wheelchair primary mode of locomotion d.<br>*NONE OF ABOVE* e. |
| 6. | MODES OF TRANSFER | ***(Check all that apply** during **last 7 days**)*<br>Bedfast all or most of time 16 a.<br>Bed rails used for bed mobility or transfer b.<br>Lifted manually c.<br>Lifted mechanically d.<br>Transfer aid (e.g., slide board, trapeze, cane, walker, brace) e.<br>*NONE OF ABOVE* f. |
| 7. | TASK SEGMENTATION | Some or all of ADL activities were broken into subtasks during last 7 days so that resident could perform them<br>0. No 1. Yes |
| 8. | ADL FUNCTIONAL REHABILITATION POTENTIAL | Resident believes he/she is capable of increased independence in at least some ADLs 5A a.<br>Direct care staff believe resident is capable of increased independence in at least some ADLs 5A b.<br>Resident able to perform tasks/activity but is very slow c.<br>Difference in ADL Self-Performance or ADL Support, comparing mornings to evenings d.<br>*NONE OF ABOVE* e. |
| 9. | CHANGE IN ADL FUNCTION | Resident's ADL self-performance status has changed as compared to status of 90 days ago (or since last assessment if less than 90 days)<br>0. No change 1. Improved 2. Deteriorated |

**FIGURE 22-1** Physical functioning and structural problems are evaluated on the MDS 2.0. (Courtesy of the Health Care Finance Administration. Reprinted with permission of Briggs Corporation, Des Moines, IA 50306 [800]247-2343)

- Maintenance of range of motion
- Proper turning and positioning in bed and chair
- Bowel and bladder training
- Care and use of prostheses and orthoses

The Minimum Data Set (MDS) 2.0 includes a section on physical functioning and structural problems (Figure 22-1). The nurse is responsible for collecting these data, but the nursing assistants can provide valuable information about the resident's abilities.

Restorative care and rehabilitation are similar and in many cases identical. Some of the differences are that:

- **Rehabilitation** involves the skills of therapists including any or all of these individuals: physical therapist, occupational therapist, speech/language pathologist.
- Rehabilitation is more intense and is time limited. That means the resident is working harder to meet a goal with a definite time limit. Medicare covers the cost of the therapists' services for a specified period of time.
- Rehabilitation nurses coordinate the care and services of the residents in rehabilitation programs. They work with the therapists to see that the programs are carried out consistently 24 hours a day.
- Restorative care is a nursing responsibility with assistance from other members of the interdisciplinary health care team. Nurses assess the residents and plan restorative programs. The nursing assistants implement the programs.

Restorative care is successful when members of the team:

- Have a positive attitude about the residents and their capabilities
- Have confidence in their own abilities as care providers
- Are willing to learn from other care providers, residents, and their families
- Learn to think creatively to increase residents' quality of life
- Cooperate with other staff as team members
- Realize that "ideal" working situations seldom exist, but attempt to bring "ideal" and "real" closer together
- Continually learn and acquire new skills by participating in educational programs

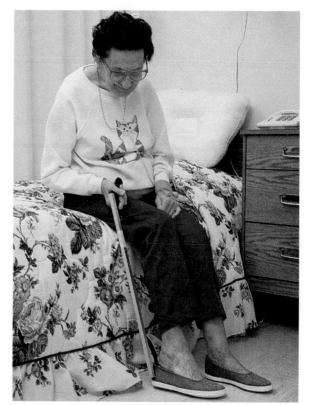

**FIGURE 22-2** This resident is using an adaptive device to increase her independence.

## PURPOSES OF RESTORATIVE CARE

The interdisciplinary health care team is concerned with:

- Increasing the resident's physical abilities. This may include **mobility skills** (the ability to move from one place to another) and the ability to care for oneself (Figure 22-2)
- Preventing complications that result from mental and physical inactivity
- Maintaining the resident's current abilities
- Helping the resident adapt to limitations imposed by a **disability** (the inability to perform certain activities because of a physical or mental impairment)
- Increasing the resident's quality of life

Most of the residents receiving rehabilitation will be discharged from the facility. Some of the residents receiving restorative care will also be able to go home.

Some of the residents living in long-term care facilities will never be able to return to their homes. For this reason, the staff may feel it is pointless to try to improve their abilities.

When residents are admitted to long-term care facilities, "good care" does not mean that the health care providers will do everything for the residents. In a short period of time, this approach will result in residents becoming helpless. In other words:

- Residents are stripped of all motivation for independence. They have no reason to act independently.
- Muscles weaken, circulation slows down, and all body systems gradually lose the ability to function. Both mind and body deteriorate.
- When residents are placed in positions of dependency, they also lose their self-esteem. They no longer see themselves as people of value.
- Residents become disinterested in what is happening around them. Life has little meaning.

People need hope and quality in their lives, even when they are living with a **chronic disease** (a disease or condition that is permanent). If residents are forced to be dependent and are not allowed to make decisions, then there is little reason for living.

Restorative care provides hope and quality by empowering the resident, that is, encouraging and allowing the resident to be as independent as possible. There may be reasons why some residents really cannot do things for themselves. In these cases, the team must do for residents what they are unable to do for themselves. However, the residents should still be allowed to make decisions regarding their care. If residents are no longer mentally competent to make decisions, the team will be responsible for all aspects of their care.

## Principles for Restorative Care

The following principles provide the foundation for restorative care:

1. **Begin treatment as soon as possible.** This means that plans for maintaining or increasing the resident's level of independence are made as soon as the resident is admitted to the facility.
2. **Stress the resident's ability, not disability.** The resident's **strengths** are used to help the resident adapt to any limitations. This means that care providers think in terms of what the resident can do, not what the resident cannot do.
3. **Activity strengthens and inactivity weakens.** Complications result from physical and mental inactivity. These can cause further disability or even be life-threatening.
4. **Treat the whole person.** It is important to attend to the residents' emotional and mental health needs as well as their physical well-being. The interdisciplinary team also works with the residents' families. Families directly influence the emotional and mental health of the residents.

## PREVENTING COMPLICATIONS FROM INACTIVITY

Restorative care attempts to prevent the complications that result from inactivity. These complications can affect elderly people more quickly than younger people because of the changes that are taking place in their bodies. Refer to the table below for a summary of possible complications and preventive nursing assistant actions.

| Complications Resulting from Inactivity | |
| --- | --- |
| **Complications by Body System** | **Prevention** |
| **Musculoskeletal System** | |
| • Muscles become weak and **atrophy**. This means that muscles that are not used shrink and become useless. | • Carry out exercise programs planned for the residents' capabilities. |

*(continues)*

## Complications Resulting from Inactivity *(continued)*

| Complications by Body System | Prevention |
|---|---|
| **Musculoskeletal System** | |
| • **Contractures** can develop, making movement impossible. The joints become stiff when they are not moved. In a short time the tissue around the joints also stiffens. Soon the joint cannot be moved at all (Figure 22-3). | • Do range of motion exercises.<br>• Use correct positioning techniques.<br>• Use splints and other devices to maintain the proper joint position. |

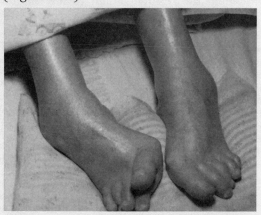

**FIGURE 22-3** Contractures are a complication of immobility.

| | |
|---|---|
| • **Osteoporosis** develops with nonuse. When the legs do not bear weight, calcium begins to leave the bones and enter the bloodstream. This causes brittle bones; fractures may occur without reason. | • Offer the resident opportunities to stand and bear weight on the legs, for example, during transfer procedures. |
| **Integumentary System** | |
| • **Pressure ulcers** develop over pressure areas. If a resident sits or lies in one spot, blood cannot circulate to that area. The cells in the skin and tissue begin to die, causing an ulcer to develop (Figure 22-4). | • Reposition the resident every 1 or 2 hours.<br>• Do range of motion exercises twice a day.<br>• Provide adequate nutrition and fluids. |

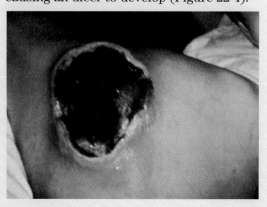

**FIGURE 22-4** Pressure sores are also a complication of immobility.

*(continues)*

## Complications Resulting from Inactivity *(continued)*

| Complications by Body System | Prevention |
| --- | --- |
| **Cardiovascular System**<br>• The heart becomes **deconditioned**. The heart is a muscle and weakens when the body is inactive. In its weakened state, the heart takes longer to return to a normal pace after activity. If this happens, the resident must rest between physical activities. | • Follow all instructions for assisting the resident with ambulation (walking) and exercise programs. |
| • Blood does not circulate as efficiently. This can lead to **embolus** and **thrombus**. A thrombus is a blood clot that forms in a blood vessel. If the thrombus breaks loose and moves through the circulatory system, it is called an embolus. | • Follow all instructions for ambulation and exercise. |
| **Respiratory System**<br>• The lungs do not expand as efficiently when a resident is immobile. Secretions collect in the lungs and bacteria grow in the secretions causing **pneumonia**, an infection of the lungs. | • Provide the resident with fluids to drink.<br>• Position the resident so the lungs can expand.<br>• Encourage the resident to take deep breaths. |
| **Gastrointestinal System**<br>• Without exercise or activity, the appetite decreases, causing weight loss.<br>• Risk of pressure ulcers increases with weight loss and lack of nutrition.<br>• Peristalsis slows down, causing indigestion and constipation (the inability to move the bowels). | • Tell the nurse if the resident likes or dislikes certain foods.<br>• Encourage resident to drink adequate fluids.<br>• Assist the resident with ambulation and exercise.<br>• Assist the resident to develop a bowel elimination schedule. Provide privacy for toileting. |
| **Urinary System**<br>• The bladder does not always empty completely if a person is not able to sit properly on the toilet or commode. This increases the risk of bladder infection.<br>• Incontinence can result from inability to get to the bathroom.<br>• Urinary stones may develop from the calcium in the bloodstream resulting from osteoporosis. | • Encourage adequate fluid intake.<br>• Assist the resident to the toilet regularly and provide privacy. |

*(continues)*

| Complications Resulting from Inactivity *(continued)* | |
|---|---|
| **Complications by Body System** | **Prevention** |
| **Psychosocial Reactions**<br>• Depression can occur from physical and mental inactivity. Depression is an emotional condition that causes the resident to be slow, unresponsive, and sad.<br>• Inactivity and **sensory deprivation** can lead to **disorientation**. Sensory deprivation occurs when there is a lack of stimulation to the senses—vision, hearing, smelling, tasting, and touching. A person who is disoriented is confused about time, place, and who he or she is. | • Cooperate with activities department to provide **sensory stimulation** programs. These are activities that increase the resident's awareness of the surroundings. |

## ACTIVITIES OF DAILY LIVING ·········

One purpose of restorative care is to increase the resident's physical abilities. This includes mobility skills and the ability to carry out **activities of daily living (ADL)**. These are the tasks that adults do throughout a day to meet their basic needs. The ADL are:

- Bathing
- Grooming—hair care, nail care, oral care, shaving, and applying makeup
- Dressing and undressing
- Eating
- Toileting
- Mobility (the ability to move about)

The ADL are taught to people when they are children. Healthy adults do these tasks automatically. If the resident cannot complete any or all of the ADL, a self-care deficit exists. A self-care deficit may be due to:

- Diseases such as multiple sclerosis, arthritis, Parkinson's disease, or Alzheimer's disease
- A stroke or injuries that have damaged the brain or spinal cord
- Vision impairment
- Emotional illness

Problems can result from these conditions that limit the resident's ability to do self-care. Examples of these problems are:

- Decreased strength
- Lack of endurance
- Limited range of motion
- **Paralysis**
- **Perceptual deficits**
- Depression
- Disorientation

Paralysis occurs because of damage to the brain or spinal cord. It means the resident cannot move one or more of the extremities. Brain damage from a stroke frequently causes **hemiplegia,** which means paralysis on one side of the body. Spinal cord injuries can cause **quadriplegia** (paralysis from the neck down) or **paraplegia** (paralysis from the waist down).

Perceptual deficits usually occur because of damage to the brain from disease or injury. Examples of perceptual deficits include the inability to:

- Organize a task. ADL cannot be completed unless the resident is able to prepare for the task, get the necessary items together, and then do the task.
- Sequence a task. A resident with this inability may put on a dress before the slip or shoes before the socks.
- Exercise judgment. This deficit may be noted if a resident puts on a wool coat in hot weather, when appropriate clothing is available.
- Identify common objects such as eating utensils and grooming items. When this occurs, the resident may look at a fork, but not know what it is.

- Use common items. The resident may be able to identify an item such as a comb or toothbrush, but be unable to pick it up and use it, even though there is no physical reason for the problem.
- Initiate or start a task without assistance.

### Instrumental Activities of Daily Living

Higher level tasks are called **instrumental activities of daily living** or **IADL.** These include skills that adults need to function independently. Examples of IADL include:

- Managing money
- Managing a household
- Driving a car

In some situations the adult may not be able to physically complete these tasks but is able to competently direct others to do so.

## SETTING UP RESTORATIVE PROGRAMS

Residents with self-care deficits are evaluated by therapists and nurses. The results of the evaluation will determine whether a resident's **functional ability** (ability to do ADL) can be increased. In other words, can the interdisciplinary team help this resident to relearn an ADL?

- This is discussed with the resident and the family. If the resident, family, and staff agree that the resident's physical abilities can be increased, then a restorative program is planned by the interdisciplinary team.
- The members of the interdisciplinary team meet together at the care plan conference (Figure 22-5). Methods for solving the resident's problems are discussed with the resident and family.

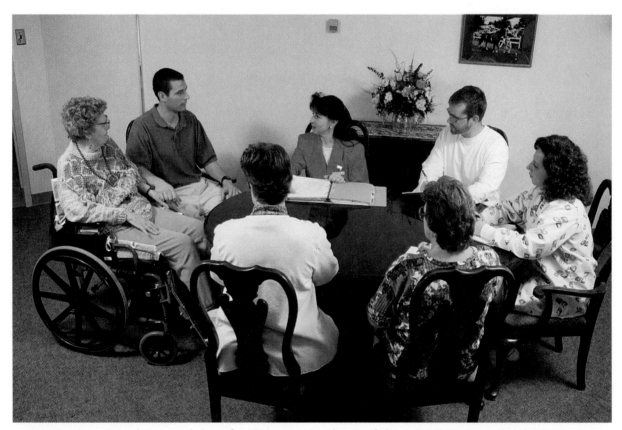

**FIGURE 22-5**   Residents and their families are members of the interdisciplinary health care team.

## Task Segmentation

| ADL | Steps of Activity | ADL | Steps of Activity |
|---|---|---|---|
| **Grooming** | • Washes, brushes, combs hair<br>• Brushes teeth<br>  • Gets equipment ready<br>  • Places paste on brush<br>  • Brushes teeth<br>  • Rinses mouth<br>  • Cleans and puts equipment away<br>• Shaves<br>  • Gets equipment ready<br>  • Shaves face<br>  • Cleans/puts equipment away<br>• Nail care<br>  • Gets equipment ready<br>  • Cleans nails<br>  • Trims nails<br>  • Cleans/puts equipment away | **Dressing/ Undressing (cont'd)** | • Manages buttons, snaps, ties, zippers<br>• Puts on/takes off skirt/pants<br>• Buckles belt<br>• Puts on/takes off shoes/socks |
| | | **Eating** | • Gets to table<br>• Uses spoon, fork, knife appropriately<br>• Opens/pours<br>• Brings food to mouth<br>• Chews, swallows<br>• Uses napkin |
| | | **Toileting** | • Gets to commode/toilet<br>• Manipulates clothing<br>• Sits on toilet<br>• Eliminates in toilet<br>• Cleans self<br>• Flushes toilet<br>• Gets clothing in place<br>• Washes hands |
| **Bathing** | • Gathers supplies<br>• Gets to tub/sink/shower<br>• Undresses<br>• Regulates water<br>• Washes/rinses upper body<br>• Washes/rinses lower body<br>• Dries body<br>• Puts away supplies | **Mobility** | • Gets self to side of bed<br>• Maintains upright position<br>• Comes to standing position<br>• Places self in position to sit in chair<br>• Locks wheelchair brakes<br>• Turns body to sit<br>• Lowers self into chair<br>• Propels wheelchair<br>• Repositions self in chair<br>• Raises self from chair<br>• Places self in position to sit on edge of bed<br>• Walks alone/with assistance<br>• Uses assistive device |
| **Dressing/ Undressing** | • Obtains/selects clothing<br>• Puts on/takes off slipover top<br>• Puts on/takes off cardigan-style top | | |

When the resident is unable to do any ADL independently, it is generally best to concentrate on relearning just one ADL at a time. The first step is to find out what the resident wants to work on first. The interdisciplinary team then works with the resident and family to plan the process. They will:

• Establish goals.
  • Each ADL consists of several steps. This is called **task segmentation** (table above).

- The resident will not be able to do all steps right away. Some residents may never be able to do all of the steps.
- Goals, therefore, are very small. For example, if the resident is in a restorative program for eating, the first goal for the resident may be to hold a glass, bring it to her mouth and drink from it.

  All goals are functional (purposeful). For example, instead of saying the resident will walk 30 feet, the goal will state: resident will walk to the dining room for breakfast.

- Plan approaches.
  - Approaches include the techniques and procedures carried out by care providers to assist resident to relearn the ADL.

The resident may participate in other physical or occupational rehabilitation programs. These programs are planned to help the resident acquire skills needed to complete a task. For example, exercises may be done that will increase range of motion, strength, or endurance.

## Approaches Used in Restorative Programs

- Setup
  - Residents with self-care deficits cannot set up or prepare for ADL. You may need to provide the setup (Figure 22-6). *Example:* The setup for mealtime includes bringing the tray to the resident and assisting with uncovering food, opening containers, removing eating utensils from package, and preparing food, if necessary.
- Verbal cues
  - Verbal cues are short, simple phrases to prompt the resident to do something. *Example:* Give the resident a prepared washcloth and then say, "Please wash your face."
- Hand-over-hand technique
  - For this technique, your hand is placed over the resident's hand to guide it (Figure 22-7). *Example:* For eating program, place a spoon with food in the resident's hand. Place your hand over the resident's hand. Guide the spoon to the resident's mouth. Eventually, the resident will be able to do this without assistance.

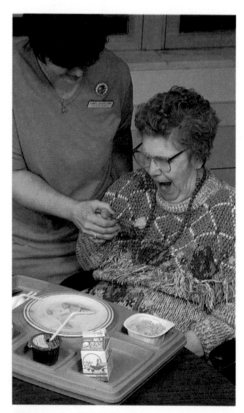

**FIGURE 22-7** The nursing assistant is using hand-over-hand techniques to help the resident regain eating skills.

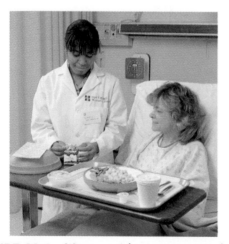

**FIGURE 22-6** Many residents can complete the activities of daily living if you set up the articles they need.

- Demonstration
    - "Act out" what you want the resident to do. *Example:* Before giving the resident a toothbrush, make the motions of brushing your teeth with the toothbrush.

The care plan will indicate the approach to be used. The decision is made by the physical therapist, occupational therapist, or restorative nurse.

**Adaptive devices** are sometimes used to simplify ADL (Figure 22-8A–C). An adaptive device is an ordinary item that is changed in some way so that it can be used by individuals with specific disabilities. These devices allow people to do things they may not otherwise be able to do. If adaptive devices are ordered, be sure they are used each time the ADL is carried out.

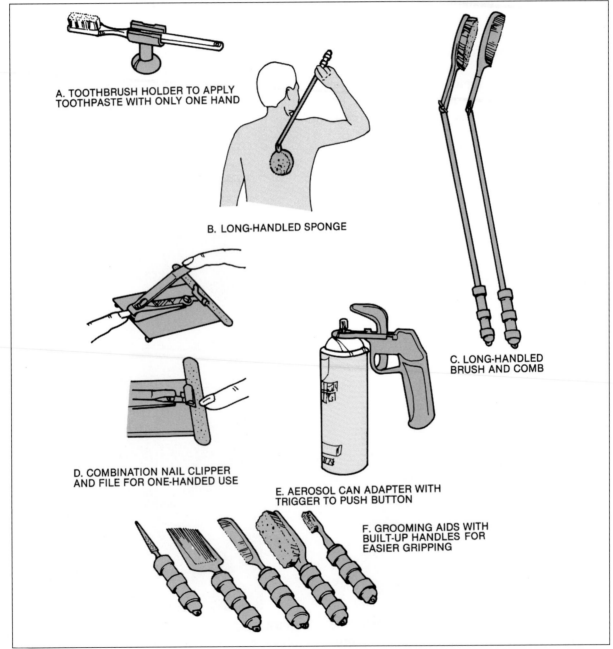

A. TOOTHBRUSH HOLDER TO APPLY TOOTHPASTE WITH ONLY ONE HAND

B. LONG-HANDLED SPONGE

C. LONG-HANDLED BRUSH AND COMB

D. COMBINATION NAIL CLIPPER AND FILE FOR ONE-HANDED USE

E. AEROSOL CAN ADAPTER WITH TRIGGER TO PUSH BUTTON

F. GROOMING AIDS WITH BUILT-UP HANDLES FOR EASIER GRIPPING

**FIGURE 22-8** A. Adaptive devices used for grooming and bathing

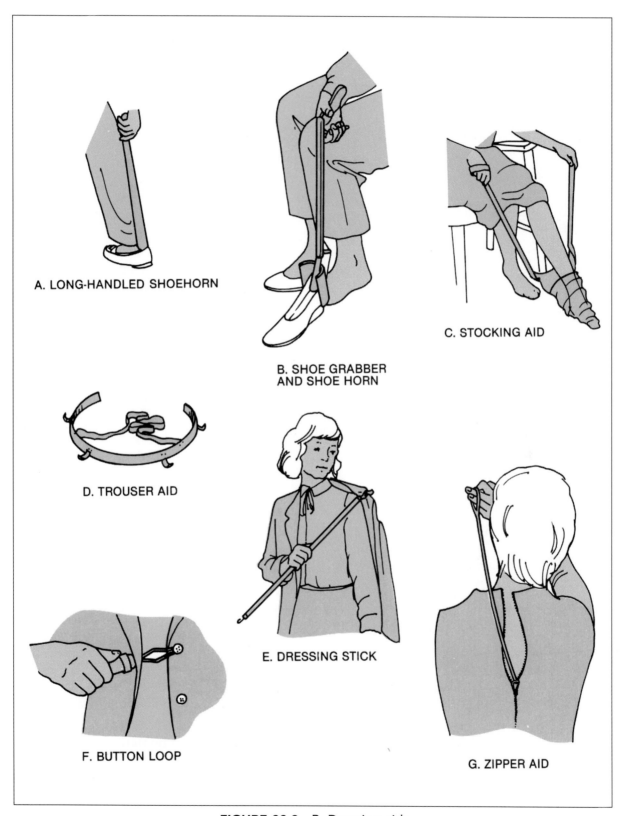

A. LONG-HANDLED SHOEHORN

B. SHOE GRABBER AND SHOE HORN

C. STOCKING AID

D. TROUSER AID

E. DRESSING STICK

F. BUTTON LOOP

G. ZIPPER AID

**FIGURE 22-8**  B. Dressing aids

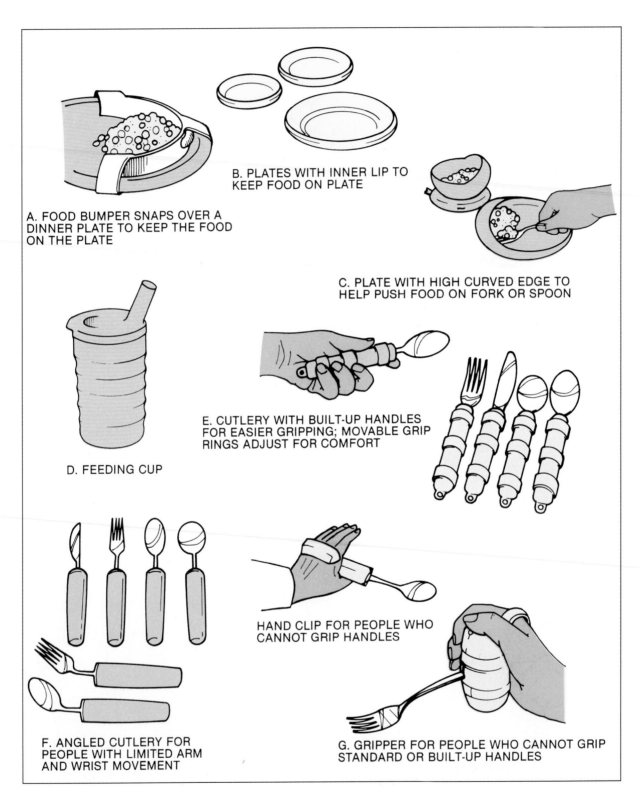

A. FOOD BUMPER SNAPS OVER A DINNER PLATE TO KEEP THE FOOD ON THE PLATE

B. PLATES WITH INNER LIP TO KEEP FOOD ON PLATE

C. PLATE WITH HIGH CURVED EDGE TO HELP PUSH FOOD ON FORK OR SPOON

D. FEEDING CUP

E. CUTLERY WITH BUILT-UP HANDLES FOR EASIER GRIPPING; MOVABLE GRIP RINGS ADJUST FOR COMFORT

F. ANGLED CUTLERY FOR PEOPLE WITH LIMITED ARM AND WRIST MOVEMENT

HAND CLIP FOR PEOPLE WHO CANNOT GRIP HANDLES

G. GRIPPER FOR PEOPLE WHO CANNOT GRIP STANDARD OR BUILT-UP HANDLES

**FIGURE 22-8** C. Adaptive devices used for eating

# *G*uidelines for

## Nursing Assistant Responsibilities in General Restorative Program

### General

1. Know the cause of the resident's self-care deficit.
2. Know the resident's goals as stated on the care plan.
3. Be consistent. Read the care plan and follow the specific approaches each time you work with the resident.
4. Keep your directions simple but not childish when you are helping the resident relearn an activity.
5. Avoid distractions. Do the ADL in a private, quiet area. Restorative programs are incorporated into the resident's daily care. For example, if the resident is in a grooming program to relearn how to comb her hair, then the program is carried out when the hair would usually be combed.
6. Use adaptive devices consistently and correctly.
7. Do not show impatience. Be encouraging and give praise.
8. Treat the resident with dignity at all times.
9. Realize that the resident's progress may be uneven and inconsistent. A resident may do better one day than another.

### Grooming

1. A grooming program may be for combing/brushing hair, applying makeup, doing nail care, shaving, or oral care.
2. The resident should sit in a comfortable chair that supports the resident's body.
3. Place the necessary items on the overbed table. Place the table in front of the resident and adjust it to the appropriate height so the resident can reach every item.
4. Avoid putting too many items on the table at once. Do not put the items close together or the resident may have trouble picking the correct item.

### Bathing

1. Residents in bathing programs should also be allowed to:
   - Wash their hands after toileting
   - Wash their face and hands after eating
   - Follow the program for AM and PM care as well as for bathing
2. A setup is usually needed:
   - Prepare the water (basin, tub, or shower).
   - Obtain all the necessary items (towels, washcloths, soap).
   - Help the resident choose clothing to put on after the bath.

### Eating

1. Assist the resident to go to the bathroom.
2. Provide opportunity for handwashing.
3. Be sure the resident has dentures in if needed and that the mouth is clean.
4. Seat the resident in a regular dining chair at a dining table.
5. Avoid distractions. Turn off televisions and radios.
6. Prepare the tray: open cartons, butter the bread, cut the meat, add seasonings as the resident wishes, and pour liquids. The resident may eventually be able to do these things independently.

### Dressing/Undressing

The following adaptations will make the program more likely to succeed:

1. Use loose-fitting styles or clothing one size larger.
2. Encourage the family to bring clothing that fastens in front rather than in back. Velcro® closings are usually easier to manipulate than zippers, buttons, or snaps.

*(continues)*

---

*G*uidelines *(continued)*

3. Suggest garments with large buttons rather than small ones. It is easier to match buttons with the right buttonholes if the resident starts to button from the bottom of a shirt or blouse rather than the top.

4. Suggest that elastic thread be used for cuff buttons so they do not need to be undone each time.
5. Encourage the resident to wear slip-on shoes or shoes with Velcro® closings.

---

Guidelines for mobility programs and toileting are presented later in this lesson.

Not all residents have potential for restorative programs. For those who do not, the goals are concerned with preventing complications and maintaining current abilities as long as possible. Restorative programs may remain in place after the resident reaches the highest goal possible. This is done to be sure that the resident does not lose the skill. Some residents with progressive diseases such as Alzheimer's reach the point where even maintenance is difficult. Preventing complications such as pressure ulcers and contractures is then the major goal.

## THE RESTORATIVE ENVIRONMENT

A restorative environment is not only for residents in restorative programs. The staff can provide an environment and act in such a manner that all residents will benefit. The interdisciplinary team can help promote this environment:

- Give residents a sense of control and the opportunity to make decisions.
- Remember that mental and physical activity are essential to the residents' well-being. Opportunities for physical exercise and various types of activities must be offered to residents.
- Encourage and assist residents to be well dressed and well groomed at all times (Figure 22-9).
- Use touch freely in appropriate ways with residents (Figure 22-10).
- Provide cues for orientation throughout the building such as large clocks, calendars, pictures, and color codes.

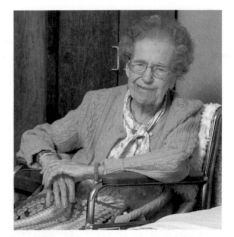

**FIGURE 22-9** All residents should be assisted to look attractive and well groomed.

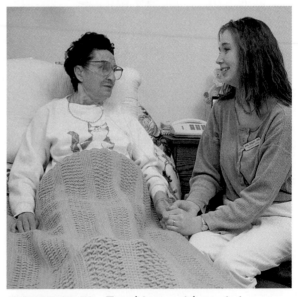

**FIGURE 22-10** Touching residents is important for restorative care.

- Respect the resident's identity, individuality, and privacy at all times.
- Respect and understand the resident's sexuality and need for intimacy.
- Give residents opportunities to do for others. All people need to feel useful.
- Encourage and assist residents to remain a part of the community and encourage the community to be a part of the facility.
- The environment should be safe, serene, and colorful.

## PROGRESSIVE MOBILIZATION

**Progressive mobilization** is a process used to increase a resident's mobility skills. Mobility includes:

- Moving in bed
- Changing position in bed
- Moving to and coming to a sitting position on the edge of the bed
- Coming to a standing position
- Transferring into a bathtub, shower, and car or out of bed and into a chair
- Ambulating or moving about in a wheelchair

Not all residents are able to complete every step of progressive mobilization. All residents should be given the opportunity to reach their own potential. Progressive mobilization, like all restorative programs, must begin at the simplest level. A resident may not be able to do any of these skills independently but may be able to do each skill with assistance.

## RANGE OF MOTION

Exercise is a basic physical need. Residents who are unable to do active exercises are exercised through passive range of motion exercises by the care provider. The physical or occupational therapist may order additional exercises to increase specific abilities or to strengthen certain muscles.

- **Passive range of motion**
  The care provider moves the joints for the resident.
- **Active assistive range of motion**
  The care provider supports the joints and assists in the movement while the resident attempts to do independent movement.
- **Active range of motion**
  The resident is able to move the joints without assistance.
- **Self range of motion**
  The resident uses the strong extremity to move the affected extremity. *Example:* A resident with a stroke may use the strong arm to passively move the paralyzed arm.

Nursing assistants in long-term care facilities may do passive range of motion exercises with residents several times a day.

---

*G*uidelines for

## Passive Range of Motion Exercises

1. Always tell the resident what you are doing and why. Have the resident help you if possible.
2. Passive exercises of the neck are not generally done on elderly people. Arthritis is a common problem and passive exercises can injure the neck. Instead, encourage the resident to move the head independently.
3. Move each joint to its fullest range. Remember that the maximum range in an elderly person may be small.
4. Never force movement or cause pain. If the resident cannot speak, watch the face for signs of pain.
5. Use gentle, physical contact. Support the extremities at the joints. Use the palms of your hands to cup the joints.

*(continues)*

## Guidelines *(continued)*

6. Do each motion at least five times. The exercises should be done at least twice a day. Do each joint unless you have been instructed to omit specific joints or a specific movement for a joint.

7. Do each motion slowly, smoothly, gently, and rhythmically. A resident's stiff joints may gradually loosen as you continue the exercises.

8. Come to a complete stop at the end of each movement before starting the next movement.

## Definitions of Joint Movements

Specific terms describe joint movements. Not all joints are capable of the same movements.

1. Flexion—bending a joint; decreasing the angle of the joint (Figure 22-11)
   - Palmar flexion—bending the hand down toward the wrist
   - Dorsiflexion—bending the hand back or bending the foot back
   - Plantar flexion—bending the foot forward toward the sole

2. Extension—the opposite of flexion—to straighten the joint out; increasing the angle of the joint (Figure 22-12)

3. Abduction—moving an extremity away from the body (Figure 22-13)
   - Horizontal abduction—bringing the arm out so the elbow is parallel to shoulder

4. Adduction—the opposite of abduction—moving the extremity back to the body (Figure 22-14)
   - Horizontal adduction—bringing the arm up and crossing it over the chest

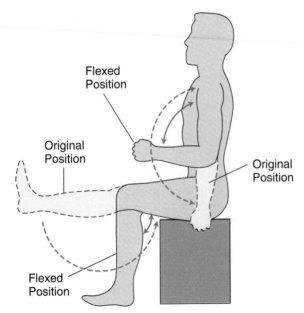

**FIGURE 22-11**   Flexion—bending a joint

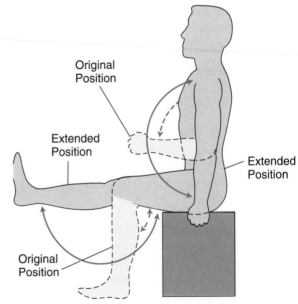

**FIGURE 22-12**   Extension—straightening a joint

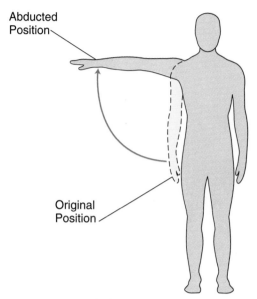

**FIGURE 22-13**  Abduction—moving an extremity away from the body

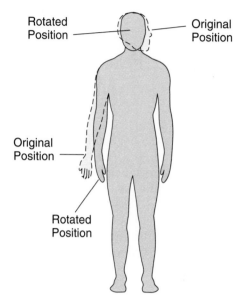

**FIGURE 22-15**  Rotation

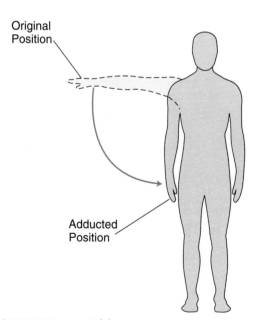

**FIGURE 22-14**  Adduction—moving an extremity back to the body

5. Rotation—turning around an axis (Figure 22-15)
   - Internal rotation—turning toward the median line
   - External rotation—turning outward from the median line
6. Pronation—turning the forearm so the palm is facing downward
7. Supination—the opposite of pronation—turning the forearm so the palm is facing upward
8. Radial deviation—lateral movement of wrist toward thumb side of hand
9. Ulnar deviation—lateral movement of wrist toward little finger side of hand
10. Inversion—turning inward
11. Eversion—the opposite of inversion—turning outward
12. Opposition—bringing palmar surface of thumb to the finger joint

It is important that you review the section on body mechanics in Lesson 9. You will need to use your muscles correctly as you help residents with their mobility. This will help prevent painful and costly injuries to both you and the residents.

# PROCEDURE 82 Passive Range of Motion Exercises

1. Carry out each beginning procedure action.
2. Position the resident in **body alignment**. This means the resident's spine is straight and the resident's extremities are straight in relation to the body. The body is straight in the bed. Bring the resident close to your side of the bed.
3. Place a bath blanket over the covers. Then bring the covers to the foot of the bed. Expose only the extremity that you are working on.
4. Remember to use correct body mechanics to avoid straining your back.
5. Lower the side rail. Do the exercises on the arm and leg on that side. Raise the side rail. Go to the other side of the bed. Do the exercises on the arm and leg on that side.
6. When all four extremities have been exercised, carry out procedure completion actions.
7. Report any unusual resident reactions or problems to the nurse.

**Shoulder**
Support the elbow and wrist during all shoulder exercises.

1. Flexion and extension
   - With shoulder in adduction, flex the resident's elbow and raise entire arm over the head (flexion) (Figure 22-16). *Note:* This movement is flexing the resident's elbow as well as the shoulder.
   - Bring arm back down parallel to body (extension) (Figure 22-17). *Note:* This movement is extending the resident's elbow as well as the shoulder.

   Repeat flexion and extension five to seven times.

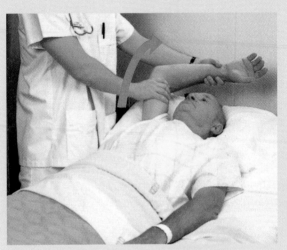

**FIGURE 22-16** Shoulder flexion. Flex elbow and raise entire arm over head.

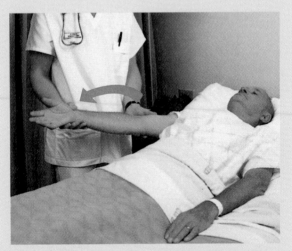

**FIGURE 22-17** Supporting the upper arm and wrist, straighten elbow.

2. Abduction and adduction
   - Bring entire arm out at right angle to body (abduction) (Figure 22-18).

*(continues)*

**PROCEDURE** *82* *(continued)*

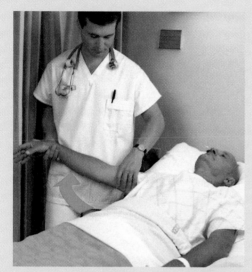

**FIGURE 22-18** Shoulder abduction and adduction. Supporting the elbow and wrist, bring the entire arm out at right angle from the body.

- Return arm to position parallel with body (adduction) (Figure 22-19).

Repeat abduction and adduction five to seven times.

**3.** Horizontal adduction and horizontal abduction

- With arm parallel to body, bring arm up and cross it over chest (horizontal adduction) (Figure 22-20).
- Bring arm back so elbow is parallel to shoulder (horizontal abduction) (Figure 22-21).

Repeat horizontal adduction and horizontal abduction five to seven times.

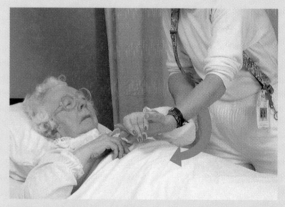

**FIGURE 22-20** Horizontal adduction of the shoulder

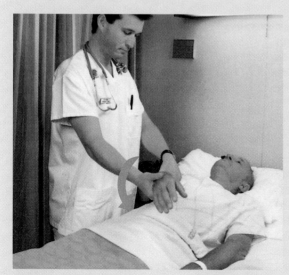

**FIGURE 22-19** Return arm to position parallel to body.

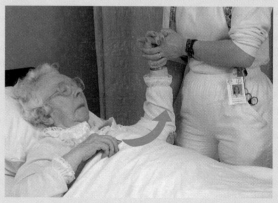

**FIGURE 22-21** Horizontal abduction of the shoulder

*(continues)*

**PROCEDURE** *82* *(continued)*

4. External rotation and internal rotation
   - With elbow parallel to shoulder, place forearm in up position with palm of hand up (external rotation) (Figure 22-22).
   - Bring forearm down with elbow and shoulder remaining stationary (internal rotation) (Figure 22-23).

   Repeat external rotation and internal rotation five to seven times.

**Elbow**

Support the resident's wrist during the elbow exercises.

1. Flexion and extension
   - With arm parallel to body and palm up, bend elbow (flexion) (Figure 22-24).
   - Return arm to position parallel with body and palm up (extension) (Figure 22-25).

   Repeat flexion and extension of elbow five to seven times.

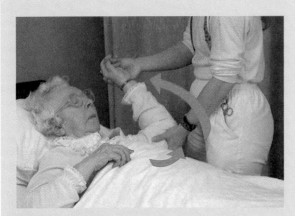

**FIGURE 22-22** External rotation of the shoulder

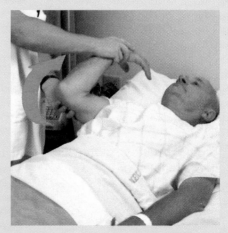

**FIGURE 22-24** Flexion of the elbow. Bring lower arm toward upper arm.

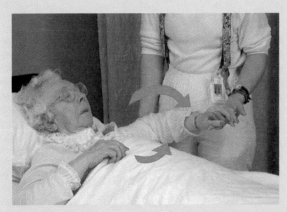

**FIGURE 22-23** Internal rotation of the shoulder

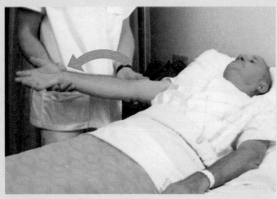

**FIGURE 22-25** Extension of the shoulder and elbow

*(continues)*

**PROCEDURE** *82*   *(continued)*

**2.** Supination and pronation
- Place your hand in resident's hand as if to shake hands. Turn resident's hand with yours so the palm is down (pronation).
- Without moving your hand, turn resident's hand with yours so resident's palm is up (supination) (Figure 22-26).

Repeat supination and pronation five to seven times.

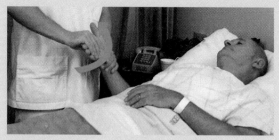

**FIGURE 22-26** Supination. Grasp resident's hand as if to shake hands; turn hand so resident's hand is palm up.

**Wrist**
Support the forearm during wrist exercises. The elbow and shoulder will rest on the bed.

**1.** Flexion (palmar flexion), extension, (dorsiflexion)
- Bend wrist forward (flexion, palmar flexion) (Figure 22-27).

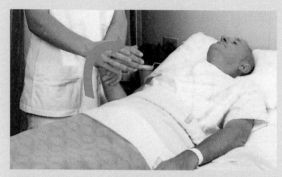

**FIGURE 22-27** Wrist flexion and extension. Place hand over resident's hand while supporting wrist and bend wrist.

- Straighten wrist so hand is even with forearm (extension) (Figure 22-28).

Repeat flexion and extension five to seven times.

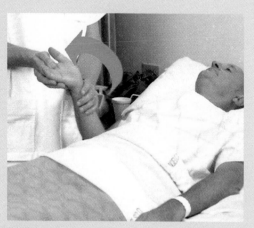

**FIGURE 22-28** Supporting arm above wrist and hand, straighten wrist.

**2.** Ulnar and radial deviation
- Move hand toward little finger side (ulnar deviation) (Figure 22-29).
- Move hand toward thumb side (radial deviation) (Figure 22-30).

Repeat ulnar and radial deviation five to seven times.

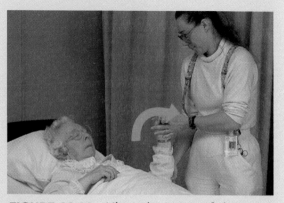

**FIGURE 22-29** Ulnar deviation of the wrist
*(continues)*

**PROCEDURE 82** *(continued)*

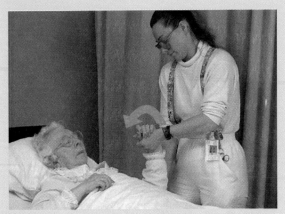

**FIGURE 22-30** Radial deviation of the wrist

**Fingers**

Support the wrist and forearm during the finger and thumb exercises.

1. Flexion and extension
   - Curl the fingers together (flexion) (Figure 22-31).
   - Straighten the fingers out (extension) (Figure 22-32).

   Repeat flexion and extension of the fingers five to seven times.

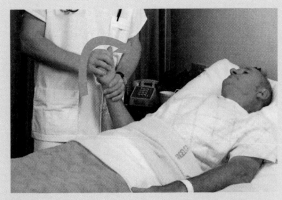

**FIGURE 22-31** Finger flexion. Supporting wrist with one hand, cover resident's fingers and curl them to make a fist.

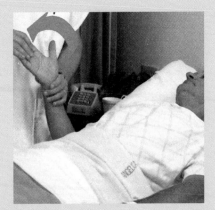

**FIGURE 22-32** Finger extension. Slip fingers over resident's flexed fingers and straighten the fingers.

2. Abduction and adduction
   - Spread each finger apart from the one next to it (abduction) (Figure 22-33).
   - Bring each finger back (adduction) (Figure 22-34).

   Repeat abduction and adduction five to seven times.

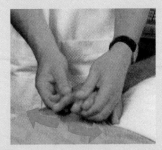

**FIGURE 22-33** Abduction of the fingers

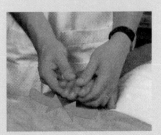

**FIGURE 22-34** Adduction of the fingers
*(continues)*

**PROCEDURE 82** *(continued)*

**Thumb**

1. Flexion and extension
   - Bend the thumb forward (flexion).
   - Straighten the thumb out (extension).

   Repeat flexion and extension of the thumb five to seven times.
2. Abduction and adduction
   - Move the thumb away from the other fingers (abduction) (Figure 22-35).
   - Move the thumb back toward the other fingers (adduction).

   Repeat abduction and adduction five to seven times.

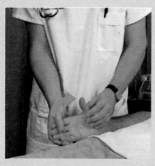

**FIGURE 22-35**   Abduction and adduction of thumb. Supporting the hand, draw the thumb toward and away from the extended fingers.

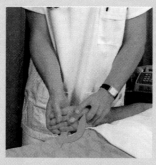

**FIGURE 22-36**   Thumb opposition. Supporting the hand, touch each finger with the thumb.

3. Opposition
   - Move the thumb to the base of each finger and then back (Figure 22-36).

   Repeat opposition five to seven times. *Note:* Opposition is an exercise for the thumb not the fingers. It is important that the thumb receive the movement.

**Hips**

Support the knee and ankle during hip exercises.

1. Abduction and adduction
   - Place the palm of your hand under the resident's knee and the other hand under the heel.
   - Move the entire leg away from the body (abduction) (Figure 22-37).
   - Move the entire leg back toward the body (adduction) (Figure 22-38).

   Repeat abduction and adduction of the hip five to seven times.

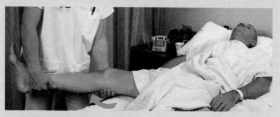

**FIGURE 22-37**   Abduction of the hip. Supporting resident's knee and ankle, move entire leg away from the body.

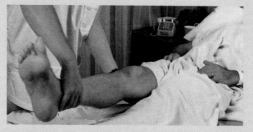

**FIGURE 22-38**   Adduction of the hip. Supporting leg, return toward center of body.

*(continues)*

**PROCEDURE** *82* *(continued)*

**2.** Flexion and extension

- Place one hand under the resident's knee. Place your other hand under the heel with the resident's foot resting against your forearm.
- Bend the resident's knee and hip toward the resident's trunk (flexion) (Figure 22-39).

*Note:* You are flexing the knee at the same time as the hip.

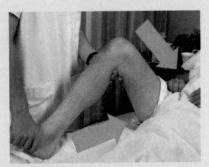

**FIGURE 22-39** Hip and knee flexion. Supporting resident's knee and ankle, flex knee and hip.

- Straighten the knee and hip (extension). Be sure to support the knee so it does not "flop" down (Figure 22-40).

*Note:* You are extending the knee at the same time as the hip. Repeat flexion and extension of the hip and knee five to seven times.

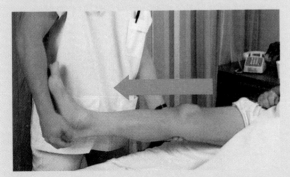

**FIGURE 22-40** Knee extension. Supporting knee and ankle, straighten knee.

**3.** Internal rotation and external rotation

- Place one hand on the resident's leg just above the knee. Place the other hand on the resident's lower leg just above the ankle.
- With the resident's leg extended, roll the leg back and forth. Rolling the leg inward is internal rotation. Rolling the leg outward is external rotation (Figure 22-41).

Repeat internal rotation and external rotation of the hip five to seven times.

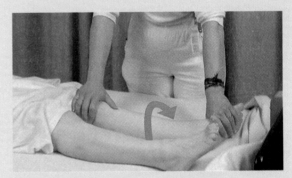

**FIGURE 22-41** External and internal rotation of the hip

**Knee**

Flexion and extension are the only knee movements. These were done with the hip.

**Ankle**

**1.** Plantar flexion and dorsiflexion

- Bend resident's knee slightly and support lower leg with your forearm and hand.
- With your other hand, bend resident's foot downward (plantar flexion) (Figure 22-42).
- Then gently bend resident's foot backward (dorsiflexion, hyperextension) (Figure 22-43).

Repeat plantar flexion and dorsiflexion five to seven times.

*(continues)*

**PROCEDURE 82** *(continued)*

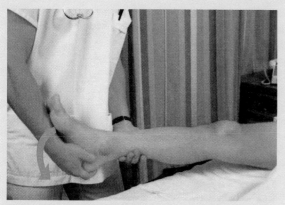

**FIGURE 22-42**  Plantar flex the ankle by drawing the foot in a downward position.

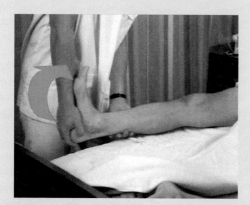

**FIGURE 22-43**  Dorsiflexion. Grasp the resident's heel with one hand, using your upper arm to support the foot. Dorsiflex the ankle by bringing the toes and foot toward the knee.

**2.** Inversion and eversion
  - Place both hands on the resident's foot. Move the foot inward (inversion) (Figure 22-44).
  - With your hands still on the resident's foot, move the foot outward (eversion) (Figure 22-45).

Repeat inversion and eversion five to seven times.

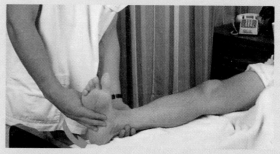

**FIGURE 22-44**  Ankle inversion. Grasp resident's foot and gently turn it inward.

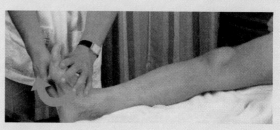

**FIGURE 22-45**  Foot eversion. Grasp resident's foot and gently turn it outward.

**Toes**
  **1.** Flexion and extension
    - Bend (flexion) and straighten (extension) each toe.

    Repeat flexion and extension of the toes five to seven times.
  **2.** Abduction and adduction
    - Move each toe away from the next toe, one at a time (abduction) (Figure 22-46).

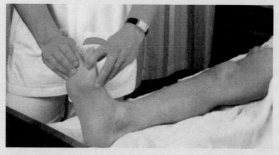

**FIGURE 22-46**  Toe abduction. Move each toe away from the next toe, one at a time.
*(continues)*

**PROCEDURE** *82* *(continued)*

- Move each toe toward the next toe, one at a time (adduction) (Figure 22-47).

Repeat abduction and adduction five to seven times.

Additional exercises can be done with the resident in the prone (lying on the abdomen) position. However, many residents cannot lie in this position. Your facility may not include these exercises. Check with your supervisor and be sure you receive instruction before doing the additional exercises.

Carry out procedure completion actions. Report to the nurse any pain or change in range of motion of the resident's joints. Position resident comfortably.

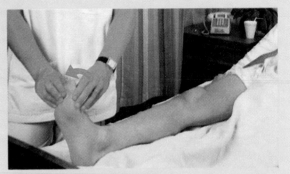

**FIGURE 22-47** Toe adduction. Move each toe toward the next toe.

## SELF RANGE OF MOTION EXERCISES

Self range of motion exercises are done by the resident. The resident can use a strong extremity to move a paralyzed or weak extremity (Figure 22-48). The physical therapist or restorative nurse will give you instructions if you are to assist a resident with self range of motion exercises.

## ACTIVE RANGE OF MOTION EXERCISES

Residents can do many exercises independently that involve movement of the joints. Many long-term care facilities have health and fitness trails within the facility that have several stations and instructions for the resident. Active range of motion exercises can also be done by residents in wheelchairs.

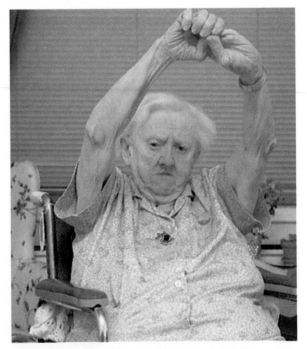

**FIGURE 22-48** The resident is using her stronger arm to raise her weak arm.

## POSITIONING THE RESIDENT··········

Residents who cannot move themselves about in bed need to be repositioned frequently. As a nursing assistant you will carry out these procedures several times a day. Three basic positions are: **supine** (lying on the back), **prone** (lying on the abdomen), and **lateral** (lying on either side). Each of these positions has variations.

Positioning procedures have several steps:

- Moving the resident's body so it is in correct body alignment
  - You may need to move the resident toward the head of the bed, the foot of the bed, or either side of the bed.
- Turning the resident to the desired position
  - To either the right or left side from the side, the back, or the abdomen
  - To the back from either side or the abdomen
  - To the abdomen from the back or other side
- Placing pillows or other supportive devices to maintain the position

### Purposes of Positioning

Positioning is done to:

- Improve circulation and respiratory function
- Maintain the resident's body alignment and good posture
- Prevent contractures, skin breakdown, pain, discomfort, thromboses, pneumonia, and edema
- Increase sensory stimulation. The sense of touch is stimulated when the assistant moves the resident. The sense of vision is stimulated when the resident is turned and sees a different part of the environment.

---

## *G*uidelines for
## Positioning

1. A firm mattress helps to maintain correct body alignment.
2. Lock the wheels of the bed before beginning the positioning procedure.
3. Raise the bed to a comfortable working height. Remember to lower the bed when the procedure is finished.
4. Raise the side rail on the other side of the bed unless there is another person helping you.
5. Use safety devices appropriately and *never* tie them to the side rails or bed frame. Tie them to the part of the bed supporting the mattress.
6. Handle the resident's body gently during mobility activities. Use the palms of your hands rather than your fingertips to support the extremities.
7. Incorporate range of motion exercises into positioning procedures. These exercises are in addition to those carried out routinely.
8. Encourage the resident's independence. Provide the assistance that is needed but avoid "overhelping."
9. Turn the resident at least every 2 hours. Inspect the skin for signs of breakdown each time. Gently massage around reddened areas with lotion. Rubbing over the area may cause further skin damage.
10. Use a turning sheet to move dependent residents in bed. This avoids friction and **shearing** the skin. Shearing occurs when the resident's body slides across the sheets; the skin moves in one direction as deeper tissues move in the opposite direction.
11. Support paralyzed extremities in extension. Prevent prolonged overstretching of weakened muscles. **Flaccid** paralysis means the extremity is limp and incapable of independent movement. **Spasticity** occurs in some paralyzed limbs. Spasticity can cause involuntary movements. It may cause the joints to assume positions

*(continues)*

## *G*uidelines *(continued)*

of flexion. Contractures can happen easily in spastic limbs.

12. Avoid dependent positions of extremities. The wrists and feet should never hang. This will cause edema (swelling).

13. Check incontinent residents each time you move them. If they have soiled the bed, cleanse them thoroughly. Change the sheets. Change clothing if soiled.

14. Tighten the sheets frequently. Wrinkles cause pressure areas on the resident's skin.

15. Items used for positioning are used only for a specific resident. Send sheets, pillows, and other washable items to the laundry as necessary. Do not let these items touch the floor.

16. Remember the privacy of the resident when completing all positioning procedures.

### Supportive Equipment

Supportive equipment may be needed to position the resident. The procedure must be adapted for residents with catheters or other tubes. You may need further instructions from the nurse for positioning residents with contractures.

**Postural supports** are devices to help maintain the resident in good posture and body alignment. Examples of postural supports include:

- Trochanter rolls
- Bath blankets
- Pillows of various sizes and shapes
- Bath towels
- Footboards
- Splints or slings, if ordered
- Turning sheet

Other postural supports are prescribed for specific residents for specific purposes (Figure 22-49). Be sure you know how to apply these devices correctly.

A trochanter roll is used to prevent external rotation of the hip. It is put in place when the resident is in supine (on the back) position. If the hip contracts in this position, the resident will be

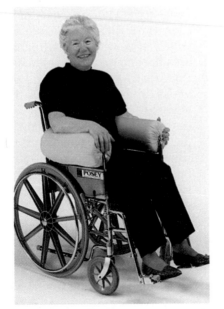
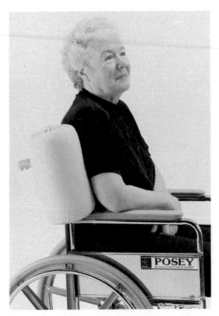

**FIGURE 22-49** Supports help position residents and maintain body alignment. (Courtesy of J. T. Posey Co., Inc., Arcadia, CA)

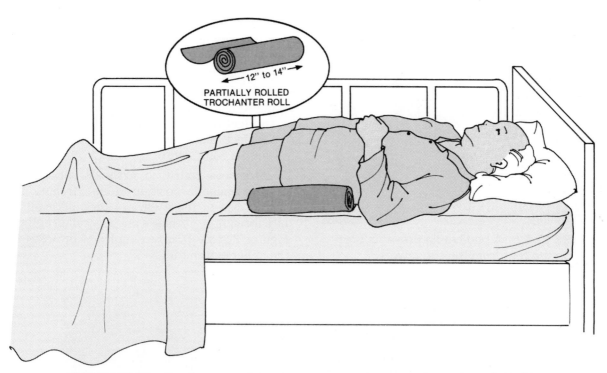

**FIGURE 22-50**   Trochanter roll in place to prevent external rotation of the hip

unable to move the leg. You can make a trochanter roll with a bath blanket:

- Fold the blanket in thirds, lengthwise. The roll needs to be 12 to 14 inches wide.
- The blanket is placed lengthwise under the resident's hips. Roll the end that is on the affected side *under* until it is firmly against the resident's body. It should extend from above the hip to just above the knee (Figure 22-50).

**Footboards** are sometimes ordered to prevent plantar flexion of the feet. This causes contracture of the ankle.

- The footboard should be well-padded, smooth, and firm.
- The footboard must extend 2 inches above the toes. This will prevent skin breakdown on the toes.
- The bottoms of the feet rest against the footboard to maintain position.

A folded pillow placed between the soles of the feet and the foot of the bed can take the place of a footboard. In some cases, a footboard may be harmful. For example, if spasticity is present in the legs, a footboard against the soles of the feet will stimulate spasticity and possibly

cause skin breakdown from the rubbing of the feet against the footboard. Special shoes worn in bed are sometimes used to maintain the feet in correct alignment (Figure 22-51). In most cases,

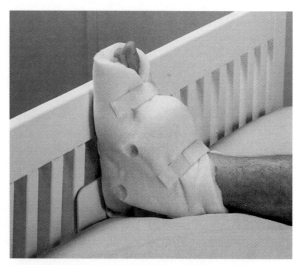

**FIGURE 22-51**   Special foot supports worn in bed prevent contractures of the ankle. (Bunny boot foot support is provided by Sammons Preston, Inc., a Bissell® HealthCare Company. Reprinted with permission.)

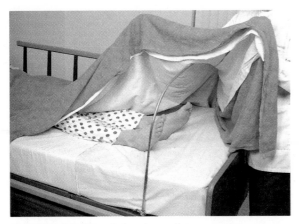

**FIGURE 22-52** A bed cradle prevents pressure on the feet from the top covers.

ankle contractures can be avoided by doing passive range of motion exercises consistently.

- A bed cradle (Figure 22-52) is placed on the bed over the resident's legs. The bed covers are placed over the bed cradle. This keeps the weight of the covers off the resident's legs and feet. It prevents the covers from forcing the feet into plantar flexion, which could cause a contracture.

A devices called an **orthosis** can also be used to maintain position of an extremity. The correct use of these devices prevents contracture formation. Orthoses are also called **splints**. Figures 22-53A–D are examples of orthoses for the upper extremities.

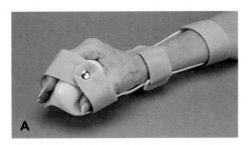

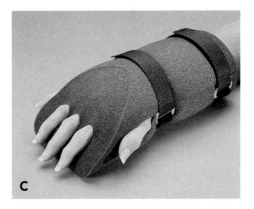

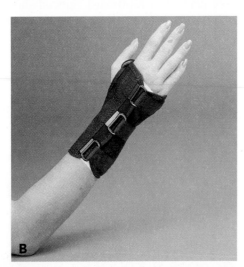

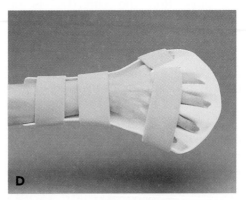

**FIGURE 22-53** A. This orthosis maintains the wrist and hand in neutral position. (Neutral Position® wrist/hand orthosis is provided by Sammons Preston, Inc. a Bissell® HealthCare Company. Reprinted with permission.) B. This is a cock-up wrist splint. (Cock-up wrist splint is provided by Sammons Preston, Inc. a Bissell® HealthCare Company. Reprinted with permission.) C. A soft, foam orthosis encourages and maintains normal extension of the wrist, fingers, and thumb joints. (Foam wrist/hand orthosis is provided by Sammons Preston, Inc. a Bissell® HealthCare Company. Reprinted with permission.) D. The antispasticity ball splint reduces spasticity by maintaining hand, fingers, and wrist in correct position. (Antispasticity ball splint is provided by Sammons Preston, Inc. a Bissell® HealthCare Company. Reprinted with permission.)

- The splint must be applied correctly. Follow the manufacturer's directions for each splint.
- Keep the splint clean. If it becomes soiled, check with the nurse to see how it should be cleaned.

The physician may also order splints or orthoses for the lower extremities. A common type is called the ankle stirrup (Figure 22-54). The stirrup provides support for an unstable ankle. The stirrup is applied to the lower leg before the shoe is put on.

When using splints:

- The splint may be ordered to be on and off the extremity at various times throughout the day. Be sure you know the correct procedure and schedule.
- Check the splint to be sure there are no pressure areas against the resident's skin.
- Folded washcloths should *never* be placed in the resident's hand. The rough surface of the cloth increases spasticity and the risk of contractures.

**Slings** are sometimes used to prevent a paralyzed arm from hanging. The force of gravity pulls on the weight of the arm, causing **subluxation**. This occurs when the shoulder joint separates (a **dislocation**). It is a permanent and

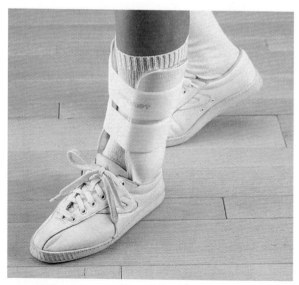

**FIGURE 22-54** This ankle stirrup reduces instability of the ankle. (Aircast® ankle stirrup is provided by Sammons Preston, Inc. a Bissell® HealthCare Company. Reprinted with permission.)

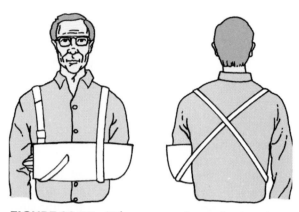

**FIGURE 22-55** When properly applied, a sling supports the wrist and does not pull on the resident's neck.

painful condition. A sling is not usually worn constantly because it forces the upper arm into a position of adduction and the elbow into flexion. If you apply a sling, remember:

- Read the manufacturer's instructions for application.
- Position the hands and fingers at about heart level.
- Support the hand and fingers with the sling. Avoid palmar flexion of the wrist.
- Check the sling for foreign bodies that may produce pressure spots.
- Position the sling to provide adequate support at the elbow so the shoulder is in good position.
- Apply the sling properly to prevent it from pulling on the resident's neck (Figure 22-55).

## TURNING THE DEPENDENT RESIDENT WITH A TURNING SHEET

A **turning sheet** is used to move a dependent resident in bed. Using a regular flat bed sheet:

- Fold the sheet in half, end to end.
- Place this on the resident's bed when the bed is made. Change it as needed.
- Place the folded side toward the head of the bed. Let the ends hang freely over the sides of the bed.
- Place it on the bed so that it extends from the resident's shoulders to knees.

## PROCEDURE 83

# Moving the Resident Toward the Head of the Bed

*Note:* A turning sheet should always be used to move dependent residents in bed. This avoids injury to the resident and the caregivers. *Always use the principles of good body mechanics to avoid injury to your back.*

1. Carry out each beginning procedure action.
   Remember to use disposable gloves if there may be contact with open lesions, wet linens, or body fluids.
2. Be sure the turning sheet is in place on the bed.
3. Two people are needed, standing on opposite sides of the bed. Three or four people may be needed if the resident is very heavy or has many restrictions (tubing, traction devices, etc.).
4. Before beginning this procedure:
   - The bed must be flat.
   - Raise it to a comfortable working height.
   - Fanfold the top covers to the foot of the bed. Do not expose the resident's bare body.
   - Remove all supportive devices from the bed.
   - Put the resident in supine position.
   - Cross the resident's arms over the chest or abdomen.
   - If the resident lacks head control, position the turning sheet to extend up under the head.
   - Remove the pillow under the resident's head and prop it against the headboard.
   - Keep your feet separated, your back straight, and your knees and hips flexed as you complete these procedures to avoid back injuries.

These directions apply to all assistants who are helping with this procedure. There are one or two assistants on each side of the bed, depending on the size of the resident.

5. Grasp the turning sheet at the level of the resident's shoulders and hips.
   - Using an overhand grasp, roll or gather the sheet until your hands touch the resident's body. Pull the sheet taut.
6. If the resident lacks head control, grasp the sheet at a level that allows you to maintain stability of the resident's head.
7. Position your body so you are facing the *foot of the bed* with your feet about 12 inches apart and your outer foot forward. (By facing the foot of the bed to move the resident to the head of the bed, you will be flexing your elbows and moving the resident toward you. This follows the principles of good body mechanics.)
   - Bend your knees and keep your back straight.
   - Get as close to the resident and bed as possible (Figure 22-56).

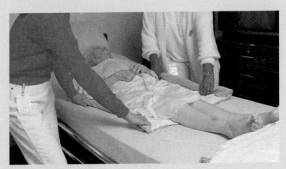

**FIGURE 22-56** Moving a resident up in bed with a turning sheet

*(continues)*

**PROCEDURE 83** *(continued)*

**8.** Before moving, place your weight on the forward foot.

- As you move, shift your weight to the other foot. (Avoid twisting. Move smoothly.)

**9.** One person gives the signal by counting to three.

- All persons move on the count of three, flexing their elbows and moving the sheet toward the head of the bed.

**10.** Position the resident according to directions and carry out procedure completion actions.

---

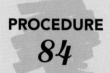

**PROCEDURE 84**

# Moving the Resident Toward the Foot of the Bed

**1.** Follow Procedure 83.
**2.** For Step 7, face the head of the bed with your outer foot forward. This allows you to flex your elbows, moving the resident toward you.

**3.** For Step 8, place your weight on the forward foot, shifting to the back foot. For Step 9, move the sheet toward the foot of the bed.
**4.** Complete Step 10.

---

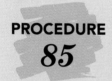

**PROCEDURE 85**

# Moving the Resident Toward the Side of the Bed

**1.** Follow Steps 1 through 6 for moving to the head of the bed (Procedure 83).
**2.** The assistant(s) on the side to which the resident will be moved has the heaviest load.

- This person places one foot forward (maintaining a broad base of support). Body weight is on this foot.

- As the resident is moved, body weight is shifted to the other foot.

**3.** The assistant(s) on the other side of the bed grasps the turning sheet to avoid dragging the resident's body. The person on this side does very little actual lifting.
**4.** Complete Steps 9 and 10.

## PROCEDURE 86   Turning the Resident to the Side

*Note:* Directions are given for turning the resident onto the right side. Reverse directions for positioning a resident on the left side.

1. Carry out each beginning procedure action.
2. Follow procedure for moving the resident to the head of the bed if necessary (Procedure 83). *Remember:* Keep your feet about 12 inches apart. Bend your knees and keep your back straight. Get as close to the bed and resident as possible.
3. Now move the resident to the left side of the bed, following Procedure 85. Assistants on both sides face the bed.
4. Move the resident's right arm away from the body.
   - Place the resident's left arm across the abdomen.
5. Cross the resident's left leg over the right leg.
6. To turn the resident without the turning sheet (turning the resident away from you):
   - The assistant on the resident's left side places the right hand so it cups the resident's left shoulder.
   - The other hand is placed so the palm is against the resident's hip (Figure 22-57).

*Note:* To turn the resident toward you, stand on the right side of the bed and place your hands as indicated (Figure 22-58).

7. If the resident is large, the assistant on the other side can place both hands beside the hands of the other assistant. On the count of three, turn the resident onto the right side.

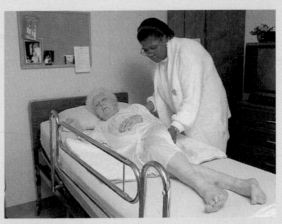

**FIGURE 22-57**   Turning the resident away from you

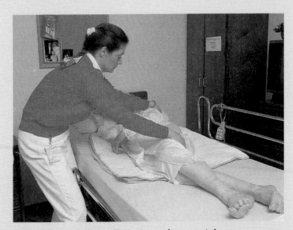

**FIGURE 22-58**   Turning the resident toward you

8. To turn the resident with the turning sheet:
   - The assistant on the resident's left side grasps the turning sheet at the shoulders and hips.
   - The other assistant reaches across the resident and grasps the turning sheet at the knees and waist.

*(continues)*

**PROCEDURE** *86* *(continued)*

9. The assistant on the right side bends elbows to pull the sheet so the resident is turned. The other assistant grasps the sheet to assist in the turn (Figure 22-59).
10. Complete positioning procedure (see Procedure 87).

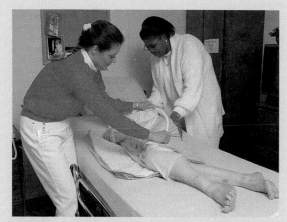

**FIGURE 22-59**   Turning the resident onto the side using a turning sheet

**PROCEDURE** *87*   Log Rolling the Resident onto the Side

*Note:* This procedure is used when the resident's spinal column must be kept straight. This technique may be used after spinal surgery or spinal injury. Directions are given for turning the resident onto the left side.

1. Carry out each beginning procedure action. Remember to use disposable gloves if there may be contact with open lesions, wet linens, or body fluids.
2. This procedure takes two or more people, depending on the size of the resident.
   • If the resident is small, two people can stand on the side to which the resident will be turning.
   • If the resident is large, another person can stand on the other side of the bed.

3. The bed is always kept flat for residents who need log rolling.
   • Elevate the bed to a comfortable working height.
   • Lower the side rails.
4. Make sure the turning sheet is in place under the resident. If the resident has poor head and neck control, the sheet should be wide enough to come up under the back of the head.
5. Place a pillow lengthwise between the resident's legs.
   • Fold the resident's arms over the chest.
   • The resident's back and legs must be straight throughout the procedure.

*(continues)*

**PROCEDURE** *87* *(continued)*

6. The assistant(s) on the left side reaches across the resident and grasps the turning sheet. The sheet should be folded until the assistants hands are close to the resident's body (Figure 22-60).

- They gently pull the sheet toward themselves until the resident is lying on the right side (Figure 22-61).
- If the resident is large and there is an assistant on the other side:
  - The assistant places one hand under the resident's left shoulder. The other hand is placed under the resident's left hip. As the other assistants move the resident onto the right side, this assistant helps by supporting the resident during the move.

7. Support the resident's body with pillows as needed. Be sure to maintain good body alignment.

8. Carry out procedure completion actions.

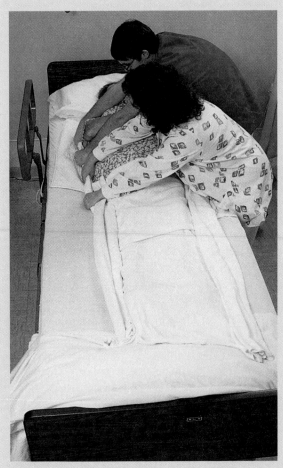

FIGURE 22-60 Begin log rolling the resident by grasping the turning sheet on the opposite side.

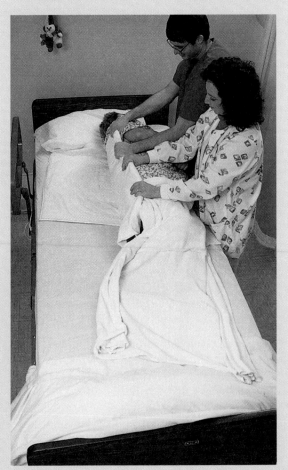

FIGURE 22-61 Pulling together, turn resident to side in one smooth movement.

# POSITIONING THE DEPENDENT RESIDENT ·····························

**PROCEDURE**

## 88   Supine Position

*Note:* This procedure should be used to position a resident who is paralyzed on one side of the body (hemiplegia). The instructions would apply to the paralyzed side. The resident should be encouraged to move the strong side. These directions are also appropriate for anyone in the supine position.

1. Carry out each beginning procedure action.
2. Refer to previous procedures for turning the resident onto the back and moving to the head of the bed. Head of bed may be slightly elevated.
3. Center a flat pillow under the resident's head. It should come down to the resident's shoulders. This will prevent too much neck flexion.
4. If the resident's leg(s) tend to fall into external rotation, place a trochanter roll under the affected hip or both hips, as directed under the section on supportive equipment.
5. Place a folded towel or small, flat pillow under each shoulder. Place the shoulders in slight abduction.
6. Place the shoulders and elbows in extension. (The arms will be straight.)
   - The forearm is pronated. (The palm of the hand is against the bed.)
7. Place a pillow under each arm that extends from the elbow to the ends of the fingers.
   - The wrist and the fingers should be extended with the fingers in slight abduction (separated).

- The hand, wrist, elbow, and shoulder on each side should be about the same distance from the bed.
8. Place a pillow under each leg, extending from the knee to the ankle. This prevents pressure on the heel.
9. Place a folded pillow between the end of the bed and the soles of the resident's feet (Figure 22-62).
10. Make sure the top covers are not pressing on the tops of the resident's feet.
11. Carry out each procedure completion action.

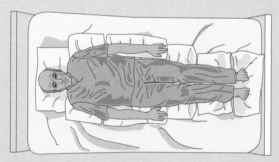

**FIGURE 22-62** Supine or dorsal recumbent position. Resident is flat on back. Bed is flat or head is slightly raised. Pillows are placed under resident's head, shoulders, arms/hands, calves, and ankles. Foot alignment is maintained. Trochanter rolls or rolled pillows placed along hips/thighs prevent external rotation.

## PROCEDURE *89*  Semisupine or Tilt Position

*Note:* Directions are given for the resident lying on the left side. This position prevents pressure on the sacrum, coccyx, and hip.

1. Carry out beginning procedure actions.
2. Gather equipment:
   - Pillows
3. Start with the resident in supine position. Roll the resident's trunk and shoulder away from you so that there is a 45° angle between the resident's back and the bed.
4. Place a pillow behind the resident's back for support.
5. Bring the resident's left shoulder forward. Flex the elbow of the left arm and place the lower left arm palm up on a pillow.
6. Flex the elbow of the right arm and bring the forearm across the chest with palm down.

7. Extend both legs. Place right leg a little behind left leg. Support right leg with two pillows. Pillows extend from groin to ankle (Figure 22-63).
8. Carry out procedure completion actions.

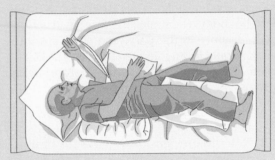

**FIGURE 22-63** Semisupine or tilt position. In this position, the resident is supported on the side with weight distributed across the shoulders. This position takes pressure off the sacrum, coccyx, and hip.

## PROCEDURE *90*  Lateral (Side-Lying) Position

*Note:* Directions are given for positioning a resident on the right side. Use the same guidelines for positioning on the left side. It is especially important that this procedure be followed when a resident with hemiplegia is positioned on the unaffected side.

1. Carry out each beginning procedure action.
2. Follow previous procedures for moving the resident to the head of the bed (Procedure 83), to the left side of the bed (Procedure 85), and onto the right side (Procedure 86).
3. Place a flat pillow under the resident's head. It should extend 3 to 4 inches beyond the resident's face.
4. When the resident is on his side, the bottom shoulder and hip should be in **protraction** (brought forward). This means

*(continues)*

**PROCEDURE 90** *(continued)*

you should not pull the shoulder and hip back. To do so will place the shoulder in **retraction** and eventually will cause contracture of those joints.

5. The right shoulder should be slightly abducted and can be in a position of internal or partial external rotation, or extension. For partial external rotation, it will need to be supported on pillows.

   • Use the position that is most comfortable for the resident.
   • Be sure the wrist and fingers are extended and fingers slightly abducted.

6. Slightly flex the right knee.
7. Support the left arm on pillows so that the resident's elbow and wrist are supported.

   • The left shoulder is protracted.
   • The elbow is very slightly flexed.
   • The hand is pronated (palm down).
   • The wrist and fingers are extended with fingers slightly abducted.
   • The shoulder, elbow, and wrist should be about the same height from the bed.

8. Support the left leg on pillows that extend from the knee to the foot.

   • Place the hip and knee in slight flexion. The hip is protracted.
   • The ankle, knee, and hip should all be about the same distance from the bed.

9. If the resident tends to fall back, place a pillow against the resident's back for support (Figure 22-64).
10. Place the top covers loosely over the resident.
11. Carry out each procedure completion action.

*Note:* The right (top) foot and hand should not dangle over the ends of the pillows.

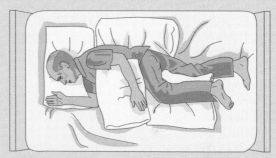

**FIGURE 22-64**   Lateral (side-lying) position. In this position, the resident's shoulders and pelvis are maintained in proper alignment.

---

**PROCEDURE 91** Lateral Position on the Affected Side

1. Follow Steps 1 through 4 in Procedure 90.
2. The affected (bottom) shoulder is protracted with elbow extended and forearm pronated.
3. The affected hip is protracted with hip and knee slightly flexed.
4. The unaffected side can be positioned as described in Procedure 90, *or*

5. If resident will be in this position only a few minutes, omit the pillows and encourage the resident to actively move these strong extremities.
6. Carry out each procedure completion action.

## PROCEDURE
## *92*  Semiprone Position

This position relieves pressure on the iliac crest and the greater trochanter. Directions are given for the resident lying on the left side.

1. Carry out beginning procedure actions.
2. Gather equipment:
   - Sheepskin
   - Pillows
   - Two foam blocks, each: $3 \times 6 \times 18$ inches
3. Place the sheepskin under the resident so it reaches from the shoulders to the knees.
4. Place the left arm in extension and tuck it slightly beneath the resident's body.
5. Place a pillow in front of and at right angles to the resident's chest.
6. Flex the resident's right knee and hip. Support with pillows that are parallel to the leg.
7. Grasp the resident's left arm from the back of the resident. Turn the resident onto the chest facing away from you. Gently pull the left arm toward you and push on resident's hip.
8. Extend the left arm upward and toward the head of the bed. Place it under the head pillow with the fingers and palm against the bed.

9. Flex the upper arm on a pillow.
10. Lift up the sheepskin and place a foam block under the sheepskin above the iliac crest.
11. Place the other foam block under the sheepskin just below the iliac crest (Figure 22-65). You should be able to slide your hand between the hip and the bed.
12. Carry out procedure completion actions.

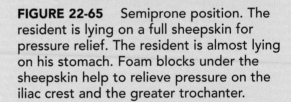

Sheepskin

**FIGURE 22-65** Semiprone position. The resident is lying on a full sheepskin for pressure relief. The resident is almost lying on his stomach. Foam blocks under the sheepskin help to relieve pressure on the iliac crest and the greater trochanter.

## PROCEDURE
## *93*  Fowler's Position

Fowler's position is a variation of supine position. In the semi-Fowler's position, the backrest of the bed is raised 30° from the horizontal position. For the Fowler's position, the backrest is raised 45° to 60° from the horizontal position. In the high Fowler's position, the backrest is at 90° from the horizontal position.

*(continues)*

## PROCEDURE *93* *(continued)*

*Note:* A resident at risk for skin breakdown along the lower spine and buttocks should not have the backrest elevated more than 30° (unless there is a nasogastric or gastrostomy tube in place or for 30 minutes after eating). A higher position causes shearing of the skin over the lower spine and buttocks.

This position is used most often for residents who have trouble breathing.

1. Carry out each beginning procedure action.
2. Use the turning sheet to move the resident's body into good alignment.
3. Raise the backrest to the desired level.
4. Place one, two, or three pillows behind the resident's head and shoulders.
5. The knees may be slightly flexed and supported with small pillows. This will prevent the resident from sliding down in bed.
6. A pillow can be placed between the resident's feet and the end of the bed.

7. Pillows may be placed under each arm. These should extend from the elbows to fingertips to support the shoulders (Figure 22-66).
8. Place top covers loosely over resident.
9. Carry out each procedure completion action.

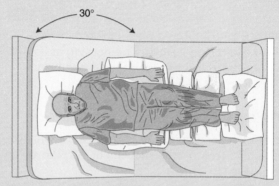

**FIGURE 22-66**   Fowler's position. In this position, the head of the bed is elevated at a low angle of 30° or 45° or at a high angle of 90°.

## Special Points for the Resident with Arthritis

Residents with **arthritis** (disease of the joints) are at risk for developing contractures. Be sure you avoid positions of flexion as much as possible.

1. Use a small, flat pillow under the head extending down to the shoulders.
2. Do not place pillows under the knees in supine position.
3. Prone position helps prevent flexion contractures of the hips and knees and should be considered for residents with arthritis.

## Special Points for the Resident with Lower Extremity Amputation

Hip flexion contractures can develop easily after a resident has a leg **amputation** (removal of a limb). Knee flexion contractures may develop in residents with below-the-knee amputations. To prevent these:

1. Avoid placing pillows under the **residual limb** (stump).
2. Keep the residual limb flat on the bed with knees extended (Figure 22-67).
3. Keep hips flat on surface of bed.
4. Keep legs adducted.

## Special Points for the Resident with Paralysis

1. If the affected extremities tend to go into flexion, use extension as much as possible when positioning.
2. If the affected extremities tend to go into extension, use flexion when positioning.
3. When paralysis is present in any resident (stroke, spinal cord injury, multiple sclerosis, etc.), use smooth, slow movements. This will avoid causing spasms.

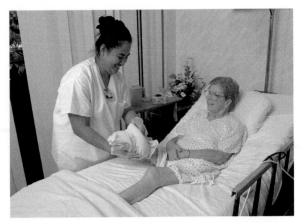

**FIGURE 22-67** Avoid placing the pillows under the residual limbs. The nursing assistant will place the residual limb flat on the bed.

## Bridging

Bridging is a technique that prevents pressure on a specific area by the placement of pillows or cushions.

1. Trochanter area
   - Place pillows under trunk and lower extremities when resident is on side, leaving trochanter area free from pressure.
2. Ankle
   - Support foot and lower leg, leaving ankle area suspended.
3. Heels
   - Support entire lower legs with pillows. Maintain good alignment of feet.
4. Sacrum
   - Support both sides of trunk and pelvis, leaving sacral area free from pressure.

## Positioning the Resident in a Chair or Wheelchair

Correct positioning for dependent residents sitting in chairs is just as important as it is when they are in bed. The resident's hips and knees should be at 90° angles. The feet should be flat on the floor (Figure 22-68). Pressure ulcers and contractures can occur just as readily in the chair. Wheelchairs are for transportation; they are not designed to be used for long periods of sitting. If this is unavoidable, be sure that the resident is allowed to stand and move about at intervals.

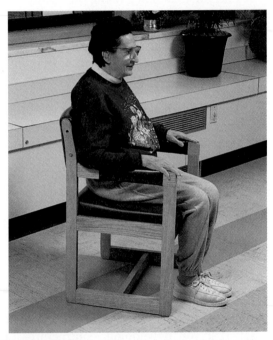

**FIGURE 22-68** Correct chair position maintains the elbows, hips, knees, and ankles at 90° angles.

**PROCEDURE**

## 94 Chair Positioning

1. Carry out each beginning procedure action.

2. Head and spine should be erect and in alignment.

*(continues)*

**PROCEDURE 94** *(continued)*

3. The resident's arms should rest on the arms of the chair or in the resident's lap. If the shoulders appear to be pushed upward:

   • Place a cushion on the chair seat. This raises the resident's body and allows for proper placement of the arms.

   If the shoulders appear to be hanging:

   • Place pillows or pads under the resident's lower arms.

4. The back of the wheelchair or other similar chair should come to the level of the resident's shoulder blades. If the back is too high:

   • Place a cushion on the chair seat to elevate the resident's body.

   If the back is too low:

   • Ask the nurse if an extension can be placed on the back of the chair to make it higher.

5. The back and buttocks should be back in the chair. The back and hips form a 90° angle.

   • A postural support may be needed to keep the hips back in the chair. Special flat pads can be placed between the resident's clothing and the chair to prevent sliding.

6. The upper and lower leg should form a 90° angle. The front edge of the seat should be about two fingers width away from the back of the knees. If the seat is touching the back of the resident's knees:

   • Place a cushion between the resident and the back of the chair. This will bring the resident forward.

7. The feet and ankles also form 90° angles. If the resident's feet do not touch the floor:

   • Place a footstool under the feet. This prevents plantar flexion of the ankle.
   • Place resident's feet on footrests of wheelchair.

8. Carry out each procedure completion action.

---

**PROCEDURE 95**

# Repositioning a Resident in a Wheelchair

Residents who slide down in a wheelchair will need to be moved back and up. You will need another assistant to help you. One stands in back of the wheelchair and one stands in front of the wheelchair.

1. Carry out each beginning procedure action.

2. Use good body mechanics: separate your feet and knees, bend your knees, and keep your back straight.

3. The assistant in back places both arms around the resident's waist.

   • He crosses his own arms in front of the resident's waist.

*(continues)*

**PROCEDURE 95** *(continued)*

- He grasps the resident's left forearm with his right hand and the resident's right forearm with his left hand.
4. The assistant in front places both arms around the resident's knees (Figure 22-69).
5. On the count of three, both assistants lift and raise the resident up and back in the chair.
6. Carry out each procedure completion action.

*Note:* It is helpful to place a lifting sheet (turning sheet) in the seats of chairs for residents who are very frail or heavy. With an assistant on each side, the sheet can be grasped to move the resident.

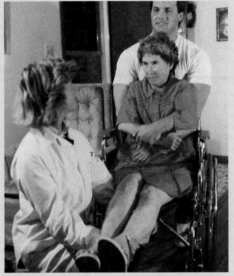

**FIGURE 22-69** Residents may need to be repositioned in their wheelchairs.

**PROCEDURE 96** Wheelchair Activities to Relieve Pressure

Residents who are in a wheelchair for longer than 1 to 2 hours need to relieve the pressure on the hips and buttocks. Teach them to do these activities. You may need to help dependent residents to do these.

**Leaning**
1. Lock the wheels.
2. Have resident lean slightly forward. (Do not let resident fall out of chair.)
3. Have resident lean from side to side, getting as much weight as possible off each hip.

**Wheelchair Pushups**
1. Raise the foot pedals. Make sure the resident does not stand on the pedals. Lock the wheels.
2. Tell the resident to place the palms of the hands on the arms of the chair. Then tell the resident to flex (bend) the elbows.
3. Have the resident lean forward, put the feet back, and spread the knees.

*(continues)*

**PROCEDURE** *96*  *(continued)*

4. Tell the resident to lift the buttocks off the chair by pushing down with the hands and straightening the knees (Figure 22-70).

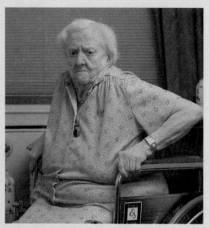

**FIGURE 22-70** Residents in wheelchairs can relieve pressure by doing wheelchair pushups.

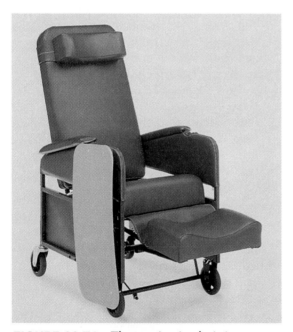

**FIGURE 22-71** The geriatric chair is designed to allow for position changes while maintaining body alignment and comfort. (Photo courtesy of Hill-Rom® Long Term Care Division)

Some long-term care facilities use geriatric chairs. These allow the resident's position to be changed (Figure 22-71).

Cardiac chairs are also frequently used for residents. These are similar to recliners. The resident may be placed in different positions. Pillows can be used to relieve pressure on the shoulders, arms, and hips (Figure 22-72).

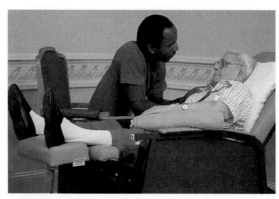

**FIGURE 22-72** Correct positioning in a chair is just as important as positioning in bed.

## INDEPENDENT BED MOVEMENT ····

The next step in progressive mobilization is to teach the resident how to move independently in bed. This provides exercise and prepares the resident to learn how to move into position to transfer out of bed.

The directions given here are for residents with hemiplegia. These directions can be used with any resident. You should not implement these procedures without instructions from the physical therapist or nurse.

---

**PROCEDURE**
**97**

# Assisting with Independent Bed Movement

1. Carry out each beginning procedure action.
2. Make sure the resident understands what you are going to do.
3. These directions are for moving to the head of the bed.
   - Instruct the resident to place his affected arm over his abdomen. Have resident grasp the side rail with his strong hand.
   - Have resident place his strong foot under his weak leg and then slide his strong foot down under his weak ankle. The weak leg will be supported by the stronger leg.
   - Tell the resident to flex the knee of his strong leg and push that foot against the mattress to help him lift his hips.
   - Have the resident raise his head and pull up with his strong arm and leg, pushing himself toward the head of the bed. (If resident is unable to support his weak leg, hold the leg off the bed while the resident moves. This avoids shearing and friction of weak leg against the sheet.)
4. Moving to the foot of the bed
   - Reverse procedure in Step 3.

5. Moving toward affected side, to side of bed
   - The resident moves segments of his body in sequence; legs and hips, head and shoulders. Order may be reversed.
   - Instruct the resident to place his affected arm over his abdomen.
   - Tell the resident to place his strong foot under the knee of his affected leg and slide it down under the affected ankle. Lift his affected leg and move it toward edge of bed on affected side.
   - Have the resident remove his strong foot and flex the knee of the strong leg. Now have the resident place his foot firmly on the bed and push down, raising his hips and moving them toward his affected side.
   - Tell the resident to raise his head and shoulders and move them toward his affected side by pushing against the mattress or side rail with his strong side. The resident can use his strong arm to push against the mattress to assist in the move.
6. Moving toward strong side, to side of bed
   - Follow above procedure, moving to strong side.

*(continues)*

**PROCEDURE *97* (continued)**

- Resident can use the strong arm to grasp side rail to assist in move.
7. Turning onto the side for lateral position.
    - If the resident is going to lie on the affected side, follow directions for moving to the *strong side first*.
    - Then have the resident use his strong arm to reach toward the opposite side rail to bring himself onto his side.
    - If the resident is going to lie on the strong side, follow directions for moving to *affected side first*. Have resident grasp his weak hand with his strong hand and raise his arms up with elbows extended. Then have resident use strong arm to "swing" body onto strong side.
8. When the procedure is completed, position the resident according to your instructions.
9. Carry out each procedure completion action.

## CONTINUING WITH PROGRESSIVE MOBILIZATION

It is important to complete passive range of motion exercises and positioning procedures correctly. This will prevent contractures and other complications that can prevent the resident from making progress in mobilization.

Transfer and ambulation activities are the next steps in progressive mobilization. Instructions for these procedures are in Lesson 23.

## BOWEL AND BLADDER PROGRAMS

Bowel and bladder programs are considered restorative/rehabilitation procedures. These programs are implemented for residents who are incontinent. **Incontinence** is the inability to control the bowel or the bladder (or both). Incontinence is not a disease and it is *never* a normal consequence of aging. There are a number of reasons why residents in the long-term care facility may be incontinent:

- The resident may be unable to get to the bathroom. This could be because of:
    - Disorientation
    - Impaired mobility
    - Physical environment—bathroom is too far away
- The resident may have a spinal cord injury.
- The resident may have problems holding urine in the bladder when coughing or laughing. This can be caused by:
    - Multiple childbirths
    - Obesity
    - Hormone deficiencies
- The resident may be unable to void and the bladder becomes full causing it to "overflow."

Incontinence causes many physical and psychological problems. It is embarrassing and may cause the resident to withdraw from all activities. Incontinence can quickly cause skin breakdown and urinary tract infections. It is difficult to avoid unpleasant odors when residents are incontinent. It is better to prevent incontinence than to try and deal with the consequences. Many different types of programs can be used for incontinence.

### Reasons for Implementing Bowel and Bladder Management Programs

1. To avoid incontinence
2. To reduce the resident's anxiety, fear, and embarrassment related to incontinence
3. To restore self-respect and dignity, which encourages the resident to participate more fully in facility activities

4. To prevent overfilling of the bladder and complications

5. To prevent urinary tract infections and skin problems

---

## Guidelines for

# Bowel and Bladder Programs

Before beginning a bowel and bladder program, the nurse will complete an assessment and then plan the program. A bladder retraining assessment form is shown in Figure 22-73. As a nursing assistant, you can help in the following ways:

1. Carry out all instructions accurately and on a timely basis.
2. Avoid the use of incontinent panties or pads during a retraining program.
3. Be consistent in carrying out the program.
4. Assist the resident to be well groomed and appropriately dressed at all times. This increases motivation to succeed.
5. Remember that comfort and privacy are important during all toileting procedures.

It may take several days for the assessment to be completed. Your responsibilities may be to:

1. Record the resident's daily fluid intake.
2. Check the resident for continence at least every 2 hours between 7:00 AM and 10:00 PM and every 4 hours during the night.
3. Record bowel eliminations and the amount of all voidings.
4. Record observations of symptoms that may indicate the reasons for the incontinence. This may include such problems as disorientation and inability to ambulate.

After the assessment is completed, the nurse will determine the type of program best suited to that resident. Program selection is based on the cause of the incontinence and the resident's:

- Mobility skills
- Orientation
- Motivation

In most cases, you will need to continue with the actions you carried out during the assessment. Different methods are used for each program. The programs may:

1. Restore a normal pattern of voiding by increasing the time between voiding.
2. Avoid incontinence by taking the resident to the bathroom according to the resident's habits. Positive reinforcement (giving praise) is important.
3. Avoid incontinence by taking the resident to the bathroom on a fixed voiding schedule, usually every 2 hours.

Other techniques are incorporated into each program. Your facility will have specific procedures to follow. It is important that all team members understand the procedures and the reasons for doing them faithfully.

Incontinence is not an inevitable problem in long-term facilities. Not all residents can be "retrained" but, in most cases, incontinence can be avoided. Catheters are not an alternative to incontinence except in very rare circumstances.

*(continues)*

*G*uidelines *(continued)*

## BLADDER RETRAINING ASSESSMENT
*(Reference tags: F315, F316)*

### CURRENT RESIDENT STATUS

DIAGNOSIS _____ RESIDENT'S AGE _____

RECENT SURGERY?  ☐ Yes  ☐ No  If Yes, date ____/____/____ and type _____

CURRENT MEDICATIONS (i.e., Diuretics, Psychotropics, etc.) _____
_____
_____

| Mental Status and Ability to Communicate | Mobility Status | Vision Status | Right | Left |
|---|---|---|---|---|
| ☐ Alert | ☐ Independent | Adequate | ☐ | ☐ |
| ☐ Aphasic | ☐ Transfer/standing ability | Adequate w/aid | ☐ | ☐ |
| ☐ Oriented x _____ | ☐ Wheelchair bound | Poor | ☐ | ☐ |
| ☐ Disoriented | ☐ Bed rest | Blind | ☐ | ☐ |
| ☐ Depressed | ☐ Contractures | **Hearing Status** | **Right** | **Left** |
| ☐ Cooperative | ☐ Other _____ | Adequate | ☐ | ☐ |
| ☐ Uncooperative | _____ | Adequate w/aid | ☐ | ☐ |
| ☐ Slow comprehension | _____ | Poor | ☐ | ☐ |
| ☐ Other _____ | _____ | Deaf | ☐ | ☐ |

### BLADDER ASSESSMENT

1. **LENGTH OF INCONTINENCE:**  _____ Days  _____ Months  _____ Years

2. **REASON FOR INCONTINENCE (if known):** _____
   **CATHETER:**  ☐ Yes  ☐ No  If Yes, specify type and size _____
   Date inserted ____/____/____ Reason for catheter _____

3. **USUAL VOIDING PATTERN:** Frequency _____ Amt./voiding _____ cc: /24 hrs. _____ cc
   Pattern:  ☐ Upon arising  ☐ After meals  ☐ No apparent pattern  ☐ Night time only
   ☐ Other (specify) _____

4. **SYMPTOMS:** (Check all that apply)
   ☐ Voids often in small amounts  ☐ Difficulty stopping stream  ☐ Urgency
   ☐ Fills bladder/voids large amount  ☐ Dribbles constantly  ☐ Burning/Pain
   ☐ Unable to void  ☐ Dribbles after voiding  ☐ Edema
   ☐ Difficulty starting stream  ☐ Dribbles while coughing  ☐ Other (specify) _____

5. **HISTORY OF:**  ☐ Urinary Disorders  ☐ Bladder Disorders  ☐ Kidney Disease  ☐ Prostate Problems
   ☐ Neurological Disorders  ☐ Fecal Impactions  ☐ Other (specify) _____

6. **RELIEF AFTER VOIDING:**  ☐ Complete  ☐ Continued desire to void

7. **BLADDER DISTENDED:**  ☐ Yes  ☐ No  **EMPTIED BY EXTERNAL STIMULI:**  ☐ Yes  ☐ No
   If Yes, Check:  ☐ Kegel Exercises  ☐ Warm water over perineum
   ☐ Other (specify) _____

8. **RESIDUAL URINE:**  ☐ Yes  ☐ No  If Yes, Amount: _____ cc

9. **PERCEPTION OF NEED TO VOID:**  ☐ Present  ☐ Diminished  ☐ Absent

10. **WELL HYDRATED:**  ☐ Yes  ☐ No  **AVERAGE FLUID INTAKE (24 HRS)** _____ cc
    **AVERAGE FLUID OUTPUT (24 HRS)** _____ cc

    Fluids Preferred _____

| NAME—Last | First | Middle | Attending Physician | Chart No. |
|---|---|---|---|---|

CFS 6-10HH  © 1992 Briggs Corporation, Des Moines, IA 50306  (800) 247-2343
Printed in U.S.A.

**BLADDER RETRAINING ASSESSMENT**
☐ Continued on Reverse

**FIGURE 22-73**  Bladder retraining assessment form (Reprinted with permission of Briggs Corporation, Des Moines, IA 50306 [800]247-2343)

*(continues)*

*G*uidelines *(continued)*

## EVALUATION FOR BLADDER RETRAINING POTENTIAL

☐ ABLE TO PARTICIPATE IN RETRAINING     EVALUATION PERIOD:_____ TO _____

PLAN: _____
_____

**PROVIDE FLUIDS:**          **FLUIDS SHOULD BE SPACED AS FOLLOWS:**

| _____ cc every 24 Hrs | ☐7AM | ☐11 | ☐3PM | ☐7 | ☐11PM | ☐3 |
| _____ cc 7-3 shift | ☐8 | ☐12N | ☐4 | ☐8 | ☐12MN | ☐4 |
| _____ cc 3-11 shift | ☐9 | ☐1PM | ☐5 | ☐9 | ☐1AM | ☐5 |
| _____ cc 11-7 shift | ☐10 | ☐2 | ☐6 | ☐10 | ☐2 | ☐6 |

OFFER NO FLUIDS AFTER ____ PM    TOILET FOR VOIDING EVERY ____ Hrs (Day and Evening)____ Hrs (Night)
(Except as needed for medications)
**RECORD RESULTS ON BLADDER RETRAINING RECORD.**

☐ UNABLE TO PARTICIPATE IN RETRAINING

REASON: _____
_____

REEVALUATION DATE: _____

COMPLETED BY: _____     __/__/__
                         Signature/Title                                                            Date

## BLADDER RETRAINING PROGRESS NOTES OR REEVALUATION NOTES

| DATE | TIME | NOTES - ALL ENTRIES MUST BE SIGNED WITH NAME AND TITLE |
|------|------|--------------------------------------------------------|
|      |      |                                                        |
|      |      |                                                        |
|      |      |                                                        |
|      |      |                                                        |
|      |      |                                                        |
|      |      |                                                        |
|      |      |                                                        |
|      |      |                                                        |
|      |      |                                                        |
|      |      |                                                        |
|      |      |                                                        |
|      |      |                                                        |
|      |      |                                                        |
|      |      |                                                        |
|      |      |                                                        |
|      |      |                                                        |
|      |      |                                                        |

| NAME—Last | First | Middle | Attending Physician | Chart No. |
|-----------|-------|--------|---------------------|-----------|

**BLADDER RETRAINING NOTES**

**FIGURE 22-73**  *(continued)*

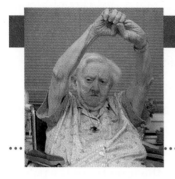

## LESSON SYNTHESIS: Putting It All Together

*Y*ou have just completed this lesson. Now go back and review the Clinical Focus. Try to see how the Clinical Focus relates to the concepts presented in this lesson. Then answer the following questions.

1. Why will you encourage Mrs. Murphy to do as much of her own care as possible?

2. If range of motion activities are not carefully and regularly carried out with her left arm and leg, what serious complication could develop?

3. When not being exercised, what is the proper position for Mrs. Murphy's affected arm and leg?

4. Before attempting to move Mrs. Murphy, what actions should the nursing assistant take?

## REVIEW

**A. Select the one best answer for each of the following.**

1. Restorative care is the responsibility of the
   a. physician
   b. nursing staff
   c. physical therapist
   d. occupational therapist

2. Activity strengthens and inactivity weakens is a principle of restorative care and means that
   a. complications result from physical and mental inactivity
   b. residents should receive several hours of bed rest each day
   c. residents are not encouraged to move about
   d. all of the above

3. Treat the whole person is a principle of restorative care and means that it is important to
   a. attend to the physical needs of the resident
   b. attend to the emotional needs of the resident
   c. attend to the mental needs of the resident
   d. all of these

4. Contractures can be prevented by
   a. doing range of motion exercises regularly
   b. using correct positioning techniques
   c. correctly applying splints
   d. all of these

5. An example of an instrumental activity of daily living is
   a. feeding oneself
   b. managing a household
   c. swimming
   d. riding a bicycle

6. A self-care deficit may be due to
   a. paralysis
   b. perceptual deficits
   c. depression
   d. all of these

7. The first step in progressive mobilization is teaching the resident to
   a. come to a standing position
   b. changing position in bed
   c. moving in bed
   d. moving about in a wheelchair

8. Passive range of motion means
   a. the care provider moves the joints for the resident
   b. the care provider supports the joints and assists in the movements while the resident attempts independent movement
   c. the resident is able to move the joints without any assistance
   d. the resident uses the strong extremity to move the affected extremity

9. An orthosis is (a, an)
   a. artificial body part
   b. sling
   c. splint
   d. none of the above

10. The purpose of an orthosis is to
    a. replace a missing body part
    b. simplify an activity of daily living
    c. help a person ambulate
    d. support a joint in correct position

11. The main purpose of bowel and bladder programs is to
    a. save time for the nursing staff so they do not have to change incontinent residents
    b. increase the resident's self-esteem and dignity
    c. save money on incontinent pads
    d. all of these

**B. Match each term (items a.–j.) with the proper definition.**

a. flexion
b. extension
c. abduction
d. adduction
e. rotation
f. pronation
g. supination
h. inversion
i. eversion
j. opposition

12. _____ bringing palmar surface of thumb to the finger joint

13. _____ bending a joint

14. _____ moving an extremity away from the body

15. _____ turning the forearm so the palm is facing downward

16. _____ straightening a joint

17. _____ turning inward

18. _____ moving an extremity back to the body

19. _____ turning around an axis

20. _____ turning the forearm so the palm is facing upward

21. _____ turning outward

**C. Answer each statement true (T) or false (F).**

22. T  F  It is a resident's right to have the staff do everything for him or her.

23. T  F  OBRA requires that restorative care be included in nursing assistant courses.

24. T  F  One purpose of restorative care is to help the resident adapt to limitations imposed by a disability.

25. T  F  Successful restorative care means that the resident always regains his or her functional abilities.

26. T  F  Restorative care generally involves training from physical therapists and occupational therapists.

27. T  F  Long-term inactivity can cause the heart to become deconditioned.

28. T  F  Restorative care is only important for residents who are planning to return to their homes.

29. T  F  Correct positioning can prevent pressure ulcers and contracture formation.

30. T  F  Incontinence is not considered a normal change of aging.

# Restoring Residents' Mobility

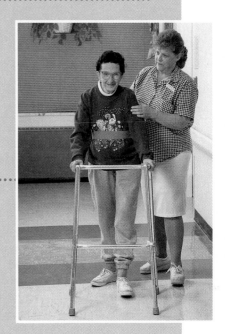

## CLINICAL FOCUS

Think about the special precautions you must take

to safeguard a resident during periods of mobility

as you study this lesson and meet:

*M*s. Peabody, who, although ambulatory with a walker since her hip surgery, is unsteady and needs assistance.

## OBJECTIVES

*After studying this lesson, you should be able to:*

- Define and spell vocabulary words and terms.
- List the guidelines for transfer procedures.
- State the contraindications to using a transfer belt.
- Describe the factors that are considered in determining the correct method of transfer.
- List the guidelines for ambulation procedures.
- Describe the purpose of assistive devices used in ambulation.
- Describe safety measures when using assistive devices.
- Demonstrate the following:
  Procedure 98   Using a Transfer Belt (Gait Belt)
  Procedure 99   Bringing the Resident to Sitting Position at the Edge of the Bed
  Procedure 100   Assisted Standing Transfer

Procedure 101   Transferring the Resident from Chair to Bed
Procedure 102   Assisted Standing Transfer/Two Assistants
Procedure 103   Wheelchair to Toilet Transfer
Procedure 104   Toilet to Wheelchair Transfer
Procedure 105   Transferring to Tub Chair or Shower Chair
Procedure 106   Transferring a Nonstanding Resident from Wheelchair to Bed
Procedure 107   Transferring Resident with a Mechanical Lift
Procedure 108   Sliding Board Transfer
Procedure 109   Ambulating a Resident
Procedure 110   Assisting Resident to Ambulate with Cane or Walker

# VOCABULARY

......................

ambulate  *(AM-byou-late)*

aneurysm  *(AN-you-rizm)*

assistive device  *(ah-SIS-tiv dih-VICE)*

colostomy  *(koh-LAHS-toh-mee)*

gait  *(gayt)*

gait belt  *(gayt belt)*

gait training  *(gayt TRAYN-ing)*

mechanical lift  *(mih-KAN-ih-kul lift)*

non-weight bearing  *(NON-wayt BAIR-ing)*

pacemaker  *(PAYS-may-ker)*

paraplegia  *(pair-ah-PLEE-jee-ah)*

partial weight bearing  *(PAR-shul wayt BAIR-ing)*

sliding board  *(SLYD-ing bord)*

transfer  *(TRANS-fer)*

transfer belt  *(TRANS-fer belt)*

weight bearing  *(wayt BAIR-ing)*

Many residents in long-term care facilities have impaired mobility. Mobility means movement. Restorative care includes assisting dependent residents with mobility and helping residents regain independent mobility.

In Lesson 22 you learned how to help residents regain independence in activities of daily living. You also learned how to perform procedures that will prevent the complications caused by immobility. The next step is to help residents get out of bed, to transfer, and to **ambulate** (walk).

Remember that restorative care is a team effort. While you are helping residents on the nursing unit, other departments are working with the residents to help them reach their goals for increasing their abilities (Figure 23-1).

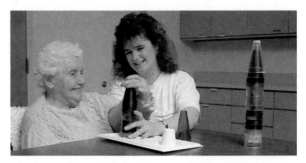

**FIGURE 23-1** Staff in occupational therapy direct the residents in activities that will help them regain the use of their hands.

The nurse or physical therapist determines the method of transfer. The method selected depends on:

1. The resident's physical condition including:
   * Paralysis of any extremity
   * Absence of an extremity due to amputation
   * Recent hip surgery
2. The resident's strength, endurance, and balance. These abilities may be affected by:
   * Respiratory disease
   * Cardiac disease
   * Neurologic disease
   * Ability to stand on one or both legs. This is called **weight bearing**. For example, a resident may not be able to bear weight on a paralyzed leg. After hip surgery the physician may order the resident to be **non-weight bearing** or to be only **partial weight bearing**.

## TRANSFERS ...................................

The word **transfer** means to move a resident from one place to another. Transfers are used to:

* Move a resident out of bed and into a chair
* Move a resident from a chair and into bed
* Move a resident from a wheelchair to a toilet or commode
* Move a resident from toilet or commode into a wheelchair
* Move a resident from a chair into a car and back
* Move a resident from a chair into a tub lift or shower chair and back into the chair

# *G*uidelines for

# Transfers

*Note:* Always use the correct transfer method as directed by the nurse or physical therapist. To disregard these instructions can result in injury to the resident or to you. If you have difficulty transferring a resident by the indicated method, consult with the nurse.

1. If the transfer requires two people, do not try to do it alone. You risk injuring yourself and the resident.
2. Use correct body mechanics for all transfers.
3. *Residents should never place their hands on your body during a transfer.* This is a dangerous practice. A resident who is disoriented or frightened can cause you to lose your balance. A resident who loses balance during transfer can pull you down. If a resident's arms are around your neck, any sudden movement can injure you.
4. *Never place your hands under a resident's arms.* Remember residents' bones

are fragile. This practice can fracture ribs and dislocate shoulders.
5. Use a transfer belt for standing transfers unless it is contraindicated (see Procedure 98).
6. The resident should wear sturdy, well-fitting shoes with nonslip soles for all standing transfers and ambulation.
7. Give the resident only the assistance needed.
8. Stand close to the resident when transferring. If the resident has a weak or paralyzed leg, brace that knee with your knee or leg.
9. Always transfer toward the resident's strongest side.
10. Allow the resident to see the surface to which the resident is being transferred. Encourage the resident to keep the head up.
11. Always explain to the resident what you are doing and how the resident can help.

3. The resident's mental condition. Can the resident understand instructions?
4. The resident's size

There are two basic types of transfer: standing and sitting. For a standing transfer, the resident

must be able to stand and have weight bearing on one leg. Examples of sitting transfers are those done with a mechanical lift or sliding board.

Several steps are involved in transferring a resident from bed to chair:

**PROCEDURE**

*98*

# Using a Transfer Belt (Gait Belt)

A **transfer belt** is a webbed belt $1\frac{1}{2}$ to 2 inches wide. It is 54 to 60 inches long. It is an assistive and safety device used to transfer or

ambulate residents who need help. When the belt is used to assist a resident with ambulation, it is called a **gait belt**.

*(continues)*

**PROCEDURE** *98* *(continued)*

1. Carry out each beginning procedure action.
2. Show the resident the transfer belt and explain that it is a safety device. Assure the resident that the belt is used only for a short time during the actual transfer or ambulation exercise.
3. The belt should never be placed over bare skin. If it is used to transfer a resident to a shower seat or tub lift, place a towel around the resident's waist and then apply the belt over it.
4. Keep the belt at the resident's waist level.
5. Buckle the belt in front—not at the back or the side (Figure 23-2A).

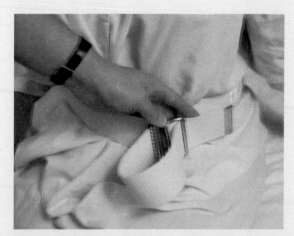

**FIGURE 23-2B** Thread the belt through the teeth side of the buckle first.

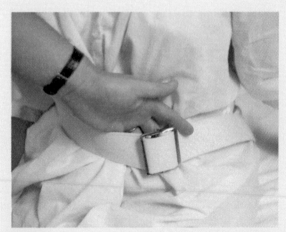

**FIGURE 23-2A** Buckle the transfer belt in front.

6. Thread the belt through the teeth side first and place belt through both openings to ensure a safe closure (Figure 23-2B).
7. Use an *underhand* grasp when holding the belt (Figure 23-3).
8. The belt should be snug but you should be able to get your fingers under it. This will prevent the belt from riding up under the breasts, rib cage, or axillae.
9. Check female residents to be sure breasts are not under the belt.

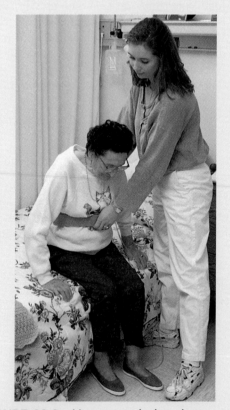

**FIGURE 23-3** Use an underhand grasp with a transfer belt.

*(continues)*

**PROCEDURE 98** *(continued)*

**10.** Avoid overusing the belt by pulling the resident up with too much force. *Remember:* The belt is not a lifting device—it is used for support and stability.

**11.** Transfer resident using correct method.

**12.** Carry out each procedure completion action.

*Note:* The transfer belt may be contraindicated for these conditions:

**1. Colostomy** located in the upper abdomen. This is a surgical opening created for the evacuation of feces.

**2. Pacemaker** located in the abdomen. This is a device used to maintain a normal heart rate.

**3.** Recent abdominal surgery

**4.** Recent back or rib fractures

**5.** Advanced cardiac disease

**6.** Advanced lung disease

**7.** Abdominal **aneurysms**. An aneurysm is a weak spot in an artery wall.

*Note:* Do not use the pants/slacks belt as a transfer or gait belt when transferring or ambulating residents. Upward movement of the belt can cause male residents severe pain in the scrotum.

- Bringing the resident to a sitting position on the edge of the bed
- Bringing the resident to a standing position
- Moving the resident to the chair
- Seating the resident

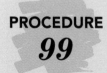

**PROCEDURE 99**

# Bringing the Resident to Sitting Position at the Edge of the Bed

**1.** Carry out each beginning procedure action.

*Note:* You may be asked to check the resident's pulse before beginning any activity. If so, take the pulse now.

**2.** If you will be transferring the resident into the chair:

- Have the chair ready to receive the resident. If it is a wheelchair, lock the brakes. Put the foot pedals up or remove them if possible. If the arm of the chair is removable, it is easier to work with it off.
- Have the resident's clothing and shoes ready.
- Have the transfer belt ready if it is to be used.

*Note:* If the resident is to transfer out of the bed, the bed must be in the low position. *Remember to use correct body mechanics.*

*(continues)*

PROCEDURE **99** *(continued)*

3. Begin with the resident lying in supine position in the center of the bed.

4. Have the resident cross arms over the abdomen or chest.

5. Cross the resident's farthest leg over the leg nearest you.

6. Stand facing the bed with your thigh that is nearest the resident's head braced against the bed. *Bend your knees and hips. Assume a broad base of support. Get close to the resident.*

7. With one hand on the resident's far shoulder and one on the far hip, turn the resident onto the side, facing you (Figure 23-4).

8. Flex the resident's hips and knees.

9. With your arm that is closest to the resident's legs, reach across the top leg and secure both legs with your arm.

10. Place your other arm so that your forearm supports the resident's shoulders. The resident's neck and head are cradled by your elbow.

11. As you shift your weight from your front to back leg, lower the resident's legs over the edge of the bed. At the same time, bring her head and shoulders to upright position (Figure 23-5).

*Note:* If the resident is able to, ask the resident to use the lower arm to support the upper body. Ask the resident to use the upper arm to push into the mattress to raise the upper body.

12. Carry out transfer as indicated in the next procedures.

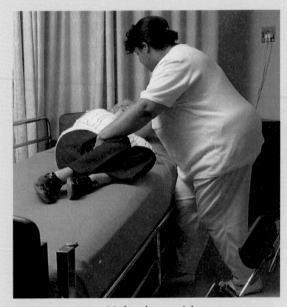

**FIGURE 23-4** Help the resident turn to the side before sitting on the edge of the bed.

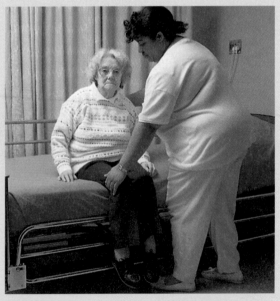

**FIGURE 23-5** Help the resident to a sitting position on the edge of the bed.

## PROCEDURE *100* Assisted Standing Transfer

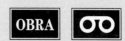

*Note:* The bed should be in the low position when you transfer a resident into or out of bed. You must use good body mechanics—keep your back straight, bend from the knees and hips, and maintain a broad base of support.

1. Carry out each beginning procedure action.
2. The chair is placed on the resident's strong side. Place it at the foot or the head of the bed and parallel to the bed.
3. If you are using a wheelchair, lock the brakes. The front casters of the chair should be straight. Put the foot pedals up or remove them from the chair.
4. Lock the wheels of the bed.
5. Check the resident's pulse if instructed to do so. Bring the resident to a sitting position on the edge of the bed as directed in Procedure 99. Allow resident to sit for a few seconds to stabilize.
6. Put a transfer belt around the resident's waist.
7. Put shoes and socks on the resident.

*Note:* If you are unsure of the resident's balance, you can put the transfer belt on while the resident is lying down. You can also put the shoes and socks on at that time.

8. Tell the resident what to do to help.
9. Assist the resident to assume the transfer position:
   - Ask the resident to lean forward ("nose over toes").
   - Have resident separate the knees for a broad base of support.
   - Have resident move the feet back.

*Note:* Be sure to check the resident's feet before transferring. Some residents are unable to tell what position their feet are in.

- Ask the resident to place the palms of the hands against the edge of the mattress. This will help the resident to "push off," (see Figure 23-3).
10. Place yourself in front of the resident. If the resident has a weak or paralyzed leg, brace that knee with your knee.
11. Place your other leg several inches back.
12. Place your hands in the transfer belt (underhand grasp) with one hand on each side of the resident's body.
13. If the resident has a weak or paralyzed arm, do not let it hang or dangle during the transfer.
    - If the resident has a sling, put this on before the transfer.
    - If there is no sling, the hand can be placed in the pants pocket or the resident can cradle the weak arm with the strong arm.
14. Before moving the resident, make sure both you and the resident are ready to move.
15. Tell the resident that on the count of three she will:
    - Use the hands (if able) to press into the mattress.
    - Straighten the elbows.
    - Straighten the knees and come to a standing position.
16. At the same time, you will use the transfer belt to gently assist the resident to stand—do not lift the resident with the belt.
    - Remember, the resident should not grasp your neck, arms, or any part of your body. You should not use your hands and arms on the resident's body.

*(continues)*

**PROCEDURE** *100* *(continued)*

**17.** If the resident cannot take any steps:
- Have resident pivot around to the front of the chair until the chair touches the back of the resident's legs.

**18.** Instruct resident to place hands on the arms of the chair and then gently lower resident into the chair (Figure 23-6).

**19.** If you took the resident's pulse before the activity, recheck it now. If there is a significant difference, report this to the nurse.

**20.** Position the resident comfortably. Place the signal light within easy reach. Be sure the resident has access to drinking water and any other items that may be needed.

**21.** Carry out each procedure completion action.

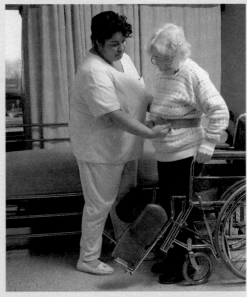

**FIGURE 23-6** Instruct the resident to place her hands on the arms of the chair and then gently lower resident into chair.

**PROCEDURE**
*101* Transferring the Resident from Chair to Bed

*Note:* Use good body mechanics—keep your back straight, bend from the knees and hips, and maintain a broad base of support with your feet.

**1.** Reverse Procedure 100.

**2.** If the resident has a weak or paralyzed side, place the wheelchair so that the resident can transfer to the strong side. Lock the brakes on the wheelchair and remove the footrests.

**3.** Lock the wheels on the bed.

**4.** Place the transfer belt around the resident's waist.

**5.** Have resident assume the transfer position as described in Procedure 100.

**6.** Follow Steps 10 through 14 in Procedure 100.

**7.** Tell the resident to place the hands on the arms of the wheelchair or chair.

**8.** On the count of three, have resident straighten both elbows and knees to come to a standing position.

*(continues)*

**PROCEDURE** *101* *(continued)*

9. Pivot around to the bed. When the resident feels the bed against the backs of the legs, have resident slowly sit down on the edge of the bed.
10. Remove the transfer belt and the resident's shoes and socks. If balance is questionable, this can be done after the resident is lying down.
11. Place your arm closest to the head of the bed around the resident's shoulders. Place your other arm around the resident's knees (Figure 23-7).
12. Guide the resident to a supine position. Position the resident comfortably.
13. Carry out each procedure completion action.

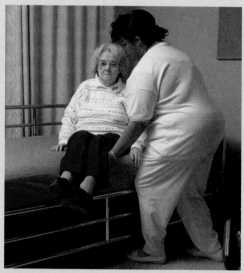

**FIGURE 23-7**   Assist the resident to lie down.

**PROCEDURE** *102*   Assisted Standing Transfer/Two Assistants

*Note:* This procedure is for a resident who is heavier, taller, has impaired balance, or only partial weight-bearing ability.

Follow your instructions when you are told that two people are required to move or transfer a resident. To disregard instructions can result in serious injury to you and the resident. *Remember:* Use good body mechanics—keep your back straight, bend from the knees and hips, and maintain a broad base of support with your feet.

1. Carry out each beginning procedure action.

This procedure is carried out the same as a one-person transfer except:

2. Both assistants stand in front of and to each side of the resident.
3. Both assistants put both hands in the transfer belt. Each assistant has one hand in the front of the belt and one in the back of the belt (Figure 23-8).

*(continues)*

**PROCEDURE 102** *(continued)*

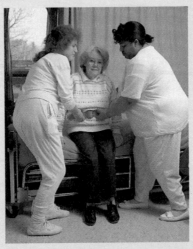

**FIGURE 23-8**  Some residents need the help of two nursing assistants. The nursing assistants have both hands in the transfer belt.

4. If the resident has a paralyzed leg, one assistant blocks that leg with her knee against the resident's knee.

It is important that both assistants and the resident clearly understand the direction of the move.

5. On the count of three, both assistants and the resident pivot around to the chair.
6. Continue procedure as with one assistant.
7. Carry out each procedure completion action.

---

**PROCEDURE 103**  Wheelchair to Toilet Transfer

*Remember:* Use good body mechanics—keep your back straight, bend from the hips and knees, and maintain a broad base of support with your feet.

1. Carry out each beginning procedure action.
2. You may need to adapt the procedure to the physical arrangement of the bathroom.
   • Grab bars should be placed securely on the wall or attached to the toilet seat (Figure 23-9). *Towel bars are not safe to use as grab bars.*
3. Most toilets are 16 inches high. Some residents may have difficulty coming to a

standing position from this level. A raised toilet seat can be added, which will raise it to 20 inches.
4. Follow all the guidelines for transfers. Use the transfer belt.
5. Place wheelchair at a right angle to the toilet. Lock the brakes. Be sure the foot pedals are up or off.
6. While the resident is still sitting, loosen clothing.
7. Bring resident to a standing position as described earlier.
   • Ask the resident to lean forward.
   • Have the resident separate knees for a broad base of support.

*(continues)*

**PROCEDURE *103* (continued)**

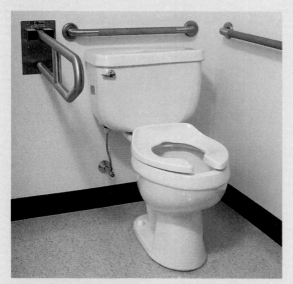

**FIGURE 23-9** Grab bars provide safety.

- Have the resident move the feet back.
- Have resident place palms of the hands on the wheelchair arms to help "push off."
- On the count of three, help the resident to a standing position (Figure 23-10).

8. Encourage the resident to stand erect. Pivot to toilet seat.
9. Have resident use the grab bars for support while you manipulate the clothing. If the resident's balance is questionable, you will need another assistant to do this while you help the resident stand.

10. With your hands in the transfer belt, assist the resident to sitting position on the toilet.
11. Remove transfer belt. Provide privacy, but remain close by. See Procedure 104.

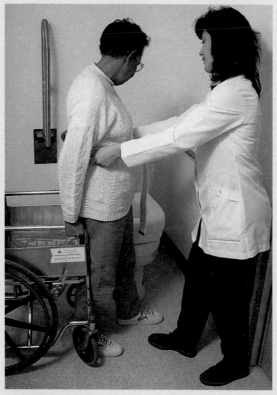

**FIGURE 23-10** Help the resident to a standing position.

**PROCEDURE *104*** Toilet to Wheelchair Transfer

*Remember:* Use good body mechanics—keep your back straight, bend from the hips and knees, and maintain a broad base of support with your feet.

*(continues)*

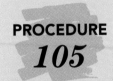

**PROCEDURE** *104* *(continued)*

1. Assemble equipment.
   - Disposable gloves
   - Wheelchair
   - Toilet tissue
   - Transfer belt
2. Follow all guidelines for transfers. Put transfer belt on resident.
3. Position wheelchair at a right angle to toilet. Lock the brakes. Be sure the foot pedals are up or off. If possible, place wheelchair on resident's strong side.
4. Have toilet tissue ready.
5. Put on gloves.
6. Bring resident to standing position. Have resident use grab bars while you clean resident's buttocks and genitalia.
   - If resident is able, provide support while the resident performs this task.

7. Arrange clothing while resident is still using the grab bars for support.
8. Assist the resident to pivot to the wheelchair.
   - Have resident put hands on the arms of the chair.
   - When resident feels the edge of the seat against the back of the legs, have the resident slowly sit in the chair.
   - Your hands are still in the transfer belt so you can provide assistance.
9. Wheel the chair to the lavatory. Assist the resident in washing and drying hands.
10. Remove your gloves. Wash and dry your hands.
11. Carry out each procedure completion action.

**PROCEDURE** *105*

# Transferring to Tub Chair or Shower Chair

*Remember:* Use good body mechanics—keep your back straight, bend from the hips and knees, and maintain a broad base of support with your feet.

The procedure for transferring a resident from a wheelchair to a tub chair or shower chair is carried out in the same manner as a transfer from a wheelchair to toilet or chair with added considerations.

1. Carry out each beginning procedure action.
2. Transport the resident to the shower or tub room by wheelchair (Figure 23-11).

3. Lock wheelchair. Remove footrests.
4. Remove the resident's top clothing while resident is seated in the wheelchair.
5. Leave the resident's shoes on until the resident has transferred to the shower or tub chair.
   - Place a large towel around the resident's shoulders to avoid chilling and exposure.
   - Place a towel around the resident's waist before applying transfer belt. Apply transfer belt.
   - Assist the resident to stand.

*(continues)*

## PROCEDURE *105* (continued)

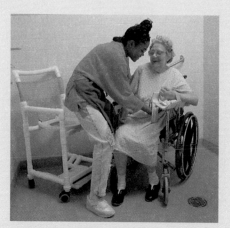

**FIGURE 23-11** Transport the resident to the shower or tub room by wheelchair.

- Have resident pivot around or take a step to the shower or tub chair.
- Loosen and bring underwear and slacks down below resident's hips.

6. Have resident sit down in shower chair or tub chair. Remove underwear, slacks, shoes, and socks.

7. Place towel over resident's lap.
8. Remove transfer belt. When shower/bath is completed, reverse procedure.
9. Dry resident while seated in tub or shower chair.
10. Help resident put on upper body clothing while seated in tub or shower chair. Then apply transfer belt.
11. Put resident's underwear and slacks on.
    - Pull up to the hips.
    - Put on socks and shoes.
12. Assist resident to stand. Pull up underwear and slacks.
13 Assist resident to pivot or step to wheelchair.
    - When the resident feels the wheelchair against the back of the legs, have resident place hands on arms of wheelchair.
    - Then have resident slowly seat self in wheelchair.
14. Carry out each procedure completion action.

---

**PROCEDURE *106***

# Transferring a Nonstanding Resident from Wheelchair to Bed

This procedure is used for residents who are unable to stand. The resident must be able to follow directions. This is not an appropriate transfer for a resident who is large. The procedure requires two assistants. It should only be done when the wheelchair has removable arms and removable footrests.

*Remember:* Use good body mechanics—keep your back straight, bend from the hips and knees, and maintain a broad base of support with your feet.

1. Carry out each beginning procedure action.

*(continues)*

**PROCEDURE** *106* *(continued)*

2. Lock wheels of bed. Put bed in lowest horizontal position.
3. Remove arms from wheelchair. Remove footrests from wheelchair. Place wheelchair at head of bed facing foot of bed. Wheelchair should be parallel to bed.
4. The first assistant stands behind the wheelchair. The second assistant stands in front of the wheelchair.
5. The first assistant places arms around resident's trunk. This assistant crosses arms and grasps the resident's left forearm with assistant's right hand. The resident's right forearm is grasped with the assistant's left hand.
6. The second assistant stands beside resident's legs, facing bed. This assistant places both arms under resident's legs.
7. Remember to use good body mechanics. On the count of three, the resident is lifted out of the chair and into bed.
8. Position resident as necessary.
9. Carry out each procedure completion action.

## USING MECHANICAL LIFTS

A **mechanical lift** may be needed to transfer certain residents. This device is used to move residents who are unable to bear weight, are heavy, or have poor trunk control. Remember these precautions when using a mechanical lift:

- *Two people are required for this procedure.*
- Be sure both people have been instructed in the correct procedure before attempting to use a mechanical lift with residents.
- The procedure may vary depending on the manufacturer of the equipment.
- Be sure the equipment is in good working order.

**PROCEDURE** *107* Transferring Resident with a Mechanical Lift

1. Carry out each beginning procedure action.
2. Get another assistant or nurse to help you. One person operates the lift. The other person guides the sling and resident.
3. Check sling and straps for frayed areas or poorly closing clasps.
4. Place a wheelchair or other chair parallel to bed, facing the head of the bed.
5. Lock the bed. Lock the wheelchair or other chair wheels.
6. Position the sling under the resident's body by rolling him first onto his left side. Place the folded sling against his body (Figure 23-12).
7. Roll resident onto his right side and straighten the sling (Figure 23-13).
8. Make sure that the sling reaches from his shoulders to his knees (Figure 23-14).

*(continues)*

**PROCEDURE** *107* *(continued)*

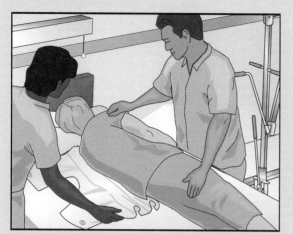

**FIGURE 23-12**  Position sling under the resident's body by rolling him first onto his left side. Place folded sling against his body.

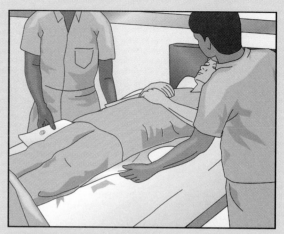

**FIGURE 23-14**  Make sure that the sling reaches from his shoulders to his knees.

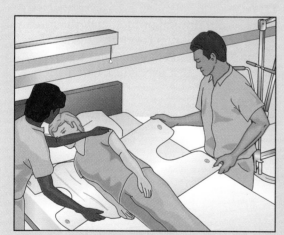

**FIGURE 23-13**  Roll resident onto his right side and straighten sling.

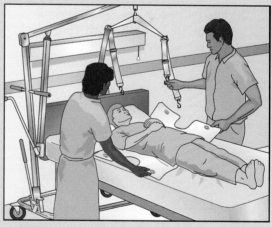

**FIGURE 23-15**  Position the lift over the bed and attach the hooks to the sling.

9. Position the lift over the bed and attach the hooks to the sling (Figure 23-15). Make sure that the open end of each hook is turned away from the resident's body (Figure 23-16).

10. Raise the lift following the directions for the specific type of lift used at your facility. Gently swing the resident to the chair. One nursing assistant can support the resident's legs (Figure 23-17).

*(continues)*

PROCEDURE *107* *(continued)*

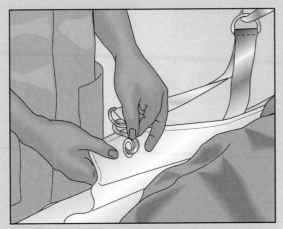

**FIGURE 23-16** Make sure that the open end of each hook is turned away from the resident's body.

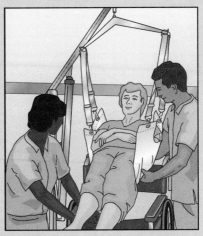

**FIGURE 23-17** Raise the lift following the directions for the type of lift used at your facility. Gently swing resident into chair.

11. Lower the lift and seat the resident in the chair. Unhook suspension straps and move lift out of the way. The sling may be left under the resident until he is ready to be lifted back into bed (Figure 23-18).

12. Position resident as necessary. Place signal light, drinking water, and other items as needed within resident's reach. Make sure resident is covered and warm.

13. Carry out each procedure completion action.

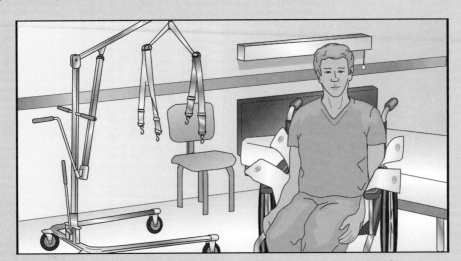

**FIGURE 23-18** Lower the lift and seat the resident in the chair. Unhook suspension straps and move lift out of the way. The sling may be left under the resident until he is ready to be lifted back into bed.

## SLIDING BOARD TRANSFER ············

A **sliding board** (Figure 23-19) is used for a sitting transfer. The board should be smooth and waxed to ease movement. This procedure is used for residents who are paralyzed in both legs (**paraplegia**) or who have had both legs amputated. It can be used for other residents who are non-weight bearing as designated by the nurse or physical therapist. The resident must have stability of the upper body for this type of transfer.

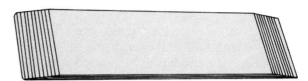

**FIGURE 23-19**  Sliding boards are used for some types of transfers.

*G*uidelines for

## Sliding Board Transfers

1. The two transfer surfaces should be at the same level.
2. The wheelchair must have removable, swing-away, or lift-off footrests and removable armrests.
3. Residents with adequate upper body strength may eventually be able to do this transfer independently.
4. The resident must be dressed for this transfer so that the buttocks and backs of the upper legs are completely covered. Never attempt to transfer a resident across the sliding board if there is a possibility that bare skin will contact the board.
5. Position wheelchair so resident can transfer toward strong side.
6. Place a transfer belt around resident's waist.
7. Lock the wheelchair and the bed.

**PROCEDURE**
*108*  Sliding Board Transfer

1. Carry out each beginning procedure action.
2. Place wheelchair at slight angle next to bed. Remove armrest and footrest on side next to bed.
3. Bring resident to sitting position on edge of bed as described in Procedure 99. Apply transfer belt.
4. Position sliding board so one end is on wheelchair and the other end is just under the resident's buttocks. *The beveled side of the sliding board is facing up.*
5. Stand in front of the resident. Assume a broad base of support with your knees and hips flexed and your back straight.

*(continues)*

**PROCEDURE 108** *(continued)*

6. Using an underhand grasp, grasp the belt on each side of the resident.
7. Slide the resident across the board and into the chair.
8. Remove the board from under the resident. Remove the transfer belt.
9. Replace the armrest and footrest.
10. Reposition resident in wheelchair if necessary. Make sure signal light and any items the resident may need are within reach.
11. Carry out each procedure completion action. To return resident to bed, reverse the procedure.

## AMBULATION

Ambulation is the process of walking. It is good exercise for the resident. The weight bearing on the legs helps prevent or delay the onset of disuse osteoporosis. Walking increases the resident's independence and provides more opportunities for socializing and activities.

The term **gait** refers to the way in which a person walks. There are many disorders that can affect a person's gait such as:

- Stroke—one side of the body is paralyzed (hemiplegia).
- Multiple sclerosis—one or both legs are weakened and balance may be disturbed.
- Huntington's disease—the resident has involuntary movements disturbing balance.
- Parkinson's disease—the resident has stiffness and slowness of movements causing shuffling.
- Arthritis—resident has pain and stiffness in joints.

### Evaluation by the Nurse or Physical Therapist

Before an ambulation program is started, the nurse or physical therapist will evaluate the resident's:

- Tolerance to movement in bed
- Ability to participate in active (as opposed to passive) exercise
- Ability to transfer safely with minimal assistance
- Ability to stand and bear weight

- Strength, endurance, and balance
- Mental state to determine if the resident can follow directions
- Ability to walk alone or whether the assistance of a person or equipment is needed

### Normal Gait Pattern

There are two phases to a normal gait (walking). The leg is on the floor during the first phase and the leg is brought forward during the second phase. Walking begins with the ankle in dorsiflexion and the heel striking the floor first (Figure 23-20), rolling onto the ball of the foot. The resident must be able to stand straight on this leg while bringing the other leg forward. The arms are normally in a slight swinging movement during walking. Each arm moves in the same direction as the opposite leg (Figure 23-21). To walk safely, the resident must have adequate joint motion in the hips and knees and strength in the muscles of the hips, buttocks, and legs. The physical therapist may work with the resident on exercises to promote movement and strength before the resident starts walking.

### Gait Training

The physical therapist may work with the resident on **gait training** (teaching the resident to walk).

The physical therapist will teach the resident how to:

- Walk correctly
- Walk on different surfaces such as linoleum floors, carpet, grass, gravel

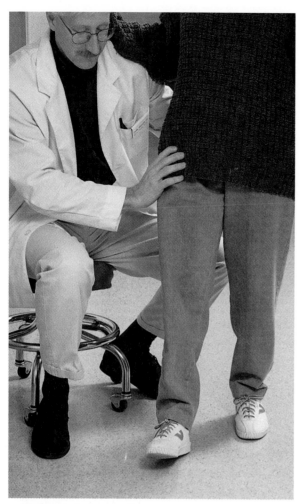

**FIGURE 23-20**  Walking begins with the ankle in dorsiflexion. The heel strikes the floor first.

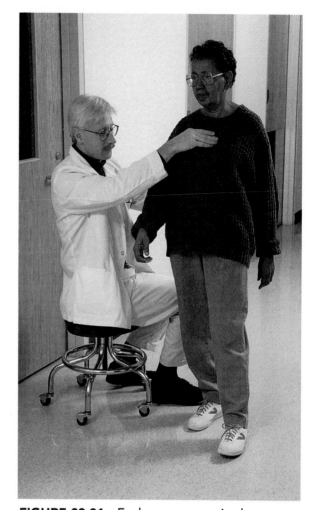

**FIGURE 23-21**  Each arm moves in the same direction as the opposite leg during walking.

- Manipulate stairs (Figure 23-22)
- Get in and out of a chair
- Use an assistive device if one is ordered

### Assistive Devices

An **assistive device** is often prescribed. These devices include crutches, canes, and walkers. An assistive device can help compensate for problems the resident has with walking. Several types of crutches, canes, and walkers are used. The needs of the resident and the cause of the problem are factors in selecting the device. The nurse or physical therapist will adjust the device to fit the resident. The gait used with the device is determined by the resident's abilities,

the cause of the impairment, and the type of assistive device. The nurse or physical therapist will select the appropriate gait. You should know the gaits that have been selected. When you walk with the resident you can then observe to make sure the resident is using the device correctly.

### Safety Guidelines for Using Assistive Devices

All canes, crutches, and walkers have rubber tips on the bottoms and rubber handgrips. (Figure 23-23). These must be replaced if the ridges are cracked, loose, or worn down. If the ridges are filled with debris, use alcohol and cotton swabs to clean them. Replace any loose

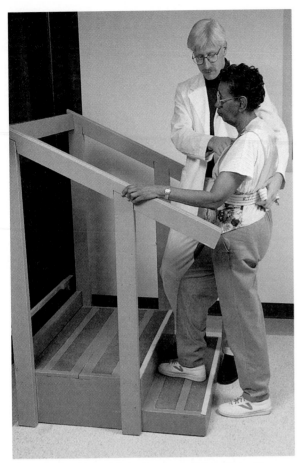

**FIGURE 23-22** The physical therapist will teach some residents how to manipulate stairs.

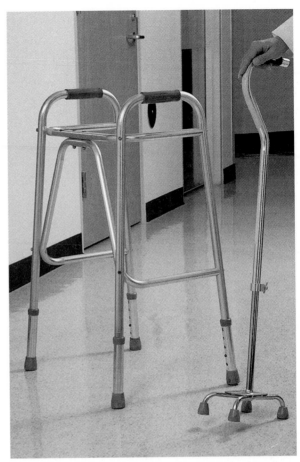

**FIGURE 23-23** All assistive devices have rubber tips on the bottoms and rubber handgrips.

or cracked handgrips. Check screws, nuts, and bolts for tightness. Do not use any device that appears unsafe. Report the problem according to facility policy.

**Use of Crutches.** Standard crutches (Figure 23-24) are seldom recommended for older adults. They can be hard to handle and require balance and two strong arms. Metal forearm or Canadian crutches may be used by residents who have weakness of both legs. The cuff of the crutch encloses the forearm so the resident can release that hand without dropping the crutch (Figure 23-25).

Forearm crutches with platforms permit weight bearing on the forearms, which provides stability. During use, the elbows are in a constant 90° angle to the shoulder (Figure 23-26). The resident may need assistance in attaching the arm straps of the platforms. If you care for residents with crutches, you will be taught the gaits the resident is to use.

**Use of Canes.** Quad canes and tripod canes provide a wide base of support. Pyramid canes are four-pronged devices with a broad base and are narrower at the top. Single-prong canes with T-handles or J-handles have straight handles with handgrip and are easier to hold than half-circle handled canes (Figure 23-27). Canes are recommended for aiding balance rather than for providing support. The cane is always held by the arm on the *strong* side of the body.

**Use of Walkers.** Walkers also come in a variety of styles (Figure 23-28). Walkers are recommended for individuals who have general weakness of both legs, partial weight bearing on one leg, or mild balance problems.

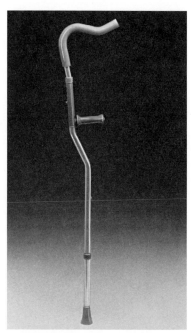

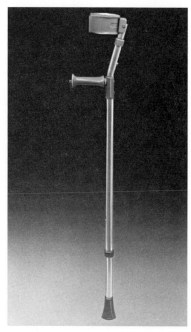

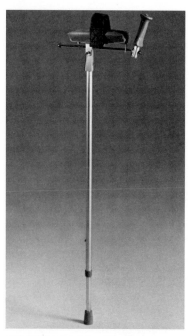

**FIGURE 23-24** Standard crutches are seldom recommended for older adults. (Courtesy of Lunex Medical Products, Bay Shore, NY)

**FIGURE 23-25** Forearm crutches will remain in place when the handle is released. (Courtesy of Lumex Medical Products, Bay Shore, NY)

**FIGURE 23-26** Platform crutches permit weight bearing on the forearms permitting stability. (Courtesy of Lumex Medical Products, Bay Shore, NY)

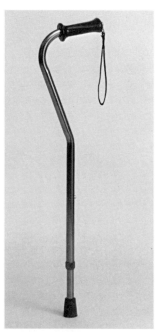

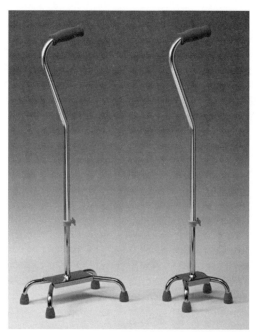

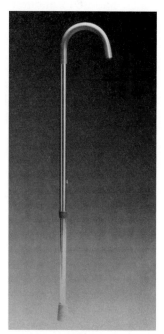

**FIGURE 23-27** Several types of canes are available. (Courtesy of Lumex Medical Products, Bay Shore, NY)

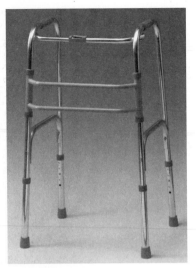
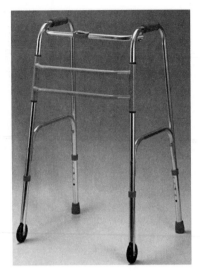
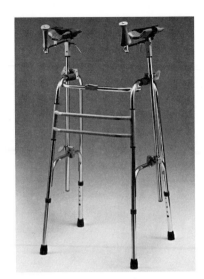

**FIGURE 23-28** Walkers come in a variety of styles. (Courtesy of Lumex Medical Products, Bay Shore, NY)

## *G*uidelines for

## Ambulation

1. Always use a transfer (gait) belt if the resident has problems with balance, coordination, or endurance.
2. If the resident's endurance is questionable, ask another person to follow behind with a wheelchair. Have the resident sit in the chair if weakness occurs.
3. If resident has balance problems, two people should ambulate the resident so counterbalance is provided.

4. The resident should wear sturdy, well-fitting shoes with nonslip soles.
5. Check clothing to be sure shoelaces or slacks are not inhibiting safe ambulation.
6. Know whether or not the resident needs an assistive device. An assistive device is anything the resident uses during ambulation, such as canes, walkers, and crutches.

## PROCEDURE
## *109*  Ambulating a Resident

 OBRA

1. Carry out each beginning procedure action.
2. Place the bed in lowest position.

3. Bring the resident to a sitting position on the edge of the bed.
4. Put the gait belt around the resident's waist.

*(continues)*

**PROCEDURE** *109*  *(continued)*

5. Using an underhand grasp on the gait belt, assist the resident to a standing position.
6. Stand on the resident's weak side. Place your hand closest to the resident in the back of the gait belt with an underhand grasp.
7. Place your other hand in front of the resident's shoulder.
8. Walk with the resident, coordinating your steps. Watch the resident for signs of weakness or faintness.
9. Encourage the resident to walk erect. Encourage normal arm swing.
10. Stop the activity before the resident becomes fatigued.
11. Assist resident back into chair or bed.
12. Carry out each procedure completion action.

---

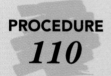 **PROCEDURE** *110*
# Assisting Resident to Ambulate with Cane or Walker

1. Carry out each beginning procedure action.
2. Get walker or cane as directed.
3. Check walker or cane for worn areas or loose parts. Be sure rubber tips and handgrips have adequate tread. If these are cracked or worn, they should be replaced.
4. Place bed in lowest horizontal position.
   - Assist resident to sitting position on edge of bed.
   - Apply transfer (gait) belt if needed.
   - If resident is sitting in a wheelchair, lock the brakes and be sure footrests are up or off. Apply gait belt if needed.
5. Place walker or cane within reach.

*Note:* Canes and walkers are not transfer devices. Never allow residents to use either device while they are getting up from the chair or bed.

6. Help resident to come to a standing position.

7. Place cane or walker within resident's reach.

**Ambulating with a Cane**
*Note:* A cane is *always* held on the strong side. For example, a person who has hemiplegia (paralysis on one side) on the right side would hold the cane with the left hand. A person who has had hip surgery on the right side would hold the cane on the left side.

1. For a three-point gait, the resident advances the cane 10 to 18 inches. Then the resident brings the weaker leg forward and then the stronger leg.
2. For a two-point gait, the resident advances the cane and weak leg at the same time. Then the resident brings the strong leg forward.
3. If resident has a gait belt on, stand slightly in back of the resident on the resident's weak side with your hand closest to the resident in the gait belt (Figure 23-29).

*(continues)*

**PROCEDURE** *110* *(continued)*

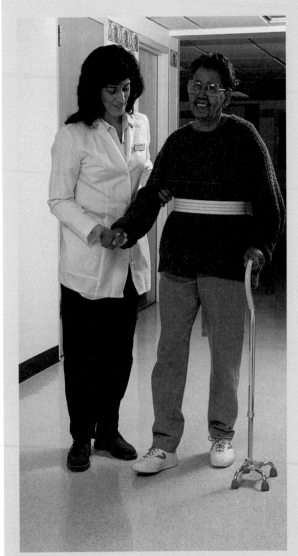

**FIGURE 23-29** The cane is held on the strong side of the body.

4. After ambulating, return resident to bed-side or chair.
   - Have resident walk within a step of bed or chair.
   - Place cane to one side and assist the resident to turn around.
   - When the resident feels the bed or chair touching the back of the legs, have the resident reach for the arm of the chair or mattress of bed and lower self into chair or bed.
5. Carry out each procedure completion action.

**Ambulating with a Walker**
*Note:* There are many different types of walk-ers. The directions given here are for a stan-dard walker.

1. Have resident advance walker 10 to 18 inches. *All four points of the walker should strike the floor at the same time.*
2. The resident then brings weaker leg forward into walker, followed by stronger leg.
3. After ambulating, return resident to bed-side or chair.
   - Have resident walk within a step of bed or chair.
   - Place walker to one side and assist resident to turn around.
   - When resident feels the bed or chair touching the back of the legs, have resident reach for arm of chair or mattress of bed and lower self into chair or bed.
4. Carry out each procedure completion action.

## USING A WHEELCHAIR

Many residents who are unable to ambulate can gain some independence with the use of a wheelchair. A wheelchair should fit the person using it. Correct fit and body alignment will pre-vent contractures. An appropriate wheelchair will have:

- About 4 inches between the top of the back upholstery and the resident's axillae
- Armrests that support the arms without push-ing the shoulders up or forcing them to hang

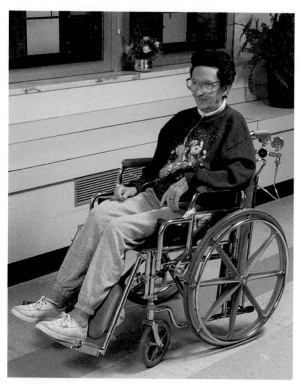

**FIGURE 23-30**   The wheelchair should fit the resident correctly.

- Two to 3 inches clearance between the front edge of the seat and the back of the resident's knee
- Enough space between the resident's hip and the chair to slide your hand between the resident's hips on each side and the side of the wheelchair; the right amount of space avoids internal or external rotation of hips.
- Two inches between the bottom of the footrests and the floor
- The feet at 90° angles to the legs whether they are on the footrests or on the floor (when the footrests have been removed) (Figure 23-30)

If the wheelchair does not fit the resident, check with the nurse or physical therapist to see how you can use pads or other devices to adapt the chair to the resident.

## Wheelchair Safety

Observe residents in wheelchairs. Remind them to:

- Place the casters in forward position for balance and stability. To do this, go forward and then back up so the casters swing to the forward position.
- Keep the wheelchair locked when not moving.
- Lift footrests out of the way when getting in or out of the wheelchair.
- Not attempt to pick up an object off the floor. If there is satisfactory trunk stability and balance, the resident may be taught to do so, but instruct resident to:
  - Remember to avoid shifting weight in the direction of the reach
  - Not move forward in the seat
  - Not reach down between the knees

The safest method is to ask for help in picking up an object from the floor. Otherwise, position the chair beside the object with casters in forward position. Lock the chair and reach only as far as the arm will extend. The resident may have an assistive reaching device that can be used to pick up objects.

The following procedures for wheelchair maneuvers are rarely implemented in a long-term care facility. However, residents may go outside the facility or be discharged. In these situations, the skills will be required. The caregiver should be evaluated on the ability to carry them out.

## SPECIAL MANEUVERS WITH WHEELCHAIRS·····························

Certain situations will require special maneuvers to be made with residents in wheelchairs. Do not attempt to use the following procedures unless you have been instructed to do so.

### Tilting a Wheelchair Backward

1. This procedure is used for curbs, single steps, ramps, and doorsills. Do not use this procedure with an indoor wheelchair.
2. Before proceeding, make sure the resident understands what you are doing. Check to see that arms, hands, fingers, and legs are in safe position. Use good body mechanics to avoid injury. Have an assistant with you the first few times you do this.
3. The purpose of the procedure is to rotate the wheelchair around the axles of the rear wheels until it reaches the balance point.

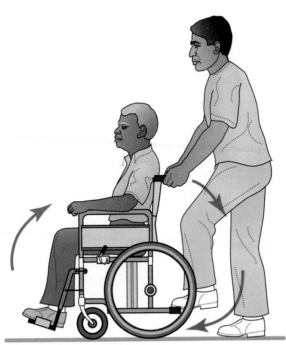

**FIGURE 23-31** With your foot on the tipping lever, apply a pushing force down and under the chair while pulling back and down on the handgrip.

4. With your foot on the tipping lever, apply a pushing force down and under the chair while pulling back and down on the handgrip (Figure 23-31).
5. Tilt back until little or no effort is required to stabilize the chair. This is the balance point, about 30°. You can now maneuver the chair on the rear wheels (Figure 23-32).
6. To return the wheelchair to the upright position, keep your foot on the tipping lever. Lower the chair, reversing the procedure. Do this slowly and smoothly and do not let the chair drop (Figure 23-33).

## Manipulating Ramps and Inclines

1. Push the resident up a ramp or incline, facing forward, with the trunk slightly forward, with or without an attendant.
2. To go down, the resident faces forward but does not lean forward.
3. It is safer if you help the resident going down the ramp. Position yourself behind the chair, place it in balance position, and slowly move it down the ramp.
4. Keep your back straight and knees bent throughout the procedure.

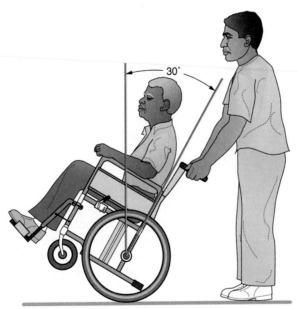

**FIGURE 23-32** You can maneuver the chair on the rear wheels when you have reached the balance point.

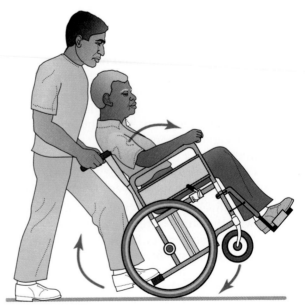

**FIGURE 23-33** Reverse the procedure to lower the chair.

## Manipulating Curbs

1. To go up, place the chair in balance position. Move forward until the front casters are on top of the curb and the rear wheels are touching the curb (Figure 23-34).
2. Lower the front of the chair to the sidewalk, making sure the wheelchair does not roll backward (Figure 23-35).
3. With your body close to the wheelchair, use one single smooth movement to lift the chair by the handles, rolling it up over the curb and pushing it forward (Figure 23-36).
4. After the wheelchair is safely on the sidewalk, step up onto the curb (Figure 23-37).
5. To go down, turn the wheelchair around and pull it to the edge of the curb.
6. Stand below the curb and allow the large wheels to slowly roll down onto the lower level.
7. After the large wheels are on the lower level, tilt the chair to its balance point while lifting the front casters off the curb.

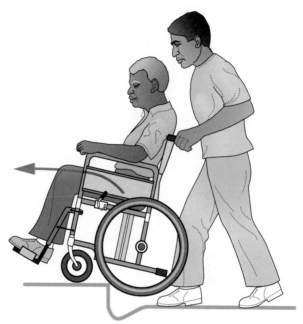

**FIGURE 23-35** Make sure the wheelchair does not roll backward.

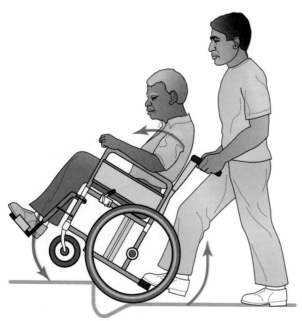

**FIGURE 23-34** Move forward until the front casters are on top of the curb and the rear wheels are touching the curb.

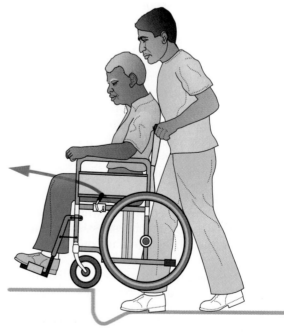

**FIGURE 23-36** Use one single smooth movement to lift the chair by the handles, rolling it up over the curb.

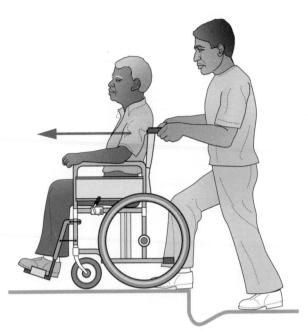

**FIGURE 23-37** Step up onto the curb after the wheelchair is on the sidewalk.

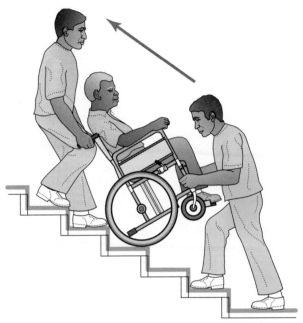

**FIGURE 23-38** The assistants lift and roll the chair up and onto the next step, keeping it at the balance point.

8. When the wheelchair is on the lower level, move backward until you can safely turn the chair around. A second assistant is needed if the curb or step is high.

## Going Up and Down Stairs

Attempt this procedure only if necessary and an elevator is not available. Never use a wheelchair on escalators. At least two people are needed who are strong enough to carry the procedure out to its completion. Check the position of the resident's extremities and inspect the handgrip for good fit on the chair.

1. To go upstairs, place the wheelchair in backward position with the rear wheels touching the first step. The strongest assistant is at the rear of the chair, standing on the second step.
2. The assistant in front grasps the chair frame on either side of the resident's lower legs, taking care not to grasp a removable part.
3. The rear assistant tilts the wheelchair to its balance point.
4. Working together, the assistants lift and roll the chair up onto the next step, keeping it at the balance point, moving themselves up with the chair (Figure 23-38).
5. This procedure is continued until the top step is reached.
6. With the chair still at the balance point, the rear assistant rolls the chair back until the assistant(s) in front are off the steps.
7. The rear assistant turns the chair around and gently returns it to upright position.
8. To go downstairs, the front assistant(s) stands on the third step from the top.
9. The rear assistant tilts the chair to the balance point and rolls it to the edge of the top step. This person is in charge of the procedure.
10. With the front assistant firmly grasping the wheelchair frame, the chair is lowered one step by rolling the large wheels over the edge of the step. All assistants move down one step (Figure 23-39).
11. Repeat the process until the chair reaches the bottom of the stairs. The rear assistant gently returns the wheelchair to the upright position.

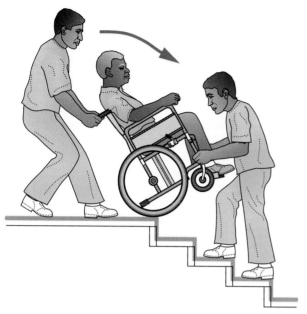

**FIGURE 23-39** All assistants move down one step.

## POSITIONING THE DEPENDENT RESIDENT IN THE WHEELCHAIR······

The dependent person may slide down in the wheelchair, requiring assistance to regain body alignment. Several procedures can be implemented to correct the dependent resident's position in the wheelchair.

*Method 1:* Stand in front of the resident and make sure the feet are in alignment and arms are on the armrests. Help resident lean forward and push with the hands and legs as you push against the resident's knees (Figure 23-40).

*Method 2:* An alternate method is to place a soft towel or small sheet under the resident's buttocks. Use this as a pull sheet to move the resident up in the chair. This requires two people (Figure 23-41).

*Method 3:* This method also requires two people. Place the transfer belt around the resident's waist. One caregiver stands

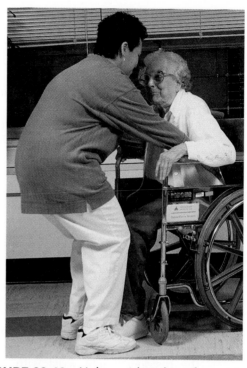

**FIGURE 23-40** Help resident lean forward and push with the hands and legs as you push against the resident's knees.

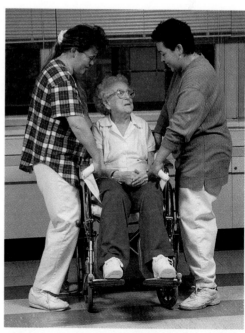

**FIGURE 23-41** A lifting sheet may be used to move the resident up in the wheelchair.

in back of the wheelchair and grasps the transfer belt with one hand on each side of the resident. The other one stands in front of the resident and places her hands and arms under the resident's knees. On the count of three this caregiver supports the lower extremities while the other one moves the resident back in the chair (Figure 23-42). This method is not recommended for a heavy resident.

*Method 4:* This method also requires two people. One assistant stands in back of the wheelchair and a second caregiver stands in front of the resident. Both caregivers work with knees and hips bent and backs straight. You are the caregiver behind the chair. Lean forward with your head over the resident's shoulder. Instruct the resident to fold the arms. Place your arms around the resident's trunk. Grasp the resident's right wrist with your left hand and grasp the resident's left wrist with your right hand. The other caregiver encircles the resident's

knees with hands and arms. On the count of three both caregivers lift and move the resident up (Figure 23-43).

*Method 5:* One person can do this procedure. The resident must be oriented and able to follow directions. Stand in front of the resident. Flex your knees and hips and keep your back straight. Position your feet, one on each side of the resident's feet. Brace your knees against the resident's knees. Have the resident lean forward. Lean forward over the resident's right shoulder with the resident's head under your right arm. Encircle your arms around the resident's trunk. The resident's arms are folded together (Figure 23-44). Rock resident forward and on the count of three, when resident's weight is over the legs, push against the resident's knees to move back in the chair.

If the resident can bear weight, it is easier and more beneficial to assist the resident to stand and then sit back down, getting the hips to the

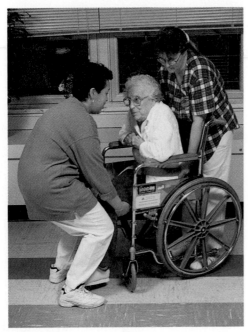

**FIGURE 23-42** A transfer belt may be used to move a lighter resident up in the wheelchair.

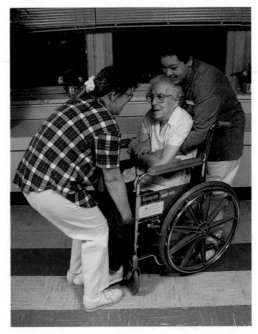

**FIGURE 23-43** On the count of three, both assistants lift and move the resident up.

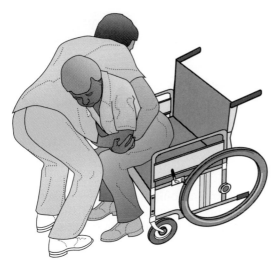

**FIGURE 23-44** Encircle your arms around the resident's trunk.

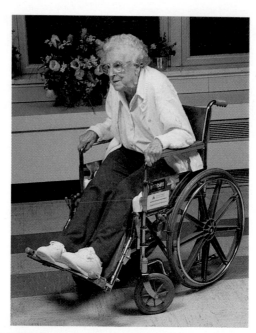

**FIGURE 23-45** Wheelchair pushups relieve pressure from sitting.

back of the chair. Wedge cushions placed in the wheelchair will prevent the resident from sliding forward.

## WHEELCHAIR ACTIVITY

Pressure over the ischia is greatly increased when the resident is sitting. Teach the resident (and provide assistance if necessary) to periodically relieve the pressure by shifting weight every 15 minutes. *Be sure wheelchair is locked before beginning any of the following activities involving the resident's movement in the chair.*

### Wheelchair Pushups

1. Teach the resident to place one hand on each armrest, keeping both elbows bent.
2. Then have resident lean forward slightly, pushing on the armrests and straightening the elbows while lifting the buttocks off the seat of the wheelchair. Have resident hold this position to the count of five if possible (Figure 23-45).

### Leaning

1. Teach the resident who cannot do pushups to place the hands on the armrests or thighs and lean forward slightly, and then to lean

to each side to relieve pressure on buttocks (Figure 23-46). Monitor the resident with balance problems to avoid falling out of the chair.

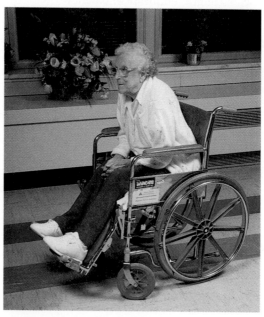

**FIGURE 23-46** Leaning forward is another method for relieving pressure.

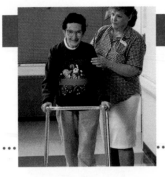

## LESSON SYNTHESIS: Putting It All Together

*Y*ou have just completed this lesson. Now go back and review the Clinical Focus. Try to see how the Clinical Focus relates to the concepts presented in the lesson. Then answer the following questions.

1. Why is it important for the person doing the transfer to always maintain a wide base of support?

2. Why are *specific instructions* written about how a resident is to be transferred?

3. The person doing the transfer should never place his or her hands under the resident's arms. Explain the reasons for this.

4. Explain why a transfer should always be toward the resident's strongest side.

## REVIEW

**A. Select the one best answer for each of the following.**

1. The method used for transferring a resident depends on the resident's
   a. size
   b. physical condition
   c. strength, endurance, balance
   d. all of these

2. A transfer belt should never be used on residents who
   a. have an abdominal aneurysm
   b. need assistance in transferring
   c. are tall
   d. all of these

3. During a transfer, the resident should never
   a. be allowed to help in the move
   b. place his hands on your body
   c. wear shoes
   d. be allowed to stand

4. When transferring a resident, you should never place your hands under a resident's arms because
   a. the resident may not want you to stand so close
   b. the resident cannot see where he is going

   c. the resident's bones are fragile
   d. the resident may be ticklish

5. Using a mechanical lift requires that
   a. there always be two persons to do the procedure
   b. the resident is able to assist in the move
   c. the resident be mentally alert
   d. all of these

6. A sliding board transfer is useful for residents who
   a. are paraplegic
   b. have cardiac problems
   c. have had a stroke
   d. have diabetes

7. A resident's gait may be affected by
   a. a stroke
   b. Parkinson's disease
   c. multiple sclerosis
   d. all of these

**B. Answer each statement true (T) or false (F).**

8. T   F   During a transfer a resident should place his or her hands on the nursing assistant's shoulders.

9. T  F  A transfer belt should always be used when ambulating a resident unless contraindicated.

10. T  F  Always transfer toward the resident's strong side.

11. T  F  During a transfer the nursing assistant should place his or her hands around the resident's trunk.

12. T  F  Always explain what the transfer person is doing and what the resident can do to help.

13. T  F  Towel bars are not safe to use as grab bars.

14. T  F  Always hold a cane on the weak side.

15. T  F  When using a walker, the front two tips of the walker should strike the floor first and then the back two tips should strike the floor.

# SECTION

# 8

# Residents with Specific Disorders

## LESSONS

**24** Caring for Residents with Cardiovascular System Disorders

**25** Caring for Residents with Respiratory System Disorders

**26** Caring for Residents with Endocrine System Disorders

**27** Caring for Residents with Reproductive System Disorders

**28** Caring for Residents with Musculoskeletal System Disorders

**29** Caring for Residents with Nervous System Disorders

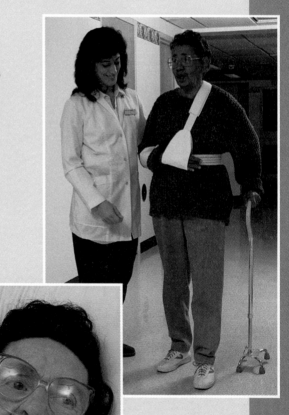

# Caring for Residents with Cardiovascular System Disorders

## CLINICAL FOCUS

Think how you might assist a resident with cardiovascular disorders as you study this lesson and meet:

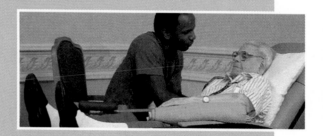

Walter Rabinowitz, who has congestive heart failure and poor circulation in his feet. He sits in a cardiac chair that supports him in an upright position comfortably. He is always complaining that his feet are cold. He has an order for elasticized stockings. During morning care, he asks for a hot water bag to put on his feet. Nursing assistants know there are safer methods of providing the comfort he needs.

## OBJECTIVES

*After studying this lesson, you should be able to:*

- Define and spell vocabulary words and terms.
- Identify the parts and function of the cardiovascular system.
- Review changes in the cardiovascular system as they relate to the aging process.
- Describe common cardiovascular disorders affecting the long-term resident.
- Correctly apply elasticized stockings.

- List observations to make when caring for residents with cardiovascular disorders.
- Describe the care given by the nursing assistant to residents with cardiovascular disorders.
- Demonstrate the following:
  Procedure 111 Applying Elasticized Stockings

## VOCABULARY

**anemia**  *(ah-NEE-mee-ah)*

**angina pectoris**  *(an-JYE-nah or AN-jih-nah PECK-tor-is)*

**aorta**  *(ay-OR-tah)*

**arteriosclerosis**  *(are-ter-ree-oh-skleh-ROH-sis)*

**artery**  *(ARE-ter-ee)*

**ascites**  *(ah-SIGH-teez)*

**atherosclerosis**  *(ath-er-oh-skleh-ROH-sis)*

**atrium (plural: atria)**  *(AY-tree-um; pl. AY-tree-ah)*

# VOCABULARY

**capillary** *(KAP-ih-lair-ee)*

**cardiac cycle** *(KAR-dee-ack SIGH-kul)*

**cardiovascular** *(kar-dee-oh-VAS-kyou-lar)*

**congestive heart failure** *(kon-JES-tiv hart FAIL-your)*

**dementia** *(dee-MEN-she-ah)*

**deoxygenated** *(dee-ock-sih-jen-AY-ted)*

**diaphoresis** *(die-ah-foh-REE-sis)*

**diastole** *(die-AS-toh-lee)*

**dyspnea** *(DISP-nee-ah)*

**edema** *(eh-DEE-mah)*

**electrocardiogram (ECG or EKG)** *(ee-leck-troh-KAR-dee-oh-gram)*

**erythrocytes** *(eh-RITH-roh-sights)*

**heart attack** *(hart ah-TACK)*

**heart block** *(hart block)*

**hemoptysis** *(hee-MOP-tih-sis)*

**hypertension** *(high-per-TEN-shun)*

**hypoxia** *(high-POCK-see-ah)*

**infarction** *(in-FARK-shun)*

**inferior vena cava** *(in-FEER-ee-or VEE-nah KAY-vah)*

**ischemia** *(is-KEE-mee-ah)*

**leukemia** *(loo-KEE-mee-ah)*

**leukocytes** *(LOO-koh-sights)*

**lumen** *(LOO-men)*

**lymph** *(limf)*

**lymph node** *(limf nohd)*

**myocardial infarction** *(my-oh-KAR-dee-al in-FARK-shun)*

**nitroglycerin** *(nigh-troh-GLIS-er-in)*

**orthopnea** *(or-thop-NEE-ah)*

**orthopneic position** *(or-thop-NEE-ick poh-ZISH-un)*

**oxygenated** *(ock-sih-jen-AT-ted)*

**pacemaker** *(PAYS-may-ker)*

**peripheral vascular disease** *(peh-RIF-er-al VAS-kyou-lar dih-ZEEZ)*

**phlebitis** *(fleh-BYE-tis)*

**plaque** *(plak)*

**plasma** *(PLAZ-mah)*

**platelet** *(PLAYT-let)*

**pulmonary artery** *(PULL-moh-nair-ee ARE-ter-ee)*

**pulmonary veins** *(PULL-moh-nair-ee vains)*

**serum** *(SEER-rum)*

**stroke** *(strohk)*

**superior vena cava** *(soo-PEER-ee-or VEE-nah KAY-vah)*

**syncope** *(SIN-koh-pe)*

**systole** *(SIS-toh-lee)*

**TED hose** *(TED hohs)*

**thrombocyte** *(THROM-boh-sight)*

**thrombophlebitis** *(throm-boh-fleh-BYE-tis)*

**transient ischemic attack (TIA)** *(TRAN-see-ent is-KEE-mick ah-TACK)*

**valve** *(valv)*

**varicose veins** *(VAIR-ih-kohs vains)*

**vasodilator** *(vas-oh-die-LAY-tor)*

**vein** *(vain)*

**ventricle** *(VEN-trih-kul)*

**venule** *(VEN-youl)*

# INTRODUCTION

The **cardiovascular** system is the transportation system of the body. It carries substances from where they are formed to where they may be used or eliminated. The cardiovascular system consists of the:

**FIGURE 24-1**   Changes in the cardiovascular system caused by aging

- Vascular walls become less flexible.
- Vascular lumens narrow.
- Blood pressure increases.
- Cardiac output decreases.
- System cannot adapt to sudden or intense changes or demands.
- Capillaries become more fragile.
- Heart rate decreases.

- Heart—a central pump
- Blood vessels—a closed circuit of arteries that lead from the heart to capillaries and then to veins that lead back to the heart
- Blood—a collection of various cells, each with a special job to perform
- Lymphatic vessels and **lymph nodes**—filter tissue fluid and return it as **lymph** back to the bloodstream

The bloodstream, spleen, liver, and bone marrow make some of the blood cells and destroy them when they are worn out.

Cardiovascular disease is the most common cause of death in the United States. Many residents in your care will suffer from disabilities caused by cardiovascular disease. Cardiovascular disease is responsible for changes that reduce the blood flow to the body tissues and result in

- Heart attack
- Peripheral vascular disease
- Hypertension (high blood pressure)
- Stroke

Reduced blood flow is called **ischemia**. Ischemia means that less oxygen is delivered to tissues, leading, eventually, to death of the tissues (**infarction**). Changes in the cardiovascular system caused by aging are summarized in Figure 24-1.

# THE HEART

The heart is a muscular organ that pumps the blood in a continuous flow through the blood vessels of the body. It is separated into a right and left side (Figure 24-2).

## Structure and Function

The *right side* of the heart:

- Receives blood from the body
- Sends blood to the lungs where carbon dioxide is removed and oxygen is picked up (Figure 24-3)

The *left side* of the heart:

- Receives blood from the lungs by way of the pulmonary veins
- Sends blood out to the body, where the oxygen is given up to the cells and the waste product carbon dioxide is picked up

Each side of the heart is divided into upper and lower parts (chambers) by **valves**. The valves permit blood flow in one direction only. The *upper chambers* are called the right **atrium** and left atrium. The *lower chambers* are the right and left **ventricles**.

The two upper chambers contract first, forcing the blood through the open valves into the two lower chambers. The ventricles fill and the valves close. The ventricles then contract, squeezing the blood up through the large blood vessels.

## Blood Vessels of the Heart

The major blood vessels of the heart are the:

- **Superior vena cava** (SVC)—returns blood to the right atrium from the upper part of the body
- **Inferior vena cava** (IVC)—returns blood to right atrium from the lower part of the body
- **Pulmonary artery**—carries blood to the lungs from the right ventricle
- **Pulmonary veins**—return blood to the left atrium from the lungs
- **Aorta** (a large artery)—carries blood to the body from the left ventricle
- Coronary arteries—nourish the heart muscle with fresh blood

Valves at the base of the pulmonary artery and aorta close as the blood moves forward, pre-

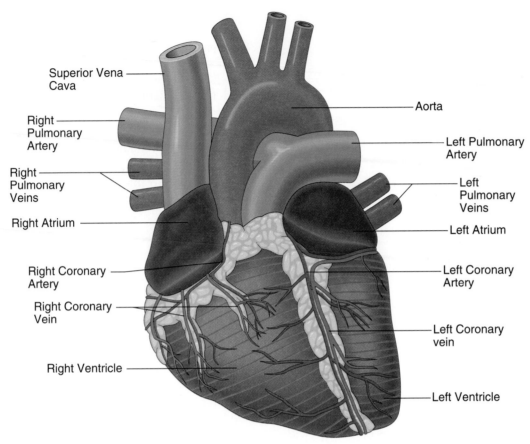

**FIGURE 24-2** External view of the heart and vessels

venting backflow of blood into the ventricles between contractions.

## Cardiac Cycle

The contractions and relaxations of the heart muscle are called the **cardiac cycle**. The cardiac cycle is controlled by special nerve tissues within the heart and by two sets of nerves:

- One set of nerves carries messages to increase the heart rate.
- The other set of nerves carries messages to slow the heart rate.

Electrical impulses passing through the nerve tissue make the muscle contract:

- **Systole** is the term meaning heart *contraction.*
- **Diastole** is the term meaning heart *relaxation.*

For a short time, the heart rests completely between beats. The pulse you feel at the radial artery corresponds to ventricular contraction. The sounds you hear when listening to the heart and when taking a blood pressure are the sounds made by the closing of the valves during the cardiac cycle.

An **electrocardiogram**, called an ECG or an EKG, is a test that traces the electrical impulses of the heart. Heart disease may be detected with this test.

## BLOOD VESSELS

There are three kinds of blood vessels:

- **Arteries**
- **Capillaries**
- **Veins**

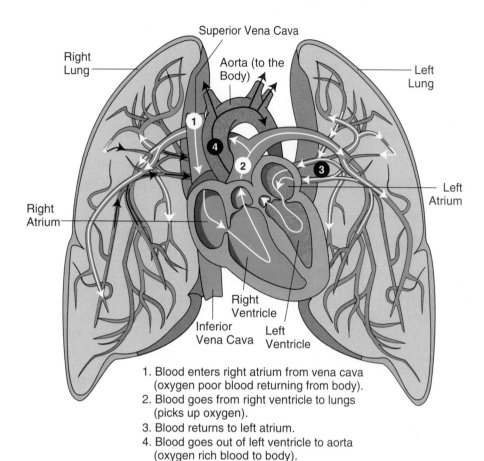

1. Blood enters right atrium from vena cava (oxygen poor blood returning from body).
2. Blood goes from right ventricle to lungs (picks up oxygen).
3. Blood returns to left atrium.
4. Blood goes out of left ventricle to aorta (oxygen rich blood to body).

**FIGURE 24-3**   Flow of blood from the heart to the lungs, to the body, and back to the heart to begin the cycle again

## Arteries

Arteries carry blood away from the heart (Figure 24-4). The blood contains oxygen picked up in the lungs. The blood is **oxygenated** and is needed to keep the body cells alive and functioning. The arteries get smaller and finally form tiny networks of vessels called capillaries.

## Capillaries

Nutrients and oxygen in the blood are exchanged through the walls of the capillaries for carbon dioxide and waste products. The capillaries form larger vessels called **venules** to begin the journey back to the heart.

## Veins

Many venules join to form larger vessels called veins (Figure 24-5). The largest veins, the supe-

rior vena cava and the inferior vena cava, return the blood to the right atrium. This blood has less oxygen and more carbon dioxide and is called **deoxygenated** blood.

The cardiovascular system is a closed system with the gases and other substances passing into and out of the blood as it passes throughout the body.

Blood vessels frequently take their names from bones nearby. For example, the radial artery and radial vein are found close to the radius, which is one of the forearm bones.

## LYMPH

Lymph is fluid that is drained from the tissues. It passes into lymphatic vessels through masses of cells called lymph nodes. Eventually, the fluid

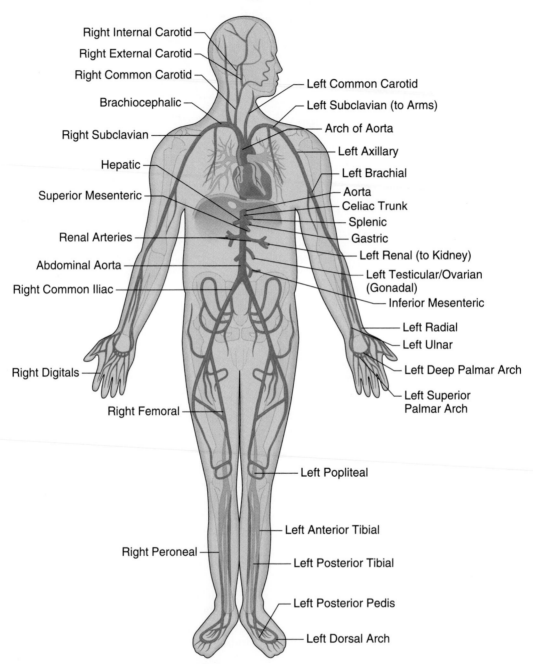

**FIGURE 24-4** Arteries of the body

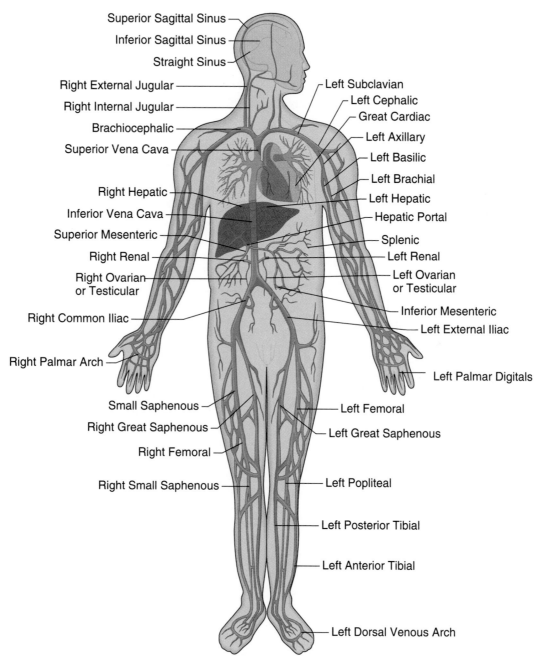

**FIGURE 24-5** Veins of the body

returns to the general circulation. The lymph nodes act as filters, removing harmful substances picked up in the tissues before they reach the general circulation.

# THE BLOOD

The blood is a red body fluid that carries the nutrients, chemicals, and waste products of the body. The average quantity of blood in the body is about 4 to 6 liters (or 4 to 6 quarts). The blood consists of two portions:

- Plasma
- Blood cells

## Plasma

The liquid part of the blood, called **plasma**, carries:

- Water
- Nutrients
- Wastes
- Proteins that help blood to clot
- Proteins that fight infection and help to move materials in and out of the bloodstream

**Serum** is the fluid that is left after the cells and some of the proteins have been removed.

## Blood Cells

Three kinds of blood cells are:

1. **Erythrocytes** (red blood cells)—carry oxygen and a small amount of carbon dioxide
2. **Leukocytes** (white blood cells)—protect the body by fighting infection
3. **Platelets** or **thrombocytes**—pieces of cells that contain a chemical important to blood clotting

# DISORDERS OF THE BLOOD

Blood abnormalities commonly seen in the elderly include:

- Cancer
- Anemia

## Cancer

Cancers of the blood include forms of **leukemia** In leukemia:

- Excessive numbers of white blood cells are formed.
- Too few platelets and red blood cells are produced.

The person with leukemia:

- Tires easily
- Is subject to infections and anemia
- Is apt to bleed

These conditions are normally treated with radiation or drugs.

## Anemia

**Anemias** are the result of a decrease in (1) the quantity or quality of red blood cells and (2) their ability to carry oxygen. People suffering from anemia have little energy. They:

- Are usually pale or jaundiced (skin is yellow)
- Complain of light-headedness
- Feel cold
- Experience dizziness
- Have an increased respiratory rate
- Suffer from poor digestion

## Special Care

Residents who have cancer or anemia require special care. You must:

- Check vital signs.
- Encourage rest and a good diet.
- See that resident avoids unnecessary exertion.
- Handle resident very gently.
- Give special mouth care because the mouth and tongue become sensitive.
- Be sure to report any signs of bleeding such as bruises or discolorations because further blood loss makes the condition worse.
- Keep resident warm.
- Protect resident from falls that may result from dizziness or weakness.
- Change the resident's position often—at least every 2 hours.

# DISORDERS OF THE BLOOD VESSELS AND CIRCULATION

Several changes can occur in blood vessels that will affect the flow of blood (circulation) through the vessels. **Arteriosclerosis** means hardening of the arteries. When this happens, the arteries lose their elasticity. It is then more difficult for the blood to flow through the vessels. **Atherosclerosis** occurs when deposits of fatty materials and calcium form roughened areas (**plaques**) on the inner walls of the arteries. As the plaques thicken, the space within the arteries (the **lumen**) narrows (Figure 24-6). This causes the blood flow to decrease. When this happens, ischemia can occur.

Arteriosclerosis and atherosclerosis are especially dangerous when they affect the arter-

ies of the brain, heart, and those leading from the body to the legs. When the vessels in the brain are affected, the risk is high for **stroke** (cerebral vascular accident or CVA). Stroke is discussed in Lesson 29. Before a stroke happens, the person may have a transient ischemic attack (TIA). The person may also get a form of **dementia** (confusion and disorientation) when the brain cells do not receive adequate oxygen. Dementia is discussed in Lesson 30.

When the vessels of the heart are affected, the person may have a heart attack (**myocardial**

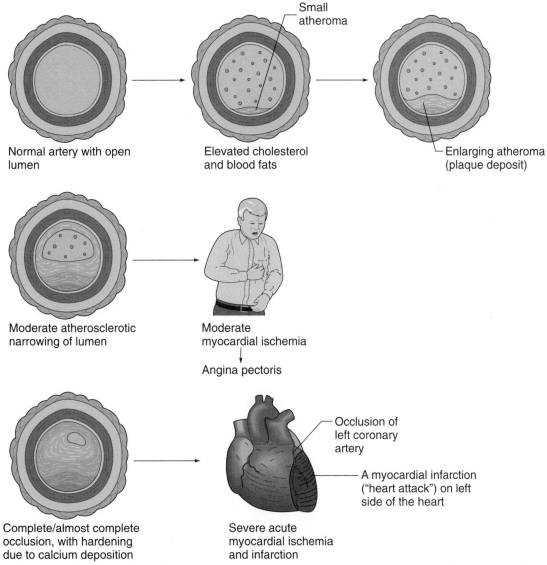

**FIGURE 24-6**  Cross sections through a coronary artery undergoing progressive arteriosclerosis and atherosclerosis

infarction). When the vessels in the legs are affected, the person has **peripheral vascular disease**. When the arteries are diseased, hypertension (high blood pressure) may occur (Figure 24-7).

The veins can also cause problems. **Varicose veins** form when the valves in the veins in the legs become weakened (Figure 24-8). This means the blood does not flow through the veins as it should. The veins then become distended and visible through the skin. The veins may become inflamed (**phlebitis**). A blood clot may form (**thrombophlebitis**). Report the signs of these disorders:

- Pain or aching in the area
- Signs of inflammation (warmth and redness)

*NEVER* rub or massage the area.

### Transient Ischemic Attack

**Transient ischemic attack (TIA)** is a temporary interruption of the blood flow to part of the brain. The resident may experience:

- Weakness or paralysis of any extremity or the face
- Vision problems
- Difficulty with speech
- Difficulty with swallowing

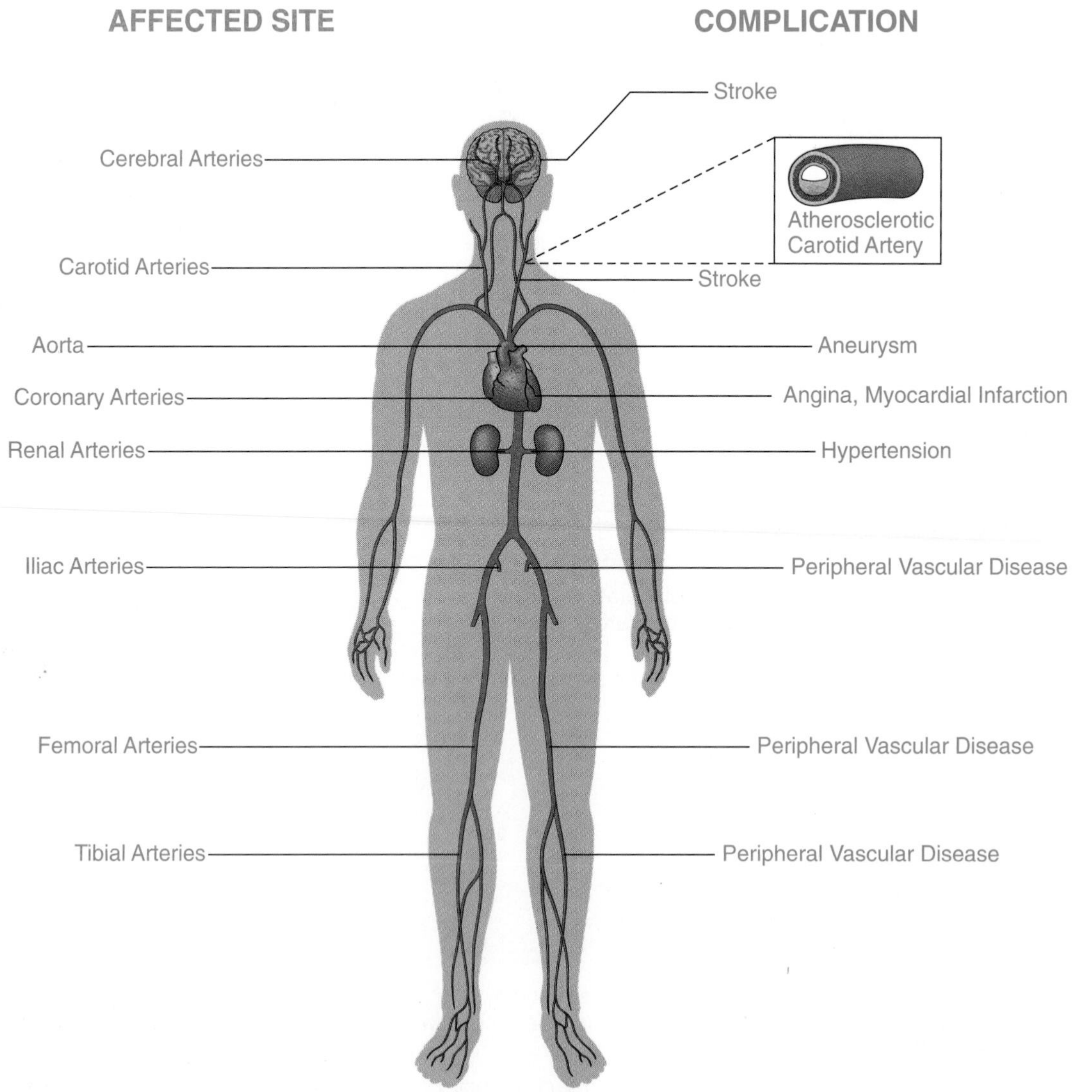

AFFECTED SITE

COMPLICATION

Cerebral Arteries — Stroke

Atherosclerotic Carotid Artery

Carotid Arteries — Stroke

Aorta — Aneurysm

Coronary Arteries — Angina, Myocardial Infarction

Renal Arteries — Hypertension

Iliac Arteries — Peripheral Vascular Disease

Femoral Arteries — Peripheral Vascular Disease

Tibial Arteries — Peripheral Vascular Disease

**FIGURE 24-7** Atherosclerosis and arteriosclerosis can cause disease in many parts of the body.

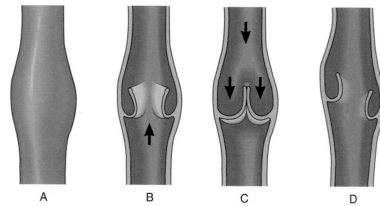

A             B             C             D

**FIGURE 24-8** Veins contain valves to prevent the backward flow of blood. A. External view of the vein shows wider area of valve. B. Internal view with the valve open as blood flows through. C. Internal view with the valve closed. D. Vein with weakened valve causing a varicose vein

These symptoms come on quickly and may last from just a few minutes to 24 hours. There are no permanent effects. However, a TIA is usually a warning that a stroke will occur at some time. If a resident has any of the above symptoms you should report them to the nurse immediately.

## Peripheral Vascular Disease

Peripheral vascular disease may be caused by:

- Diseases of the arteries (arteriosclerosis and atherosclerosis)
- Abnormalities of the veins (varicose veins)

The signs and symptoms of peripheral vascular disease include:

- Burning pain during exercise
- Hair loss over feet and toes
- Thick and rigid toenails
- Dusky red skin or cyanotic, brownish skin
- Dry and scaly or shiny skin
- Chronic edema of the feet and legs
- Cool skin temperature of feet and legs
- Difficulty with ambulation

When the arteries are affected, the blood flow may be seriously interrupted. This condition requires immediate medical treatment. Vascular ulcers may occur. These are sores that start because of the poor circulation of the blood in the legs. These ulcers are difficult to treat and may take months to heal.

When residents have peripheral vascular disease, it is important that:

- Circulation is maintained. Complications such as ulcers may then be prevented.
- The feet and legs receive excellent skin care

## *G*uidelines for

## Caring for Residents with Peripheral Vascular Disease

1. Elevate the feet when the resident is sitting in a chair for prolonged periods of time. When the feet are not elevated, make sure that the resident's feet are flat on the floor. If they are not, support the feet with a footstool. Discourage the resident from crossing the legs when sitting.
2. Discourage the resident from using circular garters.
3. Discourage smoking because it interferes with circulation.

*(continues)*

## $G$uidelines *(continued)*

4. Avoid using the knee gatch on the bed.

5. Avoid the use of heating pads or hot water bottles. The resident may not feel temperatures that are too hot.

6. Maintain body warmth. Make sure the resident has warm clothes including well-fitting socks. Provide blankets for the bed.

7. Prevent injury to the feet:
   * Instruct the resident to wear shoes when out of bed.
   * Check to see that the shoes are in good repair and that they fit well.
   * Avoid pressure to the legs and feet from any source.

8. Inspect the feet carefully when you bathe the resident or if the resident complains of any discomfort in the feet. Promptly report any signs of inflammation, injury, or circulatory problems (Figure 24-9).
   * Broken skin
   * Color change—redness, white, or cyanotic
   * Heat or coldness
   * Cracking between toes
   * Corns or calluses
   * Swelling
   * Pain
   * Loss of function
   * Drainage

9. Bathe the feet regularly.
   * Dry thoroughly and gently between the toes.
   * Use a moisturizing lotion to the feet and legs if the skin is dry.

10. Do not cut the toenails of residents with peripheral vascular disease without instructions from the nurse.

| **FIGURE 24-9**   Signs indicative of peripheral vascular disease |
| --- |
| • Broken skin |
| • Coldness or heat |
| • Color change |
| • Cracking between toes |
| • Corns or callouses |
| • Pain |
| • Loss of function |
| • Drainage |
| • Swelling |

## Hypertension

**Hypertension** means elevated blood pressure. Hypertension may have an unknown origin or follow disease of the:

* Blood vessels
* Kidneys
* Liver

Diseases of the blood vessels increase the overall blood pressure. When blood vessels are narrowed due to disease, the heart attempts to make up for the resistance in the vessels by enlarging. Over a period of time, the heart eventually fails. Hypertension further increases the rate at which disease progresses in the vessels.

Elderly people usually have a somewhat higher pressure than younger people. The normal blood pressure for young adults is 120/80, but in the elderly, the norm is higher, with the highest level of normal being 140/90 mm Hg. Above this level, the probability of stroke and heart attack increases dramatically. Hypertension is dangerous because often there are no symptoms. It may be detected during a routine blood pressure check. Report any blood pressures when the systolic is over 140 or the diastolic is over 90.

**Control of Hypertension.** Control of hypertension is essential. Steps can be taken to bring the hypertension under control to avoid the serious consequences of stroke and heart attack. These steps include:

- Drugs to lower the pressure
- Weight reduction
- Dietary restrictions, such as limiting salt intake
- Discouraging smoking
- Regular exercise

Report immediately any signs or symptoms of hypertension:

- Flushed face
- Dizziness
- Nose bleeds
- Headaches
- Changes in speech patterns
- Blurred vision

# HEART DISEASE

Many residents have some form of heart disease. Heart disease often makes self-care difficult because the resident tires easily, and residents become depressed and frustrated by their limitations. Heart disease may sometimes be due to an infection, but most heart disease develops because of changes in the blood vessels. The space inside the vessels becomes smaller. These changes make it harder and harder for the heart to do its job of pumping blood.

## Heart Attack

A **heart attack** occurs when the heart is not able to function properly. There are different kinds of attacks, and some have more serious effects than others. However, every attack is serious, and each requires some form of treatment (therapy). A heart attack is often referred to as an MI (myocardial infarction).

In myocardial infarction the normal flow of blood to the heart is decreased. Narrowing of the coronary (heart) blood vessels that supply blood to the heart may occur slowly over a period of years, allowing some new circulation to develop. However, when the heart attack occurs, the flow of blood has diminished so much that not

enough blood reaches the heart and the heart muscle may die. This lack of blood flow is known as ischemia.

Sometimes the flow of blood is cut off abruptly because a blood clot lodges in a coronary artery.

## Acute Myocardial Infarction

An acute MI is a serious medical emergency. The blood flow to the myocardium is cut off suddenly. The closure of a large vessel can result in death (infarction) of that part of the heart muscle not being supplied with blood. If too much of the heart muscle dies, the resident cannot survive.

Survival depends largely on how quickly proper medical intervention occurs, (Figure 24-10). You must recognize the signs and symptoms of this type of heart attack and report to the nurse immediately.

**Signs and Symptoms.** These include:

- Crushing chest pain, spreading down the arms and up into the neck and jaw; sometimes described as "severe indigestion"

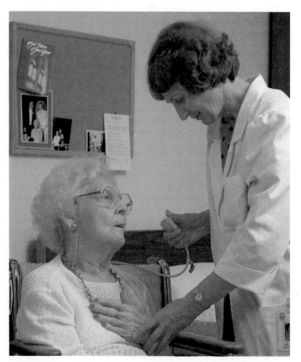

**FIGURE 24-10** If you suspect the resident is having a heart attack, summon help immediately and do not leave the resident.

- Clammy, ashen, or pale skin
- Excessive sweating (**diaphoresis**)
- Nausea
- Vomiting (sometimes)
- Anxiety and weakness
- Weak pulse
- Low blood pressure
- Shock
- Shortness of breath
- **Syncope** (fainting)
- Restlessness

**Nursing Assistant Care.**   You can help by:

- Staying with the resident
- Using the intercom or call bell to summon help
- Staying calm

The resident will usually be transferred immediately to the intensive care unit (ICU) or coronary care unit (CCU) of an acute care hospital. Early treatment is designed to reverse the shock, relieve the pain, and keep the heart functioning.

## Angina Pectoris

**Angina pectoris** is a condition in which there is decreased blood flow to the heart. Signs and symptoms of an angina heart attack that you should immediately report include:

- Pain when exercising or under stress. Stress causes a need for an immediate increase in the coronary circulation. The pain is described as dull, with increasing intensity. It is usually centered under the breast bone (sternum) spreading to the left arm and up into the neck.
- Pale or flushed face
- Resident freely perspiring

Signs and symptoms may differ with individual residents, but the symptoms are usually the same each time that a resident experiences an attack. You may assist the resident with angina pectoris by:

- Helping the resident to avoid unnecessary emotional or physical stress
- Encouraging the resident not to smoke
- Reporting any signs and symptoms of an attack to the nurse at once

Residents with a history of angina pectoris take medication called a **vasodilator** to keep the blood vessels open. **Nitroglycerin** is one type of vasodilator. It is usually administered in a patch. The nitroglycerin patch is secured to the resident's chest and the medication is absorbed slowly over a 24-hour period.

## Heart Failure

Many residents have a condition in which the heart functions less efficiently. The resident is said to be in heart failure (also called **congestive heart failure**) when certain symptoms are present, including:

- Cough
- **Dyspnea** (difficulty breathing)
- **Orthopnea** (difficulty in breathing unless sitting upright)
- Cyanosis
- **Hemoptysis** (spitting up blood)
- Fluid retained in the lungs and throughout the body
- **Edema** (fluid in the tissue spaces)
- **Ascites** (fluid collecting in the abdomen)
- Neck veins swell
- Fatiguing easily
- **Hypoxia** (inadequate oxygen levels)
- Confusion
- Irregular and rapid pulse

**Nursing Assistant Care.**   Acute heart failure is an urgent situation requiring expert care. You will assist in this care. Watch the resident carefully and report any increase in signs and symptoms at once.

Nursing care may include:

- Positioning. The resident is usually more comfortable, either sitting up in bed, in an **orthopneic position** or high Fowler's position, supported by pillows, or supported in a chair. The position must be changed frequently, but changes in position should be made slowly. Padded footboards help keep the weight of the bedding off the toes.
- Application of elasticized stockings or **TED hose**. TED hose are elastic antiembolism stockings. TED hose and Ace bandages help channel blood to the deeper vessels. They must be checked often and reapplied every 6 to 8 hours. Check the extremities carefully for adequate circulation. The skin should be pink and warm.

- Give attention to general hygiene. Complete bathing is tiring, but partial baths can stimulate circulation and provide comfort. Special attention must be given to the skin because the combination of position, edema, and poor circulation contributes to tissue breakdown.
- Assist with oxygen therapy. Oxygen therapy may be provided either by face mask or nasal cannula. Because cardiac residents often breathe through the mouth, the mouth tends to be very dry. Special mouth care may be needed.

For oxygen safety, refer to Lesson 8.

Provide for elimination. A bedside commode is convenient. The use of a commode is less tiring for the resident than using a bedpan for elimination.

- Encourage adequate nutrition. Small, easily digested meals should be encouraged. You may need to assist in feeding the resident to prevent fatigue.
- Monitor and record fluid intake. Residents with acute heart failure may be given drugs that increase the output of urine and alter the heart rate. Measuring the intake and output and taking daily weights are ways of determining if fluid is being retained. These procedures are part of the care you will give.
- Regularly check vital signs. Sometimes the force of heart contraction, which propels the blood forward into the blood vessels, does not have enough strength to make the vessels expand.

---

**PROCEDURE**

## *111* Applying Elasticized Stockings

1. Carry out each beginning procedure action.
2. Assemble equipment:
   - Elasticized stockings of proper length and size
3. With resident lying down, expose one leg at a time.

4. Grasp stocking with both hands at the top and roll toward toe end (Figure 24-11).
5. Adjust over toes, positioning opening at base of toes (unless toes are to be covered) (Figure 24-12). Remember that the raised seams should be on the outside.

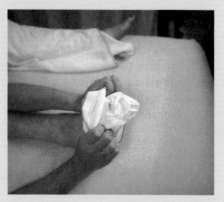

**FIGURE 24-11**   Grasp stocking with both hands at stocking top, gather, and slip over toes.

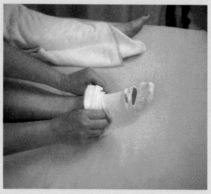

**FIGURE 24-12**   Position opening on top of foot at base of toes.

*(continues)*

**PROCEDURE** *111* *(continued)*

6. Apply stocking to leg by rolling upward toward body (Figure 24-13).
7. Check to be sure stocking is applied evenly and smoothly and there are no wrinkles (Figures 24-14 and 24-15).
8. Repeat procedure on other leg.
9. Carry out each procedure completion action.

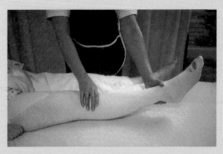

**FIGURE 24-14** Check to be sure stocking has no wrinkles.

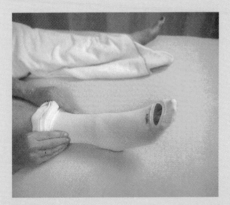

**FIGURE 24-13** Draw stocking smoothly toward knee.

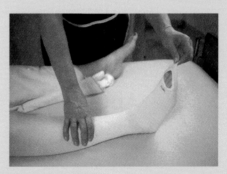

**FIGURE 24-15** Check material on toes to be sure it is not too tight.

## Chronic Heart Failure

Residents can live for years with some level of chronic heart failure. A resident with chronic heart failure needs a calm environment with planned activity that promotes mobility but not fatigue. Visiting should be limited to one or two visitors because too many visitors at one time can be tiring.

The basic care given to residents in chronic failure includes:

- Measuring fluid intake and output
- Taking apical and radial pulse
- Assisting when necessary to prevent fatigue and maintain mobility
- Reporting any change in signs and symptoms
- Reporting unusual behavior or responses

This condition requires the use of medications for long periods of time. This results in a tendency for drug levels in the body to build. Elderly people are more sensitive to drugs. Therefore, you must be alert to unusual responses or behavior that may indicate a drug reaction. Report anything unusual about the residents in your care to your supervisor.

## Heart Block

**Heart block** is a condition that develops due to interference in the electrical current through the heart. (The flow of electrical current through the heart muscle makes the normal cardiac cycle possible.)

An electronic device called a **pacemaker** (Figure 24-16) is implanted under the chest mus-

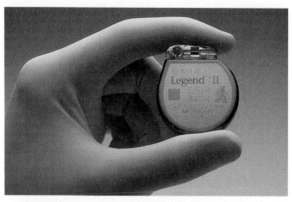

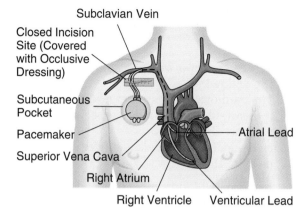

Subclavian Vein

Closed Incision
Site (Covered
with Occlusive
Dressing)

Subcutaneous
Pocket

Pacemaker

Superior Vena Cava

Right Atrium

Right Ventricle

Atrial Lead

Ventricular Lead

**FIGURE 24-16**   The electronic pacemaker sends electrical impulses to the heart muscle, causing it to contract. A. A typical pacemaker. B. The pacemaker inserted under the skin with electrode placed inside the heart, resting on the heart muscle  (Courtesy of Medtronic, Inc.)

cles or in the abdomen. An electrode carries electrical current from the pacemaker directly into the heart muscle to replace the lost control. The electrical current signals the heart to contract. Some pacemakers send messages only if normal messages carried by the conduction system are delayed. This type of pacemaker is called a demand pacemaker. Other pacemakers send regular signals to keep the heart contracting. The rate of signals is preset.

When caring for a resident who has a pacemaker:

- Count and record the pulse rate.
- Report any irregularities or changes below the present rate.
- Report any discoloration over the implant site.
- Report hiccoughing because this may indicate problems.
- Keep resident away from microwave ovens and cellular phones because they may disrupt the function of the pacemaker.

  Residents usually function very well with pacemakers so long as they are adequately monitored.

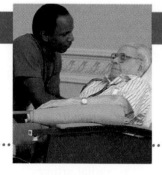

## LESSON SYNTHESIS: Putting It All Together

You have just completed this lesson. Now go back and review the Clinical Focus. Try to see how the Clinical Focus relates to the concepts presented in the lesson. Then answer the following questions.

1. Explain how a cardiac chair contributes to Mr. Rabinowitz's comfort and improved functioning of his cardiovascular system.

2. What actions can you take to increase Mr. Rabinowitz's warmth without using a hot water bag?

3. How do elasticized stockings assist the circulation in the legs?

4. What precautions should be taken when applying the elasticized stockings?

# REVIEW

**A. Select the one best answer for each of the following.**

1. The cardiovascular system includes the
   a. heart, blood, and blood vessels
   b. heart and lungs
   c. blood, blood vessels and liver
   d. all of these

2. Inadequate blood supply can lead to
   a. dementia
   b. myocardial infarction
   c. stroke
   d. all of these

3. The structures of the heart that permit blood flow in one direction only are called
   a. atria
   b. ventricles
   c. valves
   d. myocardium

4. The major artery is called the
   a. vena cava
   b. aorta
   c. pulmonary vein
   d. pulmonary artery

5. The function of the lymph system is to
   a. manufacture new red blood cells
   b. inhibit bleeding
   c. filter out harmful substances before they reach the general circulation
   d. all of these

6. Red blood cells are responsible for
   a. delivery of oxygen to all body cells
   b. protecting the body by fighting infection
   c. the blood clotting process
   d. making lymph fluid

7. Cancer of the blood includes
   a. anemia
   b. leukemia
   c. peripheral vascular disease
   d. all of these

8. The formation of plaque on the inner walls of the arteries is called
   a. atherosclerosis
   b. arteriosclerosis

c. varicose veins
d. peripheral vascular disease

9. When the valves in the veins of the legs become weakened, the result is
   a. dementia
   b. stroke
   c. varicose veins
   d. heart failure

10. When caring for persons with peripheral vascular disease, you must always:
    a. regularly inspect the feet and legs
    b. maintain appropriate hygiene of the feet and legs
    c. prevent injury to the feet and legs
    d. all of these

11. Symptoms of heart attack or MI may include
    a. crushing chest pain
    b. nausea and vomiting
    c. diaphoresis
    d. all of these

12. Persons with heart failure are more comfortable in the
    a. orthopneic position
    b. supine position
    c. side-lying position
    d. prone position

13. When caring for a resident with a pacemaker you should
    a. carefully take, record, and report the pulse rate
    b. report hiccoughing
    c. report any discoloration over the implant site
    d. all of these

**B. Match each term (items a.–i.) with the proper explanation.**

a. edema
b. myocardial infarction
c. ventricles
d. ischemia

e. radial artery
f. atria
g. valves
h. atherosclerosis
i. arteries

14. _____ upper heart chambers

15. _____ fluid in the tissue spaces

16. _____ vessels that carry blood away from the heart

17. _____ located close to the radius

18. _____ lower heart chambers

19. _____ form of vascular disease in which plaques are formed in the walls of arteries

20. _____ diminished blood flow

C. **Answer each statement true (T) or false (F).**

21. T   F   The elderly heart muscle is less effective.

22. T   F   The person with orthopnea has difficulty breathing in an upright position.

23. T   F   The anemic person must be handled very gently.

24. T   F   Leukemias are an example of a blood abnormality.

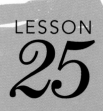

# LESSON 25

# Caring for Residents with Respiratory System Disorders

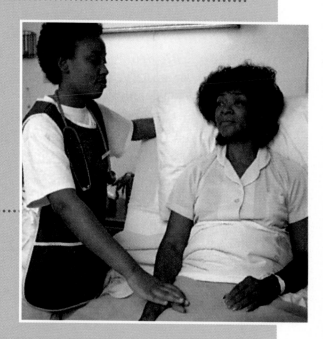

## CLINICAL FOCUS

Think about the special care needed by residents with respiratory disorders as you study this lesson and meet:

*M*ary Calcetas, who is 60 and has been a cigarette smoker for many years. Emphysema has taken its toll and now the very act of breathing is an effort. Walking the length of the corridor to the day room requires two rest periods along the way. Smoking is only permitted under supervision in the day room; so, difficult as it is, she slowly makes her way there early each morning. When an infection occurs, she requires nasal oxygen and orthopneic positioning. The nurse assigns you to collect a sputum specimen this morning.

## OBJECTIVES

*After studying this lesson, you should be able to:*

- Define and spell vocabulary words and terms.
- Identify the parts and function of the respiratory system.
- Review changes in the respiratory system as they relate to the aging process.
- Describe common respiratory conditions affecting the long-term care resident.

- Give proper care to residents in respiratory distress and receiving respiratory therapy.
- Demonstrate the following:
  Procedure 112  Collecting a Sputum Specimen
  Procedure 113  Refilling the Humidifier Bottle

# VOCABULARY

allergen  (**AL**-er-jen)

alveoli  (al-**VEE**-oh-lee)

aspiration  (**ass**-pih-**RAY**-shun)

asthma  (**AZ**-mah)

bronchi  (**BRONG**-kee)

bronchioles  (**BRONG**-kee-ohls)

bronchitis  (brong-**KEYE**-tis)

cannula  (**KAN**-you-lah)

carbon dioxide  (**KAR**-bon dye-**OCK**-side)

chronic obstructive pulmonary disease (COPD)  (**KRON**-ick ob-**STRUCK**-tiv **PULL**-moh-nair-ee dih-**ZEEZ**)

dyspnea  (disp-**NEE**-ah)

emphysema  (**em**-fih-**SEE**-mah)

endotracheal tube  (**en**-doh-**TRAY**-kee-al toob)

expectorate  (eck-**SPECK**-toh-rayt)

high Fowler's position  (high **FOW**-lerz poh-**ZISH**-un)

influenza  (**in**-flew-**EN**-zah)

larynx  (**LAR**-inks)

orthopneic position  (or-thop-**NEE**-ick poh-**ZISH**-un)

oxygen  (**OCK**-sih-jen)

oxygen mask  (**OCK**-sih-jen mask)

pharynx  (**FAR**-inks)

phlegm  (flem)

pleura  (**PLOOR**-ah)

pneumonia  (new-**MOH**-nee-ah)

regurgitate  (ree-**GUR**-jih-tayt)

sputum  (**SPEW**-tum)

tachypnea  (**tack**-ip-**NEE**-ah)

thorax  (**THOR**-acks)

trachea  (**TRAY**-kee-ah)

tracheostomy  (**tray**-kee-**OS**-toh-mee)

ventilation  (ven-tih-**LAY**-shun)

vocal cords  (**VOH**-kal kords)

## INTRODUCTION

The respiratory system exchanges gases to meet the body's metabolic needs. The two gases are:

- **Oxygen** ($O_2$)
- **Carbon dioxide** ($CO_2$)

Oxygen is brought into the lungs and carried to the cells to produce energy.

Carbon dioxide is a waste product that is carried to the lungs from the cells for excretion.

There is a close connection between the respiratory and circulatory systems. Cells depend on the bloodstream to carry gases to and from the lungs.

## THE RESPIRATORY ORGANS

The respiratory organs are shown in Figure 25-1.

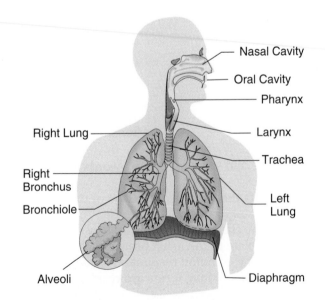

Nasal Cavity
Oral Cavity
Pharynx
Right Lung
Larynx
Trachea
Right Bronchus
Left Lung
Bronchiole
Alveoli
Diaphragm

**FIGURE 25-1**  The respiratory system

## Upper Respiratory Tract

The upper respiratory tract consists of the:

- Nose
- **Pharynx** (throat)
- **Larynx** (voice box)
- **Trachea** (windpipe)
- **Bronchi**

## The Lungs

There are two lungs, each surrounded by a double-walled membrane called the **pleura**. Between the layers of the pleura is a small amount of fluid that reduces friction as the lungs alternately expand and contract, filling with and then expelling air. The air is warmed, filtered, and moistened as it passes over the vascular mucous membrane that lines the respiratory tract, from nose to alveoli.

The bronchi join the upper respiratory tract to the lungs. Within the lungs, the bronchi branch into smaller and smaller divisions called **bronchioles**. The **alveoli** are tiny air sacs that extend from the bronchioles. The alveoli, bronchioles, and the important pulmonary blood vessels form the lungs (Figure 25-2). The way in which oxygen and carbon dioxide are exchanged between the alveoli and the capillaries is shown in Figure 25-3.

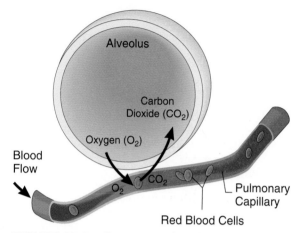

**FIGURE 25-3**   Oxygen and carbon dioxide are exchanged between the capillaries and each of the alveoli.

## The Act of Respiration

The lungs are located in the **thorax**. The size of the thorax depends on the contraction of the diaphragm and intercostal muscles. As the muscles contract, the thorax enlarges, expanding the lungs. Air carrying oxygen enters the lungs. When the muscles relax, the thorax resumes its normal size and the lungs recoil. Air carrying carbon dioxide leaves the lungs and is breathed out.

- *Inspiration* is the act of drawing air into the lungs.
- *Expiration* is the act of expelling air.
- **Ventilation** is the combination of these two actions.

## VOICE PRODUCTION

The larynx, or voice box, is part of the respiratory tract. It is important in voice production. Two membranes called the **vocal cords** stretch across the inside of the larynx. As air passes upward through the larynx, it moves through an opening in the vocal cords. Changes in the shape of the vocal cords and the size of the opening permit controlled amounts of air to reach the mouth, nasal cavities, and sinuses, where—formed by the teeth, lips, and tongue—specific speech sounds are made.

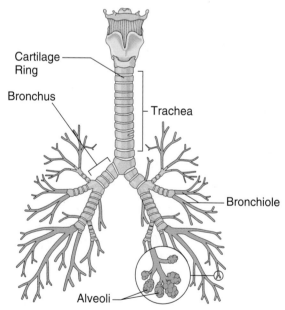

**FIGURE 25-2**   Ventral view of the structures of the lower respiratory tract

**FIGURE 25-4** Changes in the respiratory system as a result of the aging process

- Lung tissue loses elasticity
- Slower rate of gas exchange
- Breathing capacity diminished
- Diaphragm less efficient
- Rate of breathing increases
- Larynx changes make voice weaker and higher pitched
- Less efficient cough

## CHANGES IN THE RESPIRATORY SYSTEM CAUSED BY AGING

Refer to Figure 25-4. With aging, the following changes occur:
- Breathing capacity drops by one-half.
- The alveoli enlarge and lose elasticity, making recoil less effective.
- The respiratory rate increases.
- The diaphragm and intercostal muscles lose strength, so gaseous exchange is less efficient.
- Changes in the larynx make the voice higher pitched and weaker.
- Cough mechanism is less effective.

## INTRODUCTION TO PATHOLOGY

The respiratory system is affected by the same kinds of pathologies as other systems. Two of the most common pathologies are:
- Malignancies
- Infections

### Malignancies

Malignant tumors can develop in any part of the respiratory tract. Although the exact causes of malignancy are not fully understood, cigarette smoking and exposure to other cancer-producing agents in the environment are known to be contributing factors. Lung cancers are treated by surgery, radiation, or chemotherapy, or a combination of all three therapies.

### Cancer of the Larynx

Cancer of the larynx may require removal of the larynx, resulting in the loss of the voice. The resident breathes through an artificial opening in the neck and trachea. The permanent opening is called a **tracheostomy** and is a permanent stoma.

Loss of voice is a major trauma for anyone. Just think for a moment of how frustrated you would feel if you could no longer use your voice to communicate your thoughts, feelings, wants, and needs to others.

Postsurgical care is given in the acute care hospital. At this time, writing is the major form of communication available to patients. Later, the resident may be taught new ways to speak through:
- Esophageal speech
- Electronic speech

**Esophageal Speech.** The resident learns to swallow air and than bring it back up (**regurgitate**) through the esophagus into the mouth. Here it is formed by the teeth and tongue into words as it would be if it were being exhaled from the lungs. Esophageal speech is difficult to learn, but motivated residents can succeed.

**Electronic Speech.** Residents who cannot use esophageal speech may be able to use an electronic artificial larynx to create speech. Some residents may use a combination of both techniques.

Residents with laryngectomies (removal of larynx) need patience and understanding from all health care providers. Communication is possible, but the voice does not sound normal. More time is needed by the resident to formulate the sounds. A difficult psychological adjustment must be made by the resident. The loss of one's voice requires an adjustment similar to that experienced when grieving for the loss of a loved one. Expect periods of depression, anger, and hostility.

## Infections

The respiratory tract is exposed to many pathogens in the environment. Respiratory infections are common in the elderly because of reduced resistance and can be life-threatening.

Upper respiratory tract infections such as colds or sore throats are caused by viruses or bacteria. These infections are usually self-limiting and are treated by rest, fluids, and antibiotics (if caused by bacteria). Two common infections are influenza and pneumonia. Both can be life-threatening to the elderly and those with compromised immune systems.

**Influenza.**  **Influenza** is a viral respiratory infection. There is usually a sudden onset of signs and symptoms, including:

- Chills
- Fever
- Muscle pain
- Weakness
- Fatigue
- Laryngitis
- Hoarseness
- Nonproductive cough
- Runny nose and eyes

The symptoms usually last 3 to 5 days. In the elderly, however, the fatigue and cough may last for several weeks. Influenza can also lead to pneumonia. Elderly people and those with chronic illness who are not allergic to chicken, eggs, or feathers are encouraged to receive a yearly influenza ("flu") vaccine.

**Pneumonia.**  **Pneumonia** is a serious infection of the lungs that causes the alveoli to fill with fluid, affecting the exchange of gases. The causes of pneumonia include:

- Viruses
- Bacteria
- **Aspiration** of food and liquids (accidentally taking food and liquids into the trachea instead of the esophagus)
- Immobility, which allows fluid to accumulate in the lungs

The resident may have chills, fever, chest pain, and a productive cough (produces sputum). **Sputum** or **phlegm** is matter that is brought up (**expectorated**) from the lungs. Spu-

tum varies in color and character. Respiration may be labored and cyanosis may be present. Treatment includes bed rest, oxygen, and positioning to relieve breathing. Antibiotics are given for bacterial pneumonia. Drugs are also given to relieve chest pain. Residents are encouraged to take fluids. A pneumonia vaccine is available for immunization.

Residents are better able to resist respiratory tract infections when they take in adequate fluids and remain active.

## Effect of Age on the Response to Infections

As people age, their bodies may not respond as strongly to infections as those of younger people. The signs and symptoms of infection may not be as pronounced. Be sure to report:

- Changes in rate or rhythm of respirations
- Cough
- Elevated temperature
- Persistant fatigue
- Difficulty breathing (**dyspnea**)
- Rapid, shallow, or noisy breathing (**tachypnea**)
- Confusion
- Restlessness
- Changes in color of secretions
- Cyanosis
- Pallor
- Shortness of breath (SOB)

Infections are treated vigorously with:

- Rest
- Antibiotics (for bacterial infections)
- Oxygen therapy
- Drugs to keep air passageways clear
- Supportive care

Always practice standard precautions when caring for residents with respiratory infections. Remember that these infectious organisms are often airborne and found in droplets of respiratory secretions. Transmission-based precautions may be required in addition to standard precautions.

## Collecting a Sputum Specimen

You may need to collect a sputum specimen from the resident. A culture of the specimen identifies the cause of the infection.

You must be sure that the specimen comes from the lungs and is not saliva from the mouth.

If the resident cannot expectorate sputum, suctioning may be needed to obtain the speci-men. (The nurse usually performs this proce-dure.) It is easier to collect the specimen when the resident wakes up in the morning and after taking two or three deep breaths.

**PROCEDURE**
**112** Collecting a Sputum Specimen

1. Carry out each beginning procedure action.
2. Assemble equipment:
   - Disposable gloves
   - Container and cover for specimen
   - Glass of water
   - Label including:
     - Resident's full name
     - Room number
     - Resident number
     - Date and time of collection
     - Physician's name
     - Examination to be done
     - Other information as requested
   - Tissues
   - Emesis basin
   - Biohazard specimen transport bag
   - Laboratory requisition
3. Wash hands and put on disposable gloves.
4. Ask the resident to rinse mouth with water and spit into emesis basin.
5. Ask resident to breathe deeply and then cough deeply to bring up sputum. The resident spits the sputum into the con-tainer (Figure 25-5).
   - While coughing have resident cover mouth with tissue to prevent spread of infection.
   - Collect 1 to 2 tablespoons of sputum unless otherwise ordered.
   - Do not contaminate the outside of the container.
6. Remove gloves and discard according to facility policy.

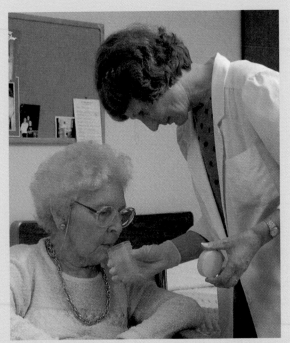

**FIGURE 25-5** After coughing deeply, the resident deposits the sputum directly into the container.

7. Wash your hands.
8. Cover container tightly and attach com-pleted label.
9. Place specimen container into biohazard transport bag and attach laboratory req-uisition.
10. Carry out each procedure completion action.
11. Follow facility policy for transport of specimen to laboratory.

# CHRONIC OBSTRUCTIVE PULMONARY DISEASE

**Chronic obstructive pulmonary disease (COPD)** is also called chronic obstructive lung disease (COLD). This term refers to conditions resulting from a prolonged impairment in the exchange of gases in the respiratory system. Several conditions can lead to COPD, including:

- Tuberculosis
- Frequent pneumonia
- Chronic asthma
- Chronic bronchitis
- Emphysema

## Asthma

**Asthma** is a breathing disorder resulting from:

- Constriction of the muscles of the bronchioles
- Swelling of the respiratory membranes
- Production of large amounts of mucus that fill the narrowed passageways

A person having an asthma attack has labored breathing and frequent coughing. An attack may result when the person contacts an **allergen** or is under emotional stress. Common allergens are:

- Pollen
- Medications
- Dust
- Feathers
- Foods such as chicken, eggs, or chocolate

If a resident has known allergies (hypersensitivity to specific items), they should be marked in the resident's health record. Long-term treatment consists of determining the allergen and eliminating it. To relieve the attack, the resident is given medication to decrease the swelling and dilate the bronchioles. Low levels of oxygen are also given.

## Chronic Bronchitis

Chronic **bronchitis** is prolonged inflammation in the bronchi due to infection or irritants. Signs and symptoms include:

- Swollen and red bronchial tissues, resulting in narrowed bronchial passageways
- Persistent cough, which may or may not produce sputum
- Respiratory distress

Treatment, in general includes:

- Antibiotics to fight the infection
- Drugs to loosen the phlegm (secretions) deep in the respiratory tract
- Techniques to improve ventilation and drainage

## Emphysema

**Emphysema** develops after chronic obstruction of the air flow to the alveoli. The air sacs:

- Become distended
- Lose their elasticity and recoil ability
- Finally become nonfunctional
- Lose ability to exchange gases

The resident can bring air into the lungs, but it becomes more difficult to expel air from the lungs. As a result, there is less and less room for air to reenter.

Several factors contribute to emphysema, including:

- Air pollutants, such as cigarette smoke, auto exhaust fumes, and insecticides
- Genetic predisposition to emphysema
- Recurrent infections, such as pneumonia and bronchitis
- Chronic asthma

People with emphysema are at greater risk for infections such as pneumonia. They experience:

- Chronic oxygen shortage and fatigue
- Increasing breathing difficulty (requires greater and greater effort)
- Productive coughing that may bring up large amounts of heavy mucous secretions (phlegm), or nonproductive coughing
- Dizziness and restlessness as carbon dioxide levels rise in the bloodstream
- Loss of appetite and weight loss
- Strain on the heart and blood vessels

# TREATMENT AND CARE OF RESIDENTS WITH COPD

The goals of treatment of the resident with COPD are to:

- Loosen and thin phlegm
- Improve ventilation
- Improve gaseous exchange
- Prevent infections

Special techniques are used to loosen the phlegm and make it easier to bring up. Removing phlegm from the passageways makes breathing easier. Some procedures will be carried out by the nurse or respiratory therapist. You may assist in:

- Positioning the resident for better ventilation
- Breathing exercises to improve respiratory efficiency
- Caring for the resident during oxygen therapy to improve gaseous exchange

## Positioning for Better Ventilation

Two positions are used to improve ventilation:

- High Fowler's position
- Orthopneic position

In the **high Fowler's position**, the resident is sitting almost upright with the knees flexed. The resident must be supported in proper alignment with pillows.

In the **orthopneic position**, an overbed table is positioned in front of the resident (Figure 25-6). The resident leans forward with arms on the table. A pillow on the overbed table supports the head. The arms may be positioned on or around the pillow. Additional pillows are used to support the resident's body and maintain proper alignment.

Most residents with COPD who are ambulatory breathe best when sitting in a chair and leaning forward with the elbows on the arms of the chair or on their legs.

## Exercises

Residents can be taught breathing exercises that improve respiration and general respiratory muscle tone. Breathing exercises stress the expiration phase of respiration. The resident is first taught the basic breathing pattern, which is to:

- Breathe in through the nose to the count of one, allowing the abdomen to rise.
- Purse the lips to the count of two and three as the abdominal wall is contracted and air is forced out of the lungs.

## Oxygen Therapy

Residents with COPD benefit by breathing low levels of oxygen. Oxygen therapy may be administered by:

- **Cannulas**—small tubes placed in the resident's nostrils and held in place by straps (Figure 25-7).
- **Oxygen mask**—placed over the resident's nose and mouth and secured in place (Figure 25-8)
- Nasal catheter—a small plastic or latex tube that is inserted into the nose

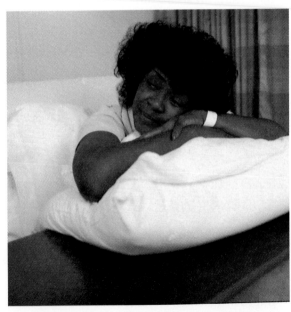

**FIGURE 25-6**  The orthopneic position

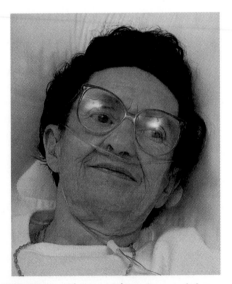

**FIGURE 25-7**  This resident is receiving oxygen through a cannula attached to the oxygen source.

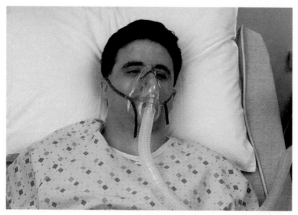

**FIGURE 25-8** The mask is placed over the resident's nose and mouth to deliver oxygen.

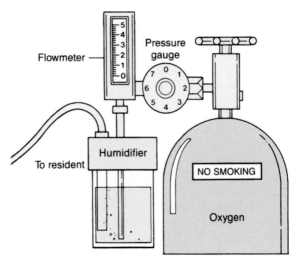

**FIGURE 25-9** Oxygen may be delivered from a tank.

The nurse will set up the oxygen equipment and will start the oxygen flow. You observe the resident for the following:

- Proper position of the catheter, cannula, or mask and the elastic band snug but not constricting
- Signs of irritation from straps, catheter, cannula, or mask
- The tubing not kinked, pinched, or restricted in any way
- Flowmeter registers volume of oxygen flow properly in liters
- Oxygen moisturized
- Resident's face free of secretions
- Safety precautions being followed (review Lesson 8)

**Source of Oxygen.**   Oxygen may be piped into the resident's room, but in long-term care facilities, tanks of oxygen may be used (Figure 25-9). If a tank is used, be sure that:

- "No Smoking" signs are in place.
- There is sufficient oxygen in the tank. Check the gauge each time you visit the resident.
- An additional tank is available.
- Empty tanks are marked and stored according to facility policy.
- The tank is upright and secure on the carrier or in the stand.
- The oxygen is moisturized.

Oxygen does not explode, but when it is present, burning is more intense and rapid. Everyone must follow oxygen safety measures. If there is a fire, sound the alarm and move the resident to safety, following facility policy.

## Oxygen Concentrator

An oxygen concentrator takes in room air and removes impurities and gases other than oxygen, allowing the oxygen to become concentrated in the unit. The air delivered to the resident from the concentrator is more than 90% oxygen. It is delivered by tubing attached to a nasal cannula or mask. The flow rate is usually 2 liters per minute (L/min). A humidifier bottle may be attached to the concentrator to offset the drying effect of the oxygen.

**General Oxygen Concentrator Precautions.** Be sure to follow these precautions when a concentrator is used to supply oxygen to a resident:

- Concentrator is placed at least 5 feet away from a heat source and at least 4 inches from the wall.
- Smoking is not permitted in the same room.
- Be sure the unit is plugged in and grounded.
- Do not use an extension cord with the concentrator.
- Never change the flowmeter setting.
- Notify the nurse if the alarm sounds.
- Be sure the fluid level in the humidifier (if used) is adequate.
- Wipe cannula or mask daily with a damp cloth (do not use alcohol- or oil-based products).
- Clean concentrator surfaces using a damp cloth only.
- Remove filter weekly. Wash in warm soapy water, rinse, squeeze dry, and replace.

**PROCEDURE**
**113**
# Refilling the Humidifier Bottle

1. Carry out each beginning procedure action.
2. Remove mask or cannula from resident or connect it to a temporary oxygen source if constant oxygen is required.
3. Turn oxygen concentrator off.
4. Remove the lid from the humidifier bottle.
5. Remove the bottle and discard any remaining water.
6. Rinse bottle well with warm water. Shake dry.
7. Refill jar with distilled water to the fill line.
8. Replace bottle and reattach lid.
9. Turn on unit.
10. Position mask or cannula on resident.
11. Wash hands.
12. Carry out procedure completion actions.

## Special Mouth Care

Breathing through the mouth and breathing oxygen are drying to the mucous membranes of the mouth and the nasal passages. The resident may complain that sputum has a bad taste. Make sure that the resident rinses his or her mouth frequently and that you provide special mouth care. This attention adds greatly to the resident's comfort. Encourage fluid intake because adequate fluids help decrease the thickness of secretions.

## Ineffective Cough

If cough is ineffective, it may be necessary to intubate the resident. An **endotracheal tube** is placed directly into the trachea through an opening (tracheotomy) in the throat. Both oxygen delivery and suctioning can take place through the tube. The tracheotomy may be made into a permanent tracheostomy.

A machine that delivers oxygen under pressure at a preset rate may be needed to assist ventilation. This technique is known as intermittent positive pressure breathing (IPPB). The machine may be attached directly to the endotracheal tube. When a resident is receiving assisted ventilation, you will check for:

- Change of color
- Signs of congestion
- Changes in vital signs
- Indications of respiratory distress

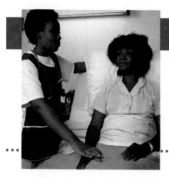

## LESSON SYNTHESIS: Putting It All Together

*Y*ou have just completed this lesson. Now go back and review the Clinical Focus. Try to see how the Clinical Focus relates to the concepts presented in the lesson. Then answer the following questions.

1. Why does Mrs. Calcetas have to rest so often when she tries to walk to the day room?

2. Why would smoking make Mrs. Calcetas' condition more difficult?

3. Why should Mrs. Calcetas rinse her mouth and then cough deeply to obtain a sputum specimen?

4. Why should the person collecting the specimen wear gloves?

5. What nursing care techniques could you use to help improve Mrs. Calcetas' breathing?

## REVIEW

**A. Select the correctly spelled word and then write its definition using the word in the definition.**

1. xpectorate  expectorate  espectarate

2. experation  xpiration  expiration

3. thorax  tharox  thorix

4. flegm  flem  phlegm

**B. Complete each statement by filling in the missing information.**

5. Another name for the windpipe is the _____.

6. As a person ages, breathing capacity diminishes by _____.

7. Changes in the larynx make the voice _____ and _____.

8. List three changes that occur in the respiratory system as a person ages.

_____  _____  _____

9. When collecting a sputum specimen, the assistant should wear _____.

10. State the two positions used to assist a resident in respiratory distress.

_____  _____

**C. Select the one best answer for each of the following.**

11. Rapid and shallow breathing is known as
   a. apnea
   b. emphysema
   c. pleura
   d. tachypnea

12. The technique of swallowing air, regurgitating it, and forming words with the teeth and tongue is called
   a. nasal speech
   b. esophageal speech
   c. electronic speech
   d. sinus speech

13. Sputum is matter from the
   a. lungs
   b. nose
   c. mouth
   d. sinuses

14. An asthma attack may occur when a sensitive person contacts an allergen such as
 a. medications
 b. feathers
 c. dust
 d. all of these

15. What is the name given to the position in which the resident is sitting almost upright with the knees flexed?
 a. orthopneic
 b. upright
 c. high Fowler's
 d. left Sims'

16. Breathing exercises for residents with COPD stress
 a. inspiratory phase
 b. expiratory phase
 c. resting phase
 d. inhalation phase

17. When a resident receives oxygen from a tank through a nasal cannula, the nursing assistant must be sure that
 a. the flowmeter registers the proper moisture content
 b. oxygen is being administered with humidification
 c. there is no irritation from the strap or cannula
 d. tank leans against the wall

**D. Identify and write the name of each structure shown in the figure.**

18. _____

19. _____

20. _____

21. _____

22. _____

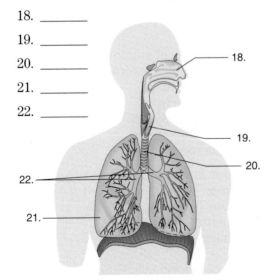

**E. Clinical Experience**
**Fill in the blanks by selecting the correct word from the list.**

| | |
|---|---|
| adjustment | gloves |
| anger | normal |
| burned | patience |
| common | report |
| cover | sputum |
| depression | strongly |

23. Mr. Drummond had a laryngectomy. He is new to your unit. He uses esophageal speech. What characteristics might you expect of him?
 a. His speech will not sound _____.
 b. He had to make a great psychological _____ to his condition.
 c. He will experience periods of _____ and _____.
 d. His care will require much _____ from staff members.

24. Mrs. Burton, who is 87, is one of the residents you care for. She said she does not have "much energy" this morning. She seems a little confused and has a slight cough. Her temperature is elevated only slightly.
 a. You know that influenza and pneumonia are _____ complications of the aging process.
 b. You also remember that as people age, they do not respond to infection as _____ as younger people.
 c. You will _____ your findings promptly.

25. Mr. Ornsteen has a respiratory infection and is confined to bed. You are assigned to care for him. What do you need to remember to protect yourself?
 a. Use _____ when handling respiratory or nasal secretions.
 b. Instruct him to _____ his nose and mouth when coughing or sneezing.
 c. Do not contaminate the outside of the specimen container when obtaining a _____ specimen.

# Caring for Residents with Endocrine System Disorders

**CLINICAL FOCUS**

Think about the special observations and care the resident with endocrine disorders needs as you study this lesson and meet:

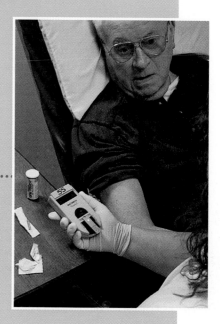

$M$r. McFarland, who is an insulin-dependent diabetic assigned to your care. He has had a cold. This morning he seems very restless and less responsive than usual. He grows increasingly confused. His 11:00 AM glucometer reading shows hyperglycemia. There are immediate actions that must be taken.

## OBJECTIVES

*After studying this lesson, you should be able to:*

- Define and spell vocabulary words and terms.
- Identify the parts and function of the endocrine system.
- Review changes in the endocrine system as they relate to the aging process.

- Explain the importance of electrolyte balance.
- Recognize reportable signs and symptoms of hypoglycemia and hypercapnia.
- Recognize reportable signs and symptoms of residents with low blood potassium levels and those with high blood sodium levels.

## VOCABULARY

**adrenal glands** *(ah-**DREE**-nal glands)*

**adrenaline** *(ah-**DREN**-ah-lin)*

**cortisone** *(**KOR**-tih-sohn)*

**diabetes mellitus** *(**die**-ah-**BEE**-teez **MEL**-ih-tus)*

**diabetic coma** *(**die**-ah-**BET**-ick **KOH**-mah)*

**diabetic ketoacidosis (DKA)** *(**dye**-ah-**BET**-ick **kee**-toh-ah-sih-**DOH**-sis)*

**electrolytes** *(ee-**LECK**-troh-lights)*

**endocrine gland** *(**EN**-doh-krin gland)*

**estrogen** *(**ES**-troh-jen)*

**gangrene** *(**GANG**-green)*

# VOCABULARY

glucagon    (*GLOO-kah-gon*)

glucose    (*GLOO-kohs*)

glycosuria    (*gligh-koh-SOO-ree-ah*)

goiter    (*GOY-ter*)

gonad    (*GOH-nad*)

homeostasis    (*hoh-mee-oh-STAY-sis*)

hormone    (*HOR-mohn*)

hyperglycemia    (*high-per-gly-SEE-mee-ah*)

hyperthyroidism    (*high-per-THIGH-roy-dizm*)

hypoglycemia    (*high-poh-gly-SEE-mee-ah*)

hypothyroidism    (*high-poh-THIGH-roy-dizm*)

insulin    (*IN-soo-lin*)

insulin-dependent diabetes mellitus (IDDM)    (*IN-soo-lin dee-PEN-dent die-ah-BEE-teez MEL-ih-tus*)

insulin shock    (*IN-soo-lin shock*)

islets of Langerhans    (*EYE-lets of LANG-ger-hans*)

ketones    (*KEE-tohns*)

metabolism    (*meh-TAB-oh-lizm*)

non–insulin-dependent diabetes mellitus (NIDDM)    (*non–IN-soo-lin dee-PEN-dent die-ah-BEE-teez MEL-ih-tus*)

ovaries    (*OH-vah-rees*)

pancreas    (*PAN-kree-as*)

parathormone    (*pair-ah-THOR-mohn*)

parathyroid glands    (*pair-ah-THIGH-royd glands*)

pineal body    (*PIN-ee-al BAH-dee*)

pituitary gland    (*pih-TOO-ih-tair-ee gland*)

polydipsia    (*pol-ee-DIP-see-ah*)

polyphagia    (*pol-ee-FAY-jee-ah*)

polyuria    (*pol-ee-YOU-ree-ah*)

progesterone    (*proh-JES-teh-rohn*)

scrotum    (*SKROH-tum*)

testes    (*TES-teez*)

testosterone    (*tes-TOS-teh-rohn*)

thyroid gland    (*THIGH-royd gland*)

thyroxine    (*thigh-ROCK-sin*)

## INTRODUCTION

The endocrine system (Figure 26-1), consists of:

- **Endocrine glands**, some of which are in pairs
- Clusters of cells

The seven distinct endocrine glands are:

- Pituitary gland
- Pineal body
- Adrenal glands
- Gonads—ovaries (women); testes (men)
- Thyroid gland
- Parathyroid glands
- Islets of Langerhans (pancreas)

The endocrine tissues are located throughout the body. They have the following functions and properties:

- Produce chemical messengers (**hormones**)
- Directly enter the bloodstream
- Regulate body activities and body chemistry

Some endocrine glands secrete more than one hormone. Hormone-producing cells may be found as part of organs that carry on other functions. For example:

- The thyroid gland produces two hormones:
    - Thyrocalcitonin
    - Thyroxine
- The **pancreas** produces two hormones:
    - Glucagon
    - Insulin

The pancreas also produces enzymes that are important in the digestive process.

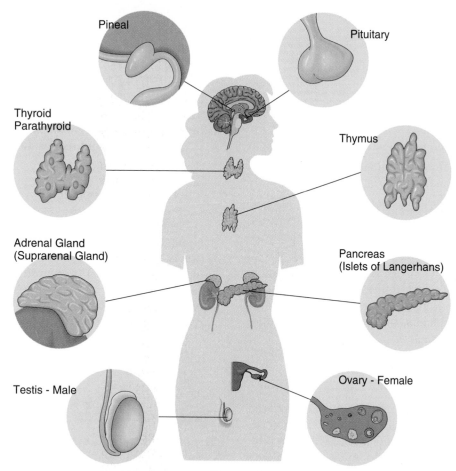

**FIGURE 26-1** The endocrine system

## ENDOCRINE GLANDS

### Pituitary Gland

The **pituitary gland** is found under the brain and secretes more than one hormone. It is sometimes called the master gland. The hormones secreted by this gland control:

- Growth
- Urine production
- Activity of most of the other glands
- Reproductive activity
- Blood chemistry

### Pineal Body

The **pineal body** is a small gland that is also located in the skull beneath the brain. It is thought to delay sexual maturity until the rest of the body is ready for reproduction. It grows smaller as we age.

### Adrenal Glands

There are two **adrenal glands**. One gland is located on top of each of the two kidneys. Each gland has two portions that secrete separate hormones. Two of these hormones, **adrenaline** (epinephrine) and **cortisone**, are often prescribed medications. In general, the adrenal hormones:

- Control the release of energy to meet emergencies
- Control water and electrolyte balance in the body

* Secrete small amounts of male and female sex hormones

## Gonads

The term **gonads** refers to the sex glands.

* Female gonads = ovaries
* Male gonads = testes

Symbols are used to indicate the different sexes:

* ♀ indicates female (woman)
* ♂ indicates male (man)

**Ovaries (♀).** The paired **ovaries** are located within the pelvis on either side of the uterus. When stimulated by the pituitary gland, they produce the hormones:

* **Progesterone**—helps to maintain pregnancy
* **Estrogen**—responsible for the development of female characteristics such as:
  * Enlargement of the female reproductive organs
  * Appearance of pubic and axillary hair
  * Enlargement of the breasts
  * Onset and regulation of menstruation

**Testes (♂).** The paired **testes** are located outside of the body in a pouch called the **scrotum**. They produce the hormone **testosterone**, which regulates the development of male secondary characteristics, including:

* Muscular development
* Deepening voice
* Growth of hair on body and face
* Growth and maturity of the reproductive organs

The male and female gonads also produce special cells, the female ovum and the male sperm, that unite during conception to form a human embryo.

## Thyroid Gland

The **thyroid gland** is located in the neck, in front of the larynx. The thyroid gland produces two hormones:

* **Thyroxine**—helps regulate the metabolic rate of all body cells
* Thyrocalcitonin—helps regulate the levels of calcium and phosphates in the blood. These are two of the electrolyte minerals involved in electrolyte balance (discussed later in this lesson).

**Metabolism** is the production of heat and energy by the cells. Energy production is related to the ability of the cells to take up and use oxygen.

Disorders of the thyroid gland include:

* **Hyperthyroidism** (exophthalmic **goiter** or toxic goiter) results from overproduction of thyroxine. The resident shows:
  * Irritability and restlessness
  * Nervousness
  * Rapid pulse
  * Increased appetite
  * Weight loss
  * Sensitivity
* **Hypothyroidism** results from underproduction of thyroxine. The lack of iodine can result in a low thyroxine production. This is known as simple goiter. A severe lack of thyroxine results in a condition called myxedema. The resident with hypothyroidism shows:
  * Slow responses
  * Lethargy
  * Weight gain
  * Slow pulse

## Parathyroid Glands

The **parathyroid glands** are several tiny glands embedded in the back of the thyroid gland. They produce the hormone **parathormone** that also helps control the use of calcium and phosphorus by the body.

## Islets of Langerhans

The **islets of Langerhans** are small groups of cells found within the pancreas. Two very important hormones produced by these cells are insulin and glucagon. These hormones help regulate blood sugar.

Blood sugar is called **glucose**. Glucose is needed by all cells for *all* body work. Glucose metabolism is discussed later in this lesson.

## AGING CHANGES

Changes in the endocrine system caused by aging include:

* Decreased glucose tolerance
* Increased levels of parathormone

- Decreased vaginal secretions
- Increased blood sugar level due to slower release of insulin by pancreatic cells
- Decreased metabolic rate resulting from changes in the thyroid

## ELECTROLYTE BALANCE

**Electrolytes** are substances that are essential to the chemical functioning of the body. The electrolytes in the body fluids must be balanced for proper functioning. You may be familiar with electrolytes as solid substances such as sodium chloride (table salt) and sodium bicarbonate, an antacid used to relieve indigestion.

In the body fluids, the electrolytes break apart to form ions that take part in the body's chemical reactions. Two important electrolytes contain the ions of:

- Sodium
- Potassium

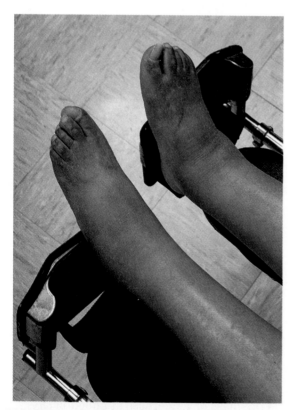

**FIGURE 26-2** Edema of the feet and legs as a result of electrolyte imbalance

| **FIGURE 26-3**  Observations to be reported for the resident with electrolyte imbalance |
| --- |
| • Swelling of feet and legs |
| • Respiratory distress |
| • Slower than normal pulse rate |
| • Lack of interest in surroundings |
| • Feelings of weakness |
| • Intake and output (if ordered) |

The **homeostasis** (balance) of body functions depends on many body activities. The endocrine system plays an important part in this process.

When there is an electrolyte imbalance in the body, many problems—sometimes serious—can occur.

Two common problems are:

- Increased levels of sodium in the blood. The sodium causes body tissues to hold fluid, resulting in swelling or edema. This is often seen in the feet and legs of elderly residents (Figure 26-2). Fluid may also accumulate in the lungs, causing respiratory distress.
- Decreased levels of potassium in the blood. This leads to a slower heart rate, feelings of weakness, and a lack of interest in surroundings.

Figure 26-3 lists observations to report for residents with electrolyte imbalance.

## GLUCOSE METABOLISM

Glucose is the primary energy source for all of the work done by the body. The level of glucose is an important factor in proper functioning. Various hormones and enzymes maintain this level and help the body to use (metabolize) glucose for energy. Two of these hormones are:

- **Glucagon**—raises the blood sugar level by converting stored sugar (glycogen) to glucose.

- **Insulin**—lowers the blood sugar level by causing glucose to move from the bloodstream into the cells. It also helps to convert glucose to glycogen (stored sugar).

  Abnormal blood sugar levels are called:

- **Hyperglycemia**—the blood sugar level is too high.
- **Hypoglycemia**—the blood sugar level is too low.

  Diabetes mellitus is a major disorder of glucose metabolism. It is usually caused by:

- Insufficient insulin in the body
- Inability of the cells to use the available insulin

## DIABETES MELLITUS

In **diabetes mellitus** the body cannot use glucose normally to meet the energy needs of the body. This disease is common in older people. In fact, in people over age 65, one of every 20 requires treatment for diabetes.

The two forms of diabetes are:

- **Insulin–dependent diabetes mellitus (IDDM)**
- **Non–insulin-dependent diabetes mellitus (NIDDM)**

Both forms may be seen in older people, but the non–insulin-dependent form is more common.

### Insulin-Dependent Diabetes Mellitus

IDDM is more often seen in younger people. Signs and symptoms include:

- Abrupt onset
- Excess thirst (**polydipsia**)
- Excess urine elimination (**polyuria**)
- Excessive hunger (**polyphagia**)
- Sugar in the urine (**glycosuria**)
- Excess blood sugar (hyperglycemia)

This form of diabetes is more difficult to control. Diabetic persons may experience periods of hypoglycemia (**insulin shock**) or hyperglycemia (**diabetic coma**). These people require:

- Regular injections of insulin to balance their blood sugar
- Regulation of food intake
- Planned exercise (which uses sugar for energy) as part of the treatment program

### Non–insulin-Dependent Diabetes Mellitus

NIDDM is also known as old-age diabetes. The older the person, the more likely that diabetes will develop. This form of diabetes is more stable than IDDM, with fewer incidents of diabetic coma or insulin shock.

**Signs and Symptoms.** Often only one or two symptoms appear in the elderly person. The person is usually overweight and may have constant fatigue or a sore or infection that takes an unusually long time to heal. About half of those with diabetes show the obvious signs (Figure 26-4). The rest have less well-defined symptoms such as:

- Fatiguing easily
- Skin infections
- Slow healing
- Itching
- Burning on urination
- Pain in fingers and toes
- Vision changes

### Complications of Diabetes

Complications, which can be severe and nonreversible in the elderly, include:

- Renal disease
- Vision changes
- Cardiovascular damage
- Hyperglycemia
- Hypoglycemia

| **FIGURE 26-4** Signs of diabetes mellitus |
| --- |
| • Polyuria (excessive urine) |
| • Polydipsia (excessive thirst) |
| • Polyphagia (excessive hunger) |
| • Weight loss |
| • Blurring of vision |
| • Complaints of itching |
| • Burning on urination |
| • Redness or tenderness at injection site |
| • Slow healing of infections or injuries |

**Vision Changes.** This is particularly common in long-term diabetes. Serious vision changes are often thought to be due to general aging. However, they may really be related to diabetes. Complications include:

- Glaucoma
- Cataracts
- Retinitis proliferans
- Blindness

**Cardiovascular Damage.** The consequences of hypoglycemia (insulin shock) or hyperglycemia (diabetic coma) can be severe in the elderly resident and may include:

- Heart attacks
- Strokes
- Peripheral vascular disease
- Amputation

Because injuries heal poorly, an ingrown toenail or improperly cut nails can lead to serious problems. Vascular changes can interfere with the normal circulation to the legs and feet. Damage may be so extensive that the tissues of the toes, feet, and legs may die. As a result, they need to be removed (amputated). **Gangrene** (death of tissue) (Figure 26-5) followed by amputation is a common problem for the older resident with diabetes. Careful observations and care can help prevent this serious condition.

**Hyperglycemia.** This condition occurs when too little insulin is available for metabolic needs. Sugar and acid compounds (**ketones**) build up in the blood. The condition is known as **diabetic ketoacidosis (DKA)** and can lead to death. Sugar and ketones then spill over into the urine.

A sudden, unexpected need for insulin brought about by stress, illness, injury, or curtailed activity may bring on DKA. It usually develops slowly, sometimes over a 24-hour period. The first symptoms may be headache, drowsiness, and confusion. The resident seems less responsive, irritable, confused, and drowsy and may slip slowly into unconsciousness (coma).

Signs and symptoms of hyperglycemia include:

- Thirst
- Blurred vision
- Nausea and vomiting
- A sweet odor to the breath
- Dry, flushed skin

It is important to note these signs early so that treatment can begin right away. Learn the signs and symptoms of diabetic coma (Figure 26-6). If these signs are noted in a resident, report them immediately. The treatment for hyperglycemia is insulin and fluids, which will be given intravenously by the nurse.

**Hypoglycemia.** Hypoglycemia or low blood sugar is far less common when oral antidiabetic

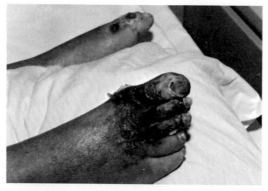

**FIGURE 26-5** Gangrene of the toes and feet often results in amputation.

| FIGURE 26-6 Signs and symptoms to be reported for diabetic coma and insulin shock | |
|---|---|
| **Diabetic Coma (Hyperglycemia)** | **Insulin Shock (Hypoglycemia)** |
| Gradual onset | Sudden onset |
| Drowsiness | Nervousness |
| Deep, difficult breathing | Shallow breathing |
| Nausea | Hunger |
| Hot, flushed, dry skin | Moist, pale skin |
| Mental confusion | Mental confusion Vision disturbance |
| Loss of consciousness | Loss of consciousness |
| Sweet odor to breath | |

agents are given than when insulin is given by injection. When hypoglycemia results from an overdose of insulin, it is known as *insulin reaction* or insulin shock. Hypoglycemia can be brought on by:

- Not eating planned snacks or eating less food (as a result of decreased appetite)
- Unusual activity
- Stress
- Vomiting
- Diarrhea
- Interaction of oral drugs with other medications being taken

In contrast to DKA, which develops slowly, hypoglycemia may occur rapidly.

Signs and symptoms of hypoglycemia include:

- Hunger
- Sweating
- Dizziness
- Drowsiness
- Blurred vision
- Erratic behavior
- Staggering gait
- Mental confusion
- Disorientation
- Pale and moist skin

Learn the signs and symptoms of hypoglycemia (see Figure 26-6). Report immediately to the nurse if you observe them in a resident.

The resident with hypoglycemia is treated with sugar in some form. A food containing sugar is given orally if the resident is conscious. If the resident is unconscious, glucagon (a hormone) may be given by injection. Orange juice or other easily absorbed sources of sugar are usually kept on the unit where they are easily accessible for the nurse to use in an emergency. Every staff member should be aware of the storage location.

## Treatment of Diabetes

For people with diabetes living independently, the control of the disease depends on self-care. For a resident with diabetes, the self-care is assisted. Residents should be encouraged to take part in their own care as much as possible.

The goals for the care of the person with diabetes, whether at home or in a facility, are the same:

- Maintain a proper metabolic balance
- Prevent complications

Although uncommon, the less stable form of diabetes (IDDM) may appear in later years. If you notice any of the acute signs, they should be reported at once. A few elderly diabetic residents are insulin dependent. The treatment is then the same as for any insulin-dependent person. Some people who have had diabetes since youth will continue to require regular insulin injections.

Three factors must be balanced in each diabetic's life:

- Diet
- Exercise
- Drugs

Note that some people with diabetes are able to manage the disease by diet and exercise and do not require drug therapy.

**Diet.** Most residents with diabetes receive specially balanced diabetic meals. Your responsibilities include:

- Checking trays carefully to be sure the correct diet is given
- Serving the trays
- Assisting in feeding
- Noticing and recording how much and what food was eaten
- Returning trays after meals
- Informing the nurse if food is not eaten
- Giving supplemental foods as ordered

If concentrated sugars such as jellies or jams are on the tray, be sure to check with the nurse before feeding the resident (concentrated sugars usually are never permitted in a diabetic diet). You must know what is allowed for each resident with diabetes in your care.

**Exercise.** The more a person exercises, the more sugar is needed for energy. The increased need for sugar usage increases the need for insulin. Less exercise decreases the need. A resident's activity will influence the need for both food and insulin. Be sure to report unusual activity or unusual inactivity.

**Drugs.** Drugs used in the treatment of diabetes are called antidiabetic drugs. Some of these may be taken by mouth (oral hypoglycemics). Insulin must be injected. The nurse will administer the drugs, but you also have some responsibilities. For oral hypoglycemics, be sure to report if the drugs are not taken. For example, if a pill is given to the resident and then is spit out after the nurse leaves the room, report this to the nurse immediately.

If the resident is receiving insulin, check the injection site and report:

- Redness
- Pain
- Itching

## Nursing Assistant Responsibilities

Residents who experience emotional stress or have an infection of any kind are at greater risk for imbalance. They need to be monitored with extra care and attention. When providing routine care for the resident with diabetes you must:

- Know the signs of insulin shock and diabetic coma.
- Be alert for the signs of diabetic coma or insulin shock and report them immediately to the nurse.
- Know the storage location of juice or other easily absorbed carbohydrates.
- When food trays are delivered, check that the resident receives the proper diet.
- Give extra nourishments only as ordered.
- Keep a record of the food consumed on the resident's chart.
- Report uneaten meals to the nurse.
- Give special attention to the care of the diabetic resident's feet.
  - Wash daily, carefully drying between toes.

- Inspect feet closely for any breaks or signs of irritation.
- Report any abnormalities to the nurse.
- Do not allow moisture to collect between toes.
- Apply lotion to dry feet.
- Toenails of a diabetic are cut only by a podiatrist, a specialist in foot care.
- Shoes and stockings should be clean, free of holes, and fit well. Anything that might injure the feet or interfere with the circulation must be avoided.
- Do not allow the resident to go barefoot.
- Prevent pressure over the toes and feet by not tucking in bedding tightly.
- Inspect the skin regularly for signs of infection.
- Avoid very warm or cold applications to the skin.

## Testing to Monitor Control of Diabetes

Drugs for hypoglycemia and insulin are prescribed according to how well the body uses sugar for energy. For this reason, blood tests for sugar are performed regularly and treatment is adjusted as necessary. This is a licensed nursing procedure.

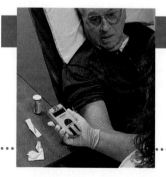

## LESSON SYNTHESIS: Putting It All Together

You have just completed this lesson. Now go back and review the Clinical Focus. Try to see how the Clinical Focus relates to the concepts presented in the lesson. Then answer the following questions.

1. How might Mr. McFarland's cold have affected his condition?

2. Explain what is meant by the fact that the resident is demonstrating hyperglycemia.

3. What action should the nursing assistant take after noting the change in Mr. McFarland's behavior?

4. What actions might the nurse decide would be appropriate?

5. What general actions should the nursing assistant take when caring for the resident with diabetes mellitus?

# REVIEW

**A. Match each term (items a.–j.) with the proper definition.**

a. thyroxine
b. hypoglycemia
c. electrolytes
d. polyuria
e. glycosuria
f. hormone
g. obesity
h. hyperglycemia
i. glucose
j. gangrene

1. _____ internal secretion produced by glands

2. _____ death of tissue

3. _____ low blood sugar

4. _____ sugar in the urine

5. _____ compounds essential to body chemistry

6. _____ blood sugar

7. _____ produced by the thyroid gland

8. _____ excessive urine output

9. _____ overweight

10. _____ excessive blood sugar

**B. Provide brief answers for each of the following.**

11. List three changes in the endocrine system due to aging.

12. What is an important sign of increased sodium levels in the blood?

13. What effect does a low level of potassium in the blood have on the heart rate?

14. List the names of the two forms of diabetes mellitus.

15. What is the most common form of diabetes mellitus?

16. List four signs of insulin–dependent diabetes mellitus.

17. List four signs of non–insulin-dependent diabetes mellitus.

18. List three factors that must be balanced for the resident with diabetes.

**C. Select the one best answer for each of the following.**

19. Endocrine glands
    a. release secretions into tubes that reach the body surface
    b. are all located in the abdomen
    c. each secrete one hormone only
    d. release secretions directly into the bloodstream

20. Hormones produced by the ovaries help
    a. urine production
    b. enlarge breasts
    c. control electrolyte balance
    d. regulate the levels of calcium

21. Which of the following is the male gonad?
    a. pituitary gland
    b. ovary
    c. testes
    d. thyroid

22. What sign or symptom is most often seen in a person with IDDM?
    a. abrupt onset
    b. skin infections
    c. itching
    d. pain in fingers and toes

23. What sign or symptom may be shown by an elderly person with NIDDM?
    a. excessive hunger
    b. burning on urination
    c. abrupt onset
    d. excessive thirst

24. The nursing assistant entered Mr. Lanzo's room and noted that he did not seem well. His skin was dry and flushed and he said he was thirsty. She reported to the nurse right away. What other symptom did she note that made her suspect the resident was hyperglycemic?
    a. complaint of hunger
    b. disorientation
    c. sweet odor to his breath
    d. pale, moist skin

25. When taking care of residents who have diabetes mellitus, the nursing assistant must remember to
   a. administer insulin on time
   b. wash the feet only occasionally so they will not get too dry
   c. avoid applying lotion to the feet
   d. make sure to serve the proper diet

26. If a resident with diabetes is receiving insulin the nursing assistant should check the injection site for
   a. redness or itching
   b. blueness
   c. coldness
   d. puncture marks

27. The nursing assistant notices that a resident with diabetes has long toenails. Her proper action is to
   a. cut the nails
   b. let the resident cut his own nails
   c. report to the nurse so the podiatrist can be called to cut the nails
   d. ignore the matter because the resident wears shoes to protect his feet

**D. Clinical Experience**

28. Mrs. Barker, a diabetic, has not eaten all the food on her tray. She is on a diabetic diet. What action should the nursing assistant take?
   a. Ignore it because it is not important.
   b. Insist the resident eat every spoonful.
   c. Report and record the amount of food eaten.
   d. Throw the food away so no one knows.

29. Mr. Samuels, a diabetic, has a darkened area on the little toe of his left foot. The nursing assistant reports this because she knows that a complication of diabetes is
   a. glaucoma
   b. renal disease
   c. cataracts
   d. gangrene

30. Mr. Lorenzo, who has IDDM, has an unpleasant visit with his daughter and her husband and now seems very upset. The nursing assistant will watch him closely for signs of hyperglycemia because she knows that this can be brought on by
   a. stress
   b. illness
   c. injury
   d. all of these

# Caring for Residents with Reproductive System Disorders

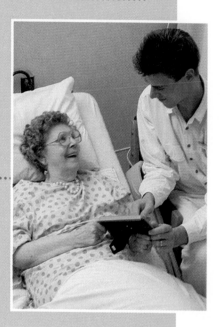

## CLINICAL FOCUS

Think about the special care required by residents with disorders of the reproductive system as you study this lesson and meet:

*B*essie Shutt, who is the mother of seven and grandmother to 23 children and 14 great grandchildren. She suffers from congestive heart failure and chronic obstructive pulmonary disease. She has a prolapsed uterus and complains of itching in the vaginal area. She is also occasionally incontinent of urine.

## OBJECTIVES

*After studying this lesson, you should be able to:*

- Define and spell vocabulary words and terms.
- Identify the parts and functions of the male and female reproductive systems.
- Review changes in the reproductive systems of men and women caused by aging.
- Describe conditions of the reproductive tract affecting long-term residents.

- Perform female breast self-examination.
- Identify and describe common sexually transmitted diseases.
- Demonstrate the following:
  Procedure 114 Breast Self-Examination

## VOCABULARY

**benign prostatic hypertrophy** (*bee-****NINE*** *pros-****TAT****-ick high-****PER****-troh-fee*)

**chlamydia** (*klah-****MID****-ee-ah*)

**climacteric** (*kligh-****MACK****-ter-ick*)

**clitoris** (***KLIT****-or-is*)

**Cowper's glands** (***KOW****-perz glands*)

**ejaculatory duct** (*ee-****JACK****-you-lah-****toh****-ree duct*)

**endometrium** (*en-doh-****MEE****-tree-um*)

**epididymis** (***ep****-ih-****DID****-ih-mis*)

**estrogen** (***ES****-troh-jen*)

**foreskin** (***FOR****-skin*)

# VOCABULARY

genitalia   (*jen-ih-TAY-lee-ah*)

gonorrhea   (*gon-or-REE-ah*)

hysterectomy   (*his-teh-RECK-toh-mee*)

labia majora   (*LAY-bee-ah mah-JOR-ah*)

labia minora   (*LAY-bee-ah mih-NOR-ah*)

menopause   (*MEN-oh-pawz*)

menstruation   (*men-stroo-AY-shun*)

ovulation   (*oh-vyou-LAY-shun*)

ovum (plural: ova)   (*OH-vum; plural: OH-vah*)

penis   (*PEE-nis*)

perineum   (*pair-ih-NEE-um*)

progesterone   (*proh-JES-ter-ohn*)

prostate   (*PROS-tayt*)

pruritus   (*prew-RYE-tus*)

puberty   (*PYOU-ber-tee*)

scrotum   (*SKROH-tum*)

seminal vesicles   (*SEM-ih-nal VES-ih-kuls*)

sperm   (*spurm*)

syphilis   (*SIF-ih-lis*)

testes   (*TES-teez*)

testicles   (*TES-tih-kuls*)

testosterone   (*tes-TOS-teh-rohn*)

transurethral prostatectomy   (*trans-you-REE-thral pros-tah-TECK-toh-mee*)

trichomonas vaginitis   (*trick-oh-MOH-nas vaj-ih-NIGH-tis*)

urethra   (*you-REE-thrah*)

uterine tubes   (*YOU-ter-in toobs*)

uterus   (*YOU-ter-us*)

vagina   (*vah-JYE-nah*)

vaginitis   (*vaj-ih-NIGH-tis*)

vas deferens   (*vas DEF-er-ens*)

venereal warts   (*vee-NEE-ree-al warts*)

vulva   (*VUL-vah*)

## INTRODUCTION

The male and female reproductive systems share some features as follows. They:

- Consist of gonads, tubes, and accessory structures
- Contribute to the reproductive process
- Provide the sex hormones
- Bring pleasure

Remember, human sexuality is the interaction between the physical and emotional needs of an individual. Sexuality is intimately involved with the individual's sense of identity. You may wish to return to Lesson 13 and review human sexuality.

## THE MALE REPRODUCTIVE SYSTEM

The male reproductive system consists of the primary organs (**genitalia**) and the accessory glands (Figure 27-1).

The primary organs are the:

- Penis
- Testes
- Epididymis
- Vas deferens
- Ejaculatory duct

The accessory glands include the:

- Seminal vesicles
- Prostate
- Cowper's glands

### Penis

The male **penis** is the organ used for sexual intercourse (also called coitus or copulation). When the special tissues of which the penis is made become filled with blood, the penis becomes enlarged and firm. The outer portion of the glans of the penis is covered by a loose skin fold called the **foreskin**.

The male **urethra** serves two purposes. It carries:

- Reproductive fluid during intercourse
- Urine during voiding

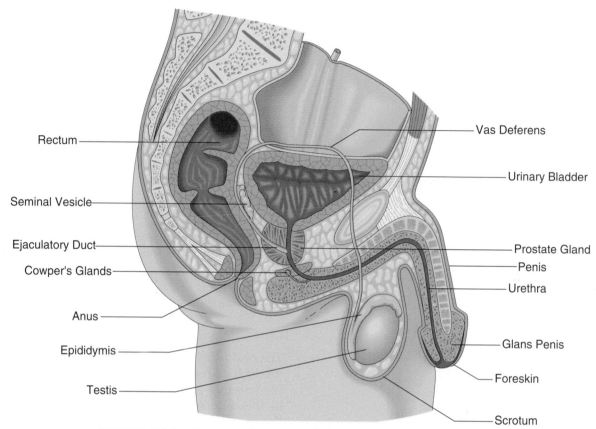

**FIGURE 27-1**   Cross-section view of the male reproductive system

The two activities cannot occur at the same time because they are under the control of different parts of the nervous system.

## Testes

The **testes (testicles)** are found in a pouch-like structure called the **scrotum**, which is located outside the body. The testes produce **sperm** throughout life and the male hormone **testosterone**. Testosterone is responsible for the male characteristics.

## Epididymis

The **epididymis** is a tube 20 feet long coiled on the back of each testis, which stores the sperm. The epididymis is the beginning of a pathway that moves the sperm upward and out of the body. This pathway includes the:

* Epididymis
* Vas deferens
* Ejaculatory duct
* Urethra

## Vas Deferens

The **vas deferens** that transports the sperm passes behind the urinary bladder, joining with the ejaculatory duct and entering the urethra.

## Ejaculatory Duct

The **ejaculatory duct** carries the fluid produced in the **seminal vesicles**. Fluids are added as the sperm are propelled forward. The sperm and fluid form the seminal fluid or ejaculate. The fluid contains nutrients and other substances needed by the sperm.

Glands that contribute to the seminal fluid are the:

* Seminal vesicles—the ejaculatory duct carries the fluid from the vesicles into the urethra.

- **Prostate** gland—surrounds the neck of the bladder and adds its secretions to the fluid.
- **Cowper's glands**—two small glands located beside the urethra. They produce mucus for lubrication.

### Accessory Glands

The seminal fluid or ejaculate is released as the result of a rhythmic series of muscular contractions. These force the fluid through the urethra to the outside. The process is called ejaculation and occurs during sexual intercourse. Ejaculation may also occur spontaneously at other times.

# THE FEMALE REPRODUCTIVE SYSTEM

The female reproductive system consists of the internal organs, (Figures 27-2A and 27-2B) and the external genitalia (the **vulva**) (Figure 27-3). The internal organs are the:

- Ovaries
- Fallopian (uterine) tubes
- Uterus
- Vagina

### Vulva

The outside of the vulva is made up of two folds called the **labia majora** (see Figure 27-3). The labia majora:

- Are covered with hair
- Surround the openings of the female urethra and vagina
- Enclose two hairless lips, the **labia minora**

The area between the vagina and anus is called the **perineum**.

**Clitoris.** The **clitoris** is an organ similar to the male penis. It:

- Is found near the union of the labia
- Is a sensitive structure
- Functions during sexual stimulation to begin the rhythmic series of contractions associated with female climax, or orgasm

### Ovaries

The two ovaries, which are the female gonads, produce the egg (**ovum**) and the hormones progesterone and estrogen. **Estrogen** is needed in the development of female characteristics. **Progesterone** is the hormone that maintains pregnancy.

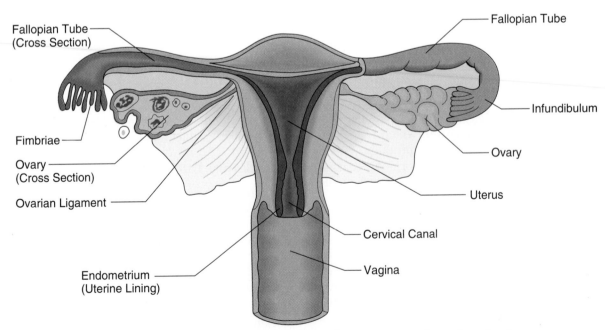

**FIGURE 27-2A** Female internal reproductive organs (anterior view)

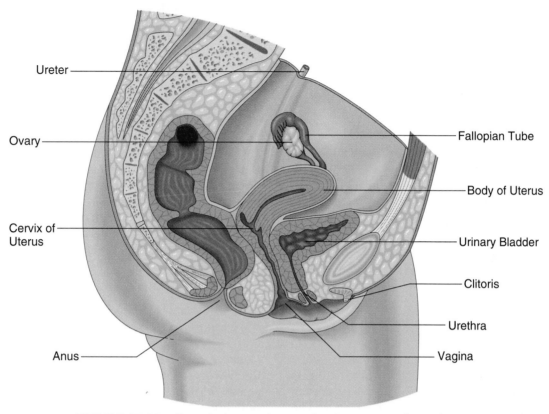

**FIGURE 27-2B** Female internal reproductive organs (lateral view)

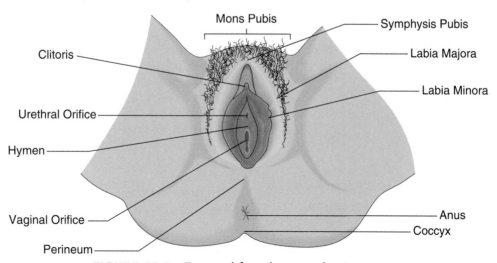

**FIGURE 27-3** External female reproductive organs

## Fallopian Tubes

The fallopian tubes (**uterine tubes** or oviducts) carry the ovum toward the uterus.

## Uterus

The **uterus** (or womb) is a hollow muscular organ about 3 inches long. It is lined with a special membrane, the **endometrium**, that:

- Is shed periodically unless pregnancy occurs
- Nourishes the growing fetus (unborn infant in the uterus) during pregnancy

## Vagina

The **vagina** is a muscular tube that serves as the output (excretory duct) for the menstrual flow and receives the penis during sexual intercourse.

# MENSTRUAL CYCLE

The menstrual cycle (female sexual cycle) begins at **puberty**. Puberty occurs in girls between the ages of 9 and 17. The cycle varies in length, usually between 25 and 30 days. The average is 28 days, which is why it is considered a monthly cycle.

During the menstrual cycle, a mature egg, or ovum (plural, **ova**):

- Is released from one of the ovaries
- Travels from the ovary to one of the fallopian tubes
- May be fertilized by a male sperm

At the same time that the ovum is being matured and expelled from the ovary (**ovulation**), the lining of the uterus (endometrium) is:

- Being built up
- Made ready to receive the fertilized ovum

If fertilization does not occur, the endometrium is:

- No longer needed
- Carried out of the body as the menstrual flow

This process is known as **menstruation**.

It is interesting that, unlike the sperm cells, all the special cells that will become the ova exist at the time that a woman is born. When the last ova are released, the menstrual cycle ceases and **menopause** begins.

# MENOPAUSE

As women age, the menstrual cycle becomes irregular and gradually ceases altogether. This is called the:

- Menopause
- **Climacteric**
- Change of life

Menopause usually occurs around the age of 55 and involves a natural series of changes that stops the menstrual cycle. These changes are not abrupt, but usually take place over a period of years. Because the ova are no longer being matured and released, pregnancy cannot occur.

Some women may undergo menopause earlier in life after surgical removal of the uterus.

# CHANGES IN THE REPRODUCTIVE SYSTEM AS A RESULT OF AGING

Changes occur in both male and female reproductive organs with aging. However, the need for sexual pleasure and sensual satisfaction does not stop.

## Changes in the Male Reproductive System

As men age, these changes occur:

- Sexual response is slower.
- Ejaculation is delayed.
- The number of sperm decreases (but number is still adequate for reproduction).
- Testosterone levels gradually decrease.
- The prostate gland may enlarge causing difficult urination.
- The scrotum becomes less firm.
- Seminal fluid thins.
- The size of the testes decreases.
- Note that usually the sex drive (libido) remains unchanged.

## Changes in the Female Reproductive System

During and after menopause, these changes occur:

- Estrogen levels decrease.
- Tissue of vulva and vaginal walls thins.

- Lubrication of vagina decreases (because of this, elderly women are more prone to vaginal infections).
- Breast tissues and muscles weaken (sagging of breasts).
- Egg production ceases.
- Ovulation and the menstrual cycle cease.
- Again, the libido remains unchanged.

## RELATED CONDITIONS

### Malignancy

Malignancies of the male and female reproductive organs are common. Be sure to report any bleeding or discharge from the reproductive tract.

In women, frequent sites for cancer development include the:

- Uterine wall
- Ovaries
- Cervix
- Breasts

In men, malignancies are often found in the:

- Prostate gland
- Testes

Radiation, surgery, and chemotherapy may be used alone or in combination to treat malignancies.

Any condition that affects the reproductive organs threatens the individual's self-concept and sense of sexual identity. In addition to the fear resulting from the diagnosis of a malignancy, the resident also fears that he or she will lose the ability to function fully as a sexual human being.

You must provide emotional support to those who are diagnosed with a malignancy of the reproductive system.

Breast tumors develop in men and women, both old and young. They are most common among mature women.

Breast tumors are often first found during self-examination or through *mammography* (x-ray examination). Most of these masses are benign tumors. The self-examination procedure should be:

- Performed by all adult women
- Carried out each month on the last day of the menstrual flow
- Carried out on one selected day of the month, after menopause
- Carried out using a procedure recommended by the American Cancer Society

---

**PROCEDURE**
## *114* Breast Self-Examination

1. Disrobe above waist and stand or sit in front of a mirror. Observe breasts for changes in shape or size (Figure 27-4).

*Note:* Some women prefer to perform breast self-examination standing in the shower.

2. Raise arms above your head and clasp hands. Press inward with hands while observing breasts, Note any "dimpling" of the breast tissue.

3. Fold a small towel.

4. Lie on the bed with the towel under the left shoulder.

5. Flex left arm and bring over your head.

*(continues)*

## PROCEDURE *114* *(continued)*

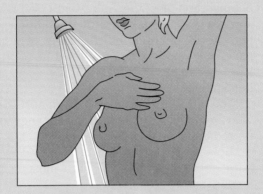

**A**

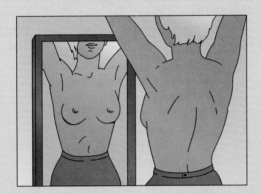

**B**

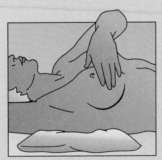
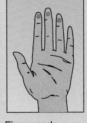

Finger pads

**C**

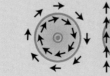
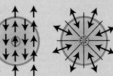

**D**

6. With the fingers of the right hand, examine the left breast.
   - Use fingertips.
   - Use a rolling motion.
   - Start at the nipple and work around the entire breast so that all tissue is examined.
7. Examine the left axilla in the same way.
8. Repeat the procedure with the opposite breast and axilla.

**FIGURE 27-4** Breast self-examination. Each breast is to be examined systematically. A. With the fingers flat, check for a knot, lump, or thickening. B. Raise your arms and compare breast shape. C. Lie down with a small pillow under the shoulder and one arm behind the head. Check again for any knot, lump, or thickening. Move fingers in a circular motion, inward toward the nipple. Use pads of fingers. D. Direction of motion of fingers over breast during examination

## Prolapsed Uterus

Prolapsed uterus is a condition that may be experienced by women who have had:

- Repeated pregnancies
- Injuries to the pelvic organs
- Injury to the muscles of the pelvic floor
- Weakening of the supportive pelvic structure due to aging

  When prolapsed uterus occurs:

- The uterus drops down from its normal position, causing pressure in the vagina.
- There is a feeling of weight in the pelvic area.
- Urinary incontinence or retention occurs.
- The person is predisposed to urinary infections.

  Prolapsed uterus is treated by repositioning the uterus or removing it (**hysterectomy**). Both treatments require surgery in an acute care facility.

## Rectocele and Cystocele

Rectoceles and cystoceles are hernias. They usually occur at the same time and are frequently seen in older women.

- A rectocele is a weakening of the wall between the vagina and rectum. This hernia frequently causes constipation and hemorrhoids (varicose veins of the rectum).
- A cystocele is a weakening of the muscles between the bladder and vagina. Cystoceles cause urinary incontinence.

These conditions are corrected by a surgical procedure that tightens the vaginal walls. It is performed in an acute care facility.

## Vaginitis

**Vaginitis** is a fairly common condition in older women because of the decrease in protection resulting from the thinner vaginal wall. This type of infection tends to be chronic and difficult to control.

A fungus infection caused by *Candida albicans* often results in vulvovaginitis. When infection is present:

- There may be a thick, white, cheesy vaginal discharge.
- Inflammation and itching are intense.
- Douches are not given for this condition.

- Special drugs and creams are prescribed to fight the infection.

  Senile vaginitis responds to estrogen therapy, vaginal suppositories, and mild douches to wash out the canal. Each treatment requires a physician's order.

## Pruritus

Itching (**pruritus**) of the vulva and anus is a common complaint of older women. Continual irritation can cause tissue breakdown and permit bacteria to enter and cause infection. Many factors can contribute to pruritus. A search must be made for the cause and steps taken to correct the condition. For example:

- If soaps are irritating, they should not be used.
- If incontinence allows acid urine to irritate the tissues, regular perineal care can often eliminate the problem.

## Benign Prostatic Hypertrophy

**Benign prostatic hypertrophy** is a common problem for elderly men. It is a nonmalignant enlargement of the prostate gland. Recall that the urethra passes through the center of this gland. Thus, as the gland enlarges it closes off the flow of urine.

Residents with this condition may have difficulty starting and stopping the stream of urine. They may not be able to empty their bladder completely, leading to bladder infections. Observe for the following:

- Frequency of urination
- Nocturia
- Poor urinary control such as dribbling

  To release the obstruction, a surgical procedure can be performed by entering through the urethra. This is called a **transurethral prostatectomy** (TURP). Although some surgical procedures on the prostate gland can cause impotence, this is not a complication of the transurethral approach.

## SEXUALLY TRANSMITTED DISEASES

Sexually transmitted diseases (STDs) affect both men and women. Although most STDs can be treated and cured, people do not develop immunity to repeated infections. In the elderly, an STD may indicate sexual abuse. The organisms causing STDs can be transmitted from:

* Mucous membrane to mucous membrane such as from genitals to mouth or genitals
* Mucous membrane to skin, such as genitals to hands
* Skin to mucous membrane, such as hands to genitals

Any disease that is transmitted mainly in this way is an STD. There are many STDs. Some are seen more commonly than others. Contact precautions should be used when caring for residents with STDs.

A complete discussion of STDs is presented here for your protection because these diseases pose a risk for health care workers as well as the people being cared for.

The most common STDs are gonorrhea, herpes simplex II, and syphilis. Other STDs are caused by chlamydia, human papilloma virus, human immunodeficiency virus, and the *Trichomonas* parasite.

It is important to realize that people may:

* Not always be aware that they have been infected
* Be too embarrassed to talk about the problem
* Not realize the serious damage these infectious diseases can do to the body

## Trichomonas Vaginitis

**Trichomonas vaginitis** is caused by a parasite, *Trichomonas vaginalis*. This condition:

* Is sexually transmitted
* May affect the male reproductive tract with no signs and symptoms
* In women, causes a large amount of white, foul-smelling vaginal discharge called leukorrhea
* Can be controlled with medication
* Requires that both sex partners receive treatment

## Gonorrhea

**Gonorrhea** is a serious STD caused by the bacterium *Neisseria gonorrheae*. The disease causes an acute inflammation.

* In men:
  * Greenish yellow discharge appears from the penis within 2 to 5 days after contact.
  * There is a burning on urination.
  * The disease can spread throughout the reproductive tract, causing sterility (inability to reproduce).
* In women:
  * Eighty percent of women infected may have no signs or symptoms until after the disease spreads.
  * Pelvic inflammatory disease can lead to formation of abscesses and sterility.
  * The disease can be spread before a woman is aware of being infected.
  * All sex partners must be treated with antibiotics.
  * When a pregnant woman has gonorrhea, her baby's eyes may be permanently damaged if they are contaminated by the disease during birth. As a preventive measure, all babies' eyes are routinely treated with silver nitrate drops or antibiotics shortly after birth.

## Syphilis

**Syphilis** is caused by the microorganism *Treponema pallidum*. Both sexes show the same effects of the disease. It is treated with antibiotics. If untreated, the disease may pass through three stages.

1. First stage—a sore (chancre) develops within 90 days of exposure. The chancre heals without treatment. Because it is not painful, it may go entirely unnoticed.
2. Second stage—a rash, sore throat, or other mild symptoms suggestive of a viral infection may occur. Again, the signs and symptoms disappear without treatment. The disease is infectious during the first and second stages and may be transmitted to a sexual partner. By this time, the microorganisms have entered vital organs such as the heart, liver, brain, and spinal cord.
3. Third stage—the stage in which permanent damage is done to vital organs. It may not appear for many years or at all.

If an infected woman is pregnant the microorganisms can attack the fetus, causing it to die or be seriously deformed.

## Herpes

Herpes simplex II (genital herpes) is an infectious disease caused by the herpes simplex virus. It is transmitted primarily through direct sexual contact. The person who has herpes:

- May develop red, blister-like sores on the reproductive organs
- Has sores that are associated with a burning sensation
- Usually has sores that heal in about 2 weeks
- Must remember that the fluid in the blisters is infectious
- May shed organisms even when an outbreak is not present

People infected with herpes may have only one episode or repeated attacks. In many cases, repeated attacks are milder. Other consequences of a herpes infection include:

- A greater incidence of cancer of the cervix and miscarriages in infected women compared to women who are not infected.
- Newborn children can be infected during the birth process.
- The mother with an active case of herpes simplex II usually delivers by cesarean section.

Treatment with the drug acyclovir reduces the discomfort and degree of communicability. There is no cure at the present time.

## Venereal Warts

**Venereal warts** are caused by a virus. Characteristics of the infection include:

- Lesions on the genitals on both skin and mucous membranes
- Cauliflower-shaped, raised, and darkened warts
- Warts may be removed by ointments or surgery but often recur.
- Venereal warts may cause discomfort during intercourse and may cause bleeding when dislodged.
- They predispose to development of cancerous changes.

- The infection rate for venereal warts is the most rapidly growing for all STDs.

## Chlamydia Infection

**Chlamydia** are small infectious organisms that invade mucous membranes of the body. These organisms are:

- Introduced into the eyes infecting the conjunctiva. This causes inflammation (conjunctivitis) and a more serious condition called trachoma. Trachoma can lead to blindness.
- Sexually transmitted and commonly cause infections of the reproductive tract
- The cause of pelvic inflammatory disease with scarring and systemic infections. The scarring can result in sterility.
- Responsible for signs and symptoms similar to those of gonorrhea, except that the discharge is usually yellow to whitish in color
- Treated with antibiotics

People with pelvic infections are usually checked for gonorrhea. If they test negative for gonorrhea, they are frequently diagnosed with nonspecified urethritis because many different organisms may cause the infection. However, chlamydia organisms are the most common cause.

## Personal Precautions

An individual can practice certain actions to lessen the risk of contracting STDs. These include:

- Abstaining from sex
- Knowing your sexual partner well before engaging in sexual activity
- Limiting the number of sexual partners
- Using a latex condom throughout sexual contact
- Washing well following sexual intercourse
- Using approved germicides that can be applied to the vagina, penis, and condom
- Providing to your partner and being provided with a negative test result covering the 3-month period before sexual activity

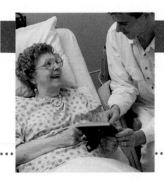

## LESSON SYNTHESIS: Putting It All Together

*Y*ou have just completed this lesson. Now go back and review the Clinical Focus. Try to see how the Clinical Focus relates to the concepts presented in the lesson. Then answer the following questions.

1. What change occurs in the lubrication of the vagina in the aging woman?

2. What increased risk does this change pose for Mrs. Shutt?

3. Do Mrs. Shutt's periods of incontinence contribute to her pruritus?

4. What special care can you give to make Mrs. Shutt more comfortable?

5. If Mrs. Shutt does not tell you of her discomfort, how may you be alerted to her problem?

6. Which of Mrs. Shutt's diagnoses might contribute to her incontinence?

## REVIEW

**A. Match each term (items a.–e.) with the proper definition.**

a. chlamydia    d. pruritus
b. climacteric    e. vaginitis
c. hysterectomy

1. _____ itching

2. _____ small infectious organisms

3. _____ menopause

4. _____ inflammation of the vagina

5. _____ removal of the uterus

**B. Select the one best answer for each of the following.**

6. The male organ used for intercourse is the
   a. vas deferens
   b. testis
   c. penis
   d. prostate

7. The male gland that may enlarge and obstruct the flow of urine is the
   a. prostate
   b. seminal vesicles
   c. Cowper's glands
   d. penis

8. The female gonads are the
   a. uterus
   b. ovaries
   c. vagina
   d. perineum

9. As men age
   a. ejaculation is more rapid
   b. sperm count increases
   c. testosterone levels decrease
   d. sexual response is more rapid

10. One characteristic of female menopause is
    a. loss of egg production
    b. reduced libido
    c. regular menstrual periods
    d. thickening of vaginal walls

**C. Fill in the blanks by selecting the correct word or phrase from the list.**

abuse    testes
cystocele    vulva
genitalia

11. The primary sexual organs are known as the _____.

12. An STD in the elderly may be a sign of sexual _____.

13. The female external genitalia is called the _____.

14. The male glands that produce the sperm are called the _____.

15. A weakening of the wall between the vagina and bladder is called a _____.

## D. Brief Answers

16. List three functions of both the male and female reproductive systems.

17. List three changes resulting from aging for the male reproductive system and three changes for the female reproductive system.

18. List five common STDs.

19. List four precautions to take to avoid getting an STD when caring for residents with an STD.

## E. Clinical Experience

20. Mr. Fazzio is acting very withdrawn this morning. When Starr, the nursing assistant, reports to her supervisor she learns that the physician has told Mr. Fazzio that he has a "lump" in his prostate gland that must be treated.
    a. Could this knowledge explain Mr. Fazzio's behavior?
    b. What fears may Mr. Fazzio be feeling?
    c. How can you help Mr. Fazzio at this time?

21. Mrs. Wells was admitted to your facility this morning. She has a diagnosis of mild confusion, malnutrition, congestive heart failure, and pelvic inflammatory disease. A culture was ordered to determine the cause of her infection. What type of precautions should be used with this resident?

# Caring for Residents with Musculoskeletal System Disorders

**CLINICAL FOCUS**

Think of the special challenge required to provide nursing assistant care to a resident with disorders of the musculoskeletal system as you study this lesson and meet:

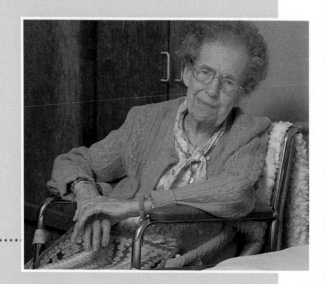

*E*ssie Branch, who suffers from osteoarthritis and osteoporosis. These conditions affect both her ability to provide self-care and to enjoy full mobility. Her osteoporosis has caused compression fractures of her spine so she is no longer able to hold her head erect easily.

## OBJECTIVES

*After studying this lesson, you should be able to:*

- Define and spell vocabulary words and terms.
- List the functions of the voluntary muscles.
- List the functions of the bones.
- Describe the changes of aging that affect the musculoskeletal system.

- Identify the symptoms related to common musculoskeletal system disorders.
- Describe the appropriate nursing care for residents with musculoskeletal disorders.

## VOCABULARY

**amputation**  *(**am**-pyou-**TAY**-shun)*
**arthritis**  *(are-**THRY**-tis)*
**atrophy**  *(**AT**-roh-fee)*
**bursae**  *(**BUR**-see)*
**bursitis**  *(bur-**SIGH**-tis)*

**cartilage**  *(**KAR**-tih-lij)*
**cast**  *(kast)*
**external fixation**  *(eks-**TER**-nal fix-**AY**-shun)*
**fracture**  *(**FRACK**-shur)*

# VOCABULARY

joint *(joynt)*

kyphosis *(kigh-FOH-sis)*

ligament *(LIG-ah-ment)*

open reduction/internal fixation (ORIF)— *(OH-pen ree-DUCK-shun/in-TER-nal fix-AY-shun)*

osteoarthritis *(os-tee-oh-are-THRY-tis)*

osteoporosis *(os-tee-oh-poor-OH-sis)*

phantom pain *(FAN-tom payn)*

podiatrist *(poh-DYE-ah-trist)*

prosthesis *(pros-THEE-sis)*

rheumatoid arthritis *(REW-mah-toyd are-THRY-tis)*

tendon *(TEN-don)*

traction *(TRACK-shun)*

## THE MUSCULOSKELETAL SYSTEM

The musculoskeletal system is composed of:

- Bones
- Skeletal muscles
- Joints
- Tendons
- Ligaments
- Bursae

The bones form a framework for the body that is called a skeleton. The muscles are formed of tissue that has the ability to contract and relax and allow movement. The muscles lie over the bones. Together, the bones and muscles have many functions, including:

- Giving shape and form to the body
- Protecting and supporting vital body organs such as the brain and heart
- Permitting movement
- Producing some of the red blood cells
- Storing calcium and phosphorus

### Bones

The human body has 206 bones (Figure 28-1). All of the bones are not alike. Some are:

- Longer bones—bones of the arms and legs
- Short bones—bones of the fingers and toes
- Irregular bones—bones that form the spinal column
- Flat bones—pelvic bones and shoulder blades

Each bone has a name. Many other body structures take their names from that of the nearby bone. For example, the radius is a bone in the forearm. Close by are the:

- Radial nerve
- Radial artery
- Radial vein

Learning the names of the bones is not difficult. Draw a line down the center of the skeleton in Figure 28-1, dividing it in half. Note that the bones on one side of the line are matched by bones in the other side.

### Muscles

The body contains more than 500 muscles (Figure 28-2). They work in groups to bring about body movement. There are three types of muscles:

- Cardiac muscle—found only in the heart wall
- Skeletal muscles—also called voluntary muscles because you can control their actions of contraction and relaxation
- Visceral or smooth muscles—also called involuntary muscles because we do not usually control them consciously

Involuntary muscles make up the walls of organs like the stomach and guard body openings like those of the digestive and urinary tracts. A special part of the brain controls involuntary muscles automatically.

Muscles are named by location, shape, or action. The quadriceps femoris, for example, is

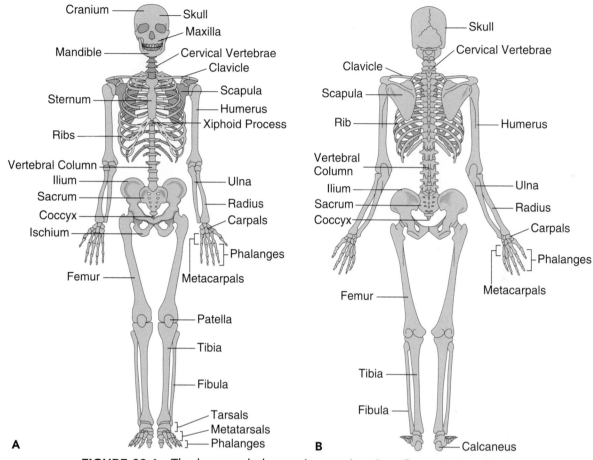

**FIGURE 28-1**  The human skeleton: A. anterior view, B. posterior view

located near the femur (thigh bone). Muscles have three parts:

- Origin, or beginning
- Body, or middle part
- Insertion, or ending

The origin and body of a muscle are found on one side of a joint and the insertion is attached to the other side. Skeletal muscles are attached to the bones by tough, fibrous bands called **tendons**.

When the muscle shortens (contracts), it pulls the point of insertion toward the point of origin, changing the position of the bone (Figure 28-3).

This relationship between muscles and bones permits movements such as walking, sitting, or holding a pencil.

Muscles that are not used will **atrophy**. This means they become weaker and smaller. Lack of

joint movement may cause a **contracture** to form. The muscle shortens, causing the joint to become fixed, making further movement difficult or impossible.

### Joints

Two bones meet or come together (articulate) at a **joint**. The elbows, knees, and hips are joints. **Ligaments** are fibrous bands that help support the points of articulation.

The ends of movable bones are covered with a protective substance called **cartilage**. The bones of the skull are not movable. The joints of the skull bones are called suture lines.

Joint movements depend on the way in which the joint is formed. Elbows and knees, for example, are hinge joints. The hip and shoulder are ball joints (Figure 28-4).

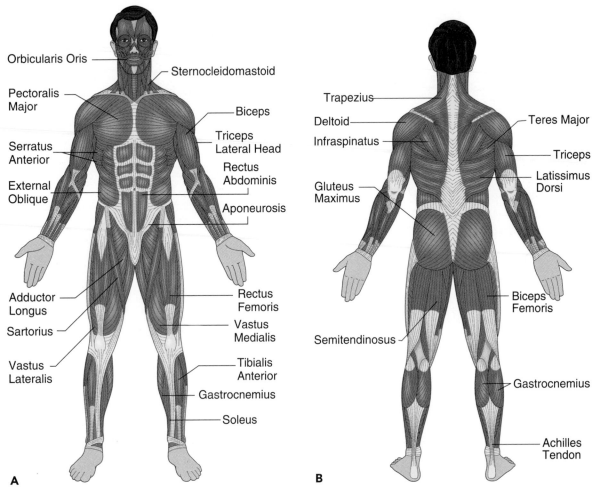

**FIGURE 28-2** Principal skeletal muscles of the body: A. anterior view, B. posterior view

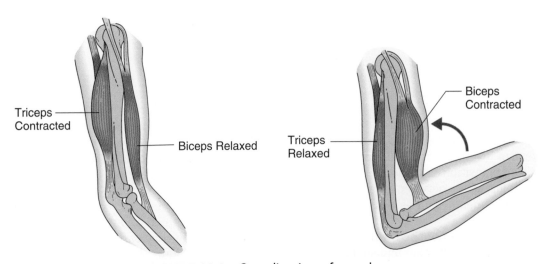

**FIGURE 28-3** Coordination of muscles

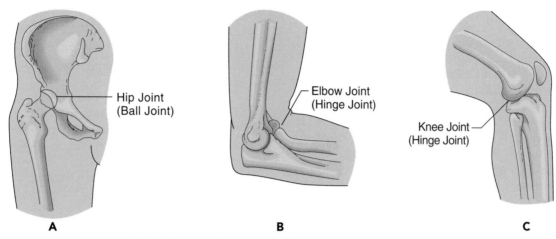

**FIGURE 28-4**   Types of joints.  A. Ball joint.  B. and  C. Hinge joints

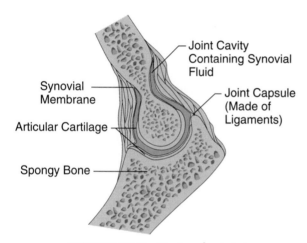

**FIGURE 28-5**   Parts of a joint

Joints are enclosed in a capsule lined with synovial membrane. The membrane secretes small amounts of fluid called synovial fluid (Figure 28-5). Small sacs of synovial fluid called **bursae** are located around joints and help reduce friction during joint movement.

## CHANGES IN THE MUSCULOSKELETAL SYSTEM CAUSED BY AGING ·····················

The aging process causes several changes in the musculoskeletal system:

- The bones become more brittle because of calcium loss.
- The joints become less flexible. The range through which the joints can be moved (range of motion) decreases.
- Muscles may become smaller because of less regular exercise. This may limit the person's strength and endurance.
- The body tends to become more flexed. It is important to avoid flexion, if possible, when positioning residents. This increases the flexion that is naturally occurring. Flexion makes movement more difficult.

Because of these changes, older adults are at risk for falling. Maintain a safe environment to prevent falls. Closely monitor residents who have a history of falling. When an older person falls, the bones may easily fracture because they are more brittle.

## CONDITIONS AFFECTING THE MUSCULOSKELETAL SYSTEM ···········

Residents with diseases or problems of the musculoskeletal system receive special care that is known as orthopedic care.

Sometimes a bursa becomes inflamed. This is called **bursitis**. The bursa is painful and movement may be reduced. Bursitis may be due to infection or excessive pressure or movement placed on the area.

## Osteoporosis

**Osteoporosis** may develop due to a lack of mobility or as a result of aging. It affects primarily women due to lack of the hormone estrogen following menopause. As osteoporosis develops, the bones lose calcium and become brittle.

The vertebrae in the spine of a person with osteoporosis may collapse without warning, resulting in a curvature of the spine called **kyphosis** (hunched back).

Fractures are common in people with osteoporosis because the bones lack strength. It is important to carry out all safety measures to prevent falls. Care must be used when moving and lifting the residents. Unsafe handling can damage the resident's joints and bones.

## Fractures

A **fracture** is a break or loss of continuity in a bone (Figure 28-6). The break may be completely through the bone *(complete fracture)* or only partially through the bone *(incomplete fracture)*. All fractures are either closed or open:

- Closed fracture
    - The bones do not protrude through the skin and are in good alignment after the fracture.
- Open fracture
    - Fragments of broken bone protrude through the skin.

Fractures are also identified according to the type of break in the bone:

- Comminuted fracture
    - The bone is broken into many pieces.
- Compression fracture
    - The internal spongy part of the bone is crushed but the hard outer covering of the bone is not broken. This type of fracture occurs most often in the vertebrae.
- Spiral fracture
    - The bone is broken in a twisted manner.

To promote the healing of fractures, the bone must be:

- In correct alignment
- Kept immobile

**Treatment of Fractures with a Cast.** A cast or splint to support the area may be all that is needed to treat a closed fracture of the arm or lower leg. A **cast** is made by applying a wet substance to the extremity, in layers. The substance is molded and shaped as it is applied so it will fit the extremity. If a resident in the facility breaks a bone, the resident may be taken to a hospital to have a cast applied. The resident may then return to the facility. After a cast is applied, follow these special precautions:

- Allow the wet cast to air dry.
- Do not put pressure on the wet cast. Any pressure can leave permanent indentations that can press against the resident's skin, causing it

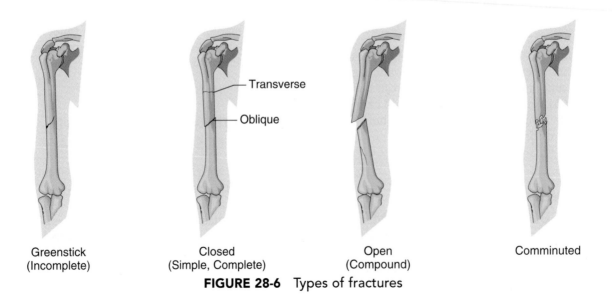

|                          |                           |                      |             |
| Transverse               |                           |                      |             |
| Oblique                  |                           |                      |             |

Greenstick (Incomplete)     Closed (Simple, Complete)     Open (Compound)     Comminuted

**FIGURE 28-6** Types of fractures

to break down. Use the palms of your hands, not your fingers, to move the casted extremity.
- Keep the casted extremity elevated and uncovered until it is dry.
- Check the skin area around the cast frequently for signs of circulatory impairment: blue color (cyanosis), cold to touch, swelling (edema), odor, drainage, and complaints of pain or tingling in the area. Report any of these signs immediately.
- Closely observe skin areas around the cast edges for signs of irritation.

- After an arm cast dries, a sling may be needed for support. Residents with a leg cast may need a wheelchair for support.

**Treatment of Fractures with Traction.** **Traction** is used to treat some fractures. This means the broken ends of the bone are pulled into normal alignment. In *skin traction* a belt or strap is applied to the body and weights are attached to the ropes (Figure 28-7). *Skeletal traction* involves the insertion of a metal pin into the bone. Weights are then attached by ropes to the pin (Figure 28-8). Traction may be used until the bone heals or it may be used only until surgery is performed or a cast is applied. When caring for a resident in traction:

- Review the placement of pulleys, ropes, and weights with the nurse so you know the purpose and correct placement of each.
- Do not disturb the weights or permit them to swing, drop, or rest on any surface.
- Keep the resident in good alignment and ensure that the body is acting properly as countertraction.
- Check under belts or straps for areas of pressure or irritation.
- Make sure that straps and belts are smooth, straight, and properly secured.

**Treatment of Fractures with External Fixation.** **External fixation** devices are some-

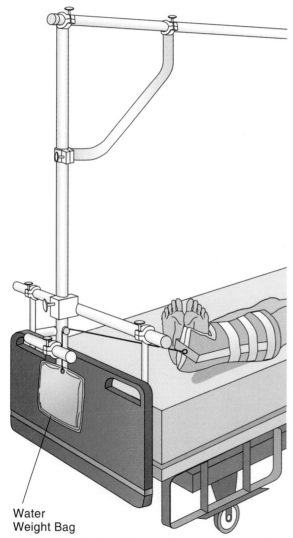

Water
Weight Bag

**FIGURE 28-7**  Buck's traction is an example of skin traction sometimes used for a fractured hip.

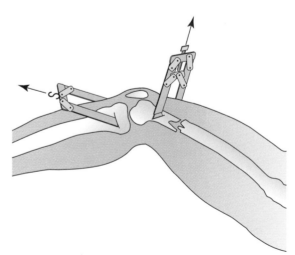

**FIGURE 28-8**  Skeletal traction immobilizes a body part by attaching weights directly to the resident's bones with pins, screws, wires, or tongs.

times used to manage fractures of the tibia (large bone in lower leg) (Figure 28-9). These devices are inserted into the bone to maintain alignment. The external part allows the orthopedic surgeon to adjust the device as necessary to promote healing.

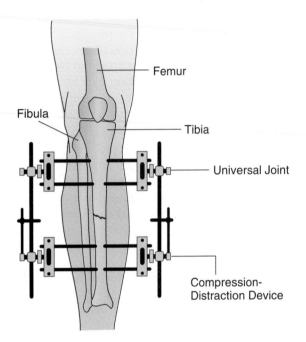

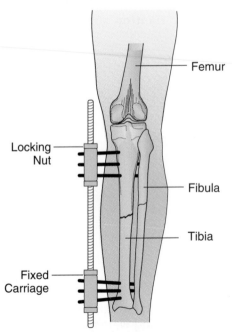

**FIGURE 28-9** External fixation devices are sometimes used for fractures of the tibia.

## Fractured Hip

The most common fracture seen in residents of long-term care facilities is a fractured hip. This term refers to any break involving the upper third of the femur (upper leg bone) (Figure 28-10). A fractured hip may occur spontaneously as a result of osteoporosis. The resident is walking and, without warning, the bone breaks, causing the resident to fall. In other cases, the resident falls causing the bone to break. Signs and symptoms of a fractured hip include:

- Pain in the hip sometimes radiating to the knee
- Feeling of pressure on the hip
- Shortening and turning outward of the leg on the injured side
- Bruising and swelling of the hip, groin, and thigh
- The resident may have heard a "snap" just before or after the fall.

If you suspect a fractured hip, *NEVER* attempt to move the resident without instructions from the nurse. The resident will be taken by ambulance to the hospital for x-rays of the affected joint and bones. If a fracture has

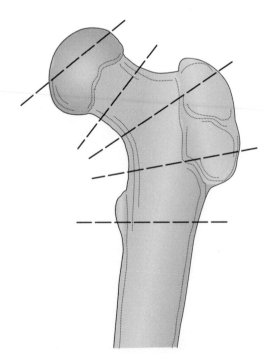

**FIGURE 28-10** The lines indicate where fractures usually occur in the femur.

occurred, the resident will be admitted to the hospital for repair of the fracture.

**Open Reduction/Internal Fixation.** Fractured hips are usually repaired by **open reduction/internal fixation (ORIF)**. This method may also be used for fractures of other large bones. The resident is given a general anesthetic and is asleep during surgery. An incision is made, the surgeon aligns the broken ends of the bone, and a nail, pin, or screw is inserted to maintain alignment. The device is usually permanent. The resident will stay in the hospital for several days and then convalesce in the long-term care facility.

**Caring for Residents with ORIF.** Residents who have had an ORIF usually have physical therapy for several weeks after. The physical therapist starts a program of progressive mobilization and teaches the resident to:

- Move independently in bed
- Transfer from bed to chair without bearing weight on the involved leg
- Stand and hold onto a bar while doing active range of motion exercises with the involved leg without weight bearing (Figure 28-11).
- Start weight bearing by standing and balancing, then walking through the parallel bars
- Walk with cane or walker

When you care for a resident with ORIF, you must:

- Know whether there are any restrictions for positioning the resident in bed
- Know whether or not the resident is allowed to bear weight on the affected leg
- Know how to transfer the resident if the resident is non-weight bearing or partial weight bearing
- Know whether you should do passive range of motion exercises on the affected leg
- Encourage the resident to do activities of daily living as independently as possible
- Encourage involvement in activities away from the nursing unit
- Report:
    - Complaints of pain
    - Changes in vital signs
    - Signs of bleeding, inflammation (redness, heat, swelling), or drainage from the incision

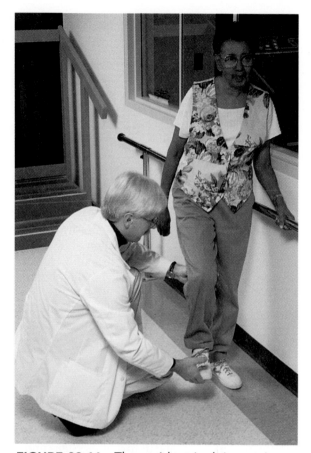

**FIGURE 28-11**   The resident is doing active range of motion exercises without weight bearing on the affected side.

- Signs of disorientation or confusion (common after hip surgery and usually temporary)

## Arthritis

**Arthritis** is a common problem in the elderly. The conditions and care are described in Figure 28-12. Many forms of arthritis exist, but the two most common forms are:

- Osteoarthritis
- Rheumatoid arthritis

**Osteoarthritis** is due to the "wear and tear" of the joints. The cartilage at the ends of the bones wears away with movement. It begins during middle age and can be very painful. This form of arthritis does not usually cause severe disability. However, for some individuals, it can

**FIGURE 28-12** Orthopedic problems in older adults

| Condition | Disease Process | Treatment | Special Care |
|---|---|---|---|
| Osteoarthritis | Breakdown (degeneration) of joints. Weight-bearing joints such as ankles, knees, and hips are most commonly involved. Movement is painful and condition is progressive. | Medication to relieve pain; physiotherapy to maintain mobility; light massage and heat; ambulatory aids to reduce pressure in joints; weight reduction; surgery in selected cases. | Give positive, emotional support; carry out heat treatments, massage, and ROM exercises, as ordered. |
| Osteoporosis | Defective bone formation and maintenance. Bones become brittle and are easily broken. Complications: fractures, kidney stones, and loss of height and posture. More common in females than males. | Keep resident as active as possible; diet adequate in protein and vitamins C and D, and calcium; maintain adequate fluid intake; hormone therapy. | Encourage food and fluid intake. Assist in exercise. Report pain; apply support as needed. Emotional support must not be overlooked. |
| Rheumatoid Arthritis | Inflammation of joint lining (synovium). Joint changes cause painful muscle spasms, flexion, and deformities. Signs and symptoms may temporarily disappear (remission). Flareups may be related to emotional stress. | Drugs to reduce pain and inflammation; heat treatments for comfort; exercise when inflammation subsides; surgery in selected cases. | Provide emotional support. Provide self-help devices such as long shoe horns and grab bars. Carry out heat treatments and ROM exercises, as ordered. |

limit their mobility. The joints, especially hip joints, may require replacement with an artificial joint (**prosthesis**) (Figure 28-13).

**Caring for Residents with a Hip Prosthesis.**
The physician usually places the resident on hip precautions for a minimum of 6 weeks after surgery. These precautions may include:

- Turn to back and unaffected hip only.
- Keep affected leg in neutral position when in bed and during activities.
- Place abductor splint or at least two pillows between the legs when turning. Keep hips abducted when in wheelchair.

- Use an elevated toilet seat to avoid hip flexion when rising.
- Report any signs or symptoms of:
  - Swelling of affected leg
  - Redness or discoloration of hip
  - Pain at the hip, groin, or thigh
  - Drainage or bleeding from incision
  - Chest pain (a blood clot in the lungs is sometimes a complication of hip surgery)
- Do not allow the resident to:
  - Adduct the legs (cross affected leg over midline) (Figure 28-14)
  - Flex legs past 90°

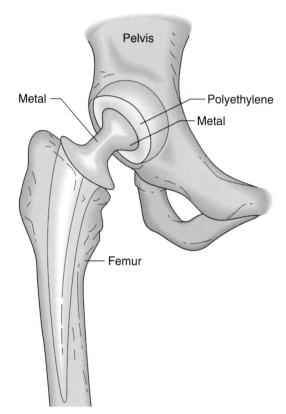

**FIGURE 28-13** Damaged hip joints can be replaced with an artificial joint (prosthesis).

- Flex hip when in side-lying position
- Bend forward at hip during transfers or other activities or when sitting up in bed (Figure 28-15)
- Sit for long periods of time
- Internally rotate affected leg (Figure 28-16)

**Rheumatoid arthritis** can begin at any age and sometimes occurs in children. This disease can be mild or progressive until it destroys the joints. In either case, severe pain is a symptom. Hand deformities from rheumatoid arthritis are shown in Figure 28-17.

The most important aspect of care for residents with arthritis is to balance activity with rest. Too much activity at one time may increase the pain. Too much rest results in stiffness and can lead to contractures. When you touch the resident's body, remember to be gentle.

## Lower Extremity Amputation

You may care for residents who have had one or both feet or legs surgically removed (amputated). When an elderly person has an **amputation**, it is usually because of circulatory problems. These problems may be due to changes in the blood vessels or because of diabetes. Gangrene may develop (the tissues die) and amputation is needed.

It is common for people to experience **phantom pain** after the removal of a limb. Residents may feel pain or tingling where the limb used to be. These feelings may persist for months. The pain is real, although it is difficult to explain.

After an amputation, some people are fitted with a prosthesis (an artificial limb). They have to learn how to walk and sit when the prosthesis is worn. If you are responsible for helping a resident put on a prosthesis, be sure you know how to attach and secure it.

Residents who have had amputations need to be positioned correctly. This is explained in Lesson 22.

## Foot Problems

As people age, foot and toenail problems develop. If these problems are not corrected, they may affect the person's ability to walk. Many people

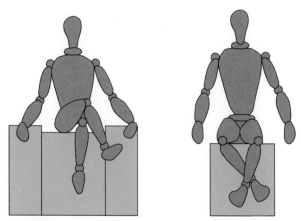

**FIGURE 28-14** The resident with a new hip prosthesis should never cross the affected leg over the midline of the body.

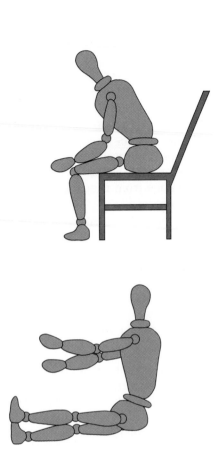

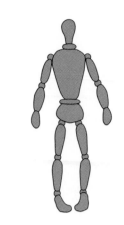

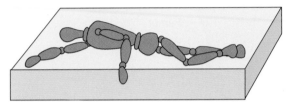

**FIGURE 28-16** The resident with a new hip prosthesis should never internally rotate the hip on the affected side.

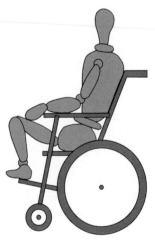

**FIGURE 28-15** The resident with a new hip prosthesis should never flex the affected hip more than 90°.

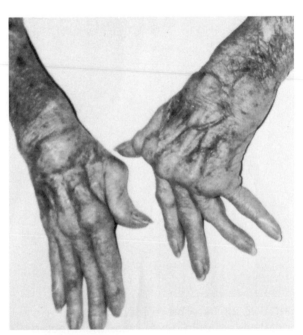

**FIGURE 28-17** Joint deformities as a result of rheumatoid arthritis

require the services of a **podiatrist** for treatment of the feet and toenails. Nursing assistants provide foot care as follows:

1. Clean the resident's feet thoroughly during the bathing procedure.
   - Wash, rinse, and dry carefully between each toe.
   - Clean the toenails.
2. Observe the feet for:
   - Bluish color
   - Swelling
   - Breaks in the skin

3. Report any changes to the nurse.
4. Protect the resident's feet.
   - Be sure the resident wears properly fitting shoes and socks when up.
   - Avoid bumping or hitting the resident's feet as you do positioning and range of motion procedures.
   - Loosen the covers over the resident's feet.
5. Do not allow the resident's feet to dangle. If the feet do not touch the floor when sitting in a chair, provide a footstool.
6. Know your facility's policy for cutting toenails.

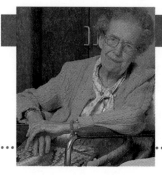

## LESSON SYNTHESIS: Putting It All Together

You have just completed this lesson. Now go back and review the Clinical Focus. Try to see how the Clinical Focus relates to the concepts presented in this lesson. Then answer the following questions.

1. What factors contribute to Essie Branch's flexed posture?

2. Why are women more prone to osteoporosis in later years compared to men?

3. Because the bones of this resident have less strength, what special precautions must be included in her care?

## REVIEW

**A. Select the one best answer for each of the following.**

1. The musculoskeletal system
   a. gives shape and form to the body
   b. permits movement
   c. produces red blood cells
   d. all of these

2. Skeletal muscles are attached to the bones by
   a. ligaments
   b. tendons
   c. cartilage
   d. bursa

3. Small sacs of synovial fluid are located around joints. They sometimes become inflamed, causing
   a. bursitis
   b. arthritis
   c. tendinitis
   d. osteoporosis

4. When osteoporosis occurs
   a. the bones become brittle and porous
   b. the bones fracture easily
   c. kyphosis may develop
   d. all of these

5. When a resident has a new cast, signs and symptoms indicating circulatory impairment include
   a. pink toes
   b. warm to touch
   c. swelling and complaints of pain and tingling
   d. all of these

6. Skin traction involves
   a. application of a belt or strap to the body and attachment of weights
   b. insertion of a metal pin into the bones and attachment of weights
   c. application of a splint
   d. application of an external fixation device

7. When a resident has had an ORIF you must know
   a. whether the resident can bear weight
   b. whether there are restrictions for positioning the resident in bed
   c. how the resident is to transfer from bed to chair
   d. all of these

8. When a resident has had a hip prosthesis inserted, you must discourage the resident from
   a. doing activities of daily living independently
   b. being out of bed
   c. adducting the legs
   d. participating in activities

9. Rheumatoid arthritis may
   a. have temporary remissions
   b. cause inflammation of the joint lining
   c. cause painful muscle spasms, flexion, and deformities
   d. all of these

10. Osteoarthritis is
    a. due to wear and tear of the joints
    b. common in children
    c. a cause of severe disability
    d. all of these

11. With any type of arthritis, the most important aspect of care is to
    a. encourage the resident to remain in bed as much as possible
    b. encourage the resident to exercise as much as possible
    c. balance rest and activity
    d. perform all activities of daily living for the resident

12. Amputation of a lower extremity may cause phantom pain. Phantom pain is
    a. due to the resident's imagination
    b. due to the resident's need for attention
    c. a type of surgical pain
    d. real and may persist for months

B.  **Answer each statement true (T) or false (F).**

13. T   F   As one ages, the joints become more flexible.

14. T   F   Movements in joints depend on the way in which the joint is formed.

15. T   F   When a person has osteoporosis, the vertebrae may collapse without warning.

16. T   F   Gangrene can be treated successfully with medication.

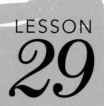

# Caring for Residents with Nervous System Disorders

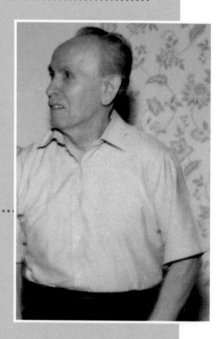

## CLINICAL FOCUS

Think of the special challenge presented in providing nursing assistant care to a resident with neurologic disorders as you study this lesson and meet:

*T*homas Raye who suffers from Parkinson's disease. This is a neurologic disorder that affects his ability to control and coordinate his voluntary movements. Although able to move, Mr. Raye cannot stop and start activities smoothly. He walks with small, shuffling steps and stands with a characteristic bent frame.

## OBJECTIVES

*After studying this lesson, you should be able to:*

- Define and spell vocabulary words and terms.
- List the functions of the nervous system.
- List the structures of the nervous system.
- Recognize the changes of aging that affect the nervous system.
- Describe the sensory deficits caused by disease.

- Identify the symptoms related to common nervous system disorders.
- Describe the nursing care for residents with nervous system disorders.
- Demonstrate the following:
  Procedure 115 Care of Eyeglasses
  Procedure 116 Applying and Removing In-the-Ear or Behind-the-Ear Hearing Aids

## VOCABULARY

**age-related macular degeneration** *(ayj-ree-* ***LAY****-ted **MAH**-kyou-lar **dee**-jen-er-**AY**-shun)*

**aneurysm** *(**AN**-you-rizm)*
**aphasia** *(ah-**FAY**-zee-ah)*

591

# VOCABULARY

atherosclerosis (**ath**-er-oh-skleh-**ROH**-sis)

auditory nerve (**awe**-dih-**TOH**-ree nurv)

brain stem (brayn stem)

cataract (**KAT**-ah-ract)

central nervous system (**SEN**-tral **NUR**-vus **SIS**-tem)

cerebellum (ser-eh-**BELL**-um)

cerebrospinal fluid (ser-eh-broh-**SPY**-nal **FLEW**-id)

cerebrovascular accident (CVA) (ser-eh-broh-**VASS**-kyou-lar **ACK**-sih-dent)

cerebrum (**SER**-eh-brum)

choroid (**KOH**-royd)

conjunctiva (kon-junk-**TIGH**-vah)

cornea (**KOR**-nee-ah)

dementia (dee-**MEN**-she-ah)

diabetic retinopathy (**die**-ah-**BET**-ick ret-ih-**NOP**-ah-thee)

embolus (**EM**-boh-lus)

emotional lability (ee-**MOH**-shun-al lah-**BILL**-ih-tee)

equilibrium (**ee**-kwih-**LIB**-ree-um)

genetic disease (jeh-**NET**-ick dih-**ZEEZ**)

glaucoma (glaw-**KOH**-mah)

hemianopsia (**hem**-ee-an-**OP**-see-ah)

hemiplegia (**hem**-ee-**PLEE**-jee-ah)

Huntington's disease (**HUNT**-ing-tonz dih-**ZEEZ**)

hypertension (**high**-per-**TEN**-shun)

intention tremor (in-**TEN**-shun **TREM**-or)

iris (**EYE**-riss)

lens (lenz)

Lhermitte's sign (**LAIR**-mits sign)

magnetic resonance imaging (MRI) (mag-**NET**-ick **REZ**-oh-nans **IM**-aj-ing)

meninges (meh-**NIN**-jeez)

motor nerve (**MOH**-tor nerv)

multiple sclerosis (MS) (**MULL**-tih-pul skle-**ROH**-sis)

myasthenia gravis (MG) (**my**-as-**THEE**-nee-ah **GRAH**-vis)

nerve impulses (nurv **IM**-pul-ses)

nerves (nurvs)

neurons (**NEW**-ronz)

neurotransmitter (**new**-roh-**TRANS**-mit-er)

nystagmus (nis-**TAG**-mus)

ophthalmologist (of-thal-**MOL**-oh-jist)

optic nerve (**OP**-tick nurv)

paralysis (pah-**RAL**-ih-sis)

paraplegia (**pair**-ah-**PLEE**-jee-ah)

Parkinson's disease (**PARK**-in-sons dih-**ZEEZ**)

peripheral nervous system (peh-**RIF**-er-al **NUR**-vus **SIS**-tem)

position sense (poh-**ZISH**-un sens)

presbycusis (**pres**-beh-**KYOU**-sis)

presbyopia (**pres**-bee-**OH**-pee-ah)

pupil (**PYOU**-pil)

quadriplegia (**kwahd**-rih-**PLEE**-jee-ah)

reflex (**REE**-flex)

retina (**RET**-ih-nah)

sclera (**SKLEH**-rah)

sensory nerve (**SEN**-sor-ee nurv)

spatial-perceptual deficit (**SPAY**-shul-per-**SEP**-tyou-al **DEF**-ih-sit)

stroke (strohk)

thrombus (**THROM**-bus)

transient ischemic attack (TIA) (**TRAN**-see-ent is-**KEE**-mick ah-**TACK**)

unilateral neglect (**you**-nih-**LAT**-er-al neh-**GLECT**)

vertigo (**VER**-tih-goh)

## COMPONENTS OF THE NERVOUS SYSTEM

The nervous system controls body functions by sending electrical messages called **nerve impulses** throughout the body. The two parts of the nervous system are the:

- **Peripheral nervous system** (PNS)—the nerves outside the brain and spinal cord
- **Central nervous system** (CNS)—the brain and spinal cord

Special sense organs and receptors receive information from the environment. The information travels along the cranial or spinal nerves to reach the brain and spinal cord, where the sensation is interpreted. Information is received by the:

- Eyes
- Ears
- Taste buds
- Receptors in the nose for smell
- Nerve endings (receptors) in the skin, muscles, joints, and tendons
- Receptors in body organs

The nerve endings in the skin pick up sensations of pain, pressure, and variations in temperature. Receptors in muscles, tendons, and joints carry information about the degree of muscle contraction and position of body parts. Receptors in the walls of body organs carry information related to hunger, thirst, and visceral (organ) pain.

### Neurons

**Neurons** are special cells that carry messages (Figure 29-1). The neurons and other cells make up the nervous tissue of the brain, spinal cord, and peripheral nerves. Neurons are composed of:

- A central area, called the body
- One or more dendrites—structures that receive messages and carry them toward the cell body
- An axon—the structure that carries messages away from the cell body

Axons and dendrites are called nerve fibers. A message or nerve impulse begins in the dendrites and is carried along the cell body and then to the axon. It takes more than one neuron to carry the message from where it begins to where it can be carried out or interpreted. The neurons

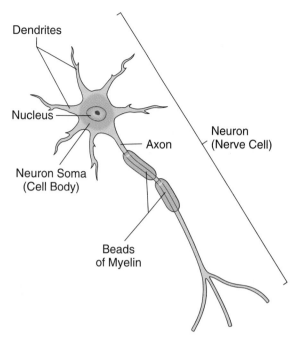

**FIGURE 29-1**   A neuron

do not actually touch each other. The little space between the axon of one neuron and the dendrites of the next is called the synapse.

### Neurotransmitters

**Neurotransmitters** are chemicals that enable messages (nerve impulses) to pass from one cell to another (Figure 29-2). If the chemicals are not produced in adequate amounts, the message pathway becomes confused or blocked.

### Nerves

**Nerves** are bundles of nerve fibers (axons and dendrites) that connect the body with the CNS. Nerves are named according to the type of message they carry and the direction in which they carry the message. The two general types of nerves are:

- Sensory nerves
- Motor nerves

**Sensory nerves** carry messages about pain, temperature change, changes in body position, taste, touch, sound, and sight. They carry messages toward the brain and spinal cord. When sensory nerves are damaged, the ability to receive messages and interpret sensations is impaired or lost.

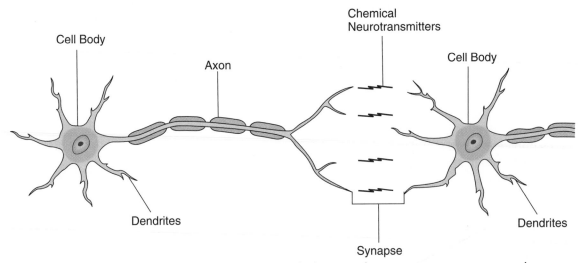

**FIGURE 29-2** Chemicals called neurotransmitters help pass the nerve message across the synapse from one neuron to the next.

**Motor nerves** carry messages from the brain and spinal cord to muscles and glands to bring about responses. When motor nerves are damaged, the person loses the ability to voluntarily control body movement. This condition is called **paralysis**. Paralysis may be complete, with no movement possible, or partial with a weaker than normal response.

Peripheral nerves carry both incoming and outgoing information. These are mixed bundles of nerves carrying both sensory and motor fibers throughout the body.

## CENTRAL NERVOUS SYSTEM

The CNS is made up of the brain and spinal cord. These organs are protected by the bones of the skull and vertebral column. A triple-layered membrane, the **meninges**, surrounds the brain and spinal column, providing additional protection.

### Spinal Cord

The spinal cord is about 18 inches long and extends from the brain to just above the small of the back. Thirty-one pairs of spinal nerves enter and leave the spinal cord, carrying messages to and from the body. The spinal cord:

- Carries messages to and from the brain and relays them to the body through the spinal nerves (Figure 29-3).
- Handles certain special responses called reflexes.

A **reflex** occurs when an incoming message becomes an outgoing command without needing to go to a higher conscious level. For example, if you touch something hot, you immediately pull your hand back. You may then realize what you have done, but pulling back your hand was a reflex response handled by the spinal column.

### The Brain

The brain is the most complex organ in the body (Figure 29-4). The neurons of the brain carry out many complex functions, including:

- Reasoning
- Thinking
- Forming and recalling memories
- Making judgments
- Controlling body functions
- Interpreting the sensations that are brought in by the nerves

Twelve pairs of cranial nerves carry messages into and out of the brain.

The **cerebrum** is the largest part of the brain. It is divided into two halves or hemispheres. The surface of the cerebrum forms lobes that have

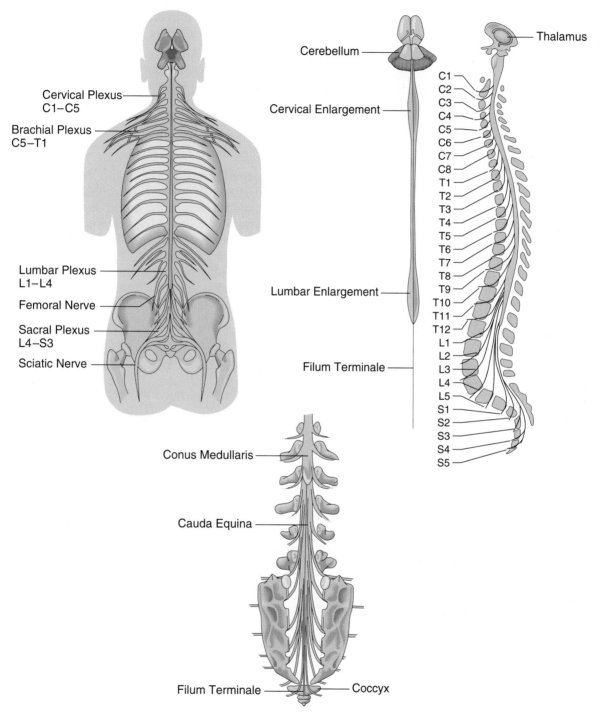

**FIGURE 29-3**   Spinal cord and nerves

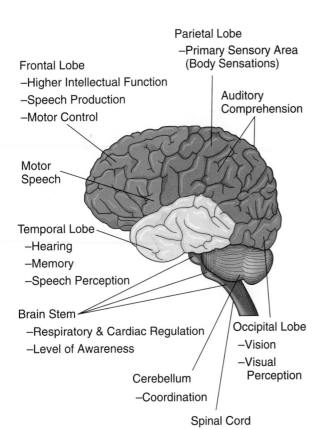

Frontal Lobe
–Higher Intellectual Function
–Speech Production
–Motor Control

Motor
Speech

Temporal Lobe
–Hearing
–Memory
–Speech Perception

Brain Stem
–Respiratory & Cardiac Regulation
–Level of Awareness

Parietal Lobe
–Primary Sensory Area
(Body Sensations)

Auditory
Comprehension

Occipital Lobe
–Vision
–Visual
Perception

Cerebellum
–Coordination

Spinal Cord

**FIGURE 29-4** Functional areas of the brain

the same names as the bones under which they are located. They are the:

- Frontal lobes
- Parietal lobes
- Temporal lobes
- Occipital lobes

(Refer to Figure 29-4.)

Different parts of the cerebrum carry out specific activities:

- Motor control of one side of the body is managed by cells in the opposite side of the frontal lobe.
- Sensations originating on one side of the body are interpreted on the opposite side of the parietal lobe.
- Vision is interpreted in the occipital lobe.
- Hearing is in the temporal lobe.

The **cerebellum** is called the little brain. It lies beneath the occipital lobes of the cerebrum. This part of the brain coordinates muscular activities and maintains balance.

The **brain stem** is the portion of the brain that is connected to the spinal cord. It is composed of special groups of nerve cells that control the vital (living) functions of the body. These vital functions include:

- Respiration
- Heart rate and rhythm
- Size of the blood vessels
- Functioning of internal body organs such as the organs of the digestive tract

Most of the twelve pairs of cranial nerves are attached to the brain stem.

**Cerebrospinal Fluid.** The **cerebrospinal fluid** (CSF) is a clear, colorless fluid derived from the plasma of the blood. It fills cavities in the brain called ventricles and circulates in the central canal of the spinal cord. It acts as a watery cushion around both the brain and spinal cord. CSF is continuously produced. It is also reabsorbed at the same rate back into the bloodstream.

## AUTONOMIC NERVOUS SYSTEM

The autonomic nervous system is part of the PNS. It controls heart rate, the secretions of glandular cells, and the contraction of the smooth muscular walls of organs.

## SENSE ORGANS

The sense organs carry messages about the external world to the brain. Sense organs carry messages about:

- Touch
- Temperature
- Pain
- Vision
- Hearing
- Taste
- Smell
- Equilibrium

### The Eye

Each eye is located in a bony cavity of the skull. Muscles move the eyes in a coordinated way.

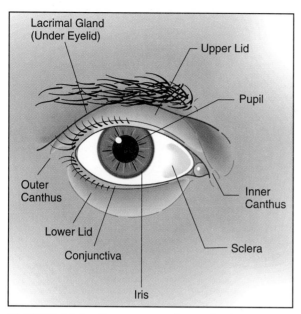

**FIGURE 29-5** Tears come from the lacrimal gland and exit from the eye through the nasolacrimal duct.

The eyelids and eye are covered by a clear mucous membrane called the **conjunctiva**. Mucus and tears from the lacrimal gland keep the eye moist (Figure 29-5). Excess tears drain into the nose and sometimes from the outside of the eyes.

The eye is a ball-shaped, fluid-filled organ made up of three layers:

- **Sclera**—the outer white protective cover. The front of the sclera forms the transparent **cornea**.
- **Choroid**—the middle layer that contains the **iris** (the colored part of the eye). The iris lies behind the cornea. The center of the iris is the **pupil**, which is an opening that changes size to control the amount of light entering the eye. The **lens** behind the iris bends and directs light rays.
- **Retina**—the innermost layer containing nerve receptors (Figure 29-6)

**Vision.** Light rays are reflected from the object being seen. The rays pass through the cornea and pupil and are bent to focus on the retina. The image on the retina is then transmitted by the **optic nerve** to the brain for vision interpretation. (The optic nerve is one of the cranial nerves.)

## The Ear

The ear enables us to hear and also assists in controlling **equilibrium**. This allows us to maintain our sense of balance. The ear is made up of the:

- Outer ear
- Middle ear
- Inner ear (Figure 29-7)

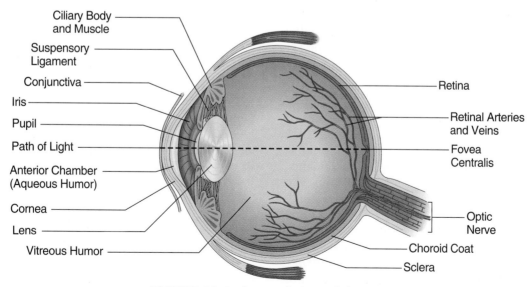

**FIGURE 29-6** Internal view of the eye

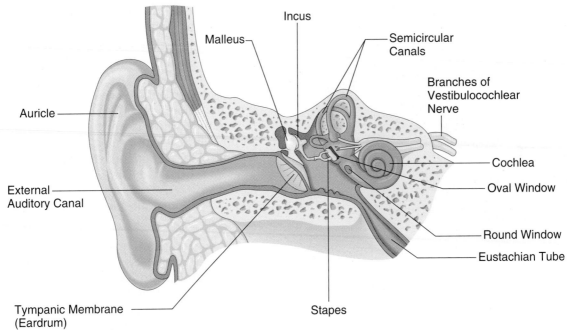

**FIGURE 29-7** Internal view of the ear

**Hearing.** Sound waves enter the ear and are carried toward the eardrum (tympanic membrane). This structure separates the outer and middle ear. The sound waves make the eardrum vibrate. Three tiny bones stretch across the middle ear. The first bone is attached to the eardrum. It begins to vibrate as the eardrum moves. The second bone is attached to the first and the third to the second. Each little bone vibrates in turn at the same rate as the eardrum moves. The third bone attaches to the membranous opening of the inner ear. Vibrations against this membrane set up fluid vibrations in the inner ear. The inner ear is made up of the:

- Semicircular canals
- Vestibule
- Cochlea

The three semicircular canals pick up information about starting and stopping movements. The vestibule picks up information about the position of the head. Deep within the snail-shaped cochlea are the special hearing receptors that are stimulated by the fluid vibrations. When these receptors are stimulated, the message is picked up and transmitted to the **auditory nerve** and then to the brain for interpretation of sounds that are heard.

## CHANGES IN THE NERVOUS SYSTEM CAUSED BY AGING ·········

The effects of aging on the nervous system are not as noticeable as they are on some of the other body systems. It is important to remember that intelligence does not decrease. Any change in mental status is an indication of a disease process.

Aging affects the senses of vision, hearing, taste, and smell. Most people have visual changes that make it difficult to read and see close objects. This is because the elasticity of the lens decreases with age. This condition is called **presbyopia** (also called farsightedness). Glasses will correct this problem. Many older people have glasses with *bifocal* or *trifocal* lenses. These lenses correct more than one visual impairment. Some residents are not able to care for their own glasses. You must remember to do this for them.

## CAUSES OF SEVERE VISION IMPAIRMENT ··············

Several disorders of the eye may result in severely impaired vision or blindness. These changes are

## PROCEDURE
# 115
## Care of Eyeglasses

1. Carry out each beginning procedure action.
2. Assemble equipment:
   - Resident's eyeglasses
   - Cleaning solution
   - Clear water
   - Soft cleaning tissues
3. Provide only the assistance that the resident needs.
4. Handle glasses only by the frames.
5. Clean lenses with cleaning solution or clear water. Check the condition of the frames and lenses. Report any damage to the frames and ear pieces and serious scratching of the lenses.
6. Dry with tissues.
7. Help resident put glasses on or return glasses to case and place in drawer of bedside table. If the resident puts the glasses on, note how well the glasses fit. Report any looseness or slipping. If the glasses have nose pieces, check that they are not irritating the resident's skin.
8. Carry out each procedure completion action.

---

not due to normal aging. Some of these disorders can be treated and are reversible. Others lead to severe vision impairment or blindness.

### Cataracts

The lens is normally clear. Sometimes the lens becomes cloudy and is called a **cataract**. The cataract causes vision to become blurred and hazy. A person with a cataract has problems judging distance. Color vision may disappear and glare from bright lights is annoying.

The only treatment for a cataract is surgery to remove the lens. The surgeon will usually put in an artificial lens during the surgery. If this is not done, the person must wear very strong glasses or contact lenses.

Some residents may have cataract surgery while they are in the long-term care facility. They generally return to the facility immediately after surgery. Be sure you know what to do for these residents. Pressure must not be placed on the eye. Thus, the residents should avoid bending over, coughing, or excessive physical activity.

### Glaucoma

**Glaucoma** exists when the pressure in the eyeball is higher than normal. This occurs when the meshwork between the iris and cornea thickens, obstructing the flow of the fluid in the eyeball. If not treated, the pressure eventually damages the optic nerve, causing blindness.

Glaucoma has few symptoms. Everyone over the age of 35 years should be tested for eye pressure routinely. The disease process can be stopped by using eyedrops prescribed by the **ophthalmologist** (eye physician).

### Age-Related Macular Degeneration

**Age-related macular degeneration** is the leading cause of visual loss in the United States. Millions of older people are affected. The cause is unknown. The macula is located on the retina. The macula is damaged when abnormal blood vessels form and leak fluid. Laser treatments may help some people with this condition.

# Guidelines for

## Assisting Visually Impaired Residents

1. Make sure the resident knows the location of all personal articles in the room. If the resident has a system for organizing belongings, do not attempt to make changes.
2. Always put things back where they were.
3. Do not rearrange furniture unless it is absolutely necessary. Then tell the resident what changes have been made.
4. Help orient the resident to a new room by teaching the resident to locate various objects from a point of reference. Just inside the door may be the reference point. Then say, for example, "The bathroom is to your right."
5. When you walk with a visually impaired resident, ask the resident to take your arm just above the elbow. You will walk slightly behind and to one side of the resident. Describe changes that require the resident's attention. For example, "We need to go up five steps now." Some residents may use special canes as "feelers" as they ambulate.
6. To help the person locate a chair, place the person's hand on the chair's back or arm. The seat should be located before sitting.
7. The floor should be dry and free of clutter and throw rugs.
8. Never leave doors partially open.
9. At mealtime, the resident's dishes should always be arranged in the same way. Describe the location and type of food using a clock system. For example. "The roast beef is at 12:00, mashed potatoes and gravy are at 3:00, and there are peas at 9:00."
10. Offer to cut meat, pour beverages, butter bread, and open cartons. Some residents may be able to do this.
11. Advise the resident to sprinkle salt and pepper into the hand rather than directly on the food. It is easier to know how much is being used.
12. Advise the resident to use a small piece of bread in one hand to help push food on the fork. This also prevents the food from being pushed off the plate.

## Diabetic Retinopathy

People with diabetes are at risk for **diabetic retinopathy**. It is caused by the deterioration of small blood vessels that nourish the retina. Laser treatments may interrupt the disease process. However, vision loss that has already occurred cannot be restored.

There are many things nursing assistants can do to improve the quality of life for residents with severe visual impairments.

Review Lesson 4 for communicating with persons with vision and hearing loss.

# HEARING LOSS

Hearing loss is common in later years. It usually results from progressive deterioration of the cochlea. This condition is called **presbycusis**. Some residents will wear hearing aids. The devices are expensive, so they must receive proper care.

## Hearing Aids

All types of hearing aids are basically the same. A battery provides the power for the hearing aid to work. The battery is contained in a battery case. The microphone picks up the sound. The amplifier makes the sound louder. The volume control adjusts the level of sound. The receiver is a tiny speaker that conveys sound to the ear. Some models have a "T" switch. This is a telephone switch that activates a telecoil. This is used when hearing over a telephone. The telephone must be compatible with the telecoil. There are several types of hearing aids:

- The canal aid is the smallest type and fits deep into the ear canal.
- The in-the-ear aid is the most commonly used. It fills the ear and is flush with the outer part of the ear (Figure 29-8).
- The behind-the-ear aid consists of an aid worn behind the ear and an earmold that directs sound into the ear canal.
- Eyeglass types of hearing aids are similar to behind-the-ear aids except that the amplification device is contained in an eyeglass frame.
- The body aid is enclosed in a case that can be carried in a pocket or attached to clothing. The hearing aid receiver attaches directly to an earmold inserted into the ear canal. The receiver is powered through a cord connected to the case of the body aid.

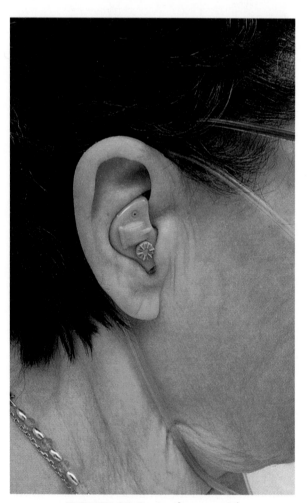

**FIGURE 29-8**　In-the-ear aid

**Caring for Hearing Aids.**

1. Store hearing aids at room temperature when not worn. Temperature extremes can damage hearing aids. They should not be worn for more than a few minutes in very cold weather. Avoid exposing them to hair dryers.
2. Keep hearing aids dry. If an aid is worn accidentally in the shower ask the nurse how to dry it. Never try to dry the aid with a hair dryer.
3. Store extra batteries in a cool, dry place. Remove batteries from the hearing aid at night or open the battery compartment. This allows air to circulate in the compartment and helps dry it out. The battery will last longer.
4. Keep hearing aids safe. They break easily if dropped on a hard floor or bumped against a hard surface.
5. Remove the hearing aid if hair spray is being used. The spray may clog the microphone, causing damage.
6. Turn the hearing aid off when not in use. Turn the aid off before removing it.
7. Wipe in-the-ear aids daily with a dry tissue.
8. Check regularly to make sure the opening of the aid or earmold is wax free. In-the-ear types come with a cleaning tool. This should be used only by someone who has been shown how to use it to remove the wax.

**Troubleshooting for Hearing Aids.** If the aid is not producing sound, before inserting in resident's ear:

- Check to make sure that the "+" (positive) side of the battery is next to the "+" inside the hearing aid battery case or compartment.
- Try a new battery—the old one may be dead.
- Check the earmold to see if it is plugged with wax.
- Make sure the hearing aid is set on "M" (microphone) not "T" (telephone switch).

  If the hearing aid is making squealing sounds:

- Determine if the earmold fits properly. It should be completely in the ear. If it does not fit well, report it to the nurse.
- Check the volume on the aid. If it is too high, turn it down until the squealing stops.
- Check the plastic tubing on a behind-the-ear aid. If it is cracked or split, it must be replaced.

**PROCEDURE**
### *116*  Applying and Removing In-the-Ear or Behind-the-Ear Hearing Aids

1. Carry out each beginning procedure action.
2. Assist resident to comfortable position with head turned so that the ear needing the hearing aid is closest to you.
3. Turn the hearing aid off and turn the volume down.
4. Make sure you insert the aid in the correct ear.

**Behind-the-Ear Hearing Aid**

- Place the aid over the resident's ear, allowing the earmold to hang free.
- Adjust the hearing aid behind the resident's ear (Figure 29-9).

**Behind-the-Ear Hearing Aid and In-the-Ear Hearing Aid**

- Grasp the earmold and gently insert the tapered end into the ear canal.
- Gently twist the earmold into the curve of the ear while gently pulling on the earlobe with the other hand. The hearing aid should fit snugly but comfortably, flush with the ear.
5. Turn on the control switch. To adjust the volume, talk to the resident as you increase the volume. Stop when the resident can hear you.

**Removing the Hearing Aid**

1. Wash hands and explain to resident what you plan to do.
2. Turn off hearing aid.

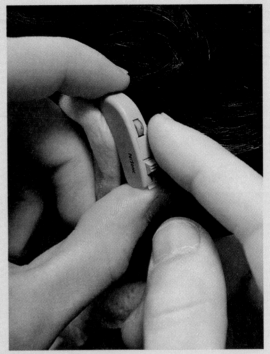

**FIGURE 29-9** Adjust the hearing aid behind the resident's ear.

3. Loosen the outer portion of the earmold by gently pulling on the upper part of the ear.
4. Lift earmold upward and outward.
5. Store in safe area.
6. Carry out each procedure completion action.

## NERVOUS SYSTEM DISORDERS

Several diseases can affect the nervous system. Some of these are due to an imbalance in neurotransmitters. Other neurologic problems are caused by damage to brain cells or the spinal cord.

Diseases affecting the nervous system often have different signs and symptoms. Some common problems that may exist with these diseases include:

- Impaired mobility because of damage to the brain, spinal cord, or nerves in the legs

- Difficulty swallowing due to damage to the brain or damage to the nerves of the face and mouth
- Communication disorders due to damage to the brain or damage to the nerves of the face and mouth

## Parkinson's Disease

**Parkinson's disease** is a chronic illness that is often progressive. It is due to a decrease in a neurotransmitter that passes messages between cells in the cerebrum and the gray matter of the brain. These cells affect movement, balance, and walking (Figure 29-10).

The signs and symptoms of Parkinson's disease include:

- Tremors
- Muscular rigidity
- Difficulty and slowness in carrying out voluntary activities

Tremors of the hands commonly affect the fingers and thumbs so that the resident appears to be rolling a pill between them. The tremors begin in the fingers, then involve the entire hand and arm, and finally affect the entire side of the body. Starting on one side, the tremors eventually involve both sides of the body.

The muscular rigidity makes the person more prone to falls and injury. The joints may develop contractures if appropriate care and treatment are not given. The rigidity also affects muscles used in breathing. This increases the risk of respiratory infections.

Persons with advanced Parkinson's typically have a shuffling walk and difficulty starting the process. Once started, they may have episodes of "freezing" when they appear unable to move.

Speech is affected, causing words to be slurred. The tone of voice is low and the sound is monotone. Rigid facial muscles cause the face to look expressionless.

The resident with Parkinson's may drool and become incontinent or constipated. Depression is a common problem. Some residents with Parkinson's may undergo mental changes known as **dementia**.

There is no specific diagnostic test for Parkinson's disease. The physician will take a history and make a thorough neurologic examination to rule out other problems.

Parkinson's disease has no cure. In some cases the disease can be controlled with medications. In other cases, the disease may be progressive, causing severe disability.

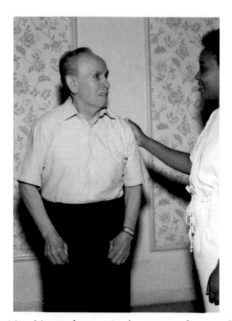
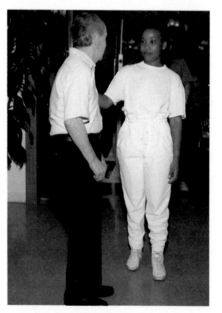

**FIGURE 29-10**   Note the typical posture from a front and side view of the resident with Parkinson's disease.

*G*uidelines for

# Caring for Residents with Parkinson's Disease

1. Give passive range of motion exercises at least twice a day. Encourage participation in active exercise if the resident is able to do so.
2. Improve walking by encouraging the resident to:
   - Bring the toes up with every step.
   - Put the foot down, heel first then toes.
   - Swing the arms.
   - Ambulate—assist by using a gait belt and walking with the resident.
3. Reposition dependent residents frequently and avoid flexion as much as possible.
4. Observe the resident closely and report:
   - Signs of respiratory infection
   - Problems with urinary elimination
   - Constipation

5. Give at least 2,000 mL fluid by mouth every day unless contraindicated.
6. Assist with activities of daily living only to the extent that is necessary.
7. Observe for drooling. Residents who are unable to control saliva may also have trouble swallowing. Watch for any problems during eating.
8. Give emotional support and encouragement. The disease usually affects the facial muscles. Because of this, the resident may have no facial expression. This lack of expression is not a true indication of what the resident is feeling.

## Stroke

**Stroke** (also called brain attack) is the fourth most common cause of death in the United States. Two-thirds of stroke victims are over age 65 years. Stroke is also called **cerebrovascular accident** or **CVA**. The word *cerebrovascular* refers to blood vessels in the brain. Major risk factors for a stroke include:

- **Hypertension** (high blood pressure)
- **Atherosclerosis** (build-up of fatty deposits in arteries)
- History of **transient ischemic attack (TIA)**
- Smoking
- Lack of exercise
- Obesity

A TIA is not a stroke, but may be a warning that a stroke is likely to occur. During a TIA, the resident may experience speech disturbances and paralysis. These symptoms last from a few minutes to 24 hours. They are never permanent.

A stroke may occur as a result of:

- Hemorrhage—This occurs when an **aneurysm** in the brain ruptures or hypertension causes a

blood vessel in the brain to rupture. An aneurysm is a thin spot on an artery wall.
- Thrombus—A **thrombus** is a blood clot. It forms when fatty deposits on the artery walls cause the walls to become roughened. This causes platelets in the blood to form a clot. When the thrombus interrupts blood flow to the brain, a stroke occurs.
- Embolus—An **embolus** is a thrombus that develops in an artery in one part of the body, breaks loose, and travels to another part of the body. In the case of a stroke, the embolus travels to an artery in the brain and blocks the flow of blood.

**Symptoms of Stroke.** The symptoms of stroke depend on the part of the brain that is damaged. If the left side of the brain is damaged, these symptoms may be noted:

- Paralysis on the right side of the body. This is called right **hemiplegia**.
- **Aphasia**—an inability to express or understand speech
- Change in personality. The individual with left brain damage becomes very slow, anxious, and cautious.

If the right side of the brain is damaged, these symptoms may be noted:

- Paralysis on the left side of the body. This is called left hemiplegia (Figure 29-11).
- **Spatial-perceptual deficits**. This means it is difficult to distinguish between left and right, up and down. The world may appear "tilted" to the person with right brain damage. The resident will have problems propelling a wheelchair, setting down items, and carrying out activities of daily living.
- Change in personality. The individual with right brain damage becomes very quick and impulsive.

Other symptoms may be present with either right or left brain damage. These include:

- Sensory-perceptual deficits.
  - Loss of **position sense**. The individual cannot tell where the affected foot is or what position it is in.
  - The inability to identify common objects. The person who has had a stroke may not recognize a comb, a fork, a pencil, or other common items.
  - The inability to use common objects. The person may know what the object is, such as a comb, but be unable to pick it up and use it appropriately even with the unaffected arm. This is not a result of paralysis but of damage to certain cells in the brain.
- **Unilateral neglect**. The resident ignores the paralyzed side of the body. For example, the affected arm may hang over the side of the wheelchair without the resident realizing where the arm is.
- **Hemianopsia**. This is impaired vision. Both eyes only have half vision. For example, if the resident has left hemiplegia, the left half of both eyes is blind (Figure 29-12).
- **Emotional lability**. Residents who have had strokes may start to cry or laugh for no apparent reason. They have very little control over this and may be embarrassed.

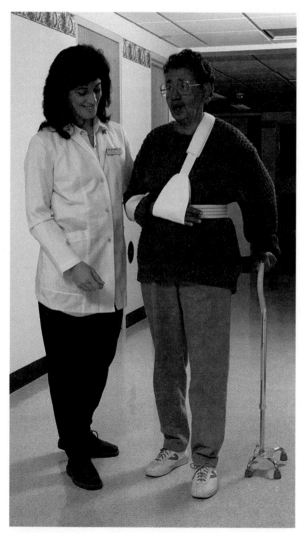

**FIGURE 29-11**  The resident had a stroke, resulting in paralysis of one side of the body.

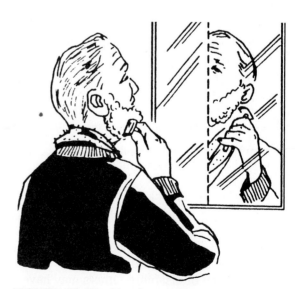

**FIGURE 29-12**  Hemianopsia causes a person to see only part of the visual field.

## *G*uidelines for

# Caring for Residents Who Have Had a Stroke

Complications following stroke can be prevented by several measures.

1. Proper positioning. Lesson 22 gives instructions for positioning residents with hemiplegia. Remember to support the paralyzed arm so that the shoulder does not become dislocated. Check the paralyzed leg and arm frequently. The resident may be unaware of injury to the extremities.
2. Passive range of motion exercises twice a day (see Lesson 22). The resident may learn to do self range of motion exercises. This also provides exercise for the unaffected arm.
3. Intake of an adequate amount of fluids each shift

4. Implementation of bowel and bladder programs
5. Maintenance of nutritional status
6. Encouraging and supporting the resident at all times
7. You can help the resident regain functional abilities by encouraging and allowing the resident to do as much as possible. Provide the help that is necessary for completing activities of daily living but avoid "over-helping." You can carry out restorative programs under the direction of the physical therapist, occupational therapist, and restorative nurse.
8. You can help the resident regain mobility skills by increasing the resident's mobility as directed by the nurse or physical therapist (Lessons 22 and 23).

**Goals of Poststroke Care.** Three major nursing goals for a resident who has had a stroke are:

1. Maintain the skills and abilities that the individual has left.
2. Prevent complications caused by immobility.
   - Contractures
   - Pressure ulcers
   - Pneumonia
   - Blood clots
3. Regain functional abilities (Figure 29-13).
   - Activities of daily living
   - Bowel and bladder control
   - Mobility
   - Communication skills

Communicating with persons with aphasia is presented in Lesson 4.

The recovery from stroke is different for each person. Some individuals recover with a minimal degree of disability. Others may have a greater degree of disability but learn to adapt and regain some independence. A few individu-

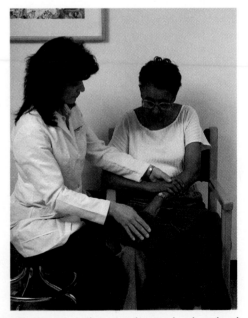

**FIGURE 29-13** The resident who has had a stroke must be retrained in activities of daily living.

als are severely impaired and will regain very little, if any, ability for self-care.

## Multiple Sclerosis

**Multiple sclerosis (MS)** is another CNS disease. The cause is unknown. The myelin sheath that covers the part of the neuron called the axon is destroyed. When the myelin sheath is destroyed, impulses are unable to travel through the axon.

MS is usually diagnosed before the age of 50. Many individuals live the usual life span even though they have this chronic disorder. Therefore, it is not unusual to see elderly residents in long-term care with this diagnosis. Most facilities also have young residents in their twenties and thirties with MS (Figure 29-14).

The symptoms are variable and may not be the same for all individuals. Symptoms may include:

- Loss of sensation with regard to temperature, pain, touch
- Feelings of numbness and tingling
- **Vertigo** (a spinning sensation)
- Loss of position sense
- **Lhermitte's sign** (a tingling, shock-like sensation that passes down the arms or spine when the neck is flexed)

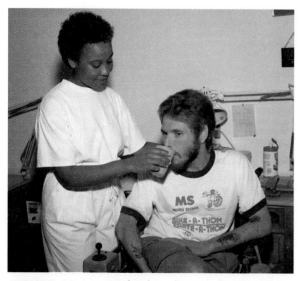

**FIGURE 29-14**   Multiple sclerosis frequently affects young people.

Problems with vision occur in almost half of the people who have MS. This problem may be permanent or temporary. Sometimes it is the first symptom that is noted. Symptoms may include:

- Blurriness, color blindness, or difficulty seeing objects in bright light
- Double vision
- **Nystagmus** (jerky eye movements)

Mobility is usually affected:

- Pain in the legs that disappears with rest
- **Paraplegia** (paralysis of both legs)
- Spasticity
- **Intention tremor** (shaking of the hands that gets worse as the individual tries to touch or pick up an object)

In severe MS, speech is affected because of the weakness of the muscles in the chest, face, and lips. The speech may be slow with poor articulation. The mind usually remains alert. Incontinence of bowel and bladder is also common.

One of the most disabling features of MS is fatigue. This very real physical symptom, not psychological, makes it impossible for the person to move about.

The diagnosis of MS is not based on a specific test. The physician takes a thorough history and performs a complete neurologic examination. **Magnetic resonance imaging (MRI)** is a test that may reveal lesions in the neurons in the brain. The person conducting the test records pictures (scans) of brain tissue beneath the bone.

MS may eventually lead to **quadriplegia** (paralysis of all four extremities). Residents with quadriplegia require total care. However, not all persons who have MS are severely impaired. At the time of diagnosis, it is seldom known what course the disease will take. It is difficult for the person to deal with this uncertainty for the future. The disease may follow one of four courses:

- *Benign course:* mild attacks with long periods of no symptoms
- *Exacerbating-remitting:* Severe attacks (exacerbations) followed by periods of partial or complete recovery (remissions). Often the periods of exacerbation get longer with shorter periods of remission.
- *Slowly progressive:* slow, steady deterioration
- *Rapidly progressive:* deterioration is rapid and progressive and may be life-threatening

# Guidelines for

# Caring for Residents with Multiple Sclerosis

1. Prevent complications.
   - Contractures can occur rapidly because of the spasticity. Range of motion exercises and position changes are important. The resident may also perform muscle stretching exercises with the help of the rehabilitation nurse or physical therapist.
   - Spasticity affects the bladder and causes incontinence. For this reason, residents with severe MS may have indwelling catheters. Scrupulous catheter care is necessary to prevent bladder infections. Make sure the resident has adequate fluid intake.
   - Residents with MS are at risk for pressure ulcers. Follow all directions for pressure ulcer prevention. Because of lack of sensation, ulcers may develop without the resident feeling discomfort or pain.
2. Encourage independence.
   - The use of adaptive devices for activities of daily living may help maintain independence for a longer period of time.
   - Mobility may be prolonged if assistive devices such as canes or walkers are used. Leg braces are helpful for some people. Many individuals (even in the facility) may use motorized scooters. This increases independence for people who are no longer able to walk.
3. Maintain a balanced schedule of rest and activity.
   - Residents with MS need exercise and activity. However, they also need rest periods to avoid becoming overtired.
   - Remember that fatigue can be a major problem. Help residents set priorities for their available energy. If a resident expects the family to visit in the evening for example, allow more rest periods during the day.
4. Provide emotional support and encouragement.
   - Residents in long-term care facilities may have access to MS support groups. Some people find these groups very helpful.
   - Not all residents with MS will be elderly. Remember the developmental stages of the residents in your care. This will allow you to be more empathic and give better care.

## Huntington's Disease

**Huntington's disease** is a hereditary disease. This means it is a **genetic disease** because it is passed from one generation to another through a defective gene. Either parent carrying the gene can transmit the disease to either sons or daughters. Each child of a parent with the defective gene for Huntington's has a 50% chance of receiving the defective gene from the parent.

The disease is progressive and affects the CNS as well as the mind and the emotions. Symptoms may become evident between the ages of 20 and 60 years. The most evident symptom is the body movements called choreiform movements. These begin early in the disease with fidgeting, twitching, clumsiness, and falling. As the disease progresses, the extremities are in constant movement during waking hours. Eventually it becomes impossible for the individual to walk or perform any activities independently.

The mind is also affected, resulting in a form of dementia. The capacity to plan and organize is lost. Impulsiveness and loss of judgment are also common. Emotional disorders such as depression, antisocial behavior, and seclusion may also develop.

---

$G$uidelines for
## Caring for Residents with Huntington's Disease

Safety is a major concern because of the constant body movements.

1. Prevent injuries by:
   - Padding side rails to avoid injury to the arms and legs
   - Using padded clothing and shoes without laces
   - Using a gait belt and having two assistants walk with the resident—providing stability and counteracting the jerky movements
   - Using alternatives to restraints, which are dangerous because of the movements

2. Prevent choking by:
   - Ensuring that all who are responsible for feeding residents are knowledgeable about the residents' abilities, if possible
   - Having all persons who feed know how to do abdominal thrusts for an obstructed airway
   - Providing a diet as tolerated

Other concerns for residents with Huntington's disease include:

3. Incontinence
   - Assist the resident to the bathroom every 2 hours or as needed. As the disease progresses this becomes impossible with the loss of ambulatory skills.
   - Catheters usually pose a danger because of the resident's involuntary movements, which may cause tearing of the urethra.
   - Incontinent pads may be necessary.
   - Careful attention to skin care is essential.

4. Nutrition
   - Additional calories may be needed because of the energy used in the involuntary movements.

---

The disease is always chronic and progressive. There may be periods of stability. As the disease progresses, the symptoms become more severe. Eventually, death occurs, usually as a result of pneumonia or an infection.

Many residents with Huntington's disease are young people. Some of them may have young children. This is a difficult situation for families as children watch a parent become progressively worse. Whether or not the children develop the disease is a major concern for all family members. Each family deals with this in its own way. Avoid passing judgment on families and the way they choose to cope with this problem. Referral for professional counseling should be made by the social services staff to all family members as well as the resident. It is the individual's decision whether or not to participate in the counseling.

## Amyotrophic Lateral Sclerosis

This disease is also known as ALS or Lou Gehrig's disease. Mr. Gehrig was a famous baseball player who died of ALS. ALS generally affects persons between the ages of 50 and 70. The nerve cells in the brain and spinal cord gradually deteriorate. The disease is chronic and progressive. There is no cure. The muscles under their control weaken and waste away. The disease eventually affects all voluntary muscles. The mind stays alert and the person is able to think clearly. The first signs and symptoms include:

- Trouble with walking—stumbling and falling
- Trouble picking up objects and frequently dropping them
- Trouble completing activities of daily living, for example, lacing shoes, buttoning, or cutting meat

## *G*uidelines for

# Caring for Residents Who Have Amyotrophic Lateral Sclerosis

1. Keep the resident upright as much as possible to avoid aspiration and to increase lung expansion. When lying down, position the resident on either side, turning at least every 2 hours. Place a cloth beneath the mouth to absorb saliva from the mouth.
2. Encourage coughing and deep breathing to prevent respiratory infections.
3. Encourage the resident to take frequent rest periods. Encourage the use of a wheelchair to save energy.
4. Use methods of communication as directed by the nurse or speech therapist. The resident may eventually have to communicate by blinking the eyes. Remember that even though the resident cannot speak, he can understand others.
5. Observe food and fluid intake. Residents with ALS may be too weak or too tired to eat. Try to have the resident rest for a half hour before meals and for 2 hours after meals. If the resident has to be fed, allow frequent breaks during the meal.
6. Report any signs of potential pressure ulcers.

Persons with ALS eventually have:
- Difficulty speaking
- Difficulty swallowing (may need a feeding tube)
- Disabling fatigue
- Shortness of breath (may need a ventilator)
- Inability to move arms or legs independently

## Myasthenia Gravis

**Myasthenia gravis (MG)** is also a chronic disease that affects the muscles. This is due to incomplete transmission of nerve impulses where the nerves and muscle join. The cause is unknown. The same muscles are not affected in

## *G*uidelines for

# Caring for Residents Who Have Myasthenia Gravis

Medications can help most people with myasthenia gravis to live productive lives. The disease affects each person differently. It is important to know for a specific resident which muscles are affected and how much activity the resident can tolerate.

1. Pace the resident's activity and allow adequate time for rest between activities.
2. Use alternative methods of communication according to the care plan.
3. Review Lesson 17 for feeding residents with swallowing problems.
4. Encourage the resident's independence but provide assistance as needed.

all people. Signs and symptoms always involve the muscles and may include:

- Weakness of the eye muscles causing double vision and drooping of the eyelid
- Inability to smile, frown, or pucker the lips if facial muscles are involved
- Voice weaker if larynx is involved

- Generalized muscle weakness:
  - Difficulty putting arms above head
  - Difficulty rising from chair or toilet and difficulty walking up stairs
  - Difficulty managing saliva
  - Mouth hangs open due to inability to close mouth

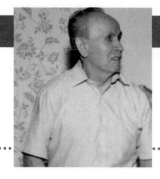

## LESSON SYNTHESIS: Putting It All Together

*Y*ou have just completed this lesson. Now go back and review the Clinical Focus. Try to see how the Clinical Focus relates to the concepts presented in the lesson. Then answer the following questions.

1. Why might self-feeding be difficult for Mr. Raye?

2. Why is it important to carry out range of motion regularly with Mr. Raye?

3. How can ambulation be encouraged and made more safe?

4. Nursing assistants must be alert to the possibility of which serious complications that could affect Mr. Raye?

5. Why do Mr. Raye and his family need the emotional support of the staff?

## REVIEW

**A. Select the one best answer for each of the following:**

1. The brain and spinal cord make up the
   a. central nervous system
   b. peripheral nervous system
   c. sensory organs
   d. all of these

2. Neurotransmitters are
   a. neurons
   b. special nerves
   c. chemicals that help pass messages from one cell to another
   d. brain cells

3. The brain stem controls
   a. voluntary movements
   b. thinking

   c. vital functions of the body
   d. emotions

4. When the lens of the eye becomes cloudy and impairs vision, it is called
   a. glaucoma
   b. macular degeneration
   c. diabetic retinopathy
   d. cataract

5. Hearing aids should be kept
   a. at room temperature
   b. dry
   c. free of wax
   d. all of these

6. Parkinson's disease is due to
   a. a decrease in a neurotransmitter
   b. brain injury

c. changes in the myelin sheath of the neuron
d. all of these

7. Persons with Parkinson's generally have
   a. tremors
   b. rigidity
   c. slowness of movement
   d. all of these

8. Nursing care for persons with Parkinson's disease includes
   a. instructions for walking
   b. positioning to avoid flexion
   c. giving adequate fluids
   d. all of these

9. A person who has had a stroke on the left side of the brain will
   a. have left hemiplegia
   b. become quick and impulsive
   c. have aphasia
   d. all of these

10. The person who has had a stroke on the right side of the brain will
    a. have left hemiplegia
    b. aphasia
    c. become slow, anxious, and cautious
    d. all of these

11. Residents with stroke
    a. need the shoulder on the affected side supported to prevent dislocation
    b. need passive range of motion exercises at least twice a day
    c. should be encouraged to do as much as possible
    d. all of these

12. Multiple sclerosis occurs because
    a. the myelin sheath of the neuron is damaged
    b. of a hemorrhage in the brain
    c. of a lack of a certain neurotransmitter
    d. muscle damage

13. Residents with multiple sclerosis may experience
    a. loss of sensation to temperature, pain, touch
    b. visual impairments

c. tremors
d. all of these

14. Spasticity of the muscles in multiple sclerosis may cause
    a. respiratory tract infections
    b. choking
    c. urinary tract infections
    d. urinary incontinence

15. Nursing care must be given to residents with multiple sclerosis to
    a. prevent contractures
    b. prevent pressure ulcers
    c. maintain mobility as long as possible
    d. all of these

16. Huntington's disease is characterized by
    a. hemiplegia
    b. aphasia
    c. chorea
    d. slowness of movements

17. Amyotrophic lateral sclerosis (ALS) causes
    a. inability to move independently
    b. disabling fatigue
    c. difficulty speaking and swallowing
    d. all of these

18. The person with ALS usually has
    a. mental impairment
    b. vision impairment
    c. shortness of breath
    d. all of these

19. Residents with ALS should
    a. be positioned upright as much as possible
    b. be kept as active as possible through the day
    c. be positioned in supine position for several hours a day
    d. communicate by writing

20. Signs and symptoms of myasthenia gravis include
    a. weakness of the eye muscles
    b. inability to keep the mouth closed
    c. drooling
    d. all of these

**B. Fill in the blanks by selecting the correct word or phrase from the list.**

age-related macular degeneration
amyotrophic lateral sclerosis
aphasia
central nervous system
dementia
equilibrium
genetic
glaucoma
hemianopsia
hemiplegia
Lhermitte's sign
neurotransmitters
nystagmus
paraplegia
position sense
presbycusis
presbyopia
quadriplegia
thrombus
unilateral neglect

21. Chemicals that help pass nerve impulses from one cell to another are called _____.

22. The brain and spinal cord make up the _____.

23. The ear is responsible for hearing and for _____.

24. Older adults often develop a vision problem called _____.

25. A condition in which the pressure within the eyeball is higher than normal is called _____.

26. The leading cause of visual loss in this country is _____.

27. Many older adults suffer hearing loss called _____.

28. Persons with Parkinson's disease may undergo mental changes referred to as _____.

29. Stroke may be caused by a blood clot called a _____.

30. Paralysis on one side of the body is called _____.

31. The inability to express or understand speech is _____.

32. If a resident with a stroke cannot tell where the affected foot is, the resident has loss of _____.

33. _____ is loss of vision of one-half of the eye in both eyes.

34. _____ means the resident ignores the paralyzed side of the body.

35. A tingling shock-like sensation that passes down the arms or spine when the neck is flexed is _____.

36. Paralysis of both legs is _____.

37. Paralysis of all four extremities is _____.

38. Jerky eye movements seen in multiple sclerosis are called _____.

39. Huntington's disease is _____.

40. The disease also known as Lou Gehrig's disease is _____.

# Residents with Special Needs

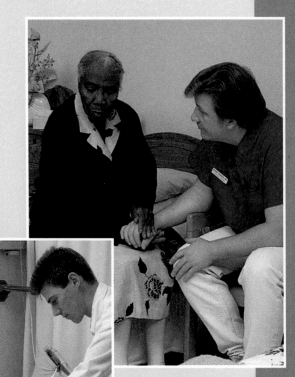

## LESSONS

**30** Alzheimer's Disease and Related Disorders (Caring for the Cognitively Impaired Resident)

**31** Caring for Residents with Developmental Disabilities

**32** Caring for the Dying Resident

**33** Caring for the Person in Subacute Care

**CLINICAL FOCUS**

Think about the nursing care required by the

resident who suffers from Alzheimer's disease

and related disorders as you study this lesson

and meet:

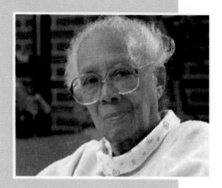

$G$race McGinnis, who has been a resident in your facility for almost 2 years. About 10 years ago, she realized that she could not remember details as well as she once had. Gradually, her mental and emotional status declined. Her husband employed a housekeeper to stay with her. Four years later, Mr. McGinnis had a heart attack and died. Family members felt admission to a long-term care facility was the only answer. Mrs. McGinnis suffers from Alzheimer's disease and is in stage 2.

## OBJECTIVES

*After studying this lesson, you should be able to:*

- Define and spell vocabulary words and terms.
- List four symptoms of Alzheimer's disease.
- Identify three approaches that are effective when working with residents with Alzheimer's disease or other dementias.

- State three guidelines for assisting residents with dementia with the activities of daily living.
- Describe four effective techniques for communicating with residents with dementia.
- Identify the concerns associated with caring for people with dementia.

# VOCABULARY

**Alzheimer's disease**  *(ALTZ-high-mers dih-ZEEZ)*

**aphasia**  *(ah-FAY-zee-ah)*

**aspiration**  *(ass-pih-RAY-shun)*

**catastrophic reaction**  *(kat-ah-STROH-fick ree-ACK-shun)*

**cognitive impairment**  *(KOG-nih-tiv im-PAIR-ment)*

**delusion**  *(dee-LEW-zhun)*

**dementia**  *(dee-MEN-she-ah)*

**depression**  *(dee-PRESH-un)*

**disorientation**  *(dis-oh-ree-en-TAY-shun)*

**hallucination**  *(hah-loo-sih-NAY-shun)*

**neurotransmitter**  *(new-roh-TRANS-mit-er)*

**organic mental syndrome**  *(or-GAN-ick MEN-til SIN-drohm)*

**pacing**  *(PAYS-ing)*

**perseveration**  *(per-sev-er-AY-shun)*

**pet therapy**  *(pet THER-ah-pee)*

**reality orientation**  *(ree-AL-ih-tee oh-ree-en-TAY-shun)*

**reminiscing**  *(reh-mih-NISS-ing)*

**sensory-perceptual changes**  *(SEN-sor-ee-per-SEP-tyou-al CHAIN-jes)*

**sundowning**  *(SUN-down-ing)*

**validation therapy**  *(val-ih-DAY-shun THER-ah-pee)*

**wandering**  *(WAN-der-ing)*

## DEFINITION OF ALZHEIMER'S DISEASE

You will care for residents who have **Alzheimer's disease** or other dementia. Alzheimer's disease is a disorder of the brain that involves thinking, memory, and judgment. Alzheimer's disease is a form of **dementia**. **Organic mental syndrome** is a general term that includes all dementias. Dementia is not a disease in itself but is a group of symptoms seen in a number of different diseases. Alzheimer's is the most common form. Other types of dementias are related to cerebrovascular disease, Parkinson's disease, and Huntington's disease. The term **cognitive impairment** means that the mental or intellectual abilities of the individual are damaged (Figure 30-1).

The information in this lesson refers to Alzheimer's disease because it is the most common form of dementia. Remember that other dementias have many of the same signs and symptoms. The treatment and care are similar regardless of the medical diagnosis.

Alzheimer's disease can begin during middle age but is more common in older persons. The disease affects people of all races, intelligence levels, education, and financial status. It is progressive and has been called a "slow death" of the mind. In the past, the term *senility* was used to describe these symptoms. We now know that it is a disease of the brain cells and is not normal aging (Figure 30-2).

Research continues into the cause of Alzheimer's disease. There is no specific test to confirm the diagnosis and no cure. When symptoms appear the individual should have a complete medical diagnostic work-up.

It is important to rule out other conditions such as diabetes and other endocrine problems, vitamin deficiencies, malnutrition, brain tumors, impaired circulation, epilepsy, depression, and medication interactions. Unlike Alzheimer's disease, these conditions may be treatable and curable. The diagnostic tests commonly include:

- Blood tests
- Electroencephalogram (EEG), a study of brain waves
- Magnetic resonance imaging (MRI)
- Brain scan
- Psychological evaluation to rule out depression
- Evaluation of all medications being taken including over-the-counter drugs
- Mental status examination

**FIGURE 30-1** Descriptions of major forms of dementia

| Disease | Features | Course |
|---|---|---|
| Alzheimer's | Lack of chemical in brain causing neurofibrillary tangles, neuritic plaques | Onset age: 60-80 Slowly progressive |
| Multi-infarct dementia | Interference with blood circulation in brain cells due to arteriosclerosis, atherosclerosis | Onset age: 55-70 Outcome depends on rate of damage to brain cells |
| Huntington's | Inherited from either parent who has gene for the disease | Onset age: 25-45 Average duration 15 years |
| Parkinson's | Deficiency of chemical in brain (dopamine) | Onset age: 55-60 Several years duration |
| Creutzfeldt-Jacob | Noninflammatory virus, changes in brain | Onset age: 50-60 Rapidly progressive |
| Syphilis | Spirochete (bacteria) causes brain damage | Occurs 15-20 years after primary infection |
| AIDS dementia | HIV-1 infection | Symptoms sometimes precede diagnosis of AIDS |

The mental status examination assesses the person's:

- Orientation to time and place
- Attention span
- Ability to recall information
- Ability to use language
- Ability to follow directions
- Ability to read and write
- Ability to copy a design

## Changes in the Brain Leading to Alzheimer's Disease

Messages are normally passed between nerve cells (neurons) in the brain by chemicals called **neurotransmitters**. People with Alzheimer's lack one of these chemicals. If an autopsy of the brain is performed after death, distinctive changes are noted. These changes are called neuritic plaques and neurofibrillary tangles—indications of the damage that has occurred to the brain.

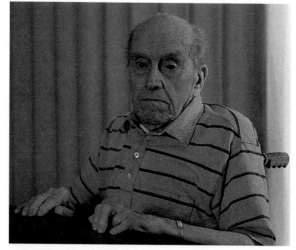

**FIGURE 30-2** The symptoms of Alzheimer's disease are not normal aging.

## Stages and Symptoms of Alzheimer's Disease

Little is certain about Alzheimer's disease. It is believed that changes in the brain may be occurring for several years before symptoms appear. The disease progresses through several stages. At first, the person appears normal to people who do not know him. In the first stage, the person is aware of the changes and realizes that something is wrong, but is helpless to change the situation. Changes in behavior are the only indication that the disease is progressing. All signs and symptoms of the person with Alzheimer's disease are related to the loss of mental abilities. The disease may last from 10 to 25 years.

### Stage 1

This stage lasts between 1 and 3 years. The person loses interest in people or activities. Little attention is paid to grooming and hygiene. Personality changes in the person cause the family to feel that a stranger has entered their home. **Depression** may be present and is marked by inactivity, withdrawal, and minimal interaction with others. Anxiety related to the inability to "figure things out" may cause the person to have angry outbursts. Changes include:

- **Short-term memory loss**
  The person may:
  - Be unable to find his way around his home
  - Get lost while driving a familiar route
  - Forget information as soon as it is given to him
- **Decreased ability to concentrate, attention span shortens**
  - If setting the table, for instance, the person may place a plate on the table and then wander off without completing the task. Directions are not followed because the person is unable to concentrate on the sequence of steps.
- **Disorientation to time and place**
  - **Disorientation** to time is the inability to determine the day, date, month, year, or season. Disorientation to place is the inability to know the building one is in (even one's home), the city, the county, or the state.

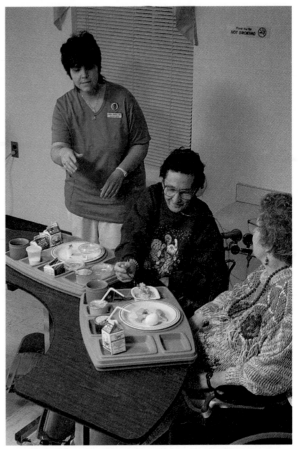

**FIGURE 30-3**  Persons with Alzheimer's disease exhibit poor judgment.

- **Poor judgment**
  - Poor judgment may be reflected in poor money management or inappropriate social behavior (Figure 30-3).
- **Delusions**
  - **Delusions** are fixed, false beliefs.

### Stage 2

Stage 2 lasts from 2 to 10 years. All of the signs and symptoms in stage 1 continue and become more intense. Some individuals may be able to remain at home if enough family members are able to provide care 24 hours a day, 7 days a week. By the end of this stage, most families are unable to give the time, energy, and emotional resources that are required. Safety is a major concern as the person's judgment is reduced further. Additional changes include:

- **Wandering and pacing**
  - **Wandering** is an aimless walking about.
  - **Pacing** is walking the same path over and over and is a result of anxiety.
- **Sundowning**
  - **Sundowning** is a term used when the person has increased disorientation in the late afternoon, evening, or during the night. Sleeplessness is often accompanied by wandering. The person may go outside and wander several miles in the middle of the night.
- **Sensory-perceptual changes**
  - The person with **sensory-perceptual changes** is unable to recognize an object and use it appropriately. This includes common objects such as eating utensils, combs, and pencils (Figure 30-4). The person is unable to distinguish right from left, up from down, left from right, hot from cold.
- **Perseveration**
  - **Perseveration** refers to repeating an action over and over. Examples are repeating the same word or phrase, lip licking, chewing, or finger tapping.
- **Catastrophic reactions**
  - **Catastrophic reactions** are characterized by increased agitation and anxiety. They may be noted by increased pacing, verbalization, and restlessness or they may result in violent behavior (Figure 30-5).
- **Hallucinations**
  - **Hallucinations** are false perceptions of sensory information (seeing, hearing, smelling) that is not real.

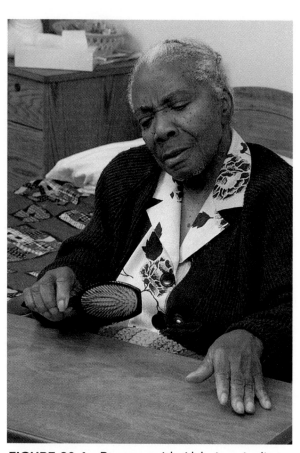

**FIGURE 30-4**  Persons with Alzheimer's disease are unable to recognize and use common items appropriately.

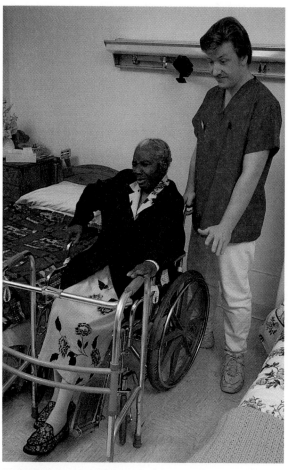

**FIGURE 30-5**  Catastrophic reactions may result in violent behavior.

- **Gait difficulties**
    - Walking becomes more difficult. The hips may appear to be internally rotated and a shuffling type gait is present.
- **Aphasia**
    - Problems with verbal communication occur. The person is unable to understand others and is unable to express speech. The person may have perseveration of speech or use words inappropriately. Aphasia also affects the ability to read and to write.
- Bowel and bladder incontinence

## Stage 3

Stage 3 lasts from 8 to 12 years. Almost all persons with stage 3 Alzheimer's disease will be in a long-term care facility. Characteristics of stage 3 include:

- Total dependence for all activities of daily living
- Verbally unresponsive
- Totally incontinent
- Minimal mobility

## CARING FOR RESIDENTS WITH DEMENTIA

Caring for residents with a dementia is challenging, rewarding, and gratifying. Caregivers must be compassionate, patient, and calm and have a sense of humor.

Providing quality care to residents with Alzheimer's disease revolves around the ability of staff members to manage the behaviors of the residents. When caring for residents with Alzheimer's disease or other dementias it is helpful to remember:

- Residents with Alzheimer's have the same needs as anyone else—physical needs, the need to feel safe and secure, and a need for love and self-esteem. They are dependent on the caregivers to meet these needs (Figure 30-6).
- All behavior has a reason even though we may not always know what the reason is.
- Behavior is neither good nor bad—it just is. Avoid using negative terms such as uncooperative, rebellious, or hostile to describe behavior.

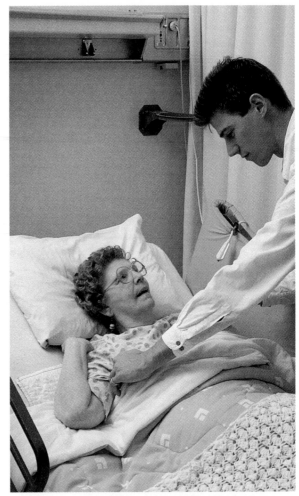

**FIGURE 30-6** People with Alzheimer's disease need love and attention.

- Realize that residents with a dementia are not responsible for what they do or say.
    - Their behavior is not intentional and they cannot change.
    - They are not aware of what they are doing.
    - They lose the ability to control their impulses. They may say or do whatever comes into their minds, whether or not it is appropriate (Figure 30-7).
- Avoid confrontation. Always allow them to "save face" and not feel belittled or embarrassed.
- Residents with Alzheimer's disease can "read" us. They respond to nonverbal communication. Their behaviors tend to reflect the behav-

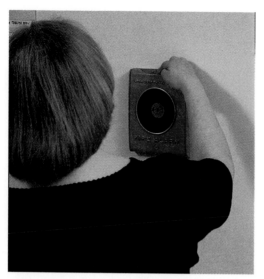

**FIGURE 30-7** People with Alzheimer's disease lose the ability to control their impulses.

iors of those around them. If staff members are anxious and abrupt, residents will tend to become anxious and agitated.

- Even though both short-term and long-term memory are eventually lost, "affective" memory tends to remain. This means that the resident may not remember certain individuals but will sense feelings of discomfort if that person was unpleasant, rude, or abusive to the resident. This may be reflected in increased verbalization or anxiety or attempts to hit that person.
- If a new behavior occurs, investigate the cause. The resident may have a physical illness or be agitated by the environment.
- Reconsider behaviors. Before attempting to modify a behavior, ask the questions:
  - "Is it interfering with the health or safety of the resident?"

---

# *G*uidelines for

# Caring for Residents with Alzheimer's Disease

1. Use eye contact with residents, if culturally appropriate (Figure 30-8).

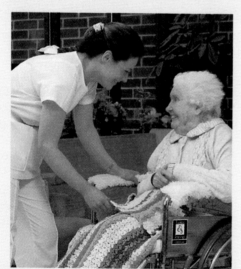

**FIGURE 30-8** Use eye contact, if culturally appropriate.

2. Use appropriate body language.
3. Accept residents as they are without being judgmental or critical.
4. Use touch appropriately. This can be soothing, but if a resident is surprised by the body contact, it can result in a catastrophic reaction.
5. Avoid using logic, "reasoning," or lengthy explanations. This will only increase the resident's agitation.
6. Remember that when the ability to use speech is lost, communication can still occur through nonverbal means.
   - Biting, scratching, and kicking may be the only way the resident can express displeasure.
   - Facial expressions, body language, and the resident's eyes may give clues to feelings and moods (Figure 30-9).
   - Learn what triggers agitation or anger and work on preventing these situations.

*(continues)*

## *G*uidelines *(continued)*

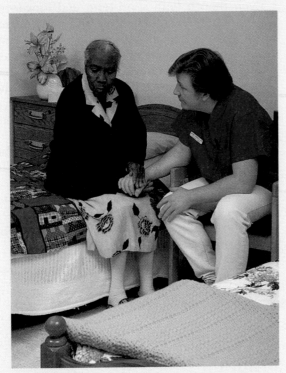

**FIGURE 30-9** Observe facial expressions and body language for clues to the resident's feelings.

7. Use techniques of diversion and distraction. These work well because of the resident's shortened attention span. Calmly take the resident by the hand and walk together or direct the resident's attention to another activity.
8. Remember that the most important qualities for caregivers are to:
   - Be creative. Be willing to look beyond the usual procedures and routines for solutions to giving care.

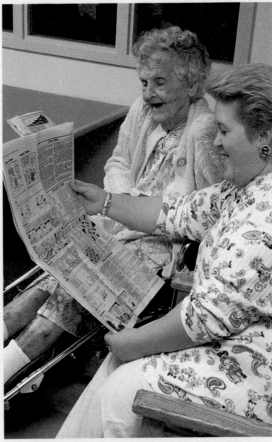

**FIGURE 30-10** A sense of humor is beneficial for staff and residents.

   - Be able to laugh with the resident (Figure 30-10). Many of them retain a keen sense of humor for a long time. Laughter is beneficial for residents and staff.
   - Be able to go back in time with the resident. If the resident is living in 1950, think of what life was like then.

- "Is it interfering with the health or safety of others?"
- "Is it infringing on the rights of other residents?"
- "Is it causing the resident to be anxious or agitated?"

If the answer to these questions is no, then the behavior probably does not need modifying.

- No one really knows what is happening in the minds of people with dementia. Never assume that they are unaware of the environment and the people around them.

## Goals for Caregiving

Always keep in mind the following goals when caring for residents with Alzheimer's disease or other dementias:

1. Protect the resident from physical injury.
2. Maintain the resident's independence as long as possible.
3. Focus on what the resident is still able to do.
4. Provide physical and mental activities within the resident's capabilities.
5. Support the resident's dignity and self-esteem at all times.

To meet these goals:

1. The care must be consistent. Procedures should be carried out in the same way, all the time. All caregivers should use the same approach.
2. The routine of care should be structured but flexible to accommodate residents when they are more responsive or less responsive.
3. The care must be given in a peaceful, quiet environment that is simple, uncluttered, and unchanged.
4. Staff members must be educated to the needs of the residents with dementia and must learn how to meet these needs.

## Residents' Rights

Residents with dementia have the same rights as other residents. They may need assistance to ensure that these rights are protected. It is important to remember that:

- Making decisions and having choices is a resident's right. However, residents with dementia may be unable to make decisions and may become overwhelmed with too many choices. This can cause the resident to become very upset.
- Staff must protect residents with dementia. Do not allow them to be taken advantage of or abused by other people.
- The rights of residents with dementia do not have priority over the rights of other residents. For example, it is upsetting to other residents to have confused residents wandering into their rooms. The resident with dementia is not aware of this. It is the staff's responsibility to resolve these issues without infringing on the rights of either resident.

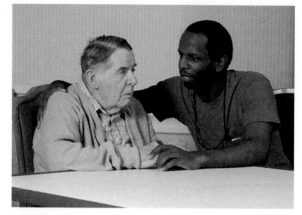

**FIGURE 30-11** Always treat the resident with dignity.

- Residents with dementia have the right to have possessions that give them pleasure as long as these do not impair the health or safety of the resident or other people. For example, if a resident receives pleasure from a doll or stuffed animal, do not take it away. Above all, do not tease or make fun of the situation. The resident deserves to be treated with dignity (Figure 30-11).

## Family Members

In most cases, family members have cared for the resident with a dementia for months or years prior to admission to the long-term care facility. By the time the decision is made to admit the individual, the family is often physically and emotionally drained. The admission is a traumatic experience. As you work with the residents with Alzheimer's or other dementias, remember:

1. The family remembers the resident as a vital family member. Acknowledge the family's presence.
2. The spouse of the resident may have no other support system. If they have children, they may be many miles away. It can be very upsetting to not be recognized by a spouse of many years. Some facilities have support groups for families.
3. Listen to the family's suggestions. They often know what will work and what will not be effective in caring for the new resident.
4. Allow the family to participate in the care, if they choose to and if it is appropriate. For example, many family members like to assist the resident at mealtime.

# Guidelines for

# Activities of Daily Living

1. Allow the resident to do as much as possible.
   - Use hand-over-hand techniques for personal care and eating.
   - Give only one short, simple direction at a time.

2. Assist the resident to maintain a dignified, attractive appearance by helping with grooming, dressing, and hygiene. Residents may be unaware of soiled or torn clothing.
   - Help them change when necessary.
   - Pick out clothing for the resident or hold out two outfits for the resident to choose from. Residents with a dementia are unable to make decisions. If you ask the resident, "What do you want to wear today?" the resident may become agitated. She cannot remember what is in her closet. Showing the resident all of the clothing is overwhelming and will also cause agitation.

3. Residents with dementia may not want to bathe.
   - Consider the resident's previous habits. Did the resident prefer a tub bath or shower? How often did the resident bathe? Was bathing done in the morning or evening?
   - Check the environment. Is the room warm enough? Is it light enough? Is there adequate privacy?
   - Do not ask the resident "Do you want to take a bath now?" The resident may say no every time you ask. Calmly walk with the resident to the bathroom. When you get there say, "I am going to help you with your bath now" and begin the bath procedure calmly and slowly. If the resident refuses, try again later.
   - Do not attempt to remove the resident's clothes right away. Many residents feel unsafe when they are nude. When the resident realizes he is going to get wet, he will usually be willing to undress.

4. Monitor food and fluid intake.
   - Too many foods at once are confusing.
   - Place one food at a time in front of the resident.
   - Do not use plastic utensils that can break in the resident's mouth.
   - Provide nutritious finger foods when the resident is unable to use utensils.
   - Avoid pureed foods as long as possible.
   - Check food temperatures before serving.
   - Prepare foods for eating by buttering the bread, cutting meat, opening cartons.
   - If you are feeding the resident, watch for swallowing. Sometimes they will appear to be chewing long after they have swallowed (perseveration).
   - Check the resident's mouth after eating. Squirreling food in the mouth can cause **aspiration** (the food goes into the trachea or windpipe).
   - Maintain adequate fluid intake. Residents with dementia may not realize when they are thirsty.
   - Weigh the resident regularly to detect patterns of weight gain or loss.
   - Maintain a quiet and calm environment for eating.

5. Residents with dementia eventually lose bowel and bladder control. Taking residents to the bathroom every 2 hours keeps them dry and prevents skin breakdown. For successful toileting:
   - Toilet regularly.
   - Evaluate wandering and pacing behavior for possible need to toilet.
   - Provide privacy.
   - Make sure the bathroom is warm, quiet, and calm.
   - Allow the resident ample time to eliminate urine or stool.
   - Provide comfort. A commode may work better than the toilet.
   - Praise success.

## Recreational Activities

Residents with dementia need activities that match their level of ability.

- Avoid large groups or competitive activities.
- In later stages, use sensory stimulation with soft touching, quiet talk, familiar odors, or old time pictures.
- Puppies or kittens (**pet therapy**) bring pleasure to severely impaired residents.
- Activities with children may also be satisfying to the residents with dementia.
- Music is an appropriate activity. Residents with dementia respond to soft music from their past. Many of them like to dance. Old hymns are also a favorite.
- "Normalizing" activities are beneficial. Consider the resident's past and provide opportunities for:
  - Folding towels and washcloths
  - Dusting
  - A hand craft such as knitting (Figure 30-12)

- Baking (with supervision)
- Using a manual carpet sweeper
- "Tinkering" with familiar tools (with supervision)

Daily exercise needs to be planned according to the resident's habits and abilities (Figure 30-13).

- The resident who wanders or paces throughout the day may need only range of motion exercises.
- Residents in the final stage will need passive range of motion exercises at least twice a day.
- Many recreational activities can be directed to the abilities of the resident:
  - Shooting baskets
  - Bowling
  - Volleyball
  - Hitting a ball with a bat

Community outings may also be enjoyable. Plan outings carefully and be sure that:

- There will be no excessive sensory stimulation. This will agitate many of the residents.
- The residents will not be fearful of wide, open spaces.
- Public places can accommodate residents with mobility problems.
- The residents will not be mistreated by others if they exhibit unusual behaviors in public.

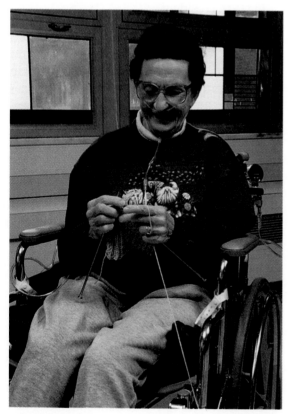

**FIGURE 30-12** Familiar tasks bring enjoyment.

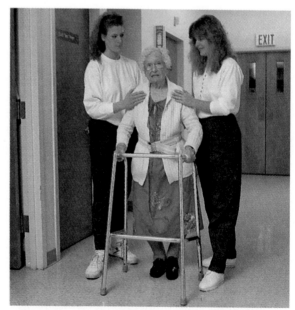

**FIGURE 30-13** Daily exercise is important.

## SPECIAL PROBLEMS ·····················

### Wandering and Pacing

Residents with Alzheimer's disease may wander or pace for hours at a time. No one knows why this occurs. Some reasons may be:

- They are looking for companionship, security, or loved ones.
- It is a way to handle stress.
- They realize they are in a strange environment and are looking for home.

When this behavior occurs:

1. Allow them to wander. The use of restraints increases their anxiety and frustration, resulting in other problems.
2. Adapt the environment to the residents, making it safe and secure. There are many types of security systems available. Getting lost, rather than falling, may be a problem. When the resident walks off, walk with the resident, gradually returning to the direction of the facility.
3. Watch wandering residents for signs of fatigue. They may have forgotten how to sit down and will need reminders and demonstrations of how to get into the chair or bed.
4. Special chairs for residents with Alzheimer's disease allow the residents to rock without tipping over. A tray table top keeps residents secure and can be used for hand activities.
5. Nutritional needs increase with wandering. Additional food intake may be necessary.

### Agitation, Anxiety, and Catastrophic Reactions

Agitation and anxiety are shown by an increase in physical activity such as pacing or perseveration. If appropriate actions are not taken in time, a catastrophic reaction is likely to occur. This is noted by any or all of the following:

- Increased physical activity
- Increased talking or mumbling
- Explosive behavior with physical violence

Not all catastrophic reactions are dramatic or violent. However, if not dealt with appropriately, the reaction may grow. To avoid catastrophic reactions:

1. Monitor behavior closely.
2. Watch for signs of increasing agitation.

3. Check to see if the resident:
   - Is hungry
   - Needs to go to the bathroom
   - Is too hot or too cold
   - Is overtired or in pain
   - Has signs of physical illness
4. Check the environment for:
   - Too much noise
   - Too many people
   - Staff anxiety
   - Television programs—people with dementia cannot distinguish fiction from reality.
5. People with dementia may not be able to make decisions. The simple question, "What do you want to wear today?" may be more than they can handle.

When agitation or catastrophic reactions occur:

1. Do not use physical restraints or force to subdue the resident. This increases agitation and can result in injury to the resident and caregivers.
2. Avoid having several staff members approach the resident at the same time. This is frightening to the resident.
3. Use a soft, calm voice. Do not try to reason with the resident. Using touch may or may not be appropriate. Some residents respond in a positive manner to the smooth stroking of the arm or back. Others may react violently if they are already agitated.

### Sundowning

Sundowning means the resident has increased confusion and restlessness in the late afternoon, evening, or during the night. It may be prevented by avoiding too much activity before bedtime and by establishing a consistent bedtime routine.

1. Overfatigue may cause sundowning. Encourage the resident to nap or rest in the early afternoon for a short time.
2. Discourage the resident from sleeping too much during the day.
3. The evening meal should be eaten at least 2 hours before bedtime. Eliminate caffeine from the diet.
4. Involve the resident in quiet evening activities with a caregiver or family member.

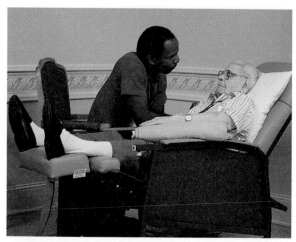

**FIGURE 30-14** A recliner may be useful for a resident with sundowning.

5. At bedtime, provide a light snack that is easily chewed and digested.
6. Take the resident to the bathroom just before bedtime. Allow enough time for bladder and bowel elimination.
7. Give a slow back massage if resident accepts touch.
8. Check with family members and continue established habits such as wearing socks to bed, using two pillows, or having a night light.
9. Check the lighting of the room. Shadows and reflections may be disturbing.
10. If the resident wakes up during the night, repeat the bedtime routine. If this is ineffective and the resident does not remain in bed, try a recliner or Alzheimer's chair (Figure 30-14). The resident may like to sit by the nurses' station.

### Delusions and Hallucinations

Delusions are fixed, false beliefs. Never argue with a resident about a delusion. This will increase the agitation and probably cause a catastrophic reaction. If the delusion is not bothering the resident, let it be. For example: a resident tells you, "I have to take care of my babies now," and is not agitated. She may be reliving a happier, more satisfying time in her life. If the delusion is causing the resident to be anxious, then you must try to assure the resident that you will keep the resident safe.

Follow the same approach with hallucinations.

### Pillaging and Hoarding

This does not present a major problem unless residents collect items from other residents' rooms (pillaging) or they hide things that are difficult to find (hoarding).

1. Label all residents' belongings.
2. If a missing item is located, note where it was found. It is likely that the resident will choose the same hiding place the next time.
3. Check the room daily for food.
4. Keep the resident's hands busy. Activities like folding washcloths or "fiddling" with keys on a ring may help.
5. Provide a "rummaging" drawer or box for the resident.

## SPECIAL MANAGEMENT TECHNIQUES

### Reality Orientation

**Reality orientation** (RO) is used for helping disoriented residents remain oriented to the environment, to time, and to themselves. When used appropriately, it decreases anxiety in the resident. RO may be effective in the first stages of dementia. In later stages, it is meaningless and increases agitation. Follow these basic guidelines for RO:

1. Always treat residents as adults, with respect and dignity, no matter how confused they may be.
2. Speak clearly and directly. Avoid the temptation to speak louder when they do not understand.
3. Give simple, brief instructions and responses.
4. Set and maintain a structured, flexible routine.
5. Be polite and sincere.
6. Allow residents to be independent as long as possible.
7. Give residents adequate time to respond.
8. Set residents' watches to the correct time.
9. Make sure they have clean eyeglasses and hearing aids if they need them.
10. Place large-numbered calendars in rooms and cross off the days as they pass.
11. Placement of large-numbered clocks around the facility helps orient residents to the time of day.

12. Call residents by name. Disoriented residents usually respond more quickly to their first names.
13. Tell residents your name, but do not expect them to remember you.
14. Use RO in conversation with residents—"It's only March fifth today, but it is very warm outside."

When using RO:

1. Do not put residents on the spot. For example, do not ask, "Do you remember who I am?" or "Do you know what day this is?" If you need to verify their orientation, ask them, "What are your plans for today?" The answer usually will tell you if the resident is oriented.
2. Answer questions honestly but avoid giving the residents information they are unable to handle. A resident whose husband is deceased may ask, "Is my husband coming today?" It is cruel to answer by saying, "Remember, your husband died 2 years ago." This response is likely to trigger a catastrophic reaction. It is better to answer by asking another question: "Emma, will you tell me about your husband?" She will receive pleasure from reminiscing and may work up to the present time on her own.
3. Never argue with a resident's reality. When a resident has a delusion, arguing increases anxiety and agitation. Many delusions are based on past life experiences. Because the resident is disoriented, the experience seems to be happening in the present. Some residents may be much happier if they are living in the past. If this is true, do not force reality on them.
4. Residents with some forms of dementia may have moments of orientation from time to time. Do not assume the resident is disoriented because you do not understand what the resident is saying.
5. Do not reinforce the resident's confusion or tease the resident about the confusion.
6. Remember that a pleasant facial expression, relaxed body language, and caring touch are the most important aspects of caring for disoriented residents.

## Reminiscing

**Reminiscing** is a natural activity for people of all ages. We tend to reminisce when we see old friends or get together with families.

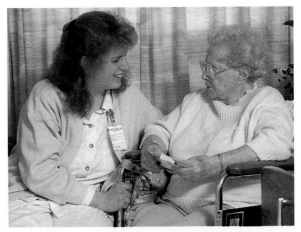

**FIGURE 30-15** Reminiscing can help recall happy times.

1. Pleasant times from the past are remembered and enjoyed.
2. As people age, the tendency to reminisce increases and is more important.
3. It is an appropriate activity for residents in early stages of dementia if long-term memory is still intact.
4. Reminiscing may serve as a life review as past life experiences are remembered. This process can also bring back unpleasant memories. If this occurs, the situation must be handled skillfully and tactfully. If these experiences are resolved, peace of mind can be found. The recall of happy memories can confirm the worth and value of the individual's life (Figure 30-15).
5. Reminiscing can help people adapt to old age. It helps to maintain self-esteem and allows them to work through personal losses.
6. When we listen to residents reminisce we understand them better.
7. Reminiscing therapy can be a group activity. The leader must be skillful and sensitive to the feelings of the members.

## Validation Therapy

**Validation therapy** was developed by Naomi Feil. It is based on the following assumptions:

1. The identity and dignity of the residents must be maintained.
2. We can help disoriented people with dementia feel good about themselves.

3. There is a reason for all behavior. What seems like disoriented behavior may be an acting out of memories.

4. Feelings and memories can be acknowledged.

5. Disoriented people have the right to express feelings when they are no longer able to be oriented to reality.

6. Living must be resolved to prepare for dying.

7. Elderly persons may have experienced so many losses during a lifetime that they have no coping abilities left.

8. To live in reality is not the only way to live.

9. Disoriented people have worth. We can give them joy by allowing them to express themselves.

10. Within each disoriented person is a human being who was once a child and later an adult with hopes, joys, sadness, failures, and successes. They deserve to be cared for and loved in their final years.

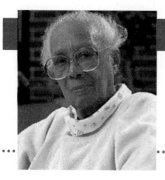

## LESSON SYNTHESIS: Putting It All Together

*Y*ou have just completed this lesson. Now go back and review the Clinical Focus. Try to see how the Clinical Focus relates to the concepts presented in the lesson. Then answer the following questions.

1. Why do people think of Alzheimer's disease as a "slow death"?

2. Why do the families of residents with Alzheimer's disease need special understanding and support?

3. Because Mrs. McGinnis is in stage 2, what special safety precautions must be observed?

4. What special characteristics are needed in a nursing assistant who cares for residents suffering from Alzheimer's disease?

## REVIEW

**A. Select the one best answer for each of the following.**

1. Alzheimer's disease is
   a. curable
   b. preventable
   c. progressive
   d. congenital

2. Alzheimer's disease is more common in
   a. young people
   b. older people
   c. middle-aged people
   d. the white race

3. One of the first symptoms of Alzheimer's disease is
   a. short-term memory loss
   b. long-term memory loss
   c. aphasia
   d. sundowning

4. Delusions are
   a. false perceptions of sensory information
   b. an example of sensory-perceptual changes
   c. false, fixed ideas
   d. the result of catastrophic reactions

5. Goals for giving care to residents with Alzheimer's include
   a. protecting the resident from physical injury
   b. maintaining the resident's independence as long as possible
   c. focusing on what the resident can do
   d. all of these

## B. Answer each statement true (T) or false (F).

6. T  F  There are many types of dementia.

7. T  F  There is no specific test for diagnosing Alzheimer's disease.

8. T  F  Alzheimer's disease is the result of poor circulation in the brain.

9. T  F  Residents who wander should be restrained.

10. T  F  Catastrophic reactions may result from too much stimulation in the environment.

11. T  F  Residents with Alzheimer's disease are unable to feel emotion.

12. T  F  Residents with Alzheimer's disease frequently exhibit bad behavior.

13. T  F  The best way to manage behavior is to use logic to reason with the resident.

14. T  F  Many residents with Alzheimer's disease have a keen sense of humor.

15. T  F  Reminiscing is healthy and beneficial.

16. T  F  Residents' rights do not apply to residents with Alzheimer's disease.

17. T  F  A dignified, attractive appearance is important for residents with Alzheimer's disease.

18. T  F  Residents with Alzheimer's disease enjoy large group activities.

19. T  F  Baking is an example of a "normalizing" activity.

20. T  F  Some residents are happier if they are living in the past.

# Caring for Residents with Developmental Disabilities

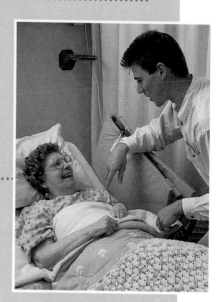

## CLINICAL FOCUS

Think about the special care needs of the resident who is developmentally disabled as you study this lesson and meet:

*T*eresa Michaels, who is developmentally disabled and unable to care for herself. Her mind is bright and keen. She is unable to use her hands for self-care because of the spastic paralysis related to her cerebral palsy.

## OBJECTIVES

*After studying this lesson, you should be able to:*

- Define and spell vocabulary words and terms.
- List the characteristics present in a developmental disability.
- List four examples of developmental disabilities.
- Describe three possible causes of a developmental disability.
- Define the three classifications of mental retardation.
- Describe different types of seizures.

## VOCABULARY

**adaptive behavior**  *(ah-**DAP**-tiv bee-**HAYV**-yur)*

**anoxia**  *(ah-**NOX**-ee-ah)*

**ataxic cerebral palsy**  *(ah-**TACK**-sick **SER**-eh-bral **PAWL**-zee)*

**athetoid cerebral palsy**  *(**ATH**-eh-toyd **SER**-eh-bral **PAWL**-zee)*

**behavior modification**  *(bee-**HAYV**-yur **mod**-ih-fih-**KAY**-shun)*

**cerebral palsy**  *(**SER**-eh-bral **PAWL**-zee)*

**developmental disability**  *(dee-**vel**-op-**MEN**-tal dis-ah-**BILL**-ih-tee)*

**diplegia**  *(die-**PLEE**-jee-ah)*

**electroencephalogram (EEG)**  *(ee-**leck**-troh-en-**SEF**-ah-loh-gram)*

**epilepsy**  *(**EP**-ih-**lep**-see)*

**grand mal seizure**  *(grand mahl **SEE**-zhur)*

**hemiplegia**  *(**hem**-ee-**PLEE**-jee-ah)*

# VOCABULARY

• • • • • • • • • • • • • • • • • • • • • • •

**intelligence quotient (IQ)** *(in-TELL-ih-jens KWOH-shent)*

**mental retardation** *(MEN-tal ree-tar-DAY-shun)*

**petit mal seizure** *(peh-TEE mahl SEE-zhur)*

**quadriplegia** *(kwahd-rih-PLEE-jee-ah)*

**seizure** *(SEE-zhur)*

**spastic cerebral palsy** *(SPAS-tick SER-eh-bral PAWL-zee)*

## CHARACTERISTICS OF A DEVELOPMENTAL DISABILITY • • • • • • • • • •

Long-term care facilities often provide care for residents with developmental disabilities. A **developmental disability** has specific characteristics. It is:

• Caused by a mental or physical impairment or a combination of both
• Apparent before 22 years of age (some states indicate before 18 years of age)
• Likely to continue indefinitely

In addition, the disability must result in functional limitations in three or more of these life activities:

• Self-care
• Use of receptive and expressive language
• Learning
• Mobility
• Self-direction
• Independent living
• Economic self-sufficiency

Because of these limitations, the person who is developmentally disabled requires lifelong care, treatment, or services (Figure 31-1).

Some residents in your facility who have developmental disabilities did not acquire these as adults. Federal legislation forbids the admission of persons with developmental disabilities to skilled nursing facilities unless the facilities are licensed to care for them. However, there may be residents who were in the facility before this law was implemented. They may also be admitted if they have another medical problem that requires skilled nursing care.

A developmental disability may be caused by:

• A condition that impairs the development of the brain or body before birth (Figure 31-2)

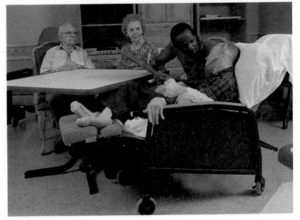

**FIGURE 31-1** The resident on the right has needed assistance with activities of daily living throughout his life.

• A condition that causes damage to the newborn infant during the birth process
• A disease or injury that causes damage to the brain or body after birth, before the age of 22 years, or the age specified by state regulations

At one time, people with developmental disabilities often died before reaching adulthood. Today they frequently live a normal life span. During childhood they go to school and attend classes that meet their needs and abilities. After graduating, they may work in a sheltered workshop or obtain a job that they are capable of doing. They may be able to live independently with assistance or in supervised group homes. Some people with milder disabilities may marry and have children.

People with developmental disabilities also experience the aging process. Sometimes the changes of aging combined with the disability make it increasingly difficult for them to function.

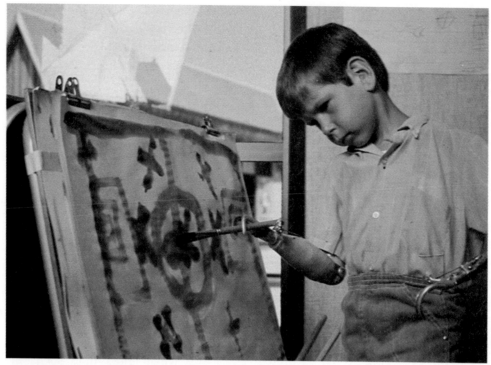

**FIGURE 31-2**   This child with phocomelia has no hands because a drug taken by his mother during early pregnancy interfered with limb development. (Courtesy of the March of Dimes Birth Defects Foundation)

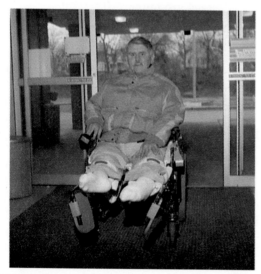

**FIGURE 31-3**   This man is developmentally disabled but is not mentally impaired.

Of the many types of developmental disabilities, some affect physical function, some affect mental function, and some affect both. Persons with mental retardation are developmentally disabled. However, not all persons who are developmentally disabled are mentally retarded (Figure 31-3).

## MENTAL RETARDATION

Children and adults with mental retardation are limited in their ability to learn. They are generally socially immature and sometimes have special emotional and physical needs. **Mental retardation** is a condition that occurs before age 22 and refers to significantly below average mental function. In addition, deficits in adaptive behavior exist. **Adaptive behavior** is the degree to which the person meets standards of personal independence and social responsibility appropriate for the person's age and culture. These standards apply to:

* Physical self-care
* Communication skills
* Social skills
* Economic abilities
* Holding a job
* Capability for self-direction

## Causes of Mental Retardation

Some disorders in which mental retardation may be present are:

- Down syndrome (a chromosomal disorder)
- Cerebral palsy (not all people with cerebral palsy are mentally retarded)
- Phenylketonuria (PKU)—a metabolic disorder present at birth

Mental retardation may also be caused by:

- Environmental influences such as poor nutrition
- Lack of oxygen (**anoxia**) before, during, or after birth
- Complications of diseases during childhood such as encephalitis or meningitis
- Premature birth (lack of developmental maturity)

## Testing for Level of Impairment

People with mental retardation do not all have the same degree of disability. Screening tests may be performed during infancy if a delay in development is noted. Later, **intelligence quotient (IQ)** tests can be given. Intelligence includes the:

- Ability to solve problems appropriate to one's age
- Ability to adapt appropriately to the demands of environment
- Ability to understand abstract relationships

The results of the IQ test alone do not confirm the absence or presence of mental retardation. Intelligence is not constant. It is variable and influenced by emotions and the environment. IQ tests are considered along with other test results.

An Adaptive Behavior Scale measures a person's behaviors as they relate to activities of daily living, self-help skills, physical and social development, language ability, and time and number concepts. The scale also examines inappropriate behaviors such as violence and self-abuse. The results are compared to the expected behavior of people of the same chronological age.

Diagnosis and evaluation should be conducted by an interdisciplinary team of specialists in the field. The IQ level used for classification varies somewhat with the test being used.

Usually, mental retardation is classified on the following basis:

- Mild retardation
  - IQ is 52 to 67.
  - Development is slow.
  - Children are educable within limits.
  - Adults with training can achieve social and vocational skills adequate for minimum self-support.
  - Adults may need guidance and assistance when under unusual social or economic stress.
  - Most persons with mental retardation are in this category.
- Moderate retardation
  - IQ is 36 to 51.
  - Development is slow.
  - Persons can be taught to complete activities of daily living.
  - Adults need to work and live in sheltered environment.
  - Supervision and guidance are needed when under mild social or economic stress.
- Severe retardation
  - IQ is 20 to 35.
  - Motor development, speech, and language are impaired.
  - The person is often, but not always, physically challenged.
  - Adults may contribute partially to self-maintenance under complete supervision.
  - Adults can develop self-protection skills to a minimal useful level in controlled environment.
- Profound retardation
  - IQ is less than 20.
  - Constant care and supervision are necessary for survival.

Many services are available to meet the needs of persons with mental retardation. Children can benefit from special education and training. A program that is started early and is consistent is most effective in meeting their special needs and helping them to enjoy a good quality of life. Remember that individuals with mental retardation have all the needs of another person of the same chronological age. They need affection, discipline, and acceptance just as all humans do. They are less able, however, to handle rejection or confusion or the demands of too high expectations.

Families, too, need support and empathy because they may be dealing with personal feelings of guilt and frustration.

If people with mental retardation are living in your facility, the care you give depends on the:

- Specific problems of the individual
- Age of the individual
- Degree of retardation
- Presence of other physical problems

Even the most profoundly retarded person responds favorably to:

- Pleasant, colorful, personalized surroundings
- The healing and comforting effect of caring persons

# OTHER FORMS OF DEVELOPMENTAL DISABILITIES ·······

## Cerebral Palsy

**Cerebral palsy** describes a large group of movement disorders of varying symptoms and severity. *Cerebral* refers to the brain and *palsy* means disorder of movement. Figure 31-4 lists several causes of cerebral palsy. These include damage to the baby before, during, or after birth that result in damage to the nervous system.

A person with mild cerebral palsy may be only a little awkward with movements but otherwise mentally and physically capable. A person with more severe cerebral palsy may be mentally retarded, subject to seizures, or physically challenged. Several terms describe the movement disturbance and effect on the limbs, as follows:

| **FIGURE 31-4** Causes of cerebral palsy |
|---|
| • Cerebral anoxia |
| • Hemorrhage |
| • Maternal infection |
| • Cord around infant's neck |
| • Meningitis |
| • Difficult delivery |

- **Diplegia**
  - The legs are primarily affected.
- **Hemiplegia**
  - Both the arm and leg on one side are affected.
- **Quadriplegia**
  - Both arms and both legs are affected.
- **Spastic cerebral palsy**
  - The muscles are tense, contracted, resistant to movement.
  - The lower legs may turn in and cross at the ankle.
  - The movements of the legs are stiff and resemble the crossed blades of a pair of scissors (scissors gait).
- **Athetoid cerebral palsy**
  - Involuntary, slow, and incessant movements (athetosis) of the parts of the body that are affected.
  - Facial grimacing and drooling may be present.
- **Ataxic cerebral palsy**
  - The principal movement disturbance is a lack of balance and coordination (ataxia).

In some cases, symptoms of each type of palsy may be mixed. Persons with cerebral palsy may also have problems in speaking, chewing, and swallowing. They may be unable to focus their eyes. Drooling and loss of bowel or bladder control also occur.

**Caring for the Resident with Cerebral Palsy.** Care may include:

- Assisting with transport to special education classes
- Caring for and applying splints and braces
- Performing range of motion exercises
- Providing emotional support
- Assisting with activities of daily living

Other problems associated with cerebral palsy are seizure disorders, mental or emotional impairment, hearing loss, and visual handicaps.

## Seizure Disorder (Epilepsy)

**Epilepsy** may be considered a developmental disability if it meets the criteria described at the beginning of this lesson. It is not a disease with a single cause. It is a set of symptoms that arise from abnormal nerve cell activity in the brain. Normally, the nerve cells (neurons) generate small bursts of electrical impulses. These impulses

**FIGURE 31-5**  Some causes of seizures

- Neoplasms
- Trauma
- Cerebral anoxia
- Metabolic imbalances
- Congenital malformations
- High temperature

move between neurons, communicating with muscles, sense organs, and glands. In epilepsy, the nerve cell activity is disturbed. This may result in a **seizure** (convulsion). The type of seizure that occurs depends on the part of the brain that is affected by the disrupted nerve cell activity. Some causes of seizures are listed in Figure 31-5.

Partial or generalized seizures may occur. Partial seizures are classified as follows. For each type, the general symptoms are listed:

1. Simple partial (sensory type) seizure
   - Feelings are distorted
   - Seeing flashing lights, hallucinations
   - Smelling foul odors
   - Dizziness
   - Tingling sensations
2. Simple partial (jacksonian motor type) seizure
   - Localized motor seizure
   - Tingling, jerking in one extremity
   - No loss of consciousness
   - May progress to generalized tonic-clonic convulsions
3. Complex partial (psychomotor or temporal lobe) seizure
   - Signs and symptoms vary
   - Purposeless behavior such as chewing movements and uncontrolled speech
   - Glassy stare
   - Aimless wandering
   - Mental confusion
   - Loss of memory following episode
4. Secondary generalized partial seizure
   - Either simple or complex
   - May experience an aura
   - Immediate loss of consciousness

Generalized seizures are classified as follows, with general symptoms listed:

1. Generalized tonic-clonic seizure (**grand mal seizure**) (Figure 31-6)
   - Early changes in sensation (aura)
   - Entire body involved
   - Sudden cry
   - Loss of consciousness
   - Involuntary contraction of the muscles producing contortions of body and limbs
   - Saliva forms around the mouth causing the appearance of "foaming at the mouth"
   - Incontinence of bowel or bladder or both may occur during the seizure
   - Person generally sleeps after the seizure
   - Lasts 2 to 5 minutes
2. Absence seizure (**petit mal seizure**)
   - No convulsion
   - Occurs most often in children without warning
   - Lasts 1 to 10 seconds
   - Vacant facial expression, staring eyes
   - No recall of episode
3. Myoclonic seizure
   - Brief involuntary jerking movements of body and extremities
   - Convulsions may occur in rhythmic waves.
   - No loss of consciousness
4. Akinetic Seizure
   - Uncommon
   - General loss of postural tone may cause resident to "drop" to the floor.
   - Temporary loss of consciousness
   - Lasts 1 to 2 minutes

When seizure activity occurs so frequently that consciousness is not gained between seizures, it is called status epilepticus.

In some people, epilepsy begins during adulthood. This may be the result of:

- An accident causing brain injury
- Brain tumor
- Stroke
- Dementia

The diagnosis of epilepsy is made by performing an **electroencephalogram (EEG)**. A computed tomography (CT) scan or magnetic resonance imaging (MRI) is also performed during the EEG. Electrodes are attached to the scalp to record the brain's electrical activity. The test can determine the presence and type of

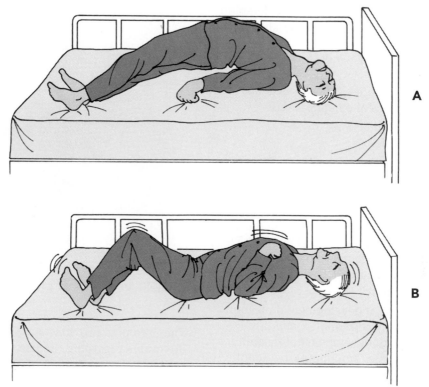

**FIGURE 31-6** Generalized seizures. These may be accompanied by A. rigid posturing or B. uncontrolled movements.

seizures. The test is painless. The CT scan and MRI permit visualization of the brain structures.

Many medications are able to control seizures. Sometimes the medication dosage needs to be readjusted.

Care of the resident who is experiencing a seizure is covered in Lesson 9.

## CARING FOR RESIDENTS WITH DEVELOPMENTAL DISABILITIES

Residents with developmental disabilities may be placed in a long-term care facility for the following reasons:

- The resident may have lived in a facility most of his or her life because family members were not able to provide care.
- The resident may have been admitted as an adult to the facility when the parent(s) became elderly or died (before federal laws were changed).

- The resident may have a medical problem that cannot be treated in the resident's home.

Young adult residents are often admitted for medical problems. Their parents may have devoted all their energies to the lifelong care of their child. It is difficult in these situations for the parents to "turn over" the care of the resident to staff members. It is important to:

- Acknowledge that the parents have learned much about how to care for their child in the years they have provided care.
- Listen to the parents' suggestions and their concerns.
- Answer their questions.
- Allow the parents to participate in the care as much as possible and as much as they wish.

In some cases, the resident may be admitted after one parent has died and the other is no longer able to provide total care. In these situations, the remaining parent may be suffering from guilt for placing the child in the facility. Feelings of anger at the deceased spouse may exist for "leaving" them with this problem. Attempt to understand what the parent is going through. Be kind, considerate, and nonjudgmental.

The care you give depends on the types of problems experienced by the residents with developmental disabilities. These residents are at risk for many physical complications:

- Respiratory tract infections
- Urinary tract infections
- Contractures
- Pressure ulcers

You must study the care plan to learn exactly what approach and procedures you must use.

Physical therapy and occupational therapy may be a part of the plan of care (Figure 31-7).

You may have residents who go out of the facility every day to attend a sheltered workshop. These workshops:

- Train persons with a developmental disability to acquire job skills within their abilities
- Train persons with developmental disabilities to get around in the community by adapting their abilities to the situation
- Provide opportunities for socializing with other people of the same age

Behavior problems may occur. **Behavior modification** is an approach to overcoming these problems that is based on:

- Rewarding positive behaviors
- Initiating corrective actions for negative behaviors

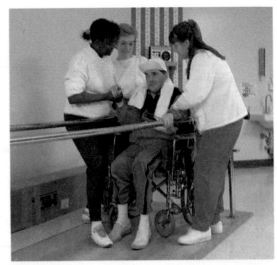

**FIGURE 31-7** Residents with developmental disabilities may need physical therapy.

The care plan provides specific approaches and directions regarding the use of behavior modification. Behavior modification will succeed only if all staff members are consistent and follow the plan exactly as it is written.

Persons with developmental disabilities have the same physical and emotional needs as everyone else. When they are in the long-term care facility, it is the responsibility of the staff to provide for these needs so that persons with developmental disabilities will enjoy a life of quality.

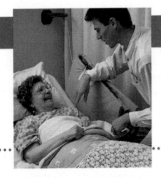

## LESSON SYNTHESIS: Putting It All Together

*Y*ou have just completed this lesson. Now go back and review the Clinical Focus. Try to see how the Clinical Focus relates to the concepts presented in the lesson. Then answer the following questions.

1. How do you think Teresa's disability affects the way people view her until they get to talk with her and know her?

2. Do all people with cerebral palsy have a low IQ?

3. What parts of Teresa's body are affected by her condition?

4. How are Teresa's special needs being met?

## REVIEW

**A. Fill in the blanks by selecting the correct word or phrase from the list.**

cerebral palsy
developmental
  disability
diplegia

hemiplegia
mental
  retardation
twenty-two

1. A severe, chronic disorder present before the age of _____ best describes a _____.

2. When a person has a significantly below average mental function with deficits in adaptive behavior, he is said to have _____.

3. A person with mild _____ may be only a little awkward with movements but otherwise be mentally and physically capable.

4. _____ describes the fact that the legs of a person with cerebral palsy are affected.

5. A person with cerebral palsy whose arm and leg on one side are affected has _____.

**B. Provide brief answers for each of the following.**

6. List three characteristics a disorder must have to be classified as a developmental disability.

7. List seven functional limitations, three of which must be present in addition to those characteristics listed in question 6.

8. Name three possible causes of developmental disabilities.

9. Name four examples of developmental disabilities.

10. List the IQ values for each level of mental retardation: mild, moderate, severe, profound.

11. Describe five activities that may occur during a grand mal seizure.

**C. Select the one best answer for each of the following.**

12. Children and adults with mental retardation are
    a. socially mature
    b. emotionally secure
    c. persons over 25 years of age when the disability developed
    d. limited in their ability to learn

13. Mental retardation may be associated with
    a. Down syndrome
    b. phenylketonuria
    c. premature birth
    d. all of these

14. A person with mild mental retardation
    a. has an IQ of 52 to 67
    b. requires constant care and attention
    c. is always physically challenged
    d. is not able to be educated

15. During a generalized tonic-clonic seizure the resident
    a. loses consciousness
    b. remains conscious
    c. may wander aimlessly
    d. remembers the event clearly

**D. Clinical Experience**

16. Rachel is 37, has spastic paralysis, and an IQ of 20. She has been a resident in your facility since her mother died. Her father visits infrequently and seems very upset when he sees her. What can you do to help reduce his stress?

17. Lea is a teenage girl who is acting out her frustration with the staff who are following the care plan. The team decides that a behavior modification approach is the way to handle the situation. On what principles is this approach based?

18. Brett is 14 and recently admitted to your facility. His mother, his primary care giver, died and his father is unable to provide care. Brett was injured when hit by a car 11 years ago. What can you do to ease the anxiety expressed by Brett's father?

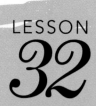
# 32

# Caring for the Dying Resident

## CLINICAL FOCUS

Think about the very special sensitivity the nursing assistant needs as he or she assists residents and their families during the period when death is drawing near as you study this lesson and meet:

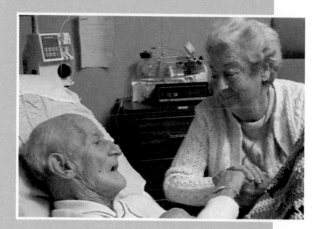

*E*rnie Sperling and his family. Mr. Sperling, a Roman Catholic, suffers from terminal cancer. His malignancy originated in his prostate gland and quickly spread throughout his pelvis and into his vertebral column. Despite surgery, radiation, and a course of chemotherapy, the progress of the disease could not be stopped. Mrs. Sperling had been separated from her husband for several years, but since his illness has visited him regularly. Mr. Sperling is often angry and uncooperative with the staff and his wife.

## OBJECTIVES

*After studying this lesson, you should be able to:*

- Define and spell vocabulary words and terms.
- Define a terminal diagnosis.
- Identify the stages of grieving as described by Elisabeth Kübler-Ross.
- Describe how different people handle the death/dying process.

- Respect the resident's cultural and religious practices during the dying process.
- Recognize at least five signs of approaching death.
- Demonstrate the following:
  Procedure 117 Giving Postmortem Care

## VOCABULARY

**acceptance**  *(ack-SEP-tans)*
**anger**  *(AYN-ger)*

**bargaining**  *(BAR-gan-ing)*
**code blue order**  *(kohd bloo OR-der)*

# VOCABULARY

comatose *(KOH-mah-tohs)*

denial *(dih-NIGH-al)*

depression *(dee-PRESH-shun)*

last rites *(last rights)*

moribund *(MOR-ih-bund)*

mottling *(MOT-ling)*

postmortem *(post-MOR-tem)*

postmortem care *(post-MOR-tem kair)*

resuscitation *(ree-sus-eh-TAY-shun)*

rigor mortis *(RIH-gor MOR-tis)*

Sacrament of the Sick *(SACK-rah-ment of the sick)*

terminal illness *(TER-mih-nal ILL-ness)*

## INTRODUCTION

The residents you care for may live in the long-term care facility for several months or years. As you get to know them, you may develop special relationships and friendships. Losing a friend through death is a sad experience.

Death, however, is a universal experience that we all share. As a nursing assistant in long-term care, you will often work with dying residents and their families. For the elderly with significant health problems, death is not unexpected. The death of younger residents may be more difficult to accept because they are closer in age to the caregivers. The role you play in providing care to dying residents is important and one you can perform with dignity.

Death occurs in various ways:

- A resident may be unresponsive for a long time before dying.
- Some residents develop an acute illness and are unable to recover.
- Others die quietly in their sleep.

## THE DYING PROCESS

Nursing assistants provide continuing care to residents through the dying (**moribund**) period and into the after-death period (**postmortem**). Accepting the idea that death is the natural result of the life process may help you respond to the resident's and family's needs more generously.

Each person will have a different response to the dying process and death (Figures 32-1

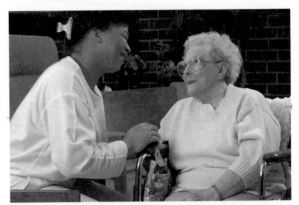

**FIGURE 32-1** People react differently as they deal with approaching death.

and 32-2). Reactions to the diagnosis of a **terminal** (life-ending) **illness** include the following:

- Some residents may have had time to prepare psychologically for death. They may accept or be resigned to it (Figure 32-3).
- Some may look forward to relief from the pain and emotional burden of a long illness. They may await death calmly.
- Some may be fearful or angry and demonstrate behavior that swings from denial to depression (Figure 32-4).
- Others may reach out, trying to verbalize feelings and thoughts of an uncertain future.
- In others, despair and anxiety may give way to moments of active hostility or periods of searching questions.

The residents will not all react in the same way to the prospect of death. They will not all

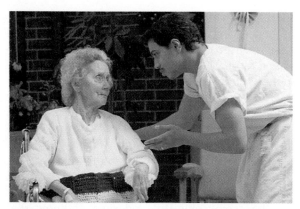

**FIGURE 32-2**   Some residents are unable to talk about their feelings and prefer to be left alone to work things out.

follow the same progression of steps in the grieving process. You must accept the resident's behavior with understanding (Figure 32-5). You must also understand the dying resident's need for support, both from caregivers and family. Finally, you will need to support the family in meeting their own needs during the adjustment period.

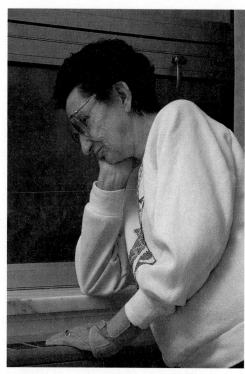

**FIGURE 32-4**   Depression and withdrawal are a natural part of the grieving process.

All staff members should know what the resident has been told about his or her condition. The amount of information given to the resident is a medical decision, with family input where possible. All staff members must abide by it.

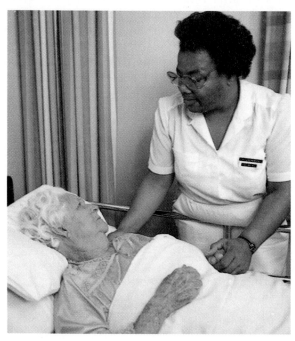

**FIGURE 32-3**   Even though the resident seems to have accepted her diagnosis, she still needs support and caring.

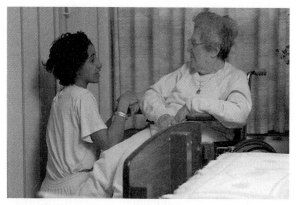

**FIGURE 32-5**   In coming to terms with the diagnosis of a terminal illness, the resident needs the support and understanding of the nursing assistant.

## Resuscitation

Unless otherwise ordered, every effort must be made to keep the resident alive. Be prepared to assist with cardiopulmonary **resuscitation** (CPR). In some facilities, nursing assistants who have had appropriate training are permitted to start this technique.

When a resident requires resuscitation, a **code blue order** is called. Staff work quickly to attempt to revive the resident. Unless you have specific responsibilities in the resuscitation effort, you should:

- Stay out of the way.
- Be prepared to assist, if asked.
- Help keep other residents calm and out of the way.

## Stages of Grieving

After a terminal diagnosis is made and the resident and the family are advised of the diagnosis, they will usually progress through a series of steps known as the stages of grieving* (Figure 32-6). These are:

- Denial
- Anger
- Bargaining
- Depression
- Acceptance

*Elizabeth Kübler-Ross has done much of the pioneer work in the understanding of the grieving process. See her book *On Death and Dying*, published by Macmillan.

Both the resident and family members will experience the grieving process. Some people will progress through all steps and reach an acceptance of death as a natural part of the life experience. Other people will not reach acceptance but will stop at some intermediate step. Some people may go back and forth between steps before moving on to acceptance. The experience is not the same for all people.

As an example of the grieving process, Mrs. Bloomberg has been told of her terminal diagnosis. In the beginning she refuses to accept it. She seems cheerful and says, "I know that there are other therapies that could help. I'm too young to die. I still have much to accomplish." She may even tell you about her future plans. She is in the stage of **denial**.

As time passes and her health does not improve, she says, "It's all so unfair. I don't deserve this!" In **anger** Mrs. Bloomberg strikes out verbally at you and her family. Then, the anger gives way to **bargaining**. She spends time in prayer and visiting the chapel. You hear her say, "If only God (nature, or the doctors) can do something, I will be a better person from now on."

When the bargaining fails, then **depression** sets in. Mrs. Bloomberg speaks of past errors and says how sorry she is that there was not time to do or say certain things. She reviews her life, mourns the losses, and is saddened by things that will be left unfinished. The last step is **acceptance**. She seems calmer and more in control. She starts to put her affairs in

**FIGURE 32-6**   Remember that residents with a terminal diagnosis move back and forth from one stage to another and may never progress to final acceptance before death.

| | Stages of Grief |
|---|---|
| **Denial** | Resident refuses to accept the truth. |
| **Anger** | Resident may act out feelings, directing anger to caregivers and family. |
| **Bargaining** | Resident attempts to "make deals" for more livable time. |
| **Depression** | Resident comes to full realization that situation cannot change and feels saddened over things that will be left unfinished. |
| **Acceptance** | Resident recognizes that death is part of the natural progression of life. |

order and may begin giving personal possessions away.

Residents at any stage of the grieving process need the emotional support of a caring, understanding staff.

## Family Dynamics

Remember that the family and friends of the resident are also going through a grieving process of their own. The relationships that exist between them and the resident are strained by the recognition that little time is left to enjoy each other or to resolve problems.

Each person has feelings of guilt, anger, frustration, and powerlessness over the inability to avoid the final separation. Feelings that were hidden in everyday activities escape when people must also deal with the stress of terminal illness and death.

As a nursing assistant, you must:

- Be aware that this is a stressful period for family and friends as well as the resident
- Know that sometimes unexpected interactions occur
- Not offer advice or take sides
- Listen quietly and be supportive
- Remember not to repeat to either the resident or the family or friends information that has been shared with you

## Caregivers and the Grieving Process

The staff must deal with their feelings about death, the loss of the resident, and their own mortality at the same time that they must be providing support to the resident and the family. Staff members who have developed close relationships with residents will also experience the grieving process.

When caregivers first encounter the process of dying and death, the experience can be frightening and stressful. This is especially true if the caregiver has a close relationship with the resident or if the resident is young. The loss of a young person is especially difficult to understand and accept. With experience, the caregiver realizes that supporting and caring for the dying resident is an important service.

There is no one way to prepare yourself completely for the first experience of death, but some things you can do may help:

- Discuss your feelings about life and death with colleagues in a private setting.
- Discuss your thoughts about death with a member of the clergy of your faith.
- Give yourself permission to feel the grief and sadness that accompanies the loss of a resident.
- Believe that the tasks will become easier with experience.
- Offer whatever physical comfort you can to visitors by advising them of the location of rest areas, rest rooms, and sources of nutrition.

It may be helpful to family members if they can be permitted to participate in simple caregiving activities that give them the sense of being needed and assisting the resident's comfort.

## Religious Practices Related to the Dying Process and Death

Many residents who have a terminal illness gain strength and peace through the practice of their religious beliefs. Each religion has practices related to death. For example, for gravely ill Roman Catholic residents a priest will be summoned to perform **last rites**, also known as the **Sacrament of the Sick** (Figure 32-7).

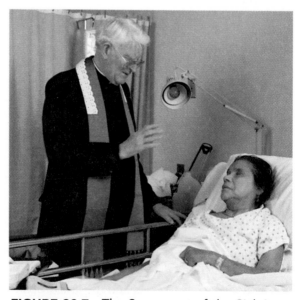

**FIGURE 32-7** The Sacrament of the Sick is administered to gravely ill Roman Catholic residents.

Residents of other religious groups may desire the spiritual support of the clergy of their own faith. Spiritual readings may provide some comfort. Be open to their needs and requests.

Figure 32-8 shows a sampling of practices related to death and dying for major religions.

## Nursing Assistant Responsibilities

You have a special opportunity to be of service to the resident with a terminal diagnosis and to his or her family. Because of your day-to-day contact, you are in a position to provide the emotional and physical support needed. Make an effort to build and maintain a trusting relationship with each resident. Make sure the resident feels secure and knows you will not abandon him. Watch carefully for verbal and nonverbal clues as to what the resident feels and needs. Use your own special touch to comfort the resident.

You can help the moribund resident by:

- Making frequent contact with the resident
- Increasing contact as death approaches
- Keeping the resident comfortable and clean
- Changing resident's position every 2 hours
- Providing proper mouth care
- Using moistened applicators on the lips and inside the mouth
- Meeting basic physical needs
- Monitoring vital signs carefully
- Keeping the room quiet but well lit

You can help the family by:

- Giving proper care to the resident
- Treating the resident with respect and ensuring the resident's dignity
- Listening quietly to their concerns
- Providing privacy

## SIGNS OF APPROACHING DEATH ···

Approaching death is signaled by a slowing of body functions and a loss of control. Signs and symptoms include:

- The body seems to relax and the jaw drops.
- Breathing becomes labored.
- Control of bowels and bladder or both may be lost (incontinence).

- Circulation slows.
- Blood pressure drops.
- Extremities become colder.
- Profuse perspiration is common.
- Respirations become labored (dyspnea) or temporarily cease (apnea).
- Periods of dyspnea followed by apnea, known as *Cheyne-Stokes respirations*, may occur.
- The pulse becomes more rapid and weaker.
- The skin pales and **mottling** (discoloration) may occur.
- The eyes do not respond to light.
- Hearing is the last sense to be lost. Do not assume that the resident can no longer hear. You must be careful in what you say. Always remember to treat the dying person with dignity and respect. This also holds true for handling the body after death.

Continue to talk to the resident in a normal tone even if the resident is **comatose** (unconscious).

Gradually, breathing becomes more labored and then stops. If the nurse is away from the bedside, note the time that breathing ceases and inform the nurse when the vital signs are lost. If the resident's family is present at the time of death, they will be asked to step outside while the nurse examines the resident and then calls the physician. Under no circumstances is the nursing assistant to inform the family that death has occurred. This is the responsibility of the nurse or physician.

Provide a comfortable, private area for the family and stay with them unless they prefer to be alone. It is appropriate to let the family know how much the resident meant to you, so do not be embarrassed if you feel like crying. Do, however, try to control your emotions because the family members will need your support.

## POSTMORTEM CARE ···············

The care given immediately after death is called **postmortem care**. The changes in the resident's body after death are listed in Figure 32-9. Make sure the resident is positioned naturally, with limbs straightened. This is important because **rigor mortis** (stiffening of the body muscles)

**FIGURE 32-8** Beliefs and practices related to dying and death for major religions

Different religions vary in beliefs and practices related to dying and death

| Religion | Autopsy | Organ Donation | Beliefs and Practices |
|---|---|---|---|
| Judaism (Orthodox) | Only in special circumstance | With consultation of Rabbi | Visits to the dying are a religious duty. <br> Witness must be present if death occurs to protect family and commit soul to God. <br> Torah and Psalms may be read and prayers recited. <br> Conversation is kept to a minimum. <br> Someone should be with the body after death until burial usually within 24 hr. <br> Body must not be touched 8–30 minutes after death. <br> Medical personnel should not touch or wash body unless death occurs on Jewish Sabbath; then care may be given by nurse wearing gloves. <br> Water is emptied from the room. <br> Mirrors may be covered at family's request. |
| Hinduism | Permitted | Permitted | Priest ties thread around neck or wrist of deceased and pours water in the mouth. <br> Only family and friends touch body. |
| Buddhism | Personal preference | Permitted | Buddhist priest is present at death. <br> Last rites are chanted at the bedside. |
| Islam (Muslim) | Only for medical or legal reasons | Not permitted | Before death read Koran and pray. <br> Resident confesses sins and asks forgiveness of family. <br> Only family touches or washes body. <br> After death body is turned toward Mecca. |
| Roman Catholic | Permitted | Permitted | Sacrament of sick administered to ill residents, to residents in imminent danger, or shortly after death. |
| Christian Scientist | Unlikely | Not permitted | No ritual is performed before or after death. |
| Church of Christ | Permitted | Permitted | No ritual is performed before or after death. |
| Jehovah's Witness | Only if required by law | Not permitted | No ritual is performed before or after death. |
| Baptist | Permitted | Permitted | Clergy ministers through counseling and prayers. |
| Episcopalian | Permitted | Permitted | Last rites are optional. |
| Lutheran | Permitted | Permitted | Last rites are optional. |
| Eastern Orthodox Christian | Not encouraged | Not encouraged | Last rites are mandatory and handled by ordained priest. |

| FIGURE 32-9   Postmortem signs |
| :--- |
| Postmortem signs include: |
| • Gradual cooling of body temperature |
| • Loss of circulation |
| • Body discoloration with pressure |
| • Evacuation of bowel or bladder or both |
| • Rigor mortis (stiffening of muscles and joints) beginning with head and neck and progressing downward |

will occur some hours after death. Return dentures to the mouth if they were normally worn. Make sure the linen is clean. Family members may want to spend a little time with the body. Stay with them, if requested, but provide privacy otherwise.

After the death of a resident, your behavior should be dignified and restrained. Death in the facility is upsetting to other residents. Residents are informed of the deaths of other residents. Some will experience feelings of the loss of a friend; others will be reminded that their own lives are limited. Some residents withdraw and others may openly grieve. Let the residents

# PROCEDURE
## *117*   Giving Postmortem Care

1. Carry out each beginning procedure action.
2. Assemble equipment:
   • Disposable gloves
   • Shroud or clean sheet
   • Basin with warm water
   • Washcloth
   • Towels
   • Pads as needed
3. Put on disposable gloves.
4. Remove all appliances, tubing, and used articles, if instructed to do so.
5. Work quickly and quietly; maintain an attitude of respect.
6. With bed flat, position the body on the back, head and shoulders elevated on a pillow.
   • Close the eyes by grasping the eyelashes, gently pulling the eyelids down, and holding shut for a few seconds.
   • Remove watch and all jewelry except a wedding band, according to facility policy.
   • Straighten arms and legs and place arms by sides.

   • Make itemized list of watch and jewelry. Ask family member to check the list and sign it.
   • If used, replace dentures in the resident's mouth. If used, replace artificial eye.
7. Bathe body as necessary. Remove any soiled dressings and replace with clean ones. Groom hair.
8. Place a disposable pad underneath the buttocks.
   • Put clean gown on resident.
   • Replace top bed linen.
9. If the family is to view the body:
   • Make sure the room is neat.
   • Adjust the lights to a subdued level.
   • Place chairs around the bed for family members.
   • Remove disposable gloves. Dispose of them according to facility policy. Wash hands.
   • Allow the family to visit in private.
10. Collect all belongings and make a list. Wrap properly and label.
11. Carry out each procedure completion action.

know that you understand their feelings. Be willing to listen. Be patient if a resident seems irritable or angry. Report the resident's reactions to the nurse so the care plan will reflect the proper staff response.

As residents grieve for their deceased friend, they may want to recall their relationship. Be supportive as they express their feelings of grief (Figure 32-10).

Some facilities hold memorial services for deceased residents. Members of the family, residents, and staff are invited to celebrate the life of the resident. The services help to bring closure.

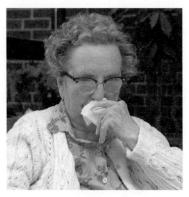

**FIGURE 32-10**  Remember that residents often form close friendships. When one dies you must be prepared to offer comfort to those who remain.

## LESSON SYNTHESIS: Putting It All Together

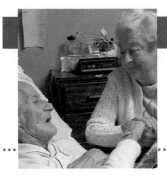

*Y*ou have just completed this lesson. Now go back and review the Clinical Focus. Try to see how the Clinical Focus relates to the concepts presented in the lesson. Then answer the following questions.

1. Why do you think Mr. Sperling is behaving the way he is?

2. How do you think the marital history of Mr. and Mrs. Sperling might affect their emotional response to this terminal condition and death?

3. How could the nursing assistant be supportive?

4. What special sacrament would be appropriate when Mr. Sperling is moribund?

## REVIEW

**A. Match each term ( items a.–e.) with the proper definition.**

   a. comatose     d. postmortem
   b. mottling      e. Sacrament
   c. moribund        of the Sick

    1. _____ discoloration

    2. _____ dying

    3. _____ last rites

    4. _____ unconscious

    5. _____ after death

**B. Provide brief answers for each of the following.**

    6. List five signs of approaching death.

    7. List the five stages of grieving.

    8. List six ways the nursing assistant can help the moribund resident.

## C. Answer each statement true (T) or false (F).

9. T  F  Death is a natural part of the life cycle.

10. T  F  Everyone responds to the thought of death in the same way.

11. T  F  A terminal illness is curable.

12. T  F  Given time, residents can move steadily forward through each stage of grieving.

13. T  F  Rigor mortis develops immediately after death.

## D. Select the one best answer for each of the following.

14. Signs of approaching death include
    a. blood pressure rises
    b. circulation speeds up
    c. extremities become warmer
    d. breathing becomes labored

15. When a resident is dying
    a. other residents are not affected
    b. staff members are not upset
    c. family members are not concerned
    d. other residents may be deeply affected

16. The Sacrament of the Sick is administered to
    a. Buddhist residents
    b. Jewish residents
    c. Roman Catholic residents
    d. residents who are members of the Church of Christ

17. After the death of a resident who belongs to the Muslim faith
    a. the nursing assistant may wash the body
    b. the body is turned toward Mecca
    c. the Bible is read
    d. none of these

18. When a resident is comatose, he
    a. may be able to see
    b. may be able to hear
    c. cannot hear
    d. is able to speak

## E. Clinical Experience

19. Liza is caring for Mr. Simms who has been comatose for 12 hours. His breathing has just ceased. The nurse is away from the bedside.
    a. What action should Liza take?
    b. Should Liza inform the family members who are in the waiting room?
    c. When the family returns to the resident's room, what should Liza do to offer them support?
    d. Mr. Simms was a resident in the facility for 18 months. Liza liked him and feels very sad about his death. Is it appropriate for her to let the family know that she will also miss him very much?

# LESSON

# 33

# Caring for the Person in Subacute Care

**CLINICAL FOCUS**

Think about the care that is required by residents in subacute units as you study this lesson and meet:

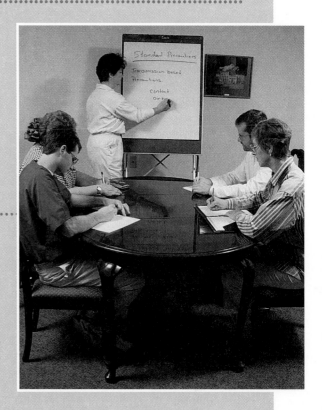

*S*teven Goldstein has been a nursing assistant for several years. He has just been hired to work in a subacute care unit of a long-term care facility. Steven will need to participate in additional in-service education to fulfill the requirements of his new job. He is looking forward to the challenge of learning and acquiring new skills.

## OBJECTIVES

*After studying this lesson, you should be able to:*

- Define and spell vocabulary words and terms.
- Describe the purpose of subacute care.
- List the differences between acute care, subacute care, and long-term care.

- Describe the responsibilities of the nursing assistant when caring for residents receiving the special treatments discussed in this lesson.

## VOCABULARY

**alopecia**  *(al-oh-PEE-shee-ah)*

**anorexia**  *(an-oh-RECK-see-ah)*

**central venous (CV) catheter**  *(SEN-tral VEE-nus KATH-eh-ter)*

**chemotherapy**  *(kee-moh-THER-ah-pee)*

**dialysis**  *(dye-AL-ih-sis)*

**enteral feedings**  *(EN-ter-al FEED-ings)*

**epidural catheter**  *(ep-ih-DOO-ral KATH-eh-ter)*

**fistula**  *(FIS-tyou-lah)*

# VOCABULARY

graft *(graft)*

hemodialysis *(he-moh-dye-AL-ih-sis)*

hyperalimentation *(high-per-al-ih-men-TAY-shun)*

intravenous (IV) therapy *(in-trah-VEE-nus THER-ah-pee)*

narcotic *(nar-KAH-tick)*

oncology *(ong-KOL-oh-jee)*

patient-controlled analgesia (PCA) *(PAY-shent kon-TROLD an-al-JEE-see-ah)*

peripheral intravenous central catheter (PICC) *(per-IH-fer-al in-trah-VEE-nus SEN-tral KATH-eh-ter)*

peritoneal dialysis *(per-ih-toh-NEE-al dye-AL-ih-sis)*

piggyback *(PIG-ee-bak)*

pulse oximetry *(puls ox-IM-ih-tree)*

radiation therapy *(ray-dee-AY-shun THER-ah-pee)*

subacute care *(sub-ah-KYOUT kair)*

total parenteral nutrition (TPN) *(TOH-tal pah-REN-ter-al new-TRIH-shun)*

tracheostomy *(tray-kee-OS-toh-mee)*

transcutaneous electrical nerve stimulation (TENS) *(trans-kyou-TAN-ee-us ee-LEK-trih-kal nerv stim-you-LAY-shun)*

transitional care *(tran-ZIH-shun-al kair)*

## DESCRIPTION OF SUBACUTE CARE

**Subacute care** is a type of "step-down" care given to persons who have been acutely ill. These individuals are out of the acute phase of illness but still need monitoring and ongoing treatment and services. Subacute care is sometimes called **transitional care**. The purpose of subacute care is to provide the care a person needs but at a lower cost than care given in an acute care facility (hospital). Subacute care units are usually located in a section of a skilled nursing facility. Most residents in subacute care units are there for 3 to 4 weeks. Residents with terminal illness or with acquired immune deficiency syndrome (AIDS) may be there for a longer time. Residents who can be discharged may go to:

- Their homes
- A skilled care or intermediate care facility
- An assisted living facility

On a subacute care unit there are:

- Highly trained nurses and nursing assistants
- More medications and treatments to administer than on a regular skilled unit

- More frequent physician's visits
- More sophisticated types of equipment

## Types of Care Provided in a Subacute Care Unit

Most subacute care units provide specialized care in one or two areas. Some examples are:

- Rehabilitation—all therapies are provided and the resident participates in rehabilitation for 5 hours a day, 6 or 7 days a week.
- Peritoneal dialysis—a method of ridding the body of wastes for a person who has kidney failure
- Ventilator weaning and tracheostomy care—for persons who have been unable to breathe without the help of a ventilator
- Cardiac monitoring—for persons who have had a myocardial infarction or acute heart failure
- Pain management and control—for persons who have acute or chronic pain
- Oncology—the care of persons with cancer who are receiving treatments such as chemotherapy or radiation
- Wound management—for persons with severe stage 3 or stage 4 pressure ulcers, ulcers

related to peripheral vascular disease, or burns

- Brain injury—for persons who have suffered brain damage resulting from trauma
- AIDS—for persons in the terminal stages of AIDS who need 24-hour-a-day care
- Hospice care—for persons in the terminal stages of any disease
- Postoperative care (care given to individuals who have had surgery) for persons who have other complicating conditions—for example, a person who has had repair of a hip fracture and who also has chronic obstructive pulmonary disease

If you work on a subacute care unit you will participate in special in-service training to meet the needs of the residents in your care. A nursing assistant on a subacute unit will be expected to:

- Work closely with registered nurses who are specialists in critical care or in a specific area of nursing such as rehabilitation or wound care
- Have extensive knowledge of the types of residents cared for on the subacute care unit
- Care for residents receiving complicated treatments
- Have excellent observational skills because of the complex conditions of the residents on the unit
- Be a member of an interdisciplinary health care team that includes highly trained professionals in areas like physical therapy, occupational therapy, speech therapy, respiratory therapy, and social services

It is important that the staff on a subacute care unit be able to provide for the resident's emotional well-being. Many of the residents on the unit will be able to return to their homes. For them, this is a time for rejoicing and for making plans for the future. Some of the residents, however, will have an uncertain future. For example:

- Will the resident receiving dialysis receive a kidney transplant in time?
- Will the cancer be cured in the resident receiving radiation or chemotherapy?
- Will the resident on the ventilator be able to be weaned off the ventilator or will it be a lifelong need?
- Will the resident receiving rehabilitation recover enough independence to be able to go home?

## SPECIAL PROCEDURES PROVIDED IN THE SUBACUTE CARE UNIT ·······

You may care for residents who are receiving special treatments because of their health problems. These treatments may require the use of equipment that is unfamiliar to you. As a nursing assistant you will not be expected to be responsible for these procedures. However, you will be providing the same personal care and procedures that you would with any residents. In addition you will need to know what observations to make for these residents.

## PULSE OXIMETRY ·······················

Residents receiving oxygen may be monitored with pulse oximetry. (See Lesson 25 for oxygen therapy.) **Pulse oximetry** is used to monitor the level of oxygen in the arterial blood. Red and infrared light are sent through an artery in the fingertip. A photodetector is placed over the finger. The photodetector measures the transmitted light as it passes through the blood (Figure 33-1). The nurse is responsible for this procedure.

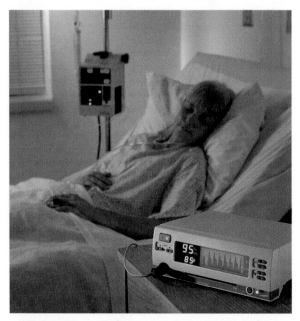

**FIGURE 33-1** Pulse oximetry monitors the level of oxygen in arterial blood. (Courtesy of Ohmeda, Louisville, CO)

# INTRAVENOUS THERAPY··················

**Intravenous (IV) therapy** refers to medication or solutions administered directly into a vein. Standard intravenous therapy is given into a peripheral vein (a large vein in the arm) (Figure 33-2). This is called an IV. The IV may consist of a single bag of solution connected to a simple tubing with a needle or small catheter on the end. Sometimes an additional small bag of fluid is attached to tubing that is connected to the main (primary) tubing. This is called a **piggyback**. This small bag contains medication such as an antibiotic that is given intermittently into the vein (Figure 33-3).

## Central Venous Insertion

Intravenous therapy can also be administered through a **central venous (CV) catheter**. A special catheter is inserted into a vein near the

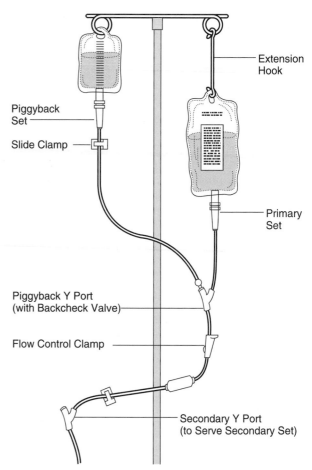

**FIGURE 33-3** The small bag (piggyback) contains medication.

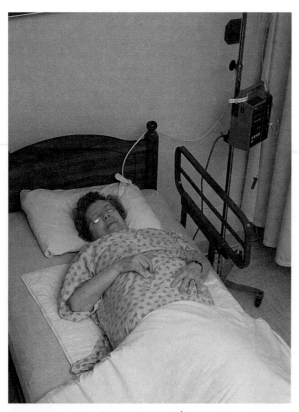

**FIGURE 33-2** Intravenous therapy is most often given through a peripheral vein in the resident's arm.

resident's collar bone (Figure 33-4). The catheter tip ends in or near the heart chamber. CV therapy is used to administer medications or to provide total parenteral nutrition.

## Peripheral Intravenous Central Catheter Line

A **peripheral intravenous central catheter** or **PICC** line consists of a catheter that is inserted into a peripheral vein and threaded upward through the vein to the jugular or subclavian vein. It is used to administer medications or to provide total parenteral nutrition.

## Total Parenteral Nutrition

**Total parenteral nutrition (TPN)** is also called **hyperalimentation**. TPN is given to a

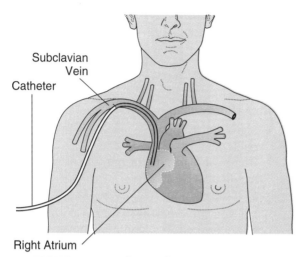

**FIGURE 33-4**  Central venous insertion

Subclavian Vein

Catheter

Right Atrium

resident whose bowel needs complete rest. All required nutrients (carbohydrates, proteins, and fats) are given directly into the vein so the bowel does not have to work to digest food. Residents receiving TPN may need to be weighed daily or every other day. This should be done at the same time of day with the resident wearing the same type of clothing. The resident may be gradually changed to **enteral feedings**. With an enteral feeding, liquid nourishment is administered through a tube inserted into the resident's stomach (Figure 33-5).

## PAIN MANAGEMENT PROCEDURES

Pain management may be the major reason why some residents are on a subacute unit. Other residents may be undergoing pain management related to other conditions such as recent surgery or pain related to cancer. Both drug and nondrug treatments can be successful in helping to prevent and control pain. Various types of relaxation techniques are frequently used for pain management.

### Patient-Controlled Analgesia

**Patient-controlled analgesia (PCA)** is used for acute, chronic, or postoperative pain. Analgesia means pain relief. A device is inserted into

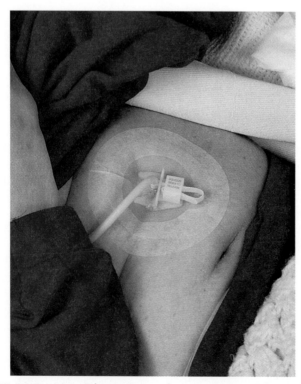

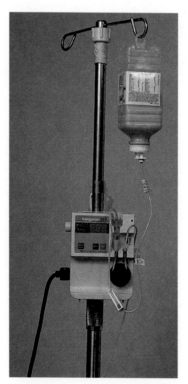

**FIGURE 33-5**  Nourishment may be given through a tube inserted into the resident's stomach.

## Guidelines for

## Caring for Residents with Intravenous Lines

The nursing assistant tasks include the following:

1. Know the drip rate in the drip chamber. Observe drip chamber for drip rate. If rate changes or drip chamber is full, notify the nurse.
2. Avoid pulling or twisting tubing. Make sure resident is not lying on tubing.
3. Observe area of needle insertion for signs of swelling, redness, or warmth.
4. Note signs of moisture that may indicate the tubing is leaking.
5. Make sure that all junctions in the tubing are securely connected.

6. Report immediately to the nurse:
   - Signs of dyspnea, cyanosis, chest, or back pain
   - Complaints of pain or burning at site of needle insertion
7. Remember that all IV procedures are sterile. If you are assisting a nurse with any of these procedures, you must never contaminate the sterile field or supplies.
8. When caring for residents with any type of intravenous therapy, *NEVER:*
   - Change drip rate
   - Disconnect any tubing
   - Manipulate needle or tubing
   - Remove, change, or manipulate dressing over site

---

**PROCEDURE**

# *118*

## Changing a Gown on a Resident with a Peripheral Intravenous Line in Place

*Note:* This procedure is to be used only when the IV is not run through an electronic pump. When a pump is used, the resident may wear a gown that snaps at the shoulder. In this case, the gown can be removed without touching the IV bag or tubing. If the resident is wearing a nonsnap gown, call the nurse if the gown is to be changed. Never disconnect the tubing from the pump.

1. Carry out each beginning procedure action.
2. Assemble equipment:
   - Clean gown

3. Make sure windows and door are closed to prevent chilling the resident.
4. Remove gown from the arm without the IV and bring gown across resident's chest to other arm.
5. Place clean gown over resident's chest to avoid exposure.
6. On the arm with the IV, gather material of gown in one hand so there is no pull or pressure on line and slowly draw gown over tip of fingers (Figure 33-6).
7. With free hand, lift IV free of standard and slip gown over bag of fluid

*(continues)*

**PROCEDURE** *118* *(continued)*

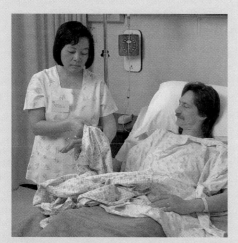

**FIGURE 33-6**  Gather material of gown in one hand so there is no pull or pressure on the line. Slowly draw gown over tips of fingers.

(Figure 33-7), removing gown from resident's body. **Never allow the bag of fluid to be lower than the resident's arm.**

 8. Take sleeve of clean gown and slip it over the bag of fluid, the tubing, and up the resident's arm.
 9. Replace bag of fluid on IV standard.
10. Remove soiled gown and place at end of bed. Finish putting clean gown on resident's other arm. Secure neck ties.

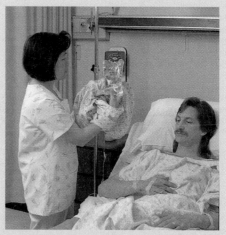

**FIGURE 33-7**  With free hand, lift IV free of standard and slip gown over bag of fluid.

11. Place soiled gown in laundry hamper.
12. Make sure IV is dripping and that tubing is not kinked or twisted.
13. Carry out each procedure completion action.

*Note:* If you are changing a gown for a resident with a centrally inserted line you will not need to lower the fluid container. Change the gown in the usual manner, taking care not to manipulate the tubing.

the resident's vein. It is connected to a solution that contains a **narcotic**. A narcotic is a drug such as morphine that is used for pain relief. The dosage is controlled by equipment that has been preset. The patient or the nurse pushes the PCA button at times of discomfort.

Report to the nurse if you note any change in the resident's:

• Level of consciousness
• Rate and pattern of respirations

• Pupil size
• Skin color

## Pain Management with an Epidural Catheter

An **epidural catheter** is implanted beneath the resident's skin. It is inserted near the spinal cord at the first lumbar (L1) space. A local anesthetic is administered either intermittently or continuously through the catheter. The resident may have leg numbness and weakness for the first 24 hours after the catheter is inserted. Report to the nurse at once if:

• Catheter becomes dislodged from the insertion site
• You note changes in respiration rate and pattern
• Resident complains of itching
• Resident vomits or complains of nausea

## Transcutaneous Electrical Nerve Stimulation

**Transcutaneous electrical nerve stimulation (TENS)** is a nondrug method of pain relief. Mild, harmless electrical current stimulates nerve fibers to block the transmission of pain to the brain. Electrodes are taped to the resident's skin. The location of the electrodes depends on the areas related to the pain. The electrodes are attached to wires that are attached to a control box (Figure 33-8). The intensity of the stimulation is set on the control box by the nurse.

## CARING FOR RESIDENTS WITH TRACHEOSTOMIES

You may care for a resident with a tracheostomy. A **tracheostomy** is a tube that is inserted into a surgical opening in the resident's trachea (windpipe). A tracheostomy is performed when the resident is unable to breathe in air through the nose. The tube allows the resident to "breathe" as air goes directly into the trachea and then into the lungs. A person who is on a ventilator for a long time will have a tracheostomy that is connected to the ventilator. The resident may have secretions coming from the chest and through the tube. The nurse will need to use suction to remove the secretions.

The tube may be made of plastic or metal. Tracheostomy tubes consist of an inner removable tube called a cannula and an outer tube called a neckplate that is held in place with neck ties. The neckplate rests between the clavicles (breastbones). There is a slot on each side. Tracheostomy ties are inserted here to secure the tube in place (Figure 33-9). Residents with tracheostomies can usually take a bath or shower but must keep the water away from the opening. Avoid using powders, sprays, or shaving cream

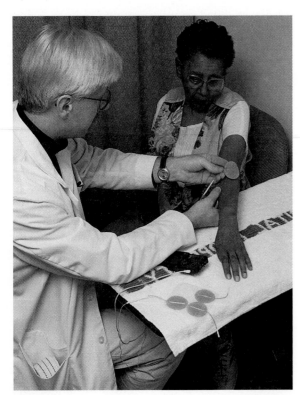

**FIGURE 33-8** A TENS unit is used to relieve pain.

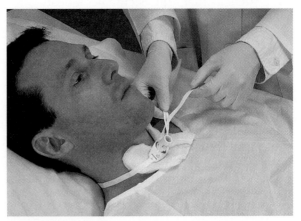

**FIGURE 33-9** Ties hold the tracheostomy tube in place.

around the tube. When you care for a resident with a tracheostomy, observe for:

- Changes in respiratory rate, depth, quality
- Changes in mental status such as confusion, restlessness, or irritability that indicate the resident is not getting enough oxygen

Report to the nurse immediately if the:

- Tube becomes dislodged from the opening
- Resident is having trouble breathing
- Resident needs suctioning

Be sure you know how the resident communicates. The incision in the trachea will interfere with the resident's ability to talk.

## CARING FOR THE RESIDENT RECEIVING DIALYSIS TREATMENTS

**Dialysis** is a process by which the blood is cleansed of liquid wastes artificially when the kidneys are unable to remove the wastes. This procedure is needed when a person has kidney failure. Without dialysis the person would die as the waste products accumulate in the bloodstream. Dialysis is usually considered a temporary treatment that is used until a suitable kidney is found for a kidney transplant. The two types of dialysis are hemodialysis and peritoneal dialysis.

### Hemodialysis

During **hemodialysis** treatment the resident's blood is circulated outside of the body into an artificial kidney machine. In the dialysis machine, the blood is cleansed with a liquid substance called dialysate and then returned to the resident's body. Most persons needing hemodialysis treatments are treated in a dialysis center. However, you may care for residents in the subacute unit who go as outpatients to the dialysis center for their treatments. Dialysis is usually done three to four times a week. Each treatment takes several hours. To do dialysis, a connection must be made between the resident's circulatory system and the artificial kidney machine. Minor surgery is done to create either a fistula or a graft. The **fistula** (Figure 33-10) is created when a vein

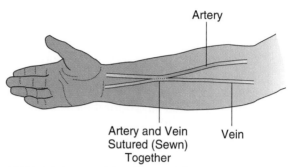

**A.V. Fistula**

Artery

Artery and Vein Sutured (Sewn) Together

Vein

**FIGURE 33-10** Fistula used for hemodialysis

is attached to an artery either in an arm or leg. When a **graft** is used (Figure 33-11), synthetic material is inserted to form a connection between an artery and a vein. Two needles are inserted for treatment with either the fistula or graft. The needles are connected to tubes that go to and from the artificial kidney machine. As a nursing assistant, you are not expected to care for the fistula or graft. You need to be aware that the resident will:

- Have fluid restrictions
- Have dietary restrictions for calories, sodium, protein, potassium, calcium, and phosphorus
- Need all fluid intake and output measured and recorded
- Need to be weighed regularly at the same time of day and with the same type of clothing
- Need to be monitored and have blood pressure taken frequently after dialysis. Remem-

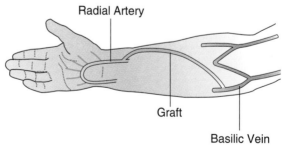

**Graft**

Radial Artery

Graft

Basilic Vein

**FIGURE 33-11** A graft used for hemodialysis

ber that blood pressure should not be taken in the arm used for dialysis.

Report to the nurse if the resident has:

- Swelling (edema) of the hands or feet
- Changes in vital signs (blood pressure, temperature, pulse, or respirations)
- A change in weight
- A change in intake and output measurements
- Shortness of breath
- Complaints of pain at the site of the fistula or graft

## Peritoneal Dialysis

**Peritoneal dialysis** is also a process of cleansing the blood. In peritoneal dialysis, the process takes place within the resident's body in the peritoneal (abdominal) cavity, rather than outside the body in a machine. During dialysis the dialysate is introduced into the abdominal cavity, allowed to stay in for some time, and then drained out. As blood flows through the vessels in the peritoneum, waste products are filtered and excess fluids are removed. The nurse instills the dialysate through a catheter that is surgically implanted through the wall of the abdomen into the abdominal cavity. This is done using sterile technique.

Nursing assistants are not expected to administer peritoneal dialysis. You may be responsible for monitoring the resident's vital signs every 10 to 15 minutes for the first 1 to 2 hours after a treatment and then every 2 to 4 hours. Notify the nurse if there are any changes in vital signs.

# ONCOLOGY TREATMENTS

**Oncology** is the care and treatment of persons with cancer. Cancer may be treated with surgery, radiation, chemotherapy, or a combination of any of these.

## Radiation Therapy

Residents receiving radiation therapy in the long-term care facility will be transported to a special cancer treatment center or to a hospital to receive the therapy as an outpatient. **Radiation therapy** is the use of high-energy radiation to kill cancer cells. It is considered a local therapy because it kills only the cancer cells in the area being treated. Residents receiving radiation may complain of fatigue and lack of appetite. When caring for residents receiving radiation therapy:

- Report signs of redness, pain, or peeling of the skin in the area being treated.
- Do not remove markings made on the skin for treatment purposes.
- Do not use any heat or cold treatments on the area being treated.
- Wash the area only with tepid water and a soft washcloth. Do not apply any soaps, powders, deodorants, perfumes, makeup, lotions, or skin preparations to the area.
- Instruct resident to avoid wearing tight clothing over area.

## Chemotherapy

**Chemotherapy** is the use of drugs to kill cancer cells within the body. The drugs may be given by mouth (orally), through the vein (IV), or in the muscle (intramuscular [IM]). The nurse or physician administers the drugs. The person receiving chemotherapy may have side effects including nausea, vomiting, **anorexia** (loss of appetite), or **alopecia** (loss of hair). Modern treatment techniques have minimized the side effects of chemotherapy. However, loss of hair is still common. The hair will usually come back after the treatments are completed. Some persons prefer to wear wigs during this time. Respect the resident's wishes regarding personal appearance.

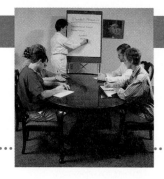

## LESSON SYNTHESIS: Putting It All Together

*Y*ou have just completed this lesson. Now go back and review the Clinical Focus. Try to see how the Clinical Focus relates to the concepts presented in this lesson. Then answer the following questions.

1. Consider the different types of care that subacute units provide. If Steven works in a unit with residents receiving dialysis, what should he know about kidney function and kidney disease?

2. Using the knowledge presented in earlier lessons in this text, what differences would you expect between acute care, subacute care, and long-term care?

3. What challenges would you expect to accept if you work in a subacute care unit?

4. How would you prepare yourself for meeting these challenges?

## REVIEW

**A. Select the one best answer for each of the following.**

1. Subacute care is given to persons who
   a. have been acutely ill
   b. have had a long, progressive illness
   c. require only custodial care
   d. require intensive care

2. The purpose of subacute care is to
   a. increase the population of long-term care facilities
   b. discharge patients from the hospital as quickly as possible
   c. provide the care a person needs at a lower cost
   d. all of these

3. Examples of the type of residents treated in subacute care include persons
   a. requiring dialysis
   b. requiring high levels of rehabilitation
   c. receiving wound care
   d. all of these

4. A nursing assistant working in subacute care would need to
   a. learn how to start intravenous feedings
   b. have excellent observational skills
   c. learn how to administer chemotherapy
   d. instruct residents in pain management techniques

5. If you accept a position in a subacute care unit, you may need to learn
   a. why hyperalimentation is given
   b. your responsibilities for residents receiving dialysis
   c. more about the rehabilitation process
   d. all of these

6. The procedure to measure the level of oxygen in arterial blood is called
   a. hemodialysis
   b. pulse oximetry
   c. total parenteral nutrition
   d. intravenous therapy

7. A central venous catheter is inserted into
   a. a vein in the resident's arm
   b. an artery in the resident's arm
   c. the jugular or subclavian vein
   d. the epidural space

8. Total parenteral nutrition (TPN) is used for residents
   a. who need to lose weight
   b. who are unconscious

c. who refuse to eat

d. whose bowel needs complete rest

9. The nursing assistant's responsibility for caring for residents with intravenous feedings is to
   a. insert the needle into the vein
   b. add medication to the bag of fluid when it is due
   c. observe for complications
   d. change the drip rate if it is going too fast or too slow

10. Patient-controlled analgesia is used
    a. for acute, chronic, or postoperative pain
    b. for administering narcotics for pain
    c. to allow the resident to receive the medication when he or she needs it
    d. all of these

11. An epidural catheter is used for
    a. pain management
    b. administering nutrition
    c. emptying the bladder
    d. intravenous feedings

12. When caring for residents with tracheostomies you should
    a. not allow the resident to take a bath or shower
    b. observe for changes in respiratory rate, depth, and quality
    c. maintain the resident on a liquid diet
    d. be responsible for changing the tracheostomy tube

13. Dialysis is a procedure for
    a. cleansing the blood of liquid wastes
    b. relieving postoperative pain
    c. administering oxygen
    d. giving total parenteral nutrition

14. A resident on dialysis will have
    a. fluid restrictions
    b. dietary restrictions
    c. frequent weights taken
    d. all of these

15. When caring for residents on dialysis you should observe for
    a. edema of the hands and feet
    b. changes in vital signs
    c. shortness of breath
    d. all of these

16. Oncology is the care and treatment of residents with
    a. severe wounds
    b. kidney failure
    c. cancer
    d. terminal illness

17. When caring for residents receiving radiation therapy you should
    a. remove the markings made on the skin for treatment purposes
    b. apply cold treatments to the area
    c. avoid applying soaps, powders, lotions, deodorants, or other substances to the treated area
    d. wrap the treatment area with an elastic bandage

**B. Fill in the blanks by selecting the correct word or phrase from the list.**

| | |
|---|---|
| dialysis | pulse oximetry |
| enteral | transcutaneous |
| hyperalimentation | electrical nerve |
| narcotic | stimulation |
| piggyback | transitional care |

18. Subacute care is also called _____.

19. A procedure for removing liquid wastes from the blood is called _____.

20. _____ is used for measuring the oxygen level in arterial blood.

21. A _____ refers to a small bag of fluid containing intravenous medication that is connected with a tube to the primary tubing.

22. Total parenteral nutrition (TPN) is also called _____.

23. A feeding administered through a tube into the resident's stomach is called an _____ feeding.

24. A _____ is a potent drug used for pain relief.

25. The use of electrical current to treat pain is done with a procedure called _____.

# Employment

## LESSONS

*34* Surviving a Survey

*35* Seeking Employment

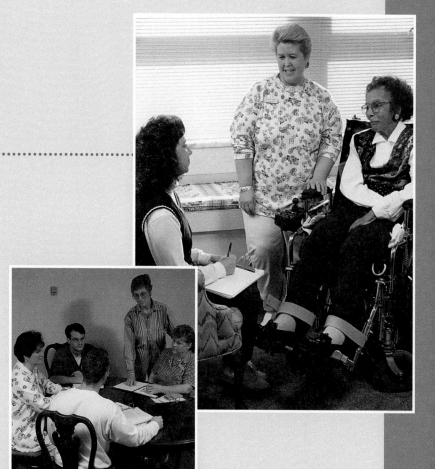

# LESSON 34

## Surviving a Survey

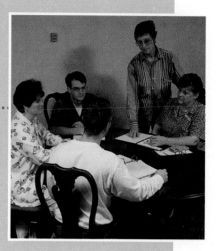

### CLINICAL FOCUS

Think about the reasons for a survey and meet:

*K*athy Bergetti, who has been a nursing assistant for almost a year. She has worked at Community Nursing and Rehabilitation Center since she finished her nursing assistant course. The facility is expecting surveyors within the next month. This is Kathy's first time to participate in a survey.

## OBJECTIVES

*After studying this lesson, you should be able to:*

- Define and spell vocabulary words and terms.
- State the purpose of a survey in a long-term care facility.

- List the information that the nursing assistants are expected to know.
- Describe the survey process.
- Briefly describe the consequences of an unsatisfactory survey.

## VOCABULARY

**certification** (*sir*-teh-feh-**KAY**-shun)

**compliance** (kom-**PLY**-ans)

**deficiency** (deh-**FISH**-en-see)

**exit conference** (**EX**-it **KON**-fer-ens)

**licensure** (**LIE**-sen-shur)

**ombudsman** (**OM**-buds-man)

**plan of correction** (plan of kor-**RECK**-shun)

**survey** (**SIR**-vay)

**surveyor** (sir-**VAY**-or)

## PURPOSE OF A SURVEY

The word **survey** means to examine, to inspect, to observe, or to scrutinize. Surveys carried out in health care facilities do all of these things.

All health care facilities undergo surveys on a regular basis. Hospitals, long-term care facilities, home health agencies, and other health care organizations all must be licensed (Figure 34-1) to provide care. The license is awarded

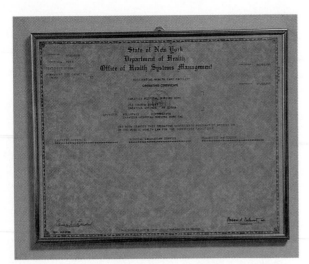

**FIGURE 34-1** All health care facilities must have a license to operate.

by the agency that regulates care. In most states this is the Department of Public Health. The license is renewed if the facility passes the survey.

Facilities that receive funds from Medicaid and Medicare participate in a **certification** process. This means that in addition to the license requirements, special criteria must be met to receive these government funds. One survey is usually done for both **licensure** and certification.

A team of health care professionals called **surveyors** is responsible for conducting the survey. The team determines if the facility is following all state and federal regulations. In other words, is the facility in **compliance** (doing what they are supposed to do)? The purpose of the survey is to:

• Review the quality of life for the residents
• Review the quality of care given to the residents
• Determine areas of deficient care
• Review policies and procedures

No one knows exactly when the surveyors will come to do the survey. Surveys can be stressful. It is like having someone in your home for several days examining your house, your activities, the meals you serve, the care you give your children, and your personal records. Being prepared can reduce the stress.

# SURVEY PREPARATION BY SURVEYORS AND STAFF

## Surveyor Preparation

Preparation for a survey begins long before the surveyors arrive. The surveyors gather information about the facility. They identify:

• Potential areas of concern
• Special features of the facility such as Alzheimer's units (Figure 34-2)
• Residents and families to interview

The **ombudsman** is contacted by the survey team before the survey. This is to find out whether complaints or problems with the facility or the staff have been reported.

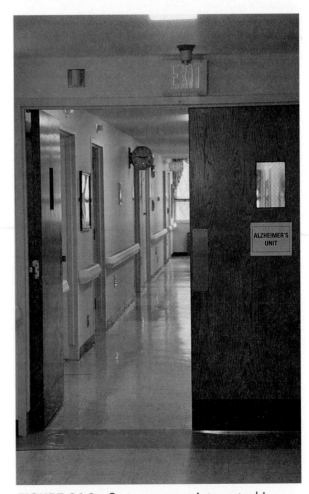

**FIGURE 34-2** Surveyors are interested in special features of a facility such as this Alzheimer's unit.

## Facility Preparation

The facility should be "survey ready" every day. Quality care is expected every day, not just during the survey. However, certain environmental and "paper" procedures need to be checked:

- Make sure that all records, policy and procedure manuals, and other documents are up to date.
- Check the environment for needed repairs and cleaning.
- Determine whether staff are following the care plans for each resident.
- Scrutinize state and federal regulations to ensure that the facility is in compliance (Figure 34-3).
- Review the results of surveys from the last few years to see that past problems have been corrected.
- Review infection control procedures and observe staff to make sure they wash their hands and use proper technique.

Many facilities will conduct a "mock" survey several times a year by their own staff to make sure that all departments are in compliance with all rules and regulations.

## SURVEY PROCESS

Surveyors make judgments about a facility by:

- Making observations
- Asking questions of staff members (Figure 34-4)
- Interviewing residents and their families
- Reviewing residents' medical records, care plans, and facility manuals and records

### Facility Tour

Employees are notified when the surveyors arrive in the facility. The surveyors will also place signs around the facility that inform everyone that a survey is taking place. The larger the facility the more surveyors are on the team. The

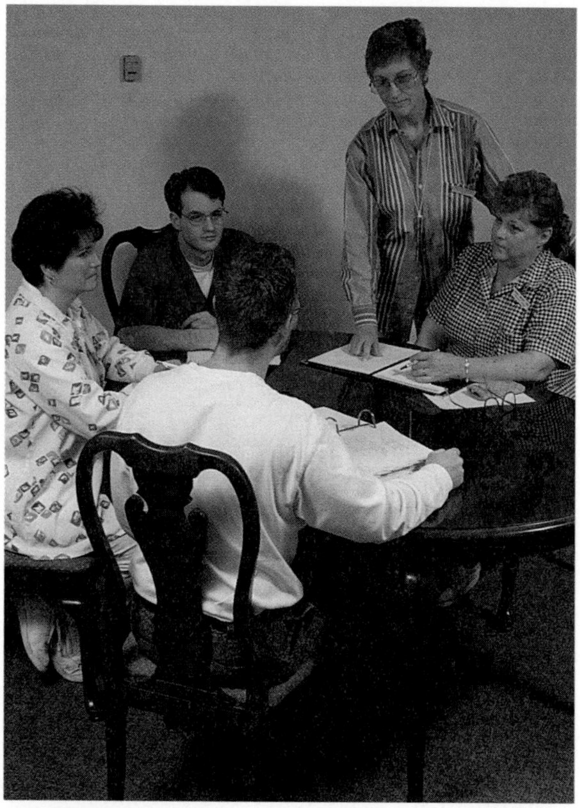

**FIGURE 34-3**   The staff must be knowledgeable about all state and federal regulations.

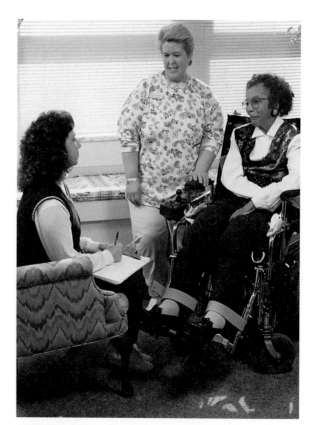

**FIGURE 34-4**   Surveyors ask questions of staff members.

first action of the surveyors is to take a tour of the facility. A staff member (a nurse manager) will accompany each surveyor. During the tour they will observe:

1. The environment for standards of:
   - Safety
     —Are the halls free of equipment and clutter?
     —Do the call lights work?
   - Infection control
     —Do staff members wash their hands?
     —Are clean and soiled linens handled appropriately?
     —Are standard precautions being followed?
     —Are isolation procedures implemented correctly?
   - General maintenance
     —Are the floors, ceilings, and walls in good repair?
     —Are there any electrical hazards?
     —Are there any plumbing, heating, or air conditioning problems?
   - Housekeeping
     —Is the facility clean?
     —Are there offensive odors?
     —Are wastebaskets emptied frequently?

2. Quality of life and quality of care issues:
   - Are the residents' rights followed?
     —Do staff knock before entering residents' rooms?
     —Are restraints being used?
     —Are residents allowed to be as independent as possible?
     —Are residents given choices when possible?
     —Is privacy provided during care?
   - Grooming, dress, and hygiene of residents
     —Are the residents wearing clean, suitable clothing, underwear, and shoes or slippers that are in good repair?
     —Are residents clean shaven?
     —Is their hair clean and combed?
     —Are fingernails clean and trimmed?
     —Are the residents receiving oral hygiene regularly?
   - Positioning of residents in bed and in chairs
     —Are the residents in good body alignment?
     —Are supportive devices used appropriately?
     —Are positioning schedules being followed? (Figure 34-5).
     —Are residents in one position for too long?
   - Number of residents with pressure ulcers
   - Number of residents with indwelling urinary catheters
   - Number of residents with physical and chemical restraints
   - Interactions between staff and residents
     —Do staff converse with residents appropriately?
     —Do staff display patience?
     —Do they tell the residents what they are doing?
     —How do staff respond to residents with emotional conduct and behavior?
   - Activities
     —Is the activity schedule being followed?
     —Are the activities appropriate to the residents' interests and abilities?

What the surveyors observe during the tour will help them determine whether they need to do further research on any specific situation. For example, if poor positioning is noted on one or two residents, they will observe many residents at different times to determine whether the problem exists throughout the facility or whether this is an isolated incident.

**TURNING SCHEDULE**

| NOC | | DAY | | EVE | |
|-----|---|-----|---|-----|---|
| 2400 | L | 0800 | chair | 1600 | R |
| 0200 | R | 1000 | L | 1800 | chair |
| 0400 | L | 1200 | chair | 2000 | L |
| 0600 | R | 1400 | L | 2200 | R |

COMMENTS:_____

_____

**FIGURE 34-5** Positioning and positioning schedules are observed by surveyors.

## Interviews

During the tour the surveyors try to find residents who would be suitable to interview. During the interview, the surveyor asks the residents questions about their care, the food, the activities, the staff, and the environment. They also ask the residents whether their questions and concerns are handled promptly and satisfactorily. Several families are also selected for interviews. The questions are similar to those asked of residents. Group interviews are held during a meeting of a residents' council. The meeting is open to all residents.

## RESPONSIBILITIES OF THE NURSING ASSISTANTS DURING SURVEY

Surveyors spend several hours making observations on the nursing units. Remember to remain calm, cool, and collected if a surveyor is observing you as you care for the residents. Carry out your assignment as you normally would. The survey process is much less stressful if you always use good work habits. This means that you make it a point to:

- Always follow the residents' rights.
- Know the residents and their care plans.
- Know the policies and procedures for your facility.
- Attend in-service sessions regularly so you know about new information or changes that occur.
- Be informed of quality assurance activities within the facility.

Surveyors are responsible for evaluating the care given by your facility. They must make observations and ask questions of the staff to do their jobs properly. They may observe:

- Meal times and feeding procedures
- Nursing assistants doing passive range of motion exercises with residents (Figure 34-6)
- Positioning procedures
- Handwashing
- Nurses doing medication passes
- Nurses doing treatments

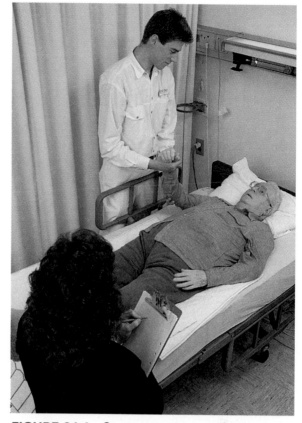

**FIGURE 34-6**  Surveyors may watch nursing assistants doing passive range of motion exercises.

In addition to making observations, surveyors may ask questions about:

- Problems listed on the residents' care plans
- Interventions or approaches that have been developed to overcome the problems
- Residents' rights
- What nursing assistants are expected to do for specific residents

If a surveyor asks you a question you cannot answer, be honest and say "I do not know the answer, but I will find out for you." Be sure you know where to find information that may be asked. Do not give excuses such as:

- "I don't usually work on this floor."
- "No one ever told me that."
- "I'm new here."

Do not try to outsmart a surveyor. They know the "tricks" that may be used to cover up for a lack of ability or information. The attitudes of the staff can go a long way to avoid problems with the survey process.

## Survey Completion

After the surveyors have collected all the information they need they complete an information analysis to determine whether any **deficiencies** (lack of compliance with all relevant standards) have been noted. They write out their findings. They present the findings at an **exit conference**. People who attend the exit conference include:

- All surveyors who were present in the facility throughout the survey
- Representatives from the residents' council
- Management staff

At the exit conference:

- The lead surveyor goes over the results of the information analysis.
- Other members of the survey team may also make comments. The team explains why and how they developed the findings.
- A written report is given to the administrator.

The findings of the surveyor may include:

- Comments about improvements that are needed in caregiving, procedures, records, or the environment
- Deficiencies that must be corrected

A deficiency can result in a monetary fine of as much as $10,000 per day if it is for a life-threatening problem.

The administrator and management staff must complete a document called the **plan of correction** after the survey. The plan of correction includes all actions the facility staff will take to correct the problems noted during the exit conference. These actions may include:

- In-service education
- Writing and implementing new policies or procedures
- Improvements to the physical environment

The survey process should be viewed as a learning experience. Although it may be stressful, the survey can help the facility staff to improve the quality of life for the residents.

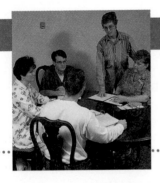

## Lesson Synthesis: Putting It All Together

*Y*ou have just completed this lesson. Now go back and review the Clinical Focus. Try to see how the Clinical Focus relates to the concepts presented in this lesson. Then answer the following questions.

1. What suggestions would you give Kathy to help her remain calm, cool, and collected during the survey process?

2. How would you relate the survey process to the quality of care within a facility?

3. What should nursing assistants know about the residents and the facility?

4. What specific actions can nursing assistants take in order to help make a successful survey?

## REVIEW

**A. Select the one best answer for each of the following.**

1. The purpose of a survey is to
   a. punish the health care facility
   b. create stress for the staff
   c. review the quality of life and the quality of care given to residents
   d. all of these

2. The survey team is made up of
   a. health care professionals
   b. nursing assistants from other facilities
   c. families of residents
   d. police officers

3. To prepare for a survey, the facility will
   a. check the environment for needed repairs and cleaning
   b. determine whether staff are following the residents' care plans
   c. go over results of surveys for the last few years
   d. all of these

4. The first thing the survey team does when they arrive at the facility is to
   a. watch nursing assistants do procedures
   b. interview residents
   c. take a tour of the facility
   d. read residents' medical records

5. Surveyors observe to see that standards are being met for
   a. safety
   b. infection control
   c. residents' rights
   d. all of these

**B. Answer each statement true (T) or false (F).**

6. T   F   All health care facilities are surveyed on a regular basis.

7. T   F   Certification is a process that is completed for facilities to receive government funds.

8. T   F   The survey team notifies facilities when they will be arriving.

9. T   F   The ombudsman is a member of the survey team.

10. T   F   Surveyors do not want staff and residents to know that they are in the building.

11. T   F   Surveyors will interview residents.

12. T   F   Nursing assistants are not expected to participate in a survey.

13. T   F   If a surveyor asks a question you cannot answer, you should respond, "I do not know the answer, but I will find out for you."

14. T   F   The survey team conducts an exit conference at the end of the survey.

15. T   F   The plan of correction may include in-service education.

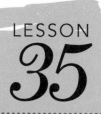

## LESSON 35

# Seeking Employment

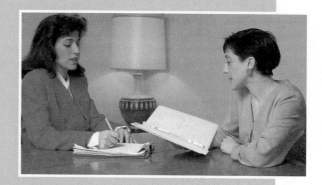

**CLINICAL FOCUS**

Think of the process involved in

successfully seeking employment

as you study this lesson and

meet:

*R*uby Stepp, who has just completed a program that has prepared her to work in a long-term care facility. She has passed all tests. Ruby is now ready to enter a field of service and personal satisfaction as she seeks her first full employment.

## OBJECTIVES

*After studying this lesson, you should be able to:*

- Define and spell vocabulary words and terms.
- List objectives to be met in obtaining and maintaining employment.

- List sources of nursing assistant employment.
- Develop a process for self-evaluation.
- Get set for a successful interview.
- Prepare a résumé and letter of resignation.

## VOCABULARY

**cross-training** *(kros-**TRAYN**-ing)*
**interview** *(**IN**-ter-vue)*
**networking** *(**NET**-werk-ing)*

**references** *(**REF**-er-en-ses)*
**résumé** *(**REH**-zoo-may)*

## CONGRATULATIONS ARE IN ORDER

You have done it! You have passed the certification tests and have proven your ability in the clinical area. You are now certified and are ready

to make your contribution to the care of residents in a long-term care facility.

You will now begin the search for available positions and prepare yourself to apply for them. You can do several things to make the search easier and more productive.

## STEP I—SELF-APPRAISAL ⋯⋯⋯

The first step is a self-appraisal—an honest look at your own strengths and limitations (Figure 35-1). You can do this by making a list.

On one side of a sheet of paper, list all the things you have to offer an employer. Be as specific as you can about personal as well as educational assets or strengths. For example, write statements about:

- Your sense of responsibility—Are you a punctual person?
- Your nursing assistant skills—How well trained and prepared are you?
- Your attitude—Are you caring and patient?
- Your personal appearance—Are you clean and neat at all times?

These are important characteristics in a successful nursing assistant.

On the other side of the paper, list any restrictions to your employment. Write statements about:

- Your availability for work—Are there hours when you cannot work, for example, when you must be home to care for children?
- Preferred location of work—Do you have to work within a specific area because you rely on public transportation?
- Personal responsibilities you may have—Do you have any responsibilities that may interfere with the performance of a job?

Think of ways to manage your responsibilities so they will not interfere with your employability. For example, if you have an elderly parent living with you and must be home to prepare meals, is there a neighbor or other family member who could prepare meals on the days or hours that you work?

Put the list away and then review it in a day or two. There may be items you will want to add or revise.

## STEP II—POSSIBILITY SEARCH ⋯⋯

You have listed your strengths and limitations. Now it is time to search for job possibilities. Where do you look?

- Start with the newspapers.
  - The classified advertisements are your best bet here (Figure 35-2). Circle those that list positions located within your desired work area and that have openings for the shift you need to work.
  - Look in the telephone book for facilities in your area.
  - List names, numbers, and addresses. Follow up and contact them.
- Investigate the facility in which you had your clinical experience. Nursing administrators

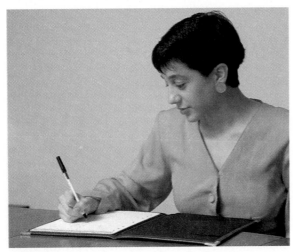

**FIGURE 35-1** Nursing assistant listing strengths and limitations

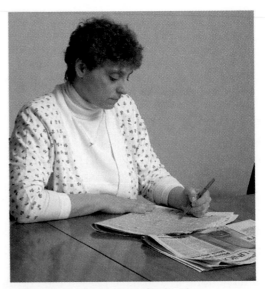

**FIGURE 35-2** The classified ads are a good place to start your job search.

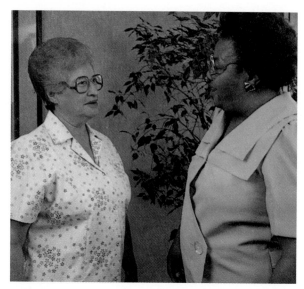

**FIGURE 35-3**  Friends, classmates, and colleagues are valuable sources of information about potential jobs.

often will invite nursing assistants who have trained in their facilities to join the staff on completion of training. There are advantages to this policy. For one thing, you have already spent time in the facility so less time is needed to orient you as a new employee. Also, the staff has had time to evaluate you while observing you during your training period.

- Networking is a valuable technique that can reveal opportunities (Figure 35-3). Let friends and colleagues know that you are looking for employment. Jobs are often located on the recommendation of a network of friends. Making connections and learning of opportunities through people one meets is called **networking**. Networking means gathering a group of people with similar needs and interests to learn about:
  - Working conditions
  - Job openings
  - Special ways of carrying out your responsibilities

## STEP III—THE RÉSUMÉ

A **résumé** is a summary of your education and prior work experience. The résumé should be neatly prepared, preferably typed. It is helpful to a prospective employer to have the résumé before and after your interview is held.

When an employer interviews many applicants, it is sometimes difficult to remember all the information given during a particular conversation. A note on your résumé by the interviewer can make all the difference between being hired and not being hired.

The résumé should include:

- Your name, address, and telephone number
- Your educational background. List your most recent education first, giving dates and a brief summary of the content.
- Your work history, especially if it shows successful experience in the same or related areas as the position for which you are applying. Include your work history over the past 5 years. List your most recent experience first.
- Other experiences you have had can be valuable. Jobs in which you have shown initiative, reliability, and trustworthiness are a plus and should be included. If you have not had paid employment, indicate how you spent your time. Worthwhile endeavors that might be included are:
  - Taking care of children
  - Finishing school
  - Doing volunteer work for your church or community
- List three references (people who know you and can comment on your character and abilities). *Note:* You must get permission from your references before using their names.
- Include some personal information, such as hobbies and other interests. It is not necessary to include your:
  - Ethnic origin
  - Religion
  - Age
  - Marital status

*Note:* Some people feel that to include personal information such as height, weight, sex, marital status, or religious affiliation is an invasion of privacy. Some of this information may be discussed in the interview, but it is not necessary to include it on your résumé.

Make several copies of your résumé. Always keep the original so that you can make more copies if necessary. Put a copy in your own file.

Carry a copy of your résumé whenever you seek employment. It is a ready reference as you fill out forms.

## STEP IV—REFERENCES

**References** are people who know you and who are willing to comment, either in writing or over the telephone, about you and your abilities. The references need to know you well enough to make an honest evaluation, but they should not be part of your family. Always get permission to use their names before listing references in your résumé. This is a matter of courtesy and ethics.

You may want to refresh the memory of your references about dates of employment or experiences that you have listed in your résumé. When listing these references be sure to include:

- Names
- Accurate titles
- Addresses
- Telephone numbers

## STEP V—TAKING THE STEP

You have made your assessment of your strengths, limitations, and needs. You have searched the market for opportunities and prepared your résumé. Now you must apply for a job:

- Select three facilities that you are most interested in.
- Call and ask for the Director of Nursing or Personnel Department (Figure 35-4).
- If you are responding to advertisements in the newspaper, follow the printed instructions about the person to contact and if your résumé must be mailed or personally delivered to the facility.
- Ask if there are any openings for a nursing assistant. If yes, ask what application procedure is to be followed.

The person in charge of hiring may ask you some questions about your education and experience, so be prepared to answer in a positive manner. He or she may set up an appointment for an **interview**. This is a specific time to meet and discuss your possible employment. Before you call, it is helpful if you know when you will

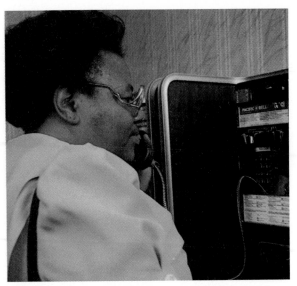

**FIGURE 35-4** Call for an appointment for an interview.

be available and how you would reach the facility to keep the appointment.

Before hanging up:

- Obtain the name of the person to whom you are speaking.
- Thank this person by name.

## STEP VI—THE INTERVIEW (PUTTING YOUR BEST FOOT FORWARD)

You must sell yourself during the interview. Prepare carefully for the interview by.

- Planning what you will wear
  - Do not overdress.
  - Be sure your clothes are neat and clean.
  - Polish your shoes.
  - Check your clothes for loose or lost buttons or stains; repair hems if necessary.
- Being sure to use deodorant
- Making sure your hair is clean and neat
- Making sure a beard or mustache is trimmed

Next, make a list of information you want to share with the interviewer (Figure 35-5). You will of course share your background and answer questions the interviewer will ask. The interviewer will want proof of citizenship. Many facil-

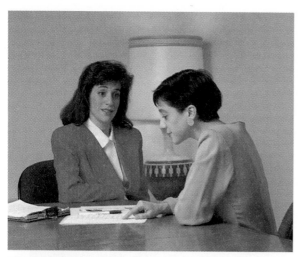

**FIGURE 35-5**   Be prepared for the interview. Know what you want to learn and what you want to share with the interviewer.

ities require drug testing and a criminal background check. Information from the certified nursing assistant registry of each state in which you were previously employed will be gathered. Be honest.

You will be asked to complete an employment application. Be sure you have a copy of your résumé for reference.

In turn, you will want to learn the following:

- Starting salary
- Schedule of raises
- Fringe benefits
    - Holiday pay or overtime
    - Health benefits
- Hours of work
- Responsibilities (ask for a job description)
- Uniform regulations
- Opportunities for growth (in-service, education, and orientation)

Make sure your interview is a success:

- Be on time for your interview. Promptness indicates interest and dependability.
- Stand until you are invited to sit down—then do so.
- Thank the interviewer(s) at the end of the interview, whether you are hired or not.
- Leave a copy of your résumé, if you have not already done so. If an opening occurs in the near future, your file is available and you will be remembered.

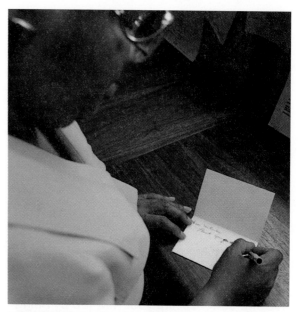

**FIGURE 35-6**   Send a thank-you note after the interview. It is considerate and helps the interviewer remember you.

After the interview:

- Go home and congratulate yourself if you were hired.
- If you were not hired, do not be discouraged. Think through the interview. Consider changes you may want to make in your answers in future interviews.
- Send a short thank-you note to the person who interviewed you. Thank the person for giving you the opportunity to be interviewed for the job (Figure 35-6).

Job hunting is not easy. It is emotionally stressful and can be physically exhausting. Keep trying and you will find a position to challenge you. Good luck!

## KEEPING THE JOB

Getting the job was only the beginning; now you must keep it. You can secure your position if you:

- Arrive on time (Figure 35-7).
- Perform your work as taught, and be flexible to change.
- Follow the rules of ethical and legal conduct.
- Maintain an open positive attitude; be ready to learn and grow. *Remember:* Learning is a lifelong challenge.

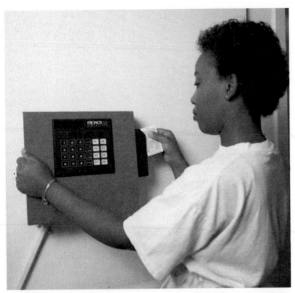

**FIGURE 35-7** Secure your new job by being prompt.

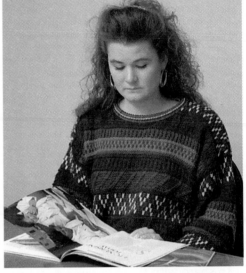

**FIGURE 35-8** Take every opportunity you can to increase your knowledge.

## GROWING

You will continue to grow if you take advantage of each new experience and the opportunities you find.

- Watch experienced staff members and learn by their example.
- Do not be afraid to ask questions at the appropriate times.
- Use the nursing and medical literature that is available to learn more about the conditions of the residents (Figure 35-8).
- Participate in the care plan conferences with an open mind so that each can become a learning experience for you.
- Listen to your periodic evaluation with an open mind and follow the suggestions for improvement.

Investigate ways of advancing your education, such as:

- A general education course offered at the high school or college in your area
- Courses in communication, listening, English, and psychology. These can be helpful in your career.
- **Cross-training** courses to increase your skills in related work. For example, you may be trained to draw blood or perform specific

respiratory care procedures. Such a program may be available in your facility, at a local community college or vocational school, or in an acute care hospital.

- Courses offered for continuing education credit for nurses. These are sometimes available, without credit and at a reduced price, for nonlicensed persons.
- Courses offered by hospitals or public health facilities on subjects of general public interest, such as hypertension, weight control, and diabetes
- Selecting books at the library about aging and the aging process
- Programs that can prepare you for professional development as a licensed practical nurse or registered nurse
- Learning about advanced positions in your own facility for which you may be qualified now or could study to qualify for at a later time

### In-Service Education

All staff members are expected to participate in in-service education programs. This is called staff development. Some of the programs will be attended by all members of the interdisciplinary team. Other programs may be presented for nursing assistants only (Figure 35-9). OBRA

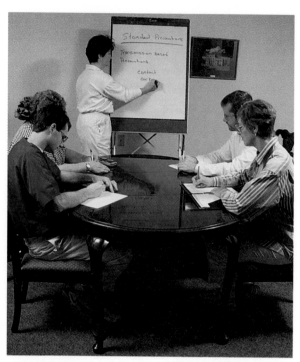

**FIGURE 35-9** In-service education helps the staff grow in their understanding of residents and their needs.

requires that all nursing assistants participate in a minimum of 12 hours of in-service education each year. At these programs, you will learn:

- New or revised state and federal regulations
- New facility policies

- New procedures for resident care
- Use of new equipment
- Care of residents with unusual diagnoses or unique problems
- Issues in health care

The more you learn, the better you can care for residents and the more you will enjoy your work.

## RESIGNING

The time may come when you find it necessary to leave your current job. To do this properly, you should give notice as early as possible and submit a letter of resignation. Appropriate notice is usually equal to the time of a pay period, or 2 weeks on the average.

Your letter of resignation should include:

- The date
- A salutation to the Director of Nursing
- A brief explanation of your reasons for leaving. *Note:* Even if you feel upset by something that happened, make your reasons positive in nature.
- The date your resignation is to be effective
- A thank-you for the opportunity to have worked and learned as an employee of the facility
- Your signature

Remember that if you do not work as a nursing assistant in long-term care for 24 months, you must recertify before you can be re-employed.

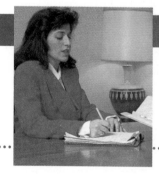

## LESSON SYNTHESIS: Putting It All Together

*Y*ou have just completed this lesson. Now go back and review the Clinical Focus. Try to see how the Clinical Focus relates to the concepts presented in the lesson. Then answer the following questions.

1. Why is honest self-appraisal the first step a nursing assistant must take when seeking employment?

2. Why should a reference be someone who is unrelated to the applicant?

3. Why is it important to dress "appropriately" for an interview?

4. Why is it important to be truthful during the initial interview about any limitations or restrictions related to employment?

## REVIEW

**A. Match each term (items a.–d.) with the proper definition.**

a. interview    c. references
b. networking    d. résumé

1. _____ gathering a group of people with similar needs and interests to learn about work-related opportunities

2. _____ specific time to meet and discuss possible employment

3. _____ summary of education and work experiences

4. _____ people who know you and are willing to comment about you and your abilities

**B. Answer each statement true (T) or false (F).**

5. T  F  The first step in preparing to find a job is to call for an interview.

6. T  F  A positive attitude is important in a person who is seeking a job.

7. T  F  Personal appearance is important in making a first impression on a prospective employer.

8. T  F  After giving a person's name as a reference you should always obtain permission from that person.

9. T  F  During the interview you should learn about the responsibilities of the job.

10. T  F  Thank the interviewer whether you are hired or not.

11. T  F  Being prompt to an interview indicates interest.

12. T  F  Before the interview, you should make a list of the information you want to share with the interviewer and the information you want from the interviewer.

**C. Provide brief answers for each of the following:**

13. List two factors that may limit the location where you can work.

14. Name three places to start looking for job opportunities.

**D. Select the one best answer for each of the following.**

15. When completing a résumé, include your
    a. ethnic origin
    b. religion
    c. educational background
    d. marital status

16. A person listed as a reference should be able to comment on your
    a. character and abilities
    b. age and marital status
    c. religion and ethnic origin
    d. height and weight

17. When listing a reference, be sure to include the person's
    a. place of employment
    b. ethnic origin
    c. marital status
    d. accurate telephone number

18. You can grow in your career if you
    a. never ask questions
    b. attend related educational courses
    c. do not attend care plan conferences
    d. read books on flower arranging

19. During the interview you will want to learn about
    a. salary
    b. benefits
    c. hours of work
    d. all of these

**E. Clinical experience**

20. Sarah has been employed by her facility for a year. She enjoys her work and the people she works with but she would like to be more challenged. What actions can she take to help her meet her needs?

21. Tilly has just received her evaluation. Her supervisor suggested several ways she can improve her performance. Tilly is upset by the evaluation and complains about her supervisor to her friend during lunch. What do you think of Tilly's response? Is it a productive response? How would you respond?

22. Charlie is going to his first in-service education meeting. What kinds of information might he learn? How many hours of in-service education must Charlie have each year?

# Glossary

**abbreviation**  shortened form of a word or phrase

**abdominal**  area of trunk between thorax and pelvis

**abdominopelvic cavity**  the body cavity extending between the diaphragm and the floor of the pelvis

**abduction**  movement away from midline or center

**accelerated**  increased motion, as in pulse or respiration

**acceptance**  favorable reception

**accuracy**  completing assignments carefully, without mistakes

**acetone**  a colorless liquid produced in the body; found in small quantities in normal urine and larger amounts in diabetic urine

**active assistive range of motion**  carrying out of specific exercises by the resident with some help from the care provider; exercises are designed to move each joint through its range of motion

**active range of motion**  resident carries out exercises without help; all joints are moved through their full range of motion

**activities of daily living (ADL)**  the activities necessary for resident to fulfill basic human needs

**adaptive behavior**  the degree to which a person meets standards of personal independence and social responsibility appropriate for the person's age and culture

**adaptive device**  ordinary items that are modified or changed in some way so that the device can be used by individuals with specific disabilities

**adduction**  movement toward midline or center

**administrator**  one who manages a facility

**adrenal glands**  two glands, located one on top of each kidney, that produce hormones

**adrenaline**  epinephrine—hormone produced by adrenal glands

**advance directive**  a document signed before the diagnosis of a terminal illness when the individual is still in good health indicating the person's wishes regarding care during dying

**advocate**  one who speaks and acts on behalf of another

**age-related macular degeneration**  cause of blindness in elderly

**agitation**  an increase in physical activity usually accompanied by anger and irritation

**aiding and abetting**  not reporting dishonest acts that are observed

**AIDS**  acquired immune deficiency syndrome; a condition caused by the HIV virus

**airborne precautions**  techniques to prevent transmission of airborne organisms

**akinesia**  abnormal absence or poverty of movement

**alignment**  proper position

**allergen**  substance that causes sensitivity or allergic reactions

**alopecia**  hair loss

**alveoli**  tiny air sacs that make up the bulk of the lungs

**Alzheimer's disease**  a disorder of the brain that involves thinking, memory, and judgment; a form of dementia

**ambulate**  to walk

**amenorrhea**  abnormal cessation or absence of the menses

**amputation**  removal of a limb or other body appendage

**amulet**  protective charm

**anatomic position**  standing erect, facing observer, feet flat on the floor; arms extended, palms forward

**anatomy**  study of the structure of the human body

**anemia**  deficiency of red blood cells in the blood

**aneurysm**  a sac formed by dilation of the wall of a blood vessel (usually an artery) and filled with blood; a weak spot in an arterial wall

**anger**  feeling of hostility or rage

**angina pectoris**  acute pain in the chest caused by interference with the supply of oxygen to the heart

**ankle-foot orthosis**  assistive device that provides medial lateral support for an unstable ankle

**anorexia**  loss of appetite

**anoxia**  lack of oxygen

**anterior**  in anatomy, in front of the coronal or ventral plane

**antibiotic**  medication to fight infection caused by bacteria

**antibodies**  proteins formed in the body that protect a person against a specific infectious organism

**antidepressant**  medication effective against depressive illness

**antigen**  a foreign or pathogenic substance that enters the body and stimulates the production of antibodies

**antihypertensive**  medication effective against hypertension (high blood pressure)

**anuria**  absence of secretions of urine by the kidneys

**anus**   the outlet of the rectum lying in the fold between the buttocks

**aorta**   the great artery arising from the left ventricle

**apathy**   indifference; lack of emotion

**apex**   the top of a cone-shaped structure, such as the heart

**aphasia**   language impairment; loss of ability to comprehend normally

**apical**   pertaining to the apex of a structure such as the heart

**apical pulse**   pulse rate taken by placing stethoscope over tip of heart

**apnea**   period of no respirations

**approach**   steps to be taken to reach a goal

**Aquamatic K-Pad®**   commercial unit for applying heat or cold

**arteriosclerosis**   general term meaning a narrowing of the blood vessels, which can result in subsequent tissue hypoxia; degeneration and hardening of the walls of arteries and sometimes of the valves of the heart

**artery**   a vessel through which the blood passes away from the heart to various parts of the body

**arthritis**   joint inflammation

**articulation**   point where two bones meet

**artificial nutrition**   ways other than eating to provide nutrition for a resident

**ascites**   fluid accumulation in the abdomen

**asepsis**   without infection

**asepto syringe**   glass syringe with rubber ball used to perform moist treatments

**aspiration**   drawing foreign material into the respiratory tract

**assault**   violent act; an unlawful threat or attempt to harm another physically

**assessment**   act of evaluating

**assignments**   a designated list of duties

**assistive device**   equipment used to help people be more effective in their physical activity; helps promote/maintain independence in performing activities of daily living

**asthenia**   weakness

**asthma**   a chronic respiratory disease characterized by bronchospasms and excessive mucus production

**ataxic cerebral palsy**   form of cerebral palsy in which the principal disturbance is a lack of balance and coordination

**atherosclerosis**   degenerative process involving the lining of arteries, in which the lumen eventually narrows and closes; a form of arteriosclerosis; primarily associated with some degree of atheroma development

**athetoid cerebral palsy**   form of cerebral palsy characterized by involuntary, slow, incessant movements of the parts of the body that are affected

**atrium (pl. *atria*)**   one of the upper heart chambers

**atrophy**   shrinking or wasting away of tissues

**attitude**   the state of mind that is indicative of feelings or opinions

**audiologist**   physician specializing in hearing problems

**auditory nerve**   nerve carrying sound from the ear to the brain

**aura**   a peculiar sensation preceding the appearance of more definite symptoms in a convulsion or seizure

**aural**   pertaining to the ear

**autoclave**   a sterilizing machine

**autoimmune**   antibodies against components of the body

**axilla**   the armpit

**bacteremia**   the presence of bacteria in the blood

**bargaining**   attempting to make a "deal" to influence the final outcome of a situation

**battery**   an unlawful threat or attempt to harm another physically

**behavioral modification**   an approach that is based on rewarding positive behaviors and initiating corrective action for negative behaviors

**benign prostatic hypertrophy**   noncancerous enlargement of the prostate gland

**bile**   a secretion of the liver needed to prepare fats for digestion

**biohazard**   contaminated with blood or body fluids and having the potential to transmit disease

**bladder**   a membranous sac containing fluid, such as the urinary bladder

**blood pressure**   pressure of blood exerted against the vascular walls

**body alignment**   correct and straight body position

**body language**   nonverbal communication signaled by behavior, facial expressions, body stance

**body mechanics**   using muscles correctly to move or lift heavy objects properly

**bowel**   intestine

**Bowman's capsule**   tubule surrounding the glomerulus of the nephron

**bradycardia**   unusually slow heartbeat

**braille**   system of raised dots representing letters A through Z and numbers 0 through 9 that allows sight-impaired residents to "read" through the sense of touch

**brain stem**   part of the brain including the medulla oblongata, diencephalon, pons, and midbrain

**bridging**   technique used to reduce pressure on ischemic areas by use of pillows and pads

**bronchi** primary divisions of the trachea

**bronchioles** one of the finer subdivisions or branches of the bronchial tree

**bronchitis** inflammation of the bronchi

**burnout** loss of enthusiasm and interest in an activity

**bursae** small synovial-filled sacs located around joints that help reduce friction

**bursitis** inflammation of a bursa

**calculi** stones or concretions

**calorie restricted diet** a diet that limits the intake of calories

**cancer** a malignant tumor; malignancy

**cannula** a small tube that may be inserted into a cavity to allow the passage of fluid

**capillary** hairlike blood vessel; the link between arterioles and venules

**carbohydrates** energy foods; used by the body to produce heat and for work

**carbon dioxide** gas that is a waste product in cellular metabolism

**cardiac arrest** sudden heart stoppage

**cardiac cycle** all the events (mechanical and electrical) that occur between one contraction and the next; the series of movements through which the heart passes in performing one heartbeat

**cardiac muscle** special tissue making up the muscular wall of the heart

**cardiogram** a record of cardiac pulsation produced by cardiograph

**cardiopulmonary resuscitation (CPR)** emergency medical procedure undertaken to restart and sustain heart and respiratory function

**cardiovascular** pertaining to the heart and blood vessels

**care plan** plan developed by the interdisciplinary health care team that describes the goals and approaches that all team members are to use in caring for the resident

**care plan conference** a meeting of team members to plan resident care

**caries** dental cavities

**carrier** a person who harbors infectious organisms that can be transmitted to others but who shows no sign of illness personally

**cartilage** type of connective tissue

**cast** rigid covering to keep a joint or other body part immobile

**cataract** opacity of the lens, resulting in loss of vision

**catastrophic reaction** response characterized by increased agitation and anxiety

**catheter** tube for evacuating or injecting fluids

**cavity** an enclosed area

**cell** basic unit in the organization of living substance

**cellular respiration** physiologic process that takes place in the cells by which cellular energy is derived

**cellulose** a basic substance of all plant foods, which can supply the body with roughage

**Celsius** scale for measuring temperature

**centimeter** one-hundredth of a meter

**central nervous system** brain and spinal cord

**central venous catheter** small tube placed in a major vein, such as the subclavian vein

**cerebellum** part of the brain responsible for balance and muscle coordination

**cerebral** pertaining to the brain

**cerebral palsy** motor disorder that results in inability to control body movement

**cerebrospinal fluid** watery, clear fluid that surrounds the brain and spinal cord

**cerebrovascular accident (CVA)** interference with the cerebral blood flow

**cerebrum** largest and main portion of the brain responsible for sensory interpretation and voluntary muscle activity

**character (of pulse)** rhythm and volume of pulse

**chart** record of information concerning resident

**cheeking** storing food in one side of the mouth

**chemical restraint** drugs used to influence or control a resident's behavior

**chemotherapy** treatment with drugs or chemicals

**Cheyne-Stokes respiration** periods of apnea alternating with periods of hyperpnea

**CHF** congestive heart failure

**chlamydia** rod-shaped microbes that can cause trachoma, a serious eye infection, and sexually transmitted infections

**choroid** the vascular layer, or coat, of the eye

**chronic** persisting over a long period

**chronic bronchitis** condition in which there is excessive mucus secretion in the bronchi

**chronic disease** a condition that continues over a long period

**chronic obstructive pulmonary disease (COPD)** any condition that causes interference with normal respirations over a prolonged period, such as emphysema

**chux** disposable pads sometimes placed under residents as a linen saver

**clear liquid diet** a diet in which all nutrients must be in the form of liquid that is clear

**clergy** ministers, priests, rabbis; religious leaders

**client** resident

**climacteric** menopause; the combined phenomena accompanying the cessation of the reproductive function in the female or diminution of testicular activity in the male

**clitoris** a small, cylindrical mass of erotic tissue; part of the external female reproductive organs analogous to the penis in the male

**CNS** central nervous system

**code blue order** a signal given when a resident is in danger of dying so that lifesaving techniques can be used

**cognitive impairment** a term used to describe any form of dementia

**colon** large intestine

**colonized** establishment of a population of micro-organisms growing on body surfaces but not necessarily causing an infection

**colostomy** a surgically established opening between the colon and the surface of the abdomen to allow elimination of feces

**comatose** unconscious; in a coma

**combining forms** parts of words that may be arranged in different ways to form new words

**comminuted fracture** fracture in which the bone is broken or crushed into small pieces

**commode** a portable toilet

**communal** pertaining to something that is shared with others

**communicable** capable of being transferred from one person to another directly or indirectly, such as infectious disease

**communicate** to make known

**communication** transmission of a message from a sender to a receiver

**community services** special services provided outside of the facility

**compensation** in psychology, the act of seeking a substitute for something unacceptable or unattainable

**compound fracture** fracture in which the broken bone protrudes through the skin

**comprehension** the capacity of the mind for understanding

**concentration** an increase in strength by evaporation

**condom** a rubber sheath used to cover the penis

**confidential** keeping what is said or written to oneself; private; nonsharing

**congestive heart failure** a chronic inability of the heart to maintain an adequate output of blood from one or both ventricles, resulting in an inadequate blood supply to the body tissues

**conjunctiva** mucous membrane that covers the eye and lines the eyelids

**connective tissue** special body tissue that holds other tissues together and provides support for organs and other structures of body

**connective tissue cells** cells that produce connective tissue

**constipation** difficulty in defecating

**constricting** making narrower

**constriction** narrowed or compressed area

**consultant** one who offers professional advice

**contact precautions** practices used to prevent the spread of pathogens by direct or indirect contact

**contagious** communicable or easily spread

**contaminated** unclean; impure; soiled with germs

**continent** able to control elimination of feces and urine

**contract** an agreement between two or more people, especially one that is written; to shorten, to decrease in size

**contracture** permanent shortening or contraction of a muscle because of spasm or paralysis

**convalescent home** long-term care facility

**convulsion** involuntary muscle spasm

**COPD** chronic obstructive pulmonary disease; for example, pulmonary emphysema

**cornea** clear (transparent) anterior covering of the eye

**coronary occlusion** closing off or blockage of a coronary artery

**corporal punishment** use of painful treatment to correct behavior

**cortex** the outer covering or portions of an organ

**cortisone** hormone produced by the adrenal cortex

**cubic centimeter (cc)** a measurement of volume equal to 1000 cubic millimeters

**culture and sensitivity** taking a sample from an infected area to discover the cause of the infection and then determine the proper antibiotic therapy; the organisms are grown and their reactions to different antibiotics determined

**cutaneous** relating to the skin

**cutaneous membrane** skin

**cuticle** area around the base of a fingernail or toenail

**CVA** cerebrovascular accident

**CVP** central venous pressure; measurement of blood pressure in the large central veins

**cyanosis** bluish skin discoloration from lack of oxygen

**cyanotic** pertaining to blueness most commonly observed under the nails, lips and skin as a result of lack of oxygen

**cystocele** bladder hernia

**cystoscopy** procedure using cystoscope for visualization of the urinary bladder, ureter, and kidney

**day care center** a place where senior citizens may go for various services

**day room** a room in a long-term care residence where residents can meet for activities and socialization at times other than meal time

**debilitating**   weakening

**debridement**   removal of foreign matter or devitalized tissue from a wound

**deconditioned**   condition in which tissue and organs become weakened from lack of use

**decubiti**   pressure sores; bedsores; decubitus ulcers

**defamation of character**   making false or damaging statements about another person that damages that person's reputation

**defecation**   bowel movement that expels feces

**defense mechanism**   psychological reaction or technique for protection against a stressful environmental situation or anxiety

**dehydration**   excessive loss of fluid from the body

**delirium**   disordered mental condition in which speech is incoherent, fever may occur, and illusions, delusions, and hallucinations may be experienced

**delusion**   a false belief

**dementia**   progressive mental deterioration caused by organic brain disease

**dendrite**   the branch of a neuron conducting impulses toward the cell body

**denial**   an unconscious defense mechanism in which an occurrence or observation is refused recognition as reality to avoid anxiety or pain

**dental hygienist**   a person licensed and specially trained to perform oral hygiene, including cleaning of teeth

**dentist**   a person licensed and specially trained to practice dentistry and/or dental surgery

**dentures**   false teeth

**deoxygenated**   to have lost oxygen

**dependability**   trustworthiness; reliability

**depressant**   something (a drug, for example) that decreases functional activity

**depression**   feelings of sadness and unresponsiveness

**dermal ulcer (decubitus)**   pressure sore or bed sore

**dermis**   corium; true skin; the layer of skin beneath the epithelium

**deteriorate**   to progressively break down or disorganize

**developmental disability**   a severe, chronic disorder apparent before age 22, caused by mental or physical impairment

**developmental disease**   condition or disease that is present at birth or early childhood and limits a person's ability to provide self-care in an independent way

**developmental tasks**   in psychology, tasks that are normally carried out as steps in personality development

**diabetes mellitus**   a disorder of carbohydrate metabolism

**diabetic coma**   a comatose state of acidosis caused by diabetes mellitus

**diabetic ketoacidosis**   state of acidosis caused by diabetes mellitus

**diabetic retinopathy**   damage to the eye and vision as a result of diabetes mellitus

**diagnosis**   determination of the specific disease or condition causing a patient's symptoms

**diagnostic-related group**   classification that limits the number of days resident can stay in facility

**dialysis**   treatment when kidneys fail to remove accumulated wastes from the blood

**diaphoresis**   profuse sweating

**diaphragm**   dome-shaped muscle that divides the ventral cavity into a thorax and an abdominopelvic cavity

**diarrhea**   watery stool

**diarthrotic**   pertains to freely movable joints

**diastole**   period during which the heart muscle relaxes and the chamber fills with blood

**diastolic**   pertains to the relaxation phase of the cardiac cycle

**diathermy**   treatment with heat

**diet**   the food and drink necessary for body nourishment

**dietetics**   systematic regulation of the diet for therapeutic purposes

**dietitian**   a person specially trained in the field of nutrition and the science of dietetics (diets)

**digestion**   the process of converting food into an assimilable form

**dilating**   enlarging

**diplegia**   movement disturbance that primarily affects the legs

**directive**   serving or qualified to direct; a statement (document) that allows families, physicians, and nurses to follow the wishes of the individual when death occurs or is imminent

**dirty**   contaminated with microbes

**disability**   persistent physical or mental defect or handicap

**discharge planner**   person who arranges for care after discharge from facility and helps resident make the transition from the facility to the community

**discharge planning**   planning for care after resident leaves facility

**disinfected**   cleaned to destroy pathogens

**disinfection**   process of destroying pathogenic organisms or agents on articles or surfaces

**dislocation**   one bone displaced from its normal alignment with another

**disorientation**   loss of recognition of time, place, location, or persons

**displacement**   an unconscious defense mechanism in which an emotion such as anger is directed at the wrong person

**distal**   farthest away from a central point, such as point of attachment of muscles

**distended**   to be stretched

**diuretics**   drugs that increase urine output

**diverticula**   small blind pouches that form in the lining and wall of the colon

**diverticulitis**   inflammation of diverticula

**diverticulosis**   presence of many diverticula

**document**   the process of recording observations and data about a resident's condition

**documentation**   substantiating statements

**do not resuscitate (DNR)**   physician order indicating that resident is not to be revived when cardiac and respiratory arrest occur

**dorsal**   posterior or back

**dorsal cavity**   the posterior body cavity consisting of the cranium and vertebral canal

**draw sheet**   a sheet folded under resident and extending from above the shoulder to below the hips

**DRG**   diagnosis-related grouping

**drip chamber**   part of the equipment used to administer parenteral fluids

**droplet precautions**   practices used to prevent the spread of microbes transmitted by droplets in the air produced by laughing, talking, singing, sneezing, or coughing

**dry sterile dressing (DSD)**   a sterile dressing that is applied dry to a wound

**duodenum**   the first part of small intestine

**durable power of attorney**   a document that permits a person to delegate to another person the power to make any health care decisions that the person is unable to make

**dyspepsia**   indigestion

**dysphagia**   difficulty in swallowing

**dyspnea**   difficult or labored breathing

**dysuria**   painful urination

**edema**   excessive accumulation of fluid in the tissues

**ejaculation**   forcible, sudden expulsion of semen from the penis

**ejaculatory duct**   part of the male reproductive tract extending from the seminal vesicles to the urethra

**EKG**   electrocardiogram; a recording of the electrical activity of the heart

**electroencephalogram**   graphic recording of the electrical activity of the brain

**electrolytes**   compounds that play an essential role in body function

**elimination**   excretion; discharge from the body of indigestible materials and of waste products of body metabolism

**embolus**   blood clot that moves through the vascular system

**emergency**   unexpected occurrence that requires immediate action

**Emergency Medical Services (EMS)**   services provided by specially trained people at the scene of the emergency and in the ambulance

**emesis**   vomitus

**emesis basin**   utensil for catching vomitus

**emotional lability**   easily upset, emotionally unstable

**empathy**   intellectual understanding of something in another person that is foreign to one's self

**emphysema**   chronic obstructive pulmonary disease in which the alveolar walls are destroyed

**empowerment**   power or authority

**endocrine gland**   gland that secretes hormonal substances directly into bloodstream; ductless gland

**endometrium**   lining of the uterus

**endotracheal**   within the trachea

**endotracheal tube**   a tube placed in the trachea to assist respiration

**enema**   the introduction of liquid into the bowel or the rectum to be returned or retained

**enteral feeding**   feeding that bypasses the mouth and goes directly into the intestinal tract

**enteric**   pertaining to the alimentary canal; intestinal

**environment**   surroundings

**environmental services**   department and workers responsible for maintaining clean and comfortable surroundings for residents and staff

**enzymes**   organic catalysts produced by living cells but capable of acting independently of the cells producing them

**epidermis**   the top layer of skin

**epididymis**   an elongated, cordlike structure along the posterior border of the testes in the ducts of which the sperm is stored

**epidural catheter**   tube inserted into spinal area for delivery of medication

**epilepsy**   a noninfectious disorder of the brain manifested by episodes of motor and sensory dysfunction, which may or may not be accompanied by convulsions and unconsciousness

**epithelial cells**   cells that produce and form epithelial tissue

**epithelial tissue**   tissue that forms the skin and parts of the secreting glands and that lines the body cavities; specialized in its ability to absorb, secrete, excrete, and protect

**epithelium**   tissues characterized by tightly packed cells with a minimum of intracellular material; forms epidermis and lines all hollow organs and passages of respiratory, digestive, and genitourinary systems

**equilibrium**   sense of balance

**ergonomics**   techniques used by workers to avoid injuries

**erythrocyte**   red blood cell

**esophagus**   a tube extending from the pharynx to stomach

**estrogen**   hormone produced by ovaries

**ethical code**   rules governing the right or wrong of professional behavior

**ethics**   the study of standards of conduct or moral judgement

**evaluation**   judgment; critical review of a situation or condition; determination of how the resident's plan of care is working

**exacerbation**   period of increased severity of symptoms

**excreta**   excretions, such as feces

**expectorant**   medication to aid in expectoration (spitting up phlegm)

**expectorate**   spit

**expiration**   exhalation

**exposure incident**   a situation in which an individual has been in possible contact with infectious material

**extended care facility**   long-term care facility

**extension**   movement by which the two ends of any jointed part are drawn away from each other

**external fixation**   method of stabilizing fractured bones

**Fahrenheit (scale)**   scale for measuring temperature

**fallopian tube**   see **oviduct**

**false imprisonment**   detaining an individual without a reason and against the individual's will

**fantasizing**   imagining

**fasting**   the act of going without food over a definite and prolonged period

**fats**   nutrient used to store energy

**fecal impaction**   feces firmly wedged in the rectum

**feces**   semi-solid waste eliminated from the body

**femur**   thigh bone

**fiber**   nondigestible part of food that adds bulk to intestinal waste

**fistula**   abnormal tubelike passageway within body tissue

**flaccid**   soft, not firm; incapable of independent movement

**flatulence**   excessive gas in the stomach and intestines

**flatus**   gas or air in the stomach or intestines; air or gas expelled via any body opening

**flexed**   bent

**flora**   community of organisms living in or on a particular body area

**flow meter**   an instrument for controlling gas flow in oxygen equipment

**flow rate**   the speed at which a fluid such as glucose and water flows into an intravenous infusion, or a gas such as oxygen flows into an oxygen mask to a resident

**footboard**   appliance placed at the foot of the bed so the feet rest firmly against it; maintains feet at 90° angle to the legs

**forced fluids**   notation meaning that resident must be encouraged to take as much fluid as possible

**foreskin**   prepuce; loose tissue covering the penis and clitoris

**Fowler's position**   head of bed is rolled up and resident is in semi-sitting position

**fracture**   break in the continuity of bone

**frequency**   occurrence often repeated

**friction**   rubbing of one surface against another surface

**full liquid diet**   a diet in which all nutrients must be a liquid form

**functional ability**   ability to carry out activities of daily living

**functional changes**   decrease in ability to carry out activities of daily living

**gait**   manner of walking

**gait belt**   belt placed around the resident's waist to assist in ambulation

**gait training**   teaching the resident to walk

**gallbladder**   small, saclike organ found on the underside of the liver, which stores bile

**gangrene**   the death and putrefaction of body tissue, caused by stoppage of circulation of blood to an area

**gastritis**   inflammation of the stomach

**gastrointestinal tract**   intestinal or digestive tract

**gastrostomy**   surgical opening into the stomach

**gastrostomy tube (GT)**   tube surgically placed through the abdomen into the stomach for feeding

**gatch bed**   bed fitted with a jointed back rest and knee rest; resident can be raised to a sitting position and kept in that position; special bed that can be raised or lowered, and allows the head and knee areas to be elevated to different positions

**gavage**   feeding through a tube

**genetic disease**   condition caused by problems with the genes

**genital**   pertaining to reproduction

**genitalia**   the reproductive organs

**geriatrics**   care of the elderly

**germs**   pathogenic microorganisms

**gerontology**   study of the aging process

**glaucoma**   increased intraocular pressure, which ultimately results in loss of vision

**glomerulus**   a ball-like bed of capillaries that forms part of the nephron

**glucagon**   a hormone formed by the Islets of Langerhans in the pancreas; raises the glucose level of blood

**glucometer**   instrument used to measure blood sugar levels

**glucose**   simple sugar; also called dextrose

**glycosuria**   sugar in the urine

**goal**   objective outcome or result

**goiter**   enlargement of the thyroid gland

**gonads**   reproductive organs; ovaries (female) and testes (male)

**gonorrhea**   a sexually transmitted disease characterized by a purulent drainage from the mucous membranes of the genital organs

**gossip**   taling about residents at lunch time or on a break

**graft**   body tissue used for transplantation

**grand mal seizure**   a convulsion that involves the whole body; the person loses consciousness and may be incontinent

**Gray Panthers**   organization working for urgent reforms needed to protect the elderly

**grievance**   a circumstance felt to be unjust or in which there is grounds for complaint

**halitosis**   bad breath

**hallucination**   idea or perception that is not based on reality

**harmony**   friendly, pleasant relations

**heart**   hollow, muscular organ lying slightly to the left of the midline of the chest

**heart attack**   condition that makes the heart unable to function properly or at all

**heart block**   partial or complete inhibition of the speed of electrical impulse conduction from the atrium to the ventricle of the heart

**Heimlich maneuver**   technique used to dislodge food from the throat of a choking person

**hematuria**   blood in the urine

**hemianopia**   blindness in one-half of the visual field of one or both eyes

**hemiplegia**   paralysis on one side of the body

**hemodialysis**   removal of toxic products and excess fluid from the blood through a membrane

**hemoptysis**   expectoration of blood

**hemorrhage**   escape of blood from blood vessels

**hemorrhoids**   varicose veins in the rectum

**hepatitis**   inflammation of the liver

**hernia**   protrusion or projection of an organ or a part of an organ through the wall of a cavity that normally contains it

**herniorrhaphy**   surgial operation for hernia

**hiatal hernia**   protrusion of a portion of the stomach through the esophageal hiatus of the diaphragm

**high density**   concentrated

**high Fowler's position**   position in which the resident is sitting almost upright with knees flexed

**high protein diet**   a diet in which the protein content is increased beyond the usual

**home health services**   help provided after an acute hospitalization

**homeostasis**   a state of balance or equilibrium

**hormone**   secretion of endocrine gland; substance produced by endocrine gland

**hospice**   special facility or arrangement to provide care of terminally ill persons

**hot-line number**   a toll-free number residents may use to reach authorities outside the facility to register complaints

**hot soak**   a treatment in which a part of the body, such as a hand, is placed in warm water as a method of applying heat

**human immunodeficiency virus (HIV)**   microorganism that causes HIV disease that may progress to AIDS

**Huntington's disease**   progressive degenerative disease of the brain that results in uncontrolled movements and mental deterioration

**hygiene**   a system of principles or rules designed for the promotion of health

**hyperalimentation**   parenteral nutrition; nutrition delivered directly into the bloodstream

**hyperglycemia**   excessive level of blood sugar

**hypertension**   high blood pressure

**hyperthyroidism**   a condition in which the thyroid gland is enlarged

**hypertrophy**   increase in size of an organ or structure, which does not involve tumor formation

**hypoglycemia**   abnormally low level of sugar in the blood

**hypotension**   low blood pressure

**hypothermia**   greatly reduced temperature

**hypothyroidism**   inadequate functioning of the thyroid gland

**hypoxia**   lack of adequate oxygen supply

**hysterectomy**   surgical removal of the uterus

**I&O**   intake and output

**ice bag**   a plastic or rubber bag filled with small pieces of ice. The bag is covered with cloth and placed against a resident's body to apply cold

**ileostomy**   surgically made opening in the ileum through the abdominal wall

**ileum**   the lower three-fifths of the small intestine, lying between the jejunum and cecum

**illusion**   a mental impression derived from misinterpretation of an actual sensory stimulus

**IM**   intramuscular

**immunity**   ability of the body to fight off disease caused by microbes

**immunization**   process of making a person more resistant to infectious agents

**immunosuppression**   failure of the body to respond to the challenge of infectious disease organisms

**impaction**   condition of being tightly wedged into a part (as feces in the bowel)

**impairment**   disability

**implementation**   put into action; process of carrying out a plan

**impotence**   inhability to perform sexually

**incident**   something of consequence that happens unexpectedly. An event that might result in harm to a resident

**incontinence**   inability to predict and control elimination of body wastes

**indwelling catheter**   a small tube that remains in the patient for an extended period to provide continuous drainage

**infarction**   death of tissue

**infection**   the invasion and multiplication of any organism and the damage caused by this in the body

**inferior**   below another part

**inferior vena cava**   large vein that returns blood to the right atrium of the heart

**inflammation**   process that brings blood and white blood cells to the area of injury or infection, characterized by heat, redness, swelling, and pain

**inflammatory response**   tissue reaction to injury whether direct or referred

**influenza**   viral disease spread by droplets

**informed consent**   permission given by one who fully understands all the facts relating to what is going to happen

**infusion**   introduction of a solution into a vein by gravity such as an intravenous infusion (IV)

**inguinal hernia**   intestines push through abdominal wall in the groin area

**inhibition**   that which restrains an action, emotion, or thought

**insertion**   distal point of attachment of skeletal muscle

**inspiration**   the drawing of air into the lungs (inhalation)

**instrumental activities of daily living**   higher level tasks performed by adults, such as money management and driving

**insulin**   the active antidiabetic hormone secreted by the Islets of Langerhans in the pancreas; promotes utilization of sugar in the body

**insulin-dependent diabetes mellitus (IDDM)**   a condition in which the person must rely on insulin injections to metabolize glucose

**insulin shock**   hypoglycemia (a decrease in blood sugar), attended by anxiety, excitement, perspiration, delirium, or coma

**intake**   refers to any nourishment or fluid taken into the body; frequently refers to intake of everything that is liquid at room temperature

**integumentary system**   body system consisting of the skin, its various layers, and its accessory structures (hair, nails, and skin glands)

**intelligence quotient (IQ)**   the ability to solve problems, adapt to the demands of the environment, and to understand abstract relationships appropriate to one's age

**intention tremor**   trembling of hands that increases with efforts to control trembling

**intercourse**   interchange or communication between individuals; an alternate term for sexual relations

**interdisciplinary health care team**   group of health care providers in different specialties who act together to plan and implement the plan of care for each resident

**intermittent positive pressure breathing (IPPB)**   a technique in which a machine is used to deliver air or oxygen and medication under pressure to a person's lungs; technique for assisting breathing

**interpersonal relationships**   how people interact with each other

**intervention**   actions that influence the eventual outcome of a situation

**interventricular septum**   dividing portion between the ventricles of the heart

**interview**   meeting with a prospective employer and discussion regarding a position

**intravenous infusion**   nourishment given through a sterile tube into the veins

**intravenous therapy (intravenous infusion)**   nutrition or medication injected by means of a sterile needle and tubing directly into a vein

**invasion of privacy**   revealing information of a private nature regarding a resident

**involuntary muscle**   type of muscle forming the walls of organs; also known as visceral or smooth muscle

**involuntary seclusion**   being kept without care and apart from others against one's will

**iris**   colored portion of eye

**ischemia**   deficient blood supply to body tissues

**Islets of Langerhans**   special cells in the pancreas that produce insulin

**isolation**   place where resident with easily transmitted diseases is separated from others

**isolation technique**   special procedures carried out to prevent the spread of infectious organisms from infected persons

**jaundice**   yellowing of the skin

**jejunum**   that portion of the small intestine between the duodenum and the ileum

**job description**   the duties and responsibilities involved in a position

**joint**   point of articulation between bones

**Kardex**   a type of file in which nursing care plans are kept

**keratoses**   roughened, scaly, wartlike lesions

**ketones**   products from fat metabolism

**ketosis**   abnormal levels of ketones in the blood; a complication of diabetes mellitus

**kidney dialysis**   see **hemodialysis**

**kidneys**   glandular organs that secrete urine

**kilogram**   1,000 grams; 2.2 pounds

**kyphosis**   extreme dorsal curvature of the spine in the thoracic area (hunchback)

**labia majora**   two large, hair-covered, liplike structures that are part of the vulva

**labia minora**   two hairless liplike structures found beneath the labia majora

**lacerations**   an injury or wound made by tearing or cutting of the flesh

**lactose**   a form of sugar found in milk

**larynx**   part of the respiratory tract found on the top of the trachea just below the root of the tongue. It is the organ of voice

**last rites (sacraments of the sick)**   special service of confession and blessing practiced by clergy for Catholic residents when gravely ill

**lateral**   to the side; away from the midline

**lateral position**   side-lying position

**laxative**   medicine to relieve constipation

**legal guardian**   one who has the legal authority to make decisions and act on behalf of another

**leisure**   time free from engagement

**lens**   portion of the eye that bends light rays

**lentigines**   elevated yellow or brown spots or patches that occur on exposed skin; "liver spots"

**lesion**   abnormal change in tissue formation

**leukemia**   malignant disease of the blood-forming organs, characterized by abnormal proliferation and distortion of the leukocytes in the blood and bone marrow

**leukocyte**   white blood cell

**Lhermitte's sign**   seen in multiple sclerosis; a feeling of tingling and pain in the spinal column when head is flexed

**libel**   any oral or written defamatory statement

**libido**   sex drive

**licensed practical nurse (LPN)/licensed vocational nurse (LVN)**   a person licensed by the state who provides direct care under the supervision of a registered nurse

**life care facility**   apartment homes that offer health care and recreational facilities for the elderly

**ligaments**   bands of fibrous tissue that hold joints together

**lipase**   a fat-splitting enzyme produced by the pancreas

**lipodystrophy**   any disturbance in fat metabolism

**living will**   a written statement, usually by those who are terminally ill, requesting not to be kept alive on life support systems when faculties have failed

**long-term care facility**   a facility that provides care for residents with long-standing disabilities; can be terminal care

**lower extremities**   pertains to the legs and feet

**low fat diet**   a diet in which the amount of fat has been reduced

**low sodium diet**   a diet that limits the amount of sodium chloride, a mineral salt

**lumen**   channel (opening) within a tubelike organ

**lymph**   fluid found in lymphatic vessels

**lymph node**   a mass of lymphatic tissue along lymph vessels; mainly acts as a filter

**malignancy**   cancerous condition which, if left untreated, leads to death

**malpractice**   poor or improper medical treatment; for example, when assistant gives improper care or gives care in which he or she has not been instructed

**manipulative behavior**   actions designed to control the responses of others

**magnetic resonance imaging (MRI)**   procedure using computer and magnetic fields to visualize inner body organs

**mastication**   the act of chewing food with the teeth in preparation for swallowing

**masturbation**   sexual gratification by self-manipulation of the genitals

**Material Safety Data Sheets (MSDS)**   information sheets on chemicals used in facility that list the health hazards, safe use, and emergency procedures for chemical exposure

**maturity**   state of full development, physically, mentally, and psychologically

**meatus**   an opening or channel

**mechanical lift**   a device used to move residents who are unable to bear weight or are very heavy

**mechanical soft diet**   a diet in which the foods are specially prepared to make them easier to chew

**medial**   close to the midline of a body or structure

**mediastinum**   the space between the lungs

**Medicaid**   federal- and state-funded program that pays for medical costs for those whose income falls below a certain level

**medical asepsis**   procedures followed to keep germs from being spread from one person to another

**medical chart**   record of pertinent legal information relating to the resident, the resident's progress, and care

**Medicare**   federal program that assists those over 65 years of age with hospital and medical costs

**medulla**   the internal portion of a gland; also refers to the lowest part of the brain stem where the vital centers for respiratory, cardiac, and vasomotor control are located

**membrane**   a thin lining or covering of cells

**memo**   brief written or electronic communication

**meninges**   three-layered serous membrane covering the brain and spinal cord

**menopause**   period when ovaries stop functioning and menstruation ceases; climacteric

**menstruation**   periodic shedding of the endo-metrium

**mental abuse**   making verbal threats to hurt, punish, or humiliate a resident

**mental retardation**   a condition that occurs before age 22 and refers to significantly subaverage mental functioning and deficits in adaptive behavior

**mercury**   a silvery metal that is liquid at room temperature; most frequently used in clinical thermometers

**metabolism**   the sum total of the physical and chemical processes and reactions taking place in the body

**metastasis**   spreading of cancer to other body parts

**meter**   metric distance measurement equaling 39.371 inches

**methicillin-resistant *Staphylococcus aureus* (MRSA)**   microbe resistant to the effect of methicillin, an antibiotic

**metric system**   a system of weights and measurements based on the meter and having all units based on some power of ten

**microbe**   tiny organism that can only be seen with a microscope; some may cause disease

**micturition**   urination

**midplane**   an imaginary line that divides the body evenly into a right and left side

**milliliter (mL)**   a measurement of capacity—volume of 1 g of water at standard temperature and pressure

**mineral**   inorganic chemical compound found in nature; many minerals are important in building body tissues and regulating body fluids

**Minimum Data Set (MDS 2.0)**   assessment completed for all residents admitted to a skilled care facility

**mitered corner**   a bedmaking technique in which the top sheet is tucked in at the front of the bed, forming a 45° angle with the perpendicular edge of the mattress

**mitosis**   division of the cytoplasm and nucleus in the cell

**mobility**   ability to move or to be moved easily from place to place

**mobility skills**   ability to move easily from place to place

**morbidity**   state of being diseased; conditions inducing disease

**moribund**   dying

**mortality rate**   the proportion of deaths to population

**motor nerve**   nerve that carries messages to muscles from the brain

**mottling**   discoloration of skin or irregular areas

**MRSA**   methicillin resistant *Staphylococcus aureus;* an important infectious bacterium

**mucolytic**   destroying or dissolving mucus

**mucous**   pertaining to or resembling mucus; also, secreting mucus

**mucous membrane**   special tissues that secrete a sticky substance called mucus; these membranes line body cavities that open to the outside

**mucus**   secretion of mucous membranes; thick, sticky fluid

**multiple sclerosis**   disease characterized by hardened patches scattered throughout the brain and spinal cord that interfere with the nerves in these areas

**muscle**   tissue composed of contractile (contracts and relaxes) fibers or cells

**muscle cell**   cells characterized by their ability to contract and bring about movement

**muscle tissue**   tissue that forms the body wall and organs and is specialized for movement

**myasthenia gravis**   disease characterized by muscular weakness caused by inadequate neurotransmitters

**myocardial infarction**   area of dead heart tissue caused by lack of blood flow

**myocardial ischemia**    lack of blood flow to the heart muscle

**myocardium**    heart muscle

**myth**    fixed idea about a group of people

**narcosis**    a stuporous state produced by drugs

**narcotic**    drug that produces abnormally deep sleep

**nasogastric tube**    soft rubber or plastic tube that is inserted through a nostril and into the stomach

**necrosis**    tissue death

**neglect**    failure to attend to duties properly; lack of proper care

**negligence**    failure to give care that is reasonably expected of an assistant

**nephron**    microscopic kidney units that produce the urine; made up of the glomerulus, Bowman's capsule, and the convoluted tubules

**nerve**    a bundle of nerve processes (axons and dendrites) that are held together by connective tissue

**nerve cell**    characterized by the ability to conduct a bioelectrical current called the nerve impulse

**nerve impulse**    an electrical wave that transmits a message

**nervous tissue**    highly specialized tissue capable of conducting a nerve impulse

**networking**    a line of communications among individuals with a common interest or goal

**neuron**    cell of the nervous system

**neurotransmitter**    chemical compound that transmits a nervous impulse across cells at a synapse

**nitroglycerin**    a vasodilator drug used mainly in angina pectoris

**no-code (DNR)**    order not to resuscitate (revive) a resident

**nocturia**    excessive urination at night

**non–insulin-dependent diabetes mellitus (NIDDM)**    relative insulin deficiency or resistance to insulin action; does not necessarily require insulin replacement

**nonverbal communication**    sending messages without the use of words

**non-weight bearing**    no weight to be borne by hip(s)/leg(s)

**nosocomial infection**    infection that occurs while the resident is in facility care

**nurse's notes**    documentation in the resident's medical record done by nursing staff

**nurse's station**    area on a resident unit where medical records and care plans are kept

**nursing assistant**    nurse's aide or orderly

**nursing diagnosis**    nursing statement of a patient problem

**nutrient**    food that supplies heat and energy, builds and repairs body tissue, and regulates body functions

**nutrition**    the process by which the body uses food for growth and repair and to maintain health

**nystagmus**    involuntary and jerky repetitive movements of the eyes

**obesity**    the condition of being overweight

**objective observation**    observations made by seeing, hearing, feeling, touching, and smelling; sign

**observation**    something that is noticed

**occupational exposure**    opportunity to come in contact with a hazard while carrying out assignments

**Occupational Safety and Health Administration (OSHA)**    federal government agency responsible for developing and enforcing health and job safety standards to protect employees

**occupational therapist**    person licensed to provide rehabilitative services to evaluate and treat persons with physical injury or illness, psychosocial problems, or developmental disabilities

**occupied bedmaking**    bedmaking while the resident is present in bed

**O.D.**    as used in text, pertains to right eye

**oil gland**    sebaceous gland that is found in the skin and secretes an oily substance into the follicles

**olfactory**    pertaining to the sense of smell

**oliguria**    scant urine

**ombudsman**    a public official designated to investigate complaints objectively

**oncology**    study of neoplasms or tumors

**open reduction/internal fixation**    method of stabilizing fractures

**ophthalmologist**    a physician who specializes in the treatment of defects and diseases of the eye

**optic nerve**    nerve carrying messages from eye to brain

**optometrist**    health care provider who specializes in measuring visual acuity

**oral**    pertaining to the mouth

**oral hygiene**    proper care of the mouth and teeth

**orally**    through the mouth

**organ**    any part of the body that carries out a specific function or functions, such as the heart

**organic mental syndrome**    a general term that includes all dementias

**origin**    proximal point of attachment to skeletal muscle

**orthopnea**    condition in which there is difficulty breathing except when sitting or standing upright

**orthopneic position**    sitting supported in an upright position to relieve respiratory distress

**orthosis** device that is used to maintain position of an extremity

**orthotic device** device such as a brace or splint that restores or improves function and prevents deformity

**O.S.** as used in text, pertains to left eye

**osteoarthritis** degenerative joint disease caused by disintegration of the cartilage that covers the ends of the bones

**osteoporosis** the most common metabolic disease of bone in the United States; characterized by a decrease in the mass of bony tissue; most commonly affects women past middle age

**ostomy** suffix word ending meaning to create a new opening, as colostomy

**output** the measured amount of fluid excreted in a given period

**ovaries** endocrine glands located in female pelvis; female gonads

**oviduct; fallopian tube** part of the female reproductive tract that carries ova from ovaries to uterus

**ovulation** a discharge of an egg from the ovary

**ovum** the female egg

**oxygen** gas essential to cellular metabolism and all life

**oxygenated** carrying oxygen

**oxygen mask** a cuplike appliance attached to an oxygen source that is placed over a resident's nose and mouth to deliver oxygen

**pacemaker (pacer)** an artificial device placed in the body to regulate heartbeat

**pacing** repeatedly walking back and forth

**palliative** relieving symptoms but not curing disease

**pallor** less color than normal of the skin

**pancreas** a gland located behind the stomach. It secretes several enzymes necessary for digestion, plus insulin and glycogen

**paralysis** loss or impairment of the ability to move parts of the body

**paranoia** a state in which one has delusions of persecution and/or grandeur

**paraplegia** paralysis of both legs

**parathormone** a hormone produced by the parathyroid glands; it is important in managing the level of body calcium

**parathyroid gland** several small glands located on the posterior thyroid gland that produce the hormone parathormone

**Parkinson's disease** progressive disease of the brain, characterized by stiffness of muscles and tremors, occurring later in life

**paroxysmal** abrupt in onset and termination

**partial weight bearing** limited amount of weight can be borne on one or both legs

**passive range of motion** movement of joints by caregiver

**pathogen** microorganism or other agent capable of producing a disease

**pathology** disease

**patient** person unable to provide self-care; resident

**patient controlled analgesia** device used by patient (resident) to control when pain medication is administered

**pelvic cavity** that portion of the ventral cavity shaped like a basin surrounded by the pelvic bones

**pelvis** the lower portion of the trunk of the body; a basin-shaped area bounded by the hip bones, the sacrum, and the coccyx

**penis** male organ of copulation

**pension** retirement income or fund

**perceptual deficit** an inability to reason, think systematically, make judgments, or use common items

**perceptual process** interpretation of information

**pericardial** pertaining to the pericardium (the sac enclosing the heart)

**pericardium** membrane that surrounds the heart

**perineal care** specific cleaning of the area between the resident's legs

**perineum** in the male, the area between the anus and scrotum; in the female, the area between the anus and vagina

**peripheral** away from the center

**peripheral intravenous central catheter** small tube inserted into vein in arm and threaded through to a larger vein such as the superior vena cava

**peripheral nervous system** nerves that carry messages to and from the brain and spinal cord

**peripheral vascular disease** disease resulting from decreased blood supply to the extremities

**peristalsis** a progressive, wavelike movement that occurs involuntarily in hollow tubes of the body, especially in the alimentary canal

**peritoneal cavity** that portion of the abdomino-pelvic cavity that is enclosed within the membranous peritoneum

**peritoneal dialysis** procedure used to remove liquid wastes from blood stream

**peritoneum** delicate serous membrane that lines the abdominal pelvic cavity and covers the organs

**perservation** the constant repetition of an action such as fingertapping, lip licking

**personal inventory** list of resident's personal belongings

**personality** sum of the ways we react to the events in our lives

**personal protective equipment** coverings such as masks, aprons, gloves, and glasses that protect the caregiver against the transmission of infectious organisms

**petite mal seizure** a type of epilepsy attack, generally short in nature; absence attack

**pet therapy** providing puppies or kittens to bring pleasure to severely impaired residents

**phalange** any bone of a finger or toe

**phantom pain** pain that seems to exist in an amputated limb

**pharynx** the muscular and membranous tube between the mouth and the esophagus

**phlebitis** inflammation of a vein

**phlebotomy** incision of a vein for the purpose of withdrawing blood

**phlegm** thick mucus found in the throat or respiratory tract

**physical abuse** any physical contact that intentionally causes pain or discomfort

**physical needs** these needs include maintaining hygiene and cleanliness and maintaining nutrition and fluid intake

**physical restraint** device used to inhibit body movement; also prevents personal access to body

**physical therapist** a person licensed by the state to provide rehabilitation sources to evaluate and treat persons with neuromuscular and musculoskeletal problems caused by disease, injury, or developmental disability

**physician** a licensed medical doctor

**physiology** the science that deals with the functioning of living organisms

**physiotherapist** a trained professional who provides therapy and exercise to maintain mobility

**piggyback** procedure used to administer medication through a vein

**piles** hemorrhoids

**pineal body** glandular structure found in the cranium connected to the thalamus; produces some hormones thought to delay puberty until an appropriate age

**pitting edema** a condition in which the tissue remains indented when pressure is applied to an edematous area

**pituitary gland** the gland located beneath the brain that serves a variety of functions, including regulation of the gonads, thyroid, adrenal cortex, and other endocrine glands

**plane** imaginary line used to describe the relationship of one body part to another

**plaque** irregular patch or flat lesion that forms on artery lining in atherosclerosis

**plasma** liquid portion of blood

**platelet** thrombocyte; involved in the blood clotting mechanism

**pleura** the membranes that surround the lungs

**pleural** pertaining to the pleura

**pneumonia** inflammation of the lungs

**PNS** peripheral nervous system

**podiatrist** a physician specializing in foot problems

**podigeriatrics** a medical specialty that deals with treatment and care of aging feet

**point of attachment** areas where arms and legs are attached to the torso

**policy book** a book that outlines the rules governing the facility and explains what will be done for the residents

**polydipsia** excessive thirst

**polyphagia** excessive ingestion of food

**polyuria** excessive excretion of urine

**pore** opening of one of the ducts leading from the sweat glands to the surface of the skin

**position sense** ability to tell how one's extremities are positioned without looking at them

**posterior** back or dorsal

**postmortem** after death

**postmortem care** care of the body after death

**postural drainage** positioning a patient to encourage drainage from the respiratory tract

**postural support** pads, pillows, or rolls used to help residents remain in proper alignment

**potassium** an element essential to the body; an electrolyte

**potency** power; especially the ability of the male to perform coitus

**potentially infectious materials** material that might possibly cause infection

**Power of Attorney for Health Care** legal document that authorizes someone other than the resident to carry out the health care wishes of the resident

**prefix** a term placed before a word that changes or modifies the meaning of the word

**prepuce** foreskin, a fold of skin covering the glans penis

**presbycusis** progressive loss of hearing due to normal aging

**presbyopia** impaired vision as a result of the aging process (farsightedness)

**pressure ulcer** also called dermal ulcers or decubitus ulcers; ulcerations that form as the result of ischemia of tissues due to pressure

**procedure** a series of steps outlining how to do something and in what order and manner

**procedure book** a reference for procedures

**progesterone** hormone produced by ovaries

**prognosis** probable outcome of a disease or injury

**progressive mobilization**   a process used to increase a resident's mobility skills

**projection**   an unconscious defense mechanism in which an individual sees his or her own defects as belonging to another

**prolapse**   the falling down or downward displacement of a body part or organ

**prone**   turning the forearm so the palm is facing downward

**proprioception**   information received from internal stimuli

**prostatectomy**   removal of all or part of the prostate gland

**prostate gland**   gland of male reproductive system that surrounds the neck of the urinary bladder and the beginning of the urethra

**prosthesis**   artificial substitute for a missing body part, such as a denture, hand, leg

**protein**   the basic material of every body cell; an essential nutrient

**protraction**   to be brought forward

**proximal**   closest to the point of attachment

**pruritus**   itching

**psychosocial**   relating social conditions to mental health

**psychotic**   completely out of touch with reality

**puberty**   the condition or period of becoming capable of sexual reproduction

**pubic**   pertaining to the pubis or pubic bone, which forms the center bone of the front of the pelvis

**pulmonary artery**   blood vessel that carries deoxygenated blood from the right ventricle to the lung

**pulmonary emphysema**   a chronic lung disorder in which the terminal bronchioles become plugged with mucus and lung elasticity is lost

**pulse**   wave of pressure exerted against the walls of the arteries in response to ventricular contraction

**pulse deficit**   difference between contractions of the heart and pulse expansions of the radial artery

**pulse oximetry**   procedure used to determine oxygen levels in blood stream

**pulse pressure**   the difference between the systolic and diastolic pressure

**pulse rate**   number per minute of impulses transmitted to the arteries by contraction of the left ventricle

**pupil**   opening in the center of the iris of the eye that allows light to enter the eye

**PVD**   peripheral vascular disease

**pylorus**   the narrow, tapered end of the stomach opening into the duodenum

**pyorrhea**   periodontitis; loosening of the teeth caused by gum disease

**quadrant**   one section when imaginary lines are drawn over the abdomen, dividing it into four equal areas

**quadriplegia**   paralysis of all four limbs

**quality assurance program**   measurement of care provided to residents

**RACE**   acronym for a series of activities to take during a fire; r = remove all residents, a = activate, c = contain, e = extinguish

**radial artery**   blood vessel carrying oxygenated blood located on the lateral anterior wrist at the base of the thumb; most often used to determine pulse rate

**radiation therapy**   diagnosis and treatment using radiation

**rales**   abnormal respiratory sound heard in auscultation of the chest

**range of motion (ROM) exercises**   series of exercises specifically designed to move each joint through its range

**rapport**   understanding between two people

**rationalization**   an unconscious defense mechanism in which one devises a logical, self-satisfying but incorrect explanation for one's behavior or feelings

**reaction**   a response to a stimulus; opposite action or counteraction

**reality orientation (R.O.)**   techniques used to help residents remain oriented to the environment, to time, and to themselves

**receptor**   peripheral nerve ending; specialized for response to a particular type of stimuli

**rectocele**   protrusion of part of the rectum into the vagina

**rectum**   the lower part of large intestine, about 5 inches long, between the sigmoid flexure and the anal canal

**references**   in a résumé, statements about abilities and characteristics; persons who give such statements

**reflexes**   involuntary response to a stimulus

**registered nurse (RN)**   a person who has completed a 2-, 3-, or 4-year program in a nursing school and is licensed by the state to assess, plan for, and evaluate the nursing care needs of residents

**regular diet**   a routine or balanced diet; sometimes called a house diet

**regularity**   routinely eliminating waste products from the body

**regurgitating**   "throwing up" undigested food from the stomach

**regurgitation**   backward flow of fluids in the body

**rehabilitation**   pertaining to a return to a former improved state

**rehabilitation aide** specially trained nursing assistant who helps residents regain lost skills or teaches new skills

**reminiscing** recalling past events

**remission** period of decreased severity of symptoms in chronic disease

**renal calculi** kidney stones

**renal pelvis** the portion of the kidney that collects the urine and directs it into the ureter

**reprisal** retaliation

**resident** patient in a long-term care facility

**resident care plan** statement of the resident's medical diagnosis, problems, and directions for resolving the problems

**Resident Council** group of residents who meet regularly; the councils give residents a method for communication with each other and with staff

**resident unit** room occupied by resident and his or her personal possessions; may be shared by other residents

**residual limb** portion of a limb left after part has been removed

**respiration** process of taking oxygen into the body and expelling carbon dioxide

**respiratory arrest** when breathing stops

**rest home** long-term care facility

**restoration** to remedy or bring up to a normal state

**restorative** describing care in which the interdisciplinary health care team assists the resident to reach an optimal level of ability

**résumé** a short account of one's career and qualifications that is prepared by an applicant for a position

**resuscitation** restoration to life of one who has cardiac and respiratory arrest

**retention** the inability to excrete urine that has been produced

**retina** innermost or third layer of the eye, which receives images

**retinopathy** noninflammatory disease of the retina

**retirement** period after leaving employment

**retraction** to be brought backward

**retroperitoneal space** area of the anterior cavity behind the peritoneum; in it are the kidneys, aorta, inferior vena cava

**rheumatoid arthritis** autoimmune response that results in inflammation of the joints

**rhythm** regularity

**ribs** the 24 long, flat bones forming the wall of the thorax

**rigor mortis** a stiffening of the body some hours after death

**rotation** the act of turning about the axis of the center of a body, as rotation of a joint

**rubra** unusual redness or flushing of skin

**rupture** the bursting of a part

**Sacrament of the Sick (last rites)** given by a clergyman to a person who is terminally ill (dying)

**safety device** a device that in some way restricts the activity of a resident to protect that resident or others

**saliva** digestive secretion produced by the salivary glands and found in the mouth

**sclera** white of the eye

**scrotum** saclike pouch that holds the male gonads

**sedative** medication that has calming effect; used to control nervousness, irritability, and excitement

**seizure** sudden attack of a disease; an epileptic fit

**self-care (functional) deficit** an inability to care for oneself in one or more areas of activities of daily living

**Self-Determination Act** a federal law passed in 1990 stating that competent adults have the right to be adequately informed about their medical conditions and the options of treatment available to them, and then to make their own decision as to their degree of participation

**self-esteem** feelings of confidence about oneself

**self range of motion** exercises done by the resident

**seminal vesicles** pouchlike sacs found on the posterior wall of the bladder that produce the bulk of the seminal fluid

**semiprone position** modified prone position in which body is supported on pillows to relieve pressure on most of the bony prominences

**semisupine position** lying partially on the back and side

**senescent** growing old

**senescent changes** normal aging changes

**senile** affected with the infirmities of age

**senile keratosis** roughened, scaly, slightly elevated wartlike lesions, believed to be related to sun damage in fair-skinned individuals

**senile lentigines** yellow or brown spots that occur on exposed skin surfaces

**senior** person over the age of 65

**senior citizen center** place where seniors can meet for social and other activities

**sensitivity** the state of acute or abnormal responsiveness to stimuli

**sensory deprivation** lack of stimulation to the sense of vision, hearing, smelling, taste, or touch

**sensory nerves** nerves that carry messages—about pain, temperature change, changes in body position, taste, touch, sound, and sight—toward the brain for interpretation

**sensory/perceptual changes**  an inability to recognize and use common objects such as eating utensils, combs, or pencils

**sensory stimulation**  activities that increase the resident's awareness of the surroundings

**sensual**  pertaining to the senses or sensation

**sensuality**  quality or state of being sensual

**sepsis**  infection

**septum**  wall or partition dividing a body cavity or space

**septicemia**  infection in the blood stream

**seropositive**  HIV positive

**serous membrane**  a special tissue that secretes a serous fluid; covers organs and lines cavities that do not open to the outside

**serum**  the clear liquid portion of the blood remaining after removal of the solid components and blood clotting elements

**sexual abuse**  using physical or verbal threats to force a resident to perform any sexual act; tormenting or teasing a resident with sexual gestures or words

**sexuality**  the attitude of a person in relation to sexual attitude and behavior

**sharps**  needles, razor, or any sharp or cutting item

**shearing (force)**  occurs when any part of the supported body is on a gradient; the deeper tissue near the bone slides toward the lower gradient while the skin remains at its point of contact; the tissues between become ischemic

**sheath**  covering

**shift report**  information regarding resident status given to on-coming shift from those going off duty

**sign**  observation apparent to examiner or viewer

**signing**  using hands and facial expression to communicate without speaking words

**simple fracture**  fracture that does not produce an open wound in the skin

**sitz bath**  bath providing moist heat to the genitals or anal area

**skeletal muscle**  muscle tissue that is attached to bone; sometimes called voluntary

**skilled nursing facility**  long-term care facility

**skin**  external covering of the body

**skin tear**  small breaks that occur in fragile skin

**slander**  a false and damaging oral statement that injures the reputation of another person

**sliding board**  a smooth waxed board used for a sitting transfer, such as bed to wheelchair

**sling**  a bandage used for support

**smooth muscle**  type of tissue that forms the walls of organs—involuntary or visceral

**social worker**  a person licensed by the state to assess and provide services for nonmedical, psychosocial needs of the residents

**society**  a group of people who have common interests

**spastic cerebral palsy**  a form of cerebral palsy in which the muscles are tense, contracted, and resistant to movement

**spasticity**  a condition of rigidity or spasm of muscle

**spatial-perceptual deficit**  difficulty in distinguishing between left and right, up and down

**specimen**  sample of body secretion, excretion or tissue used for diagnosis or determination of condition

**speech-language pathologist**  person trained and educated to diagnose and treat swallowing problems and speech and language disorders

**sperm**  the male reproductive cell

**sphincter**  a circular muscle that constricts a passage or closes a natural orifice; when relaxed, it allows passage of materials

**sphygmomanometer**  instrument for determining arterial pressure; blood pressure gauge

**spinal column**  backbone or vertebral column

**spirituality**  the state of being spiritual-minded or religious

**splint**  rigid device applied to maintain a body part in a specific position

**spouse**  a marriage partner; husband or wife

**sprain**  an injury to a ligament caused by sudden overstretching

**sputum**  expectorated matter, composed of saliva and mucus from the lungs and throat

**square corner**  a bedmaking technique in which the top sheet is tucked in at the bottom of the bed by forming a line parallel to the perpendicular edge of the mattress

**standard precautions**  infection control practices used for all people receiving care

**status**  condition or state of health

**stereotype**  characteristic assigned to entire groups of people; rigid, biased ideas about people as a group

**sterile**  free from bacteria or other microorganisms; incapable of reproducing sexually

**sterilization**  process that renders an individual incapable of reproduction

**steroids**  a group name for certain compounds that include progesterone, the adrenocortical and gonadal hormones, bile acid, and sterols such as cholesterol

**stethoscope**  instrument used in auscultation to make audible the sounds produced in the body

**stimulant** agent that produces stimulation

**stoma** an artificial, mouthlike opening

**stool** an evacuation of the bowel

**strain** an excessive stretching of a muscle resulting in pain and swelling of the muscle

**strengths** activities that an individual can perform

**stress** feelings that cause a person to be anxious about his or her well being

**stroke** cerebrovascular accident; damage to the blood vessels of the brain

**stump** the distal end of a limb remaining after amputation

**subacute care** care provided to patients with stable conditions who require skilled care

**subcutaneous** beneath the layers of the skin

**subcutaneous tissue** tissue that attaches the skin to the muscles

**subjective observation** observation based on reports of the resident (symptom)

**subluxation** incomplete dislocation of a joint

**suffix** a term added to the end of a word that changes or modifies the meaning of the word

**sundowning** a resident has increased confusion and restlessness in late afternoon, evening, or during the night

**superior** toward the head; upward

**superior vena cava** large blood vessel that drains the blood from the upper part of the body into the right atrium of the heart

**supine** turning the forearm so the palm is facing upward, lying in a face-up position in the back

**supine position** lying on the back, face up

**supportive care** providing comfort measures

**support services** services not directly involved in resident care; for example, building and ground maintenance, housekeeping, kitchen work, administration duties

**suppository** medication inserted in the rectum used to help the bowels eliminate the feces

**suppression** consciously refusing to acknowledge unacceptable feelings and thoughts

**sweat gland** sudoriferous glands, found in the skin, which produce sweat

**symbol** a mark or character that represents some quality, relationship, or word

**symptom** subjective observation

**synapse** space between the axon of one cell and the dendrites of others

**synarthrotic** pertains to an immovable joint

**syncope** faint, sudden loss of strength

**synovial membrane** special membrane that lines movable joint cavities

**synovium** joint lining

**syphilis** a sexually transmitted disease that may cause lesions in almost all tissues of the body and seriously affect the nervous septum

**system** group of organs organized to carry out a specific body function or functions, as respiratory system

**systole** contraction, or period of contraction, of cardiac muscle

**systolic** applies to the contraction phase of the cardiac cycle

**tachycardia** an unusually rapid heartbeat

**tachypnea** respiratory pattern of rapid, shallow respirations

**tact** sensitive mental perception

**tactile** pertaining to touch

**talisman** engraved stones, rings, or other objects used to ward off evil

**task segmentation** breaking down a complex task into a series of single steps

**TED hose** support hose

**tendon** fibrous band of connective tissue that attaches skeletal muscle to bone

**terminal** the end

**terminal cleaning** cleaning and sterilization of a room after resident's death or departure

**terminal illness** life-ending condition

**testes** male sex glands (gonads) found in the scrotum; produce sperm and the hormone testosterone

**testicles** testes

**testosterone** male sex hormone produced by the testes

**theft** taking that which does not belong to you

**therapeutic** pertaining to results obtained from treatment; a healing agent

**therapeutic diet** a planned intake of food and fluid to treat a specific disease condition

**therapeutic recreational specialist** person trained and educated to use physical recreation as a rehabilitation therapy

**therapy** treatment designated to eliminate disease or other bodily disorder

**thermal blanket** fluid-filled blanket, the temperature of which can be raised or lowered

**thermometer** instrument used to determine temperature

**thoracic** pertaining to the chest

**thoracic cavity** chest cavity

**thorax** the chest, the part of the body between the neck and the abdomen, encased by the shoulder girdle, ribs, and diaphragm

**thrombocyte** blood platelet that is formed in the bone marrow and is important in blood clotting

**thrombophlebitis** inflammation of a vein as a result of a blood clot

**thrombus (pl. *thrombi*)** blood clot

**thyroid gland** an endocrine gland located in anterior neck in front of and on either side of the trachea. Produces hormones thyrocalcitonin and thyroxine

**thyroxine** hormone of the thyroid gland that contains iodine

**TIA** transient ischemic attack (temporary decrease in blood flow to brain)

**tilt table** a table used to secure patients during position changes to improve chest drainage

**tipping** giving a sum of money for service rendered; not salary-connected

**tissue** a group of similar cells and fibers forming a distinct structure; piece of paper used for cleansing (e.g., toilet tissue, facial tissue, Kleenex)

**toe pleat** a bedmaking technique in which an extra fold of the top sheet is made at the foot of the bed to provide extra room for the resident's feet

**torso** the body, exclusive of the head and limbs

**total care** health care that takes into account the physical and psychosocial needs of individual residents

**total parenteral nutrition (TPN)** a technique in which high density nutrients are introduced into a large vein

**trachea** the windpipe, a tube extending from the larynx to the bronchi

**tracheostomy** opening in the anterior trachea

**traction** technique that pulls the ends of bones into normal position or alignment

**tranquilizer** agent used to calm or quiet anxious person without causing drowsiness

**transcutaneous electrical nerve stimulation (TENS)** method of pain relief

**transfer** move from one place to another

**transfer belt (gait belt)** a webbed belt $1\frac{1}{2}$ to 2 inches wide, about 54 to 60 inches long; used as a safety device to assist residents during transfers

**transient ischemic attack (TIA)** drop attacks caused by vertebrobasilar insufficiency

**transitional care** care provided between acute care and discharge

**transmission** transfer from one place or person to another

**transurethral prostatectomy** removal of the prostate through the urethra

**transverse plane** an imaginary line that divides the body into a superior and inferior part

**trapeze** a horizontal bar suspended overhead down the length of the bed

**trauma** mechanical injury

**trichomonas vaginitis** an infection of the vaginal tract by a parasitic protozoan

**trochanter roll** a rolled bath blanket positioned under the resident extending from well above to well below the hips; the roll prevents external hip rotation

**tubal ligation** tying off a fallopian tube

**tubercle** small, rounded nodule formed by infection with *Mycobacterium tuberculosis*

**tuberculosis disease** condition occurring when tuberculosis organism causing tuberculosis infection begins to spread and is not restrained

**tuberculosis infection** occurs when tuberculosis germs enter the body. The organisms may be walled off, forming a tubercle and causing the person to be unaware of the process

**tumor** neoplasm; new uncontrolled growth of cells

**tunica intima** the inner coat of the blood vessels

**turning sheet** a flat bed sheet folded in half used to move dependent residents in bed

**tyloma** a callus

**tympanic** pertaining to the ear drum

**ulcer** open sore caused by inadequate blood supply and broken skin

**ulceration** development of an ulcer

**umbilicus** the navel, marks site that gave passage to umbilical vessels in the fetal stage

**unilateral neglect** the inability to recognize the existence of one side of the body

**unoccupied bedmaking** bedmaking when the resident is out of the bed

**upper extremity** the arm and hand

**uremia** the presence of excessive amounts of urea, a waste product, in the blood

**uremic frost (snow)** secretions of perspiration containing substances normally found in urine

**ureter** narrow tube that conducts urine from the kidney to the urinary bladder

**urethra** mucus-lined tube conveying urine from the urinary bladder to the exterior of the body; in the male, the urethra also conveys the semen

**urgency** the need to urinate

**urinalysis** laboratory analysis of urine

**urination** the act of discharging urine from the bladder

**urosheath** a condomlike appliance that is used to collect urine when attached to drainage tubing

**uterine tubes** fallopian tubes or oviducts; tubes through which the ova travel from the ovary to the uterus

**uterus** muscular, hollow organ where fetus develops in the female

**vaccine** suspensions or products of infectious agents used chiefly for producing active immunity

**vagina** the tube that extends from the vulva to the uterine cervix; the female organ of copulation that receives the penis during sexual intercourse

**vaginitis** inflammation of the vagina

**validation therapy** a way of relating to residents that helps them feel secure and oriented within their own reality

**value system** setting priorities of what is important in life

**valve** a fold of membrane in a passage or tube permitting the flow of contents in one direction only

**vancomycin-resistant enterococci (VRE)** microbes resistant to the effects of vancomycin, an antibiotic

**varicose veins** weakened veins usually found in lower extremities

**vas deferens** the tube that carries sperm from the epididymis to the junction of the seminal vesicle; ductus deferens

**vasectomy** excision of part or all of the vas deferens; bilateral vasectomy results in sterility

**vasoconstriction** decrease in the caliber of the blood vessels

**vasodilation** increase in the caliber of the blood vessels

**vasodilator** a neuron or medication that causes dilation of the blood vessels

**vein** a vessel through which blood passes on its way back to the heart

**venereal warts** verruca condyloma; lesions are reddish brown and have a rough, cauliflower type surface caused by the human papilloma virus

**ventilation** process of admitting fresh air and expelling stale air; the movement of gases into and out of the lungs

**ventral** front; anterior

**ventricle** a small, bellylike cavity such as one of the lower chambers of the heart

**venule** small vein

**verbal abuse** using words to mistreat another such as using sarcasm, slang, or foul language

**verbal communication** messages sent using words

**vertigo** dizziness

**visceral muscle** smooth muscle; makes up walls of internal organs

**vital capacity** the volume of air a person can forcibly expire from the lungs after a maximal inspiration

**vital signs** measurements of temperature, pulse, respiration, and blood pressure

**vitamin** a general term for various, unrelated organic substances found in many foods in minute amounts that are necessary for normal metabolic functioning of the body

**vocal cords** membranes that stretch across the inside of the larynx and function in voice production

**voiding** the release of urine from the bladder

**volume** the capacity or size of an object or of an area; the measure of the quantity of a substance

**voluntary muscle** any part of the skeletal muscle that is under direct control

**volunteerism** the contribution of one's time and energy to helping others

**vomitus** the material vomited or brought up from the stomach

**vulva** the external female genitalia

**wandering** aimless walking about

**warm soak** warm water at a specific temperature applied to a body part

**water** liquid essential for life

**weight bearing** an ability to stand on one or both legs

**wet compress** pieces of gauze that have been moistened and wrung out, then placed against the resident to apply cold or heat

**withdrawal** the retreat from reality or from social contact that is associated with severe depression and other psychiatric disorders

**withhold** order to refrain from serving a resident certain foods or all food

**womb** another term for the female uterus

**word root** word form whose basic meaning can be used in forming new words by combining it with prefixes and suffixes

**work practice controls** specific procedures to prevent the spread of infection

# Index

....................................................................................................................................

Page numbers containing *f*, *g*, and *t* indicate figures, guidelines, and tables, respectively.

## A

Abbreviations, 67, 71–74
ABCs of emergency response, 140*g*
Abdominal aneurysm, as transfer belt contraindication, 487
Abdominal cavity, 80*f*
Abdominal distention, 328
Abdominal quadrants, 76–77, 77*f*
Abduction, 446, 447*f*
  fingers and thumb, 452, 452*f*, 453, 453*f*
  hip, 453, 453*f*
  shoulder, 449, 449*f*
  toes, 455–56, 455*f*
Abuse
  legal action and, 116
  residents' right to file complaints about, 115
  right to freedom from, 102
  *See also specific types of abuse*
Accelerated respiration, 384
Acceptance stage of grief, 646–47, 646*f*
Accidents, 122
  ergonomic techniques to reduce, 123*g*
  prevention of. *See* Safety
  risk factors for, 129
  trauma from, 198
  *See also* Emergencies
Accommodation of needs, 104–6, 104*f*, 105*f*, 106*f*
Accuracy, 32
Acquired immune deficiency syndrome (AIDS), 154, 160–62, 199
  as admission reason for younger residents, 203, 203*f*
  dementia, 619*f*
  subacute care units and, 654, 655
Active range of motion exercises, 445, 456
Activities, 218
  for dementia residents, 627, 627*f*
  residents' right to participate in, 114

Activities director, 22*f*
Activities of daily living (ADL), 5, 6, 7, 37, 39, 39*f*, 198, 199
  adaptive devices for, 25, 440–42*f*
  assistance for, 199*f*
  eating as, 297, 304
  functional changes and, 225, 227, 227*f*
  guidelines for dementia resident, 626*g*
  instrumental, 200, 200*f*, 437
  restorative care and, 436–39, 439*f*
  stroke and, 606*f*
  task segmentation for, 438*t*
Acute care hospitals, 4, 4*f*, 5*f*, 6–7, 32
Acute myocardial infarction, 531–32
Adaptive behavior, 635
Adaptive Behavior Scale, 636
Adaptive devices, 25, 432*f*, 440
  dressing, 441*f*
  eating, 442*f*
  grooming and bathing, 440*f*
Adduction, 446, 447*f*
  fingers and thumb, 452, 452*f*, 453, 453*f*
  hip, 453, 453*f*
  shoulder, 449, 449*f*
  toes, 455–56, 456*f*
ADL. *See* Activities of daily living
Administrative organization, 26–27, 27*f*
Administrator, 22*f*, 26–27
Admission to facility, 402–5, 406*f*, 407
  adapting after, 407
  anxiety about, 403
  clinical focus and objectives, 401
  explanation of residents' rights before, 100*f*
  interdisciplinary health care team and, 404, 404*f*
  personal inventory for, 405, 406*f*, 407
  procedure for, 405, 405*f*
  reasons for, 402–3, 402*f*
  summary and review questions, 415–16

Adrenal glands, 552, 553*f*, 553–54
Adrenaline, 553
Advance directives, 107–8
  Living Will form, 109–10*f*
  Power of Attorney for Health Care form, 111–12*f*
Advance practice nurse, 21
Advocates, 115
African Americans
  health/illness belief systems, 212*f*
  personal space and, 235*f*
Age-related macular degeneration, 599
Aging process, 200, 224, 223–29
  basic human needs in, 208–10, 208*f*, 209*f*
  cardiovascular system effects, 521*f*
  census bureau statistics regarding, 200
  challenges to adjustments, 215–17
  clinical focus and objectives, 207, 223
  cultural influences, 210
  defense mechanisms and, 217, 217*f*
  developmental disabilities and, 634
  digestive system effects, 293, 293*f*
  effects on skin, 253–54, 253*f*, 254*f*
  endocrine system effects, 554–55
  general conclusions about, 224
  infections and, 157, 162–63, 543
  meeting psychosocial needs in, 217–18
  musculoskeletal system effects, 581
  nervous system effects, 598
  physical effects of, 224–25, 225–26*f*, 227–28, 227*f*
  reactive behaviors and, 218–20
  religion and, 212–13, 213*f*
  reproductive system effects, 568–69
  respiratory system effects, 542, 542*f*

Aging process—*cont'd*
  sexuality and, 213–15, 214*f*, 215*f*
  spirituality and, 210, 212*f*
  stereotypes and myths about, 200–3, 201*f*, 202*f*
  stress reactions and, 218
  summary and review questions, 220–22, 228–29
  theories of, 224
  urinary system effects, 346, 346*f*
Agitation, Alzheimer's disease and, 628
AIDS. *See* Acquired immune deficiency syndrome
Air circulation, in rooms, 236, 238*g*
Air mattress, 260, 260*f*
Airborne precautions, 176–77, 177*f*
Airborne transmission, 155, 156*f*
Airway obstruction, 142–43, 147
Alcoholic beverages, diet and, 296–97
Allergens, 545
Alopecia, 662
Alternating-pressure mattress, 260, 260*f*
Alveoli, 540*f*, 541, 541*f*
  emphysema and, 545
Alzheimer's disease, 60, 198, 617–32
  ADL guidelines for, 626*g*
  care of, 622–25, 622*f*, 623–24*g*, 625*f*, 627, 627*f*
  clinical focus and objectives, 617
  definition of, 618–19
  management techniques for, 629–31, 630*f*
  as reason for admission to LTC, 402
  special problems with, 628–29, 629*f*
  stages and symptoms of, 619*f*, 620–22, 620*f*, 621*f*
  summary and review questions, 631–32
  *See also* Dementia
Ambulation, 484, 500–6
  assistive devices for, 501–2, 502*f*, 503*f*, 504*f*
  with catheter, 351
  gait pattern and training in, 500–1, 501*f*
  guidelines for, 504*g*
  leg bags and, 356

podiatrists and, 26
  procedures for, 504–6, 506*f*
Amputation
  as complication of diabetes, 557
  lower extremity, 587
  positioning considerations for, 471
  sliding board transfers for, 499–500
Amulets, 212
Amyotrophic lateral sclerosis (ALS), 609–10, 610*g*
Analgesia, patient-controlled, 657, 659
Anatomic position, 75, 75*f*
Anatomy, 75
  abbreviations, 71
  terminology, 75–77, 75*f*, 76*f*, 77*f*
Anemia, 526
Aneroid manometer, 386*f*, 388*g*
Aneurysm
  abdominal, 487
  aortic, 528*f*
  brain, 604
Anger stage of grief, 646, 646*f*
Angina pectoris, 528*f*, 532
Ankle exercises, 454–55, 455*f*
Ankle stirrup, 461, 461*f*
Anorexia, from chemotherapy, 662
Anoxia, as cause of mental retardation, 636
Anterior body surface, 75, 76*f*, 77*f*
Antibiotics, 158
  and body flora balance, 156
  tuberculosis and, 159
Antibodies, 157
Antidiabetic drugs, 558–59
Antiembolism stockings, 532, 533–34, 533*f*, 534*f*
Antigen, 157
Antihypertensives, 386
Anuria, 363
Anus, 290, 293, 565*f*, 567*f*
Anxiety, 86
  about admission to LTC, 403
  Alzheimer's disease and, 628
Aorta, 521, 522*f*, 528*f*
Apex of heart, 382–83
Aphasia, 604
  communication and, 60
  as stage of Alzheimer's disease, 622
Apical pulse, 382–84, 384*f*
Apnea, 384*f*
Appetite
  loss of, 228, 662
  observation of, 88

Appliance, colostomy, 339, 340
Approach, in care plan, 93*f*, 94
Aquamatic K-Pad®, 418*f*, 419, 421
  application procedure, 420, 420*f*
Arterial pulse points, 146, 146*f*, 382*f*
Arteries, 522, 523, 524*f*, 528*f*
Arteriosclerosis, 526–27, 526*f*, 527*f*
Arthritis, 198, 585–87
  and gait, 500
  osteoarthritis, 585–86, 586*f*
  positioning for, 471
  rheumatoid, 586*f*, 587, 588*f*
Articulation, speech, 49
Artificial hip, 586–87, 586*f*, 587*f*
Artificial nutrition, right to refuse, 101
Ascites, as heart failure symptom, 532
Asepsis
  medical, 168–70, 169*f*
  surgical, 191
Asepto syringe, 421
Asians/Asian-Americans
  health/illness belief systems, 211*f*
  personal space and, 234, 235*f*
Aspiration, 143
  as cause of pneumonia, 543
  dementia and, 626*g*
  prevention of, 134
Assault and battery, 116–17
Assessment
  for care plans, 92
  nutritional, 21
Assignments
  for nursing assistants, 32, 38, 38*f*, 49–50
  sample sheet of, 51*f*
Assistant director of nursing, 21
Assisted living facility, 8, 10
Assisted standing transfer procedures, 489–90, 490*f*, 491–92, 492*f*
Assistive devices, 501–2, 502*f*, 503*f*, 504*f*
  ambulation procedure with, 505–6, 506*f*
  for multiple sclerosis, 608*g*
  physical therapists and, 25, 25*f*
  as risk factor for accidents, 129
Asthma, 545
Ataxic cerebral palsy, 637
Atherosclerosis, 526–27, 527*f*, 528*f*, 604
Athetoid cerebral palsy, 637

Athlete's foot, 155
Atrium, heart, 521, 522*f*, 523*f*
Atrophy, 579
    prevention of, 433*t*
Attitude, nursing assistant, 33, 33*f*
Audiologist, 22*f*, 26
Auditory nerve, 598
Autoclave, 190
Autonomic nervous system, 596
Autopsy, religious beliefs and
        practices regarding, 649*f*
Axilla, bathing of, 265, 268, 269
Axillary temperature, 371
    measurement procedure,
        376–77, 377*f*, 379
    normal ranges of, 371*f*

**B**

Back injury prevention, 124, 124*f*,
        125*f*
Backrubs, 261–62, 261*f*, 262*f*
Bacteremia, 156, 162
Bacterial infections, 154, 154*f*,
        157–59, 347, 543
Baptists
    death and dying beliefs and
        practices, 649*f*
    dietary practices, 300*f*
Bargaining stage of grief, 646, 646*f*
Bathing
    adaptive devices for, 440*f*
    bed baths, 264–67, 264*f*, 265*f*,
        266*f*
    general care and safety in,
        261–63, 263*f*
    guidelines for dementia
        residents, 626*g*
    partial bath, 268–69
    of perineal area, 269–73, 270*f*,
        271*f*, 272*f*
    prevention of falls and, 134
    restorative program guidelines
        for, 443*g*
    skin breakdown prevention and,
        257*g*
    task segmentation for, 438*t*
    in tub or shower, 267–68
Bathroom assistance procedures,
        326–27, 492–94, 493*f*
Bathroom equipment, 105, 321–22,
        322*f*
    infection control and, 169, 169*f*
    odor control and, 237, 238*g*
Battery, 116–17
Bed bath procedure, 264–67, 264*f*,
        265*f*, 266*f*
Bed cradle, 260, 260*f*, 460, 460*f*

Bedmaking, 241, 242*g*
    linen handling in, 241–42*g*
    occupied bed procedure,
        247–48, 247*f*, 248*f*
    unoccupied bed procedure,
        242–47, 243*f*, 244*f*, 245*f*, 246*f*
Bedpans, 322, 322*f*, 323–25, 323*f*
Beds, 11–12, 12*f*
    comfort and safety of, 126, 235
    independent movement in,
        476–77
    moving resident in. *See* Transfer
        procedures; Positioning of
        resident
Bedside commode, 321–22, 322*f*
    assistance procedure, 326
Behavior, observations of, 89*f*,
        89–90
Behavior modification, 640
Behavioral changes
    reactive behaviors, 218–20
    restraints and, 130
    seizures and, 148
    stress reactions, 218
Belief systems
    cultural and ethnic, 210, 211–12*f*
    religious, 213*f*
Benign prostatic hypertrophy, 571
Biohazardous waste disposal,
        174*g*, 175*g*
    specimen transport bag, 187,
        188*f*, 360, 360*f*
Birth defects, 634, 635*f*
Bladder, 345, 345*f*, 565*f*, 567*f*
    catheters and, 348
    effect of aging on, 227, 346, 346*f*
    urinary retention and, 347
Bladder retraining assessment
        form, 479–80*f*
Bleeding, arterial vs. venous, 147
    *See also* Hemorrhage
Blood
    components of, 526
    loss of, recording in fluid
        output, 354, 354*f*, 355
    spills, cleanup of, 174–75*g*
    in stool, 327
Blood and body fluid precautions,
        172, 176
Blood disorders, 526
Blood pressure, 370, 385–91
    equipment, 386–87, 386*f*, 387*f*
    factors influencing, 385–86, 385*f*
    measurement procedure,
        387–88*g*, 389–91, 389*f*, 390*f*
    observation of, 88
Blood sugar testing, 559

Blood vessels, 253, 521–23, 522*f*
    disorders of, 526–31, 527*f*, 528*f*,
        529*f*
    skin breakdown and, 255, 255*f*
Bloodborne pathogens, 172*f*
Body
    anatomic terminology for,
        75–77, 75*f*, 76*f*, 77*f*
    cavities of, 80*f*, 81
    membranes of, 78, 81
    natural defenses of, 156–57,
        157*f*
    organization of, 77–78
    organs of, 78, 79*f*, 80*f*
    understanding of, 74–75
Body alignment
    for passive range of motion
        exercises, 448
    positioning and, 457
    postural supports and, 458
    wheelchairs and, 506
Body flora, 156
Body fluids
    disposal of, 175*g*
    precautions, 172, 176
Body language, 48, 49, 49*f*, 55*g*,
        56*g*
    with Alzheimer's residents,
        623*g*, 624*g*
    observations of, 86, 87*f*
    with special needs residents, 58
Body mechanics, 493
    general guidelines for, 122,
        123*g*, 124, 124*f*, 125*f*
    in transfers. *See* Transfer
        procedures
Body systems, 78, 79*f*
    observations of, 88–89, 88*f*, 89*f*
    *See also specific systems*
Boils, 154
Bones, 578, 579*f*
    fractures of, 149, 582–84, 582*f*,
        583*f*, 584*f*
Bowel and bladder programs,
        477–78, 478–80*g*
Bowel elimination, 327
    commercially prepared enema
        procedure, 334–36, 335*f*
    constipation and, 328
    enemas for, 328, 329–36
    fecal impaction checking
        procedure, 329
    fecal incontinence and, 342,
        342*f*
    observation of, 88
    oil-retention enema procedure,
        330–31, 330*f*

Bowel elimination—*cont'd*
  organs of, 328*f*
  ostomies and, 338–42, 339*f*, 341*f*
  rectal tube/flatus bag and, 337, 338, 338*f*
  soapsuds enema procedure, 331–34, 331*f*, 332*f*, 333*f*
  stoma care procedure and, 340–41, 340*f*, 341*f*
  stool specimen collection and, 343–44, 344*f*
  suppositories for, 336–37, 337*f*
Bowman's capsule, 345*f*, 346
Brachial artery, 389, 389*f*, 390*f*
Bradycardia, 383
Braille, 60
Brain, 594, 596, 596*f*
Brain damage
  from stroke, 604–5
  subacute care unit and, 655
Brain stem, 596
Breast self-examination procedure, 569–70, 570*f*
Breast tumors, 569
Breathing exercises, 546
Breathing patterns, 384*f*
  dying process and, 648
  respiration counting and, 385
Bridging, 260, 472
Bronchi, 540*f*, 541, 541*f*
Bronchioles, 540*f*, 541, 541*f*
Bronchitis, chronic, 545
Buck's traction, 583*f*
Buddhism, 213*f*
  death and dying beliefs and practices, 649*f*
  dietary practices, 300*f*
Burnout, 41
Burns, 149
Bursae, 581
Bursitis, 581
Business office, 23*f*

**C**
Call lights, 13, 13*f*, 126
Calorie restricted diet, 298*f*, 299
Cancer, 199
  of blood, 526
  diets for, 299
  of digestive system, 313
  of larynx, 542
  of reproductive system, 569
  skin, 254
  treatments for, 662
*Candida albicans*, 571
Canes, 15, 25, 501–2, 502*f*
  ambulation procedure with, 505–6, 506*f*

  assisting residents with, 105
  use of, 502
Cannulas, 546, 546*f*, 547
Capillaries, 522, 523
Carbohydrates, 294
  enzymatic breakdown of, 291, 292*f*, 293
  food groups containing, 294–96
  functions of, 292*f*
Carbon dioxide, 540, 541, 541*f*
Cardiac arrest, 141–42
  airway obstruction and, 145
  DNR orders and, 108, 142*f*
Cardiac chairs, 475
Cardiac cycle, 522
Cardiac monitoring, subacute care unit and, 654
Cardiac muscle, 78, 79*f*, 578
Cardiopulmonary resuscitation (CPR), 141, 141*f*, 646
  DNR orders and, 108
Cardiovascular disorders, 519–37
  angina pectoris, 532
  arteriosclerosis/atherosclerosis, 526–28, 527*f*, 528*f*
  circulatory, 526–31, 528*f*, 529*f*
  clinical focus and objectives, 519
  as complication of diabetes, 557
  diet for, 298, 298*f*
  edema and, 352
  elastic stockings application procedure for, 533–34, 533*f*, 534*f*
  heart attack/acute MI, 531–32, 531*f*
  heart block, 534–35
  heart disease, 531–35
  heart failure, 532–33, 534
  hypertension, 530–31
  leukemia and anemia, 526
  peripheral vascular disease, 529, 529–30*g*
  summary and review questions, 535–37
  transient ischemic attack, 528–29
  varicose veins, 528, 529*f*
Cardiovascular system, 79*f*, 520–23, 522*f*, 523*f*, 524*f*, 525*f*, 526
  effects of aging on, 226*f*, 228, 521*f*
  observations of, 88, 88*f*
  prevention of inactivity effects on, 435*t*
Care plan, 14, 52, 53*f*, 54, 92, 93*f*, 94
  communication with special needs residents and, 58

  for developmental disabilities, 640
  for discharge, 412, 412–13*f*
  documentation and, 90
Care plan conference, 20–21, 92, 93*f*, 94, 437, 437*f*
  resident and family in, 101, 101*f*
Career health, 41
Caregivers, 19–30
  administrative organization of, 26–27, 27*f*
  clinical focus and objectives, 19
  confidentiality and, 104
  ethics and, 117
  and grieving process, 645, 645*f*, 647
  hepatitis B vaccine and, 157
  interdisciplinary team members, 20–21, 20*f*, 22–23*f*, 24–26, 24*f*, 25*f*, 26*f*
  quality assurance program for, 28
  self-care and, 40–41
  staff development for, 28
  summary and review questions, 28–30
  tuberculosis test and, 159
  *See also* Nursing assistant(s)
Caries
  diet and, 296
  oral hygiene and, 278
Carriers of infection, 156
Cartilage, 579
Casts, 582–83
Cataracts, 599
Catastrophic reactions, Alzheimer's disease and, 621, 621*f*, 628
Catheter(s), 656–57, 656*f*, 657*f*
  ambulation with, 351
  care of, 37*f*, 39, 163, 348, 349–50, 350*f*
  condom, 361, 362, 362*f*
  disconnection procedure, 351–52, 352*f*
  epidural, 659–60
  infection risk and, 348, 351
  routine drainage check procedure for, 348–49, 349*f*
Catholics, 213*f*
  death and dying beliefs and practices, 647, 647*f*, 649*f*
  dietary practices, 300*f*
Cavities
  body, 80*f*, 81
  dental, 278, 296
CD4 cells, HIV and, 161
Cells, 67, 77, 78

Celsius scale, 370, 372, 372*f*

Centimeter measurements, 371, 391

Central nervous system (CNS), 593, 594, 595*f*, 596, 596*f*

Central venous (CV) catheter, 656, 657*f*

Cerebellum, 596

Cerebral palsy, 637, 637*f*

Cerebrospinal fluid (CSF), 596

Cerebrovascular accident (CVA), 527, 604
*See also* Stroke

Cerebrovascular disease, 618

Cerebrum, 595, 596, 596*f*

Certification
for facility, 668
of nursing assistants, 10–11

Certified nursing assistants, 23*f*

Cervix, 567*f*

Chain of command
administrative, 27, 27*f*
nursing, 49, 50*f*

Chain of infection, 155, 155*f*, 156*f*

Chair positioning, 472–73, 472*f*, 475, 475*f*

Chair scales, 391, 392*f*, 395

Chaplain, 22*f*

Charge nurses, 21
assignments and, 38, 38*f*
in chain of command, 50*f*

Charting guidelines, 90–92, 91*f*

Chemical hazards, 125–26

Chemical restraints, 102

Chemotherapy, 662

Chest x-rays, 159

Cheyne-Stokes respirations, 384*f*, 648

Chickenpox, 154, 157, 159
infection control and, 177, 177*f*

Childhood diseases, 154, 157
as cause of mental retardation, 636

Chlamydia infection, 573

Choking
in conscious person, emergency procedure for 142–43, 143*f*
feeding and, 309
prevention of, 134
in unconscious person, emergency procedure for 144–45, 144*f*, 145*f*

Choroid, 597, 597*f*

Christian Science
death and dying beliefs and practices, 649*f*
dietary practices, 300*f*

Chronic bronchitis, 545

Chronic disease, 198
adjustments to, 216
as reason for admission to LTC, 203, 203*f*, 402
restorative care and, 433

Chronic heart failure, 534

Chronic obstructive pulmonary disease (COPD), 545–48, 546*f*, 547*f*

Chronic renal failure, 363

Church of Christ, death and dying beliefs and practices, 649*f*

Circulation
aging and, 228
disorders of, 526–31, 527*f*, 528*f*, 529*f*
emergency response and, 140*g*
observations of, 88, 88*f*
skin breakdown and, 258

Clean-catch urine specimen procedure, 360–61

Cleanliness and order, 236

Clear liquid diet, 298

Client
definition of, 5–6
health care services for, 5*f*

Climacteric, 568

Clinical nurse specialists, 21

Clinics, 4*f*, 7

Clinitron bed, 260, 261*f*

Clitoris, 566, 567*f*

Clothing
assisting residents in choosing, 104–5, 105*f*
dressing procedures and, 284–86
prevention of falls and, 134
residents' right to, 116, 116*f*

*Coccidioides immitis*, 162

Coccidioidomycosis, 162

Code blue order, 646

Code of ethics, 117

Cognitive impairment, 618
*See also* Alzheimer's disease; Dementia

Cold applications, 418–19, 418*f*, 421–25
clinical focus and objectives, 417
dry cold, 421–24, 422*f*, 423*f*
moist cold, 425, 425*f*
safety when using, 418, 419*f*
summary and review questions, 425–26

Cold pack, 421–22, 422*f*

Colitis, diets for, 299

Colon, 291, 291*f*, 293, 339*f*
disorders of, 313
elimination from, 327, 328*f*. *See also* Bowel elimination

Colostomy, 338–39, 339*f*
location and fecal characteristics, 339*f*
stoma care, 339–41, 340*f*, 341*f*
as transfer belt contraindication, 487

Coma, 648

Combining word forms, 67, 67*f*, 68–70

Commode, 321–22, 322*f*, 326

Common cold, 154

Communicable disease, 176

Communication, 47–63
clinical focus and objectives, 47
oral, 49–51, 50*f*
process of, 48–49, 48*f*, 49*f*
with residents, 54–55, 55–57*g*
with special needs residents, 58–61, 59*f*
with staff members, 49
summary and review questions, 61–63
terminology in. *See* Terminology
through touch, 57–58, 57*f*
written, 52, 52*f*, 53*f*, 54, 54*f*

Community activities, residents' right to participate in, 114

Community health care facilities, 4–8, 4*f*, 6*f*, 7*f*, 8*f*
comparisons of, 5–6*f*
*See also* Long-term care facilities

Community nursing centers, 4*f*, 7

Community services, discharge planning and, 410–11, 412

Compensation defense mechanism, 217, 217*f*

Compliance, facility, 668

Computed tomography (CT) scan, 638, 639

Computers, 14–15, 15*f*

Condom, urinary drainage with, 361, 362, 362*f*

Confidentiality, 104
nurses' station and, 14
violation of, 117

Congestive heart failure, 532–33

Conjunctiva, 597, 597*f*

Connective cells and tissue, 78

Consciousness, seizures and, 148

Constipation, 312, 327, 328
aging and, 227, 293*f*
checking procedure for, 329
enemas for, 328, 329–36, 330*f*, 331*f*, 332*f*, 333*f*, 335*f*
rectoceles and, 363
suppositories for, 336–37, 337*f*

Constriction of blood vessels, 253

Consultants, 24–26, 25*f*
Contact precautions, 178–79, 178*f*
Contact transmission, 155, 156*f*
Contamination/contagion
    disease and, 176
    disposal and, 175*g*
    of equipment and supplies, 168
    glove, mask, and gown removal
        procedures and, 181–84 181*f*,
        182*f*, 183*f*, 184*f*
    leg bag to catheter connection
        and, 358, 358*f*
    personal care prevention
        procedures and, 239*f*, 240*f*
    tuberculosis and, 159
Continence, 321
Continuing education, 28, 42, 680
Contractures, 25, 434*f*, 579
    amputation and, 471
    arthritis and, 471
    as complication of multiple
        sclerosis, 608*g*
    positioning and, 472
    prevention of, 434*t*, 459, 459*f*,
        460, 477
    restraints and, 130
    spasticity and, 458
    wheelchairs and, 506
Convulsions. *See* Seizures
COPD. *See* Chronic obstructive
    pulmonary disease
Coping mechanisms, 217
Cornea, 597, 597*f*
Corporal punishment, 102
Cortisone, 553
Coughing, intubation and, 548
Cowper's glands, 564, 565*f*, 566
Cranial cavity, 80*f*
Creutzfeldt-Jacob disease, 619*f*
Cross-training courses, job growth
    and, 680
Crutches, 15, 501–2, 502*f*, 503*f*
Cryptosporidiosis, 162
*Cryptosporidium* protozoa, 162
Cubic centimeters measurement,
    301
Cultural and ethnic groups
    communication and, 49, 54
    dietary preferences of, 297, 299,
        301*f*
    health/illness belief systems,
        211–12*f*
    personal space in, 234, 235*f*
    residents' behavior and, 210
    touch and, 215
Culture and sensitivity test, 158
Cutaneous membrane, 81

Cuticle care, 276, 277
Cyanosis, 384
Cystoceles, 363, 571
Cytology, 67

**D**

Day care facilities, 4*f*
Day room, 13
Death and dying, 643–52
    clinical focus and objectives, 643
    postmortem care, 648, 650–51,
        650*f*
    process of, 644–48, 644*f*, 645*f*,
        646*f*, 651*f*
    religious beliefs and practices
        regarding, 647–48, 647*f*, 649*f*
    signs of, 648
    summary and review questions,
        651–52
Deconditioned heart, prevention
    of, 435*t*
Decubiti, 255
    *See also* Pressure ulcers
Defamation of character, 117
Defecation, 290
    *See also* Bowel elimination;
        Elimination needs
Defense mechanisms, 217
Deficiencies of facility, surveys
    and, 672
Dehydration, 297, 310, 352
    signs of, 310*f*
    urine production and, 346
Delusions, Alzheimer's disease
    and, 620, 629
Demanding behavior, 219
Dementia
    ADL guidelines for, 626*g*
    arteriosclerosis and, 527
    caring for residents with,
        622–25, 627, 627*f*
    as complication of HIV, 161, 162
    definition of, 618
    Huntington's disease and, 608
    increased choking risk and, 134
    major forms of, 619*f*
    Parkinson's disease and, 603
    poisonous substances and, 133
    as reason for admission to LTC,
        402
    *See also* Alzheimer's disease
Denial
    as defense mechanism, 217
    as stage of grief, 646, 646*f*
Dental caries
    diet and, 296
    oral hygiene and, 278

Dental hygienist, 22*f*, 26
Dentist, 22*f*, 26
Dentures, 253, 278–80
    procedure for care of, 282–83,
        282*f*
Deoxygenated blood, 523
Departmental abbreviations, 74
Dependability, 32, 33*f*
Depressants, 385
Depression, 219–20
    prevention of, 436*t*
    as stage of Alzheimer's disease,
        620
    as stage of grief, 646, 646*f*
Dermis, 252, 256
    burns and, 149
    skin breakdown and, 256*f*
Deterioration, mental and
    physical, 218
Developmental disabilities,
    198–99, 199*f*, 633–41
    as admission reason for
        younger residents, 203, 203*f*
    caring for residents with,
        639–40
    characteristics of, 634–35, 635*f*
    clinical focus and objectives,
        633
    facilities for, 4, 4*f*, 5–6, 7, 7*f*
    forms of, 637–39
    mental retardation, 635–37
    summary and review questions,
        640–41
Developmental tasks, 210, 210*f*
Diabetes mellitus, 198, 556–59,
    556*f*, 557*f*
    foot care and, 277
    nail care and, 276
    treatment of, 558–59
Diabetic coma, 556, 557, 557*f*
Diabetic diet, 298, 298*f*
Diabetic ketoacidosis (DKA), 557
Diabetic retinopathy, 600
Diagnosis, 21
Diagnosis-related group (DRG),
    402
Diagnostic abbreviations, 71–72
Diagnostic tests. *See* Tests
Dialysis, 363, 363*f*, 403
    caring for resident receiving,
        661–62, 661*f*
    subacute care unit and, 654
Diaphoresis, 532
Diaphragm, abdominal, 540*f*
Diarrhea, 327
    diets for, 299
    protozoan infections and, 162

Diastole, 522
Diastolic pressure, 387, 390, 391
Diathermy, 419
Dietary manual, 52
Dietitian, 21, 22f, 24f, 415
Diets
  cultural and religious practices
    and preferences, 299, 300f,
    301f
  diabetic, 558
  standard, 297–98, 297f, 298f
  therapeutic, 21, 298–99, 298f
  See also Nutritional needs
Digestion process, 291–93, 292f
Digestive system, 79f, 290–93, 291f
  diets for problems in, 299
  disorders of, 312–13
  effects of aging on, 226f, 227,
    293, 293f
  observation of, 88
  prevention of inactivity effects
    on, 435t
Dilation of blood vessels, 253
Dining room, 13
Diphtheria, 157
Diplegia, 637
Dirty equipment and supplies, 168
  See also Infection control
Disabilities
  definition of, 198–200
  environmental adaptation for,
    106–7, 106f
  restorative care and, 432
  See also Developmental
    disabilities
Disaster manual, 52
Discharge of resident, 409–15
  clinical focus and objectives,
    401
  factors to consider before,
    411–15
  interdisciplinary health care
    team and, 414–15, 414f
  post-discharge care plan,
    412–13f
  procedure for, 411
  summary and review questions,
    415–16
  wheelchair maneuvers in,
    507–10, 509f, 510f, 511f
Discharge planner, 402
Discharge planning, 410
Disinfection, 190
Dislocation, 149–50, 461
Disorientation, 220
  communication and, 60–61
  prevention of, 436t

as risk factor for accidents, 129,
  130
as stage of Alzheimer's disease,
  620
Distal anatomic location, 76, 77f
Distention, abdominal, 328
Diverticuli, 313
Diverticulitis, 313
Diverticulosis, 313
Do not resuscitate (DNR) orders,
  108, 142, 142f
Documentation, 39, 40
  clinical focus and objectives, 85
  medical chart, 54, 54f, 90–92,
    90f, 91f
  of resident care procedures, 240f
  of restraint use, 131g, 133g
  summary and review questions,
    95–96
Dorsal body surface, 75, 76f, 77f
Dorsal cavity, 80f, 81
Dorsiflexion, ankle, 454, 455f
Draw sheet, 241, 242g, 243f, 248
Dressing/undressing resident,
  284–86
  aids for, 441f
  in facility survey, 670
  guidelines for dementia
    residents, 626g
  restorative program guidelines
    for, 443–44g
  task segmentation for, 438t
Droplet precautions, 177, 177f
Droplet transmission, 155, 156f
Drugs. See Medications
Dry cold applications, 418f,
  421–24, 422f, 423f
Dry sterile dressings (DSD), 258
Dry warm applications, 418f, 419
Duodenum, 292
Dying process. See Death and
  dying
Dyspepsia, 313
Dysphagia, 312
Dyspnea, 384f
  as heart failure symptom, 532
  as sign of infection, 543
Dysuria, 363

E
Ear
  components of, 597–98, 598f
  temperature procedure in,
    380–81, 380f, 381f
Eastern Orthodox Christians,
  death and dying beliefs and
  practices, 649f

Eating
  aids for, 442f
  observation of, 88
  restorative program guidelines
    for, 443g
  task segmentation for, 438t
  See also Feeding
Edema, 299, 352
  as heart failure symptom,
    532
  as sign of electrolyte imbalance,
    555, 555f
  weight monitoring and, 391
Education
  continuing, 28, 42, 680
  in-service, 680–81, 681f
Ejaculatory duct, 564, 565, 565f
Elasticized stockings, 532, 533–34,
  533f, 534f
Elbow exercises, 450–51, 450f,
  451f
Elderly. See Aging process
Electrocardiogram, 522
Electroencephalogram (EEG),
  638–39
Electrolyte balance, 555, 555f
Electronic speech, laryngectomies
  and, 542
Electronic thermometer, 373,
  373f
  axillary temperature procedure
    with, 379
  oral temperature procedure
    with, 377–78, 378f
  rectal temperature procedure
    with, 378–79, 378f
Elimination needs
  assisting with, 321, 321f
  bathroom assistance procedure,
    326–27
  bedpan procedure for, 323–25,
    324f
  bedside commode procedure
    for, 326
  bowel. See Bowel elimination
  clinical focus and objectives,
    319–20
  equipment for, 105, 321–23, 322f
  summary and review questions,
    364–65
  typical duties for, 37f
  urinal procedure for, 325
  urinary. See Urinary catheter
    drainage; Urination
Embolus
  prevention of, 435t
  stroke from, 604

Emergencies, 139–51
airway obstruction, conscious, 142–43, 143*f*
airway obstruction, unconscious, 144–45, 144*f*, 145*f*, 147
burns, 149
cardiac arrest, 141–42, 141*f*
clinical focus and objectives, 139
fainting, 150
falls, 147, 147*f*
general response guidelines, 140, 140–41*g*
hemorrhage, 146, 146*f*, 147
orthopedic injuries, 149–50
poisoning, 150
seizures, 148–49
summary and review questions, 150–51
Emergency Medical Services (EMS), 140*g*, 141*g*, 142
Emesis
aspiration during, 143, 147
fluid output recording and, 354, 354*f*
Emesis basin, 12
Emotional health
of nursing assistants, 41
observation and, 87
residents' needs and, 208, 208*f*, 209, 209*f*
Emotional lability, 605
Empathy, 32–33
Emphysema, 545
Employee personnel handbook, 52
Employee safety
equipment and, 126, 128*f*
ergonomics and body mechanics in, 122, 123*g*, 124, 124*f*, 125*f*
hazardous chemicals and, 125–26, 127*f*
oxygen use and, 128, 128*f*
Employment, 675–83
application and interview process, 678–79, 678*f*, 679*f*
clinical focus and objectives, 675
job possibilities, 676–77, 676*f*, 677*f*
references, 678
resignation and, 681
résumés, 677–78
security and growth, 679–81, 680*f*
self-appraisal and, 676, 676*f*
summary and review questions, 681–83
Empowerment activities, 113

Endocrine disorders, 551–61
clinical focus and objectives, 551
diabetes mellitus, 556–59, 556*f*, 557*f*
electrolyte imbalance, 555, 555*f*
glucose metabolism and, 555–56
summary and review questions, 559–61
Endocrine glands, 552, 553–54, 553*f*
Endocrine system, 78, 79*f*, 552–54, 553*f*
effects of aging on, 226*f*, 228, 554–55
observation of, 88
Endometrium, 566*f*, 568
Endotracheal tube, 548
Enemas, 37*f*, 39, 328, 329–30, 334
commercially prepared enema procedure, 334–36, 335*f*
oil-retention enema procedure, 330–31, 330*f*
soapsuds enema procedure, 331–34, 331*f*, 332*f*, 333*f*
Enteral feeding, 311–12, 311*f*, 312*f*, 657, 657*f*
Enterococci, 158
Environment, 233–50
bedmaking procedures in, 242–48, 242*g*, 243*f*, 244*f*, 245*f*, 246*f*, 247*f*, 248*f*
clinical focus and objectives, 233
components of, 234, 234*f*
infection control in, 172*f*
linens in, 241, 241–42*g*
maintenance of, 235–37, 237*f*, 238*g*
personal space in, 234–35, 235*f*
and prevention of falling, 134
resident care procedures in, 237–38, 239–40*f*
residents' room, 235
in restorative programs, 444–45, 444*f*
summary and review questions, 249–50
*See also* Long-term care facilities
Environmental needs, 106–7
Environmental services, 23*f*, 26, 26*f*
Enzymes, digestive, 290, 291, 292, 292*f*, 293, 293*f*
Epidermis, 252, 256
burns and, 149
skin breakdown and, 256*f*
Epididymis, 564, 565, 565*f*
Epidural catheter, 659–60

Epilepsy, 637–39, 639*f*
Episcopalians, death and dying beliefs and practices, 649*f*
Epithelial cells and tissue, 78
Equilibrium, ear and, 597
Equipment
disinfection of, 169, 169*f*
personal, in resident rooms, 12–13, 12*f*
safety, 126
supportive, 458–61, 458*f*, 459*f*, 460*f*, 461*f*
*See also specific types*
Ergonomics, 122, 123*g*
Erikson, Erik, 208
developmental stages of, 210, 210*f*
Erythrocytes, 67, 526
*Escherichia coli*, 158
Esophageal speech, laryngectomies and, 542
Esophagus, 290, 291*f*, 291
Estrogen, 554, 566
Ethics, 117
Ethnic groups. *See* Cultural and ethnic groups
Europeans/European-Americans
health/illness belief systems of, 211*f*
personal space and, 235*f*
Evacuation routes and procedures, 135, 135*f*, 136
Evaluation, in care plan, 93*f*, 94
Eversion, 447, 455, 455*f*
Excreta, 321
Excretion. *See* Bowel elimination; Elimination needs
Exercise(s)
aging and, 227
for back injury prevention, 124, 125*f*
breathing, 546
for dementia residents, 627, 627*f*
diabetes and, 558
and infection prevention, 163
range of motion. *See* Range of motion exercises
skin breakdown prevention and, 257*g*
Exit conference, 672
Expectoration, 543
Expiration, respiratory, 541
Exposure incident, 172
Extension, 446, 446*f*
elbow, 450, 450*f*
fingers, 452, 452*f*
hip, 454, 454*f*
shoulder, 448, 448*f*, 450*f*

thumb, 453
toes, 455
wrist, 451, 451*f*
External fixation, for fractures, 583–84, 584*f*
External rotation, 447
  hip, 454, 454*f*
  shoulder, 450, 450*f*
External urinary drainage (male), 361, 362, 362*f*
Extremities, 76
Eye, 596–97, 597*f*
  *See also* Vision
Eye contact
  with Alzheimer's residents, 623*g*
  in communication, 54, 55, 55*g*
  cultural and ethnic groups and, 234, 235*f*
Eyeglasses, 598
  assisting residents with, 105
  care of, 599

**F**
Face shield, 172*f*, 173*g*
Facial hair care, 274–76, 274*f*, 275*f*, 276*f*
Facilities. *See* Acute care hospitals; Community health care facilities; Long-term care facilities; Subacute care units
Fahrenheit scale, 370, 372, 372*f*
Fainting, 150
  as sign of acute MI, 532
Fallopian tubes, 566*f*, 567*f*, 568
Falls, 147, 147*f*
  aging and, 227
  prevention of, 134
False imprisonment, 117
Family
  admissions and, 403, 407
  in care plan conference, 101, 101*f*
  dementia and, 625
  dynamics in grieving process, 647
  residents' right to visit with, 115
  restorative care plan and, 437, 437*f*, 438
Fasting, 385
Fatigue
  with multiple sclerosis, 607, 608*g*
  and nursing assistants, 41
Fats, dietary, 294
  enzymatic breakdown of, 291, 292*f*, 293
  food groups containing, 296
  functions of, 292*f*

Fax machines, 15, 15*f*
Fecal impaction, 328
  checking procedure for, 329
  constipation and, 328
  enemas for, 328, 329–36, 330*f*, 331*f*, 332*f*, 333*f*, 335*f*
  suppositories for, 336–37, 337*f*
Fecal incontinence, 342, 342*f*
Feces, 290, 291, 321, 327
  characteristics, in relation to colostomy site, 339*f*
  constipation and, 312
  enemas and, 329
Feeding, 304–5, 305*f*
  alternative methods of, 311–12, 312*f*
  assistance procedure for dependent resident, 308–9, 308*f*, 309*f*
  assistance procedure for self-feeding resident, 306–7, 306*f*, 307*f*
  checking food temperature before, 133
  choking prevention and, 134, 309
  dementia residents and, 626*g*
  digestive disorders and, 312–13
  food thickeners and, 305, 307
  mealtime responsibilities and, 304
  residents' right to refuse, 108
  supplements, 309–10
  water and, 310–11, 310*f*
  *See also* Nutritional needs
Fiber
  carbohydrates and, 294
  constipation and, 312
  food groups containing, 294–96
Finger exercises, 452, 452*f*
Fire extinguishers, 136
Fire safety, 135–36, 135*f*, 136*f*
First-degree burns, 149
Fistula, for hemodialysis, 661, 661*f*
Flaccid paralysis, 457
Flatulence, 227, 293*f*
Flatus, 327, 329, 337
Flatus bag, 337, 338, 338*f*
Flexion, 446, 446*f*
  avoidance of in positioning, 471
  elbow, 450, 450*f*
  fingers, 452, 452*f*
  hip, 454, 454*f*
  shoulder, 448, 448*f*
  thumb, 453
  toes, 455
  wrist, 451, 451*f*

Flora, body, 156
Flossing procedure, 281–82, 281*f*
Flotation mattress, 260, 260*f*
Fluid intake
  calculation of, 299, 301–2, 302*f*
  in cardiac care, 533
  guidelines for, 310
  and infection prevention, 163
  measurement and recording procedure for, 302, 303*f*
  nutrition and, 304
  urine production and, 346
Fluid output
  measurement and recording procedures for, 352–55, 353*f*, 354*f*, 355–56, 355*f*, 356*f*
  specimen collection and, 359, 359*f*, 361
  urination and, 352
Fluid retention. *See* Edema
Foam pads and pillows, 260
Food-borne illnesses, outbreaks of, 164
Food groups, 294–97
Food Guide Pyramid, 294, 295*f*
Food poisoning, 158
Food storage
  infection control and, 175*g*
  labeling of, 133
Food thickeners, 305, 307
Foot and toenail care, 277, 587, 589
  in bed bath, 266
  procedure for, 278
Foot cradles, 260, 260*f*
Footboards, 459
Forearm crutches, 502, 503*f*
Foreskin, 564, 565*f*
Fowler's position, 470–71, 471*f*
  for congestive heart failure, 532
  for COPD, 546
Fracture bedpan, 322, 322*f*
Fractures, 149, 582–84, 582*f*, 583*f*, 584*f*
Free choice, as residents' right, 101–2
Friction
  positioning and, 457
  and skin breakdown, 254, 254*f*
Functional ability, 87, 437
Functional changes, 225, 227–28, 227*f*
Functional deficits, 199, 436
  evaluation of, 437–39

Fungal infections, 155, 155f, 162
Fungi, 155

**G**

Gag reflex, 292, 293, 293f
Gait, 500
Gait belt, 485
  contraindications to, 487
  prevention of falls and, 134
  transfer procedure, 485–87, 486f
Gait difficulties, as stage of
  Alzheimer's disease, 622
Gait training, 500–1, 501f
Gallbladder disease, diet for, 298,
  298f
Gangrene, 557, 557f
Gas sterilization, 190
Gastritis, 313
Gastroenteritis
  infection control and, 178
  outbreaks of, 164
Gastrointestinal tract
  effects of aging on, 290–93, 291f
  elimination from, 327, 328f. See
    also Bowel elimination
  See also Digestive system
Gastrostomy tube feedings,
  311–12, 311f
Gel-filled mattress, 260
Genetic disease, 608
Genital herpes, 573
Genitalia
  bathing of, 266, 270–73, 270f,
    272f
  catheter care and, 349–50
  female, 566, 567f
  male, 564–65, 565f
  observations of, 89
Geriatric care, 8, 200
Geriatric chair, 475, 475f
German measles, 157
Gerontology, 75, 200
*Giardia lamblia*, 162
Giardiasis, 162
Glaucoma, 599
Glomerulus, 345f, 346
Gloves
  allergy to, 173g
  gloving and removal
    procedures, 181–82, 181f, 182f
  infection control and, 170, 178f,
    179
  as standard precaution, 172f,
    173g
Glucagon, 552, 554, 555
Glucose, 554
Glucose metabolism, 555–56

Glucose monitoring, 559
Glycosuria, 556
Goals for resident, 92, 93f, 94
  in restorative care plan, 438–39
Goiter, 554
Gonads, 552, 554
Gonorrhea, 572
Gown
  dressing procedure, 180, 180f
  infection control and, 178f, 179
  patient, changing procedure for,
    658–59, 659f
  removal procedure, 182–84,
    183f, 184f
  as standard precaution, 172f,
    173g
Grabber, 135
Graft, for hemodialysis, 661, 661f
Grand mal seizure, 638, 639f
Granulocytoma, 67
Greek Orthodox, dietary
  practices, 300f
Grievances, residents' right to
  voice, 108, 113, 113f
Grieving process, 216, 651, 651f
  caregivers and, 645, 645f, 647
  family dynamics in, 647
  stages of, 646–47, 646f
Grooming
  aids for, 440f
  assistance and, 444f
  in facility survey, 670
  guidelines for dementia
    residents, 626g
  of nursing assistants, 34, 34f
  restorative program guidelines
    for, 443g
  task segmentation for, 438t
Group homes, 4f
Growth, employment, 680–81,
  680f, 681f

**H**

Hair care, 273, 273f, 274f
  facial, 274–76, 274f, 275f, 276f
Halitosis, 278
Hallucinations, Alzheimer's
  disease and, 621, 629
Hand and fingernail care, 276
  in bed baths, 265
  procedure for, 276–77
Handwashing, 169, 170, 240f
  bedmaking and, 242f, 247, 248
  infection control and, 178f
  procedure for, 170–71, 171f
  as standard precaution, 172f,
    173g, 176

Harmony, in interdisciplinary
  health care team, 37
Hazards, work environment,
  125–26, 128, 128f
Head-tilt/chin-lift method for
  airway obstruction, 144, 144f
Health care
  language of. See Terminology
  legal aspects of, 116–17
Health care facilities
  functions of, 8f
  increase of serious infections
    in, 157
  See also Acute care hospitals;
    Community health care
    facilities; Long-term care
    facilities; Subacute care units
Health care providers; see
  Caregivers; Nursing
  assistant(s)
Hearing, mechanics of, 598
Hearing aids, 600–1, 601f
  assisting residents with, 105
  communication and, 58
  procedure for applying and
    removing, 602, 602f
Hearing impairment/loss, 600–1
  aging and, 226f, 227–28
  communication and, 58, 59f
  as risk factor for accidents, 129
Heart, 521–22, 522f, 523f
  deconditioned, 435t
  See also Cardiovascular system
Heart attack, 527–28, 527f, 531,
  531f
  as complication of diabetes, 557
Heart block, 534–35
Heart disease, 198, 531–35, 531f
Heart failure
  chronic, 534
  congestive, 532–33
Heart rate, pulse rate and, 382
Heat treatments. See Warm
  applications
Height measurement and
  recording, 391, 393
  abbreviations for, 74
  in-bed procedure, 396
  upright procedure, 394, 394f
Heimlich maneuver, 142–43, 143f,
  147, 309
Hematuria, 363
Hemianopsia, 605, 605f
Hemiplegia, 436, 604, 605, 605f
  ambulation with cane and,
    505–6, 506f
  in cerebral palsy, 637

and gait, 500
  independent bed movement
    and, 476–77
  lateral positioning and, 468–69,
    469f
  supine positioning and, 467, 467f
Hemodialysis, 363, 363f, 661–62
Hemoptysis
  as heart failure symptom, 532
  as tuberculosis symptom, 159
Hemorrhage, 147
  emergency procedure for, 146,
    146f
  stroke from, 604
Hemorrhoids, 313, 363
HEPA filter mask, 177, 177f
Hepatitis, 154, 160
  outbreaks of, 164
  vaccine for, 157
Hernias, 312–13, 571
Herpes simplex, 154, 573
Herpes zoster, 154, 159
Hiatal hernia, 312–13
High density nutrients, 312
High-efficiency particulate air
    (HEPA) filter mask, 177, 177f
High Fowler's position
  for congestive heart failure, 532
  for COPD, 546
High protein diet, 298f, 299
Hinduism, 213f
  death and dying beliefs and
    practices, 649f
  dietary practices, 300f
Hip
  exercises for, 453–54, 453f, 454f
  fractures of, 584–85, 584f
  prosthesis, 586–87, 586f, 587f
Hispanics/Hispanic-Americans
  health/illness belief systems of,
    211f
  personal space and, 235f
HIV. *See* Human
    immunodeficiency virus
Home health aide, 410
Home health care, 4–5, 4f
  comparison with other health
    care facilities, 6f
Homeostasis, 555
Hormones, 552, 553–54
Hospice, 4, 4f, 5, 6f, 107
  subacute care unit and, 655
Hospitalization, 108
Hot-line number, residents' right
    to, 115, 115f
Housekeeping, 26, 26f
  survey and, 670

Human immunodeficiency virus
    (HIV), 157, 160–62, 161f
  *See also* Acquired immune
    deficiency syndrome
Human needs, basic, 208–10, 208f,
    209f, 210f
Humidifer bottle, 547, 548
Huntington's disease, 198, 608–9,
    618
  care guidelines for, 609g
  features and course of, 619f
  and gait, 500
Hygiene
  of nursing assistants, 34, 34f
  of residents. *See* Personal
    hygiene
Hyperalimentation, 311, 312,
    656–57
Hyperglycemia, 556, 557
Hypertension, 386, 528f, 530–31,
    604
Hyperthyroidism, 554
Hypoglycemia, 556, 557–58
Hypotension, 386
Hypothermia, 421
Hypothermia blanket, 418f, 423–24
Hypothyroidism, 554
Hypoxia, as heart failure
    symptom, 532
Hysterectomy, as treatment for
    prolapsed uterus, 571

**I**

Ice bag, 418f, 421
  application procedure for,
    422–23, 423f
Ileostomy, 341–42, 341f
Ileum, 66, 292
Ilium, 66
Immunity, 157
Immunizations, 157
Immunosuppression, 157
Impairment, 198–200
  *See also* Developmental
    disabilities
Implementation, for care plan, 94
Inactivity, preventing
    complications from, 433,
    433–36t
Incidents. *See* Accidents;
    Emergencies
Incontinence, 105, 321
  bowel and bladder programs
    for, 477, 478–80g
  fecal, 327, 342, 342f
  positioning residents with, 458
  prevention of, 435t

as risk factor for accidents, 129
  seizures and, 149
  as stage of Alzheimer's disease,
    622
  urinary, 347, 352, 363
Independence, loss of, 216–17,
    217f, 403
Independent bed movement,
    476–77
Indigestion, 313
Indwelling catheter(s)
  ambulation with, 351
  care of, 348, 349–50, 350f
  disconnection procedure,
    351–52, 352f
  infection risk and, 348, 351
  routine drainage check
    procedure for, 348–49, 349f
Infarction, 521
  myocardial, 527–28, 527f, 528f,
    531, 531f
Infection control, 167–93
  clinical focus and objectives, 167
  disinfection and sterilization in,
    190–92, 191f, 192f
  environmental procedures for,
    174–75g
  in facility survey, 670
  handwashing for, 170–71, 171f
  isolation precautions for,
    176–79, 177f 178f
  mask-donning procedure for, 179
  medical asepsis in, 168–70
  self-protection in, 172
  standard precautions for, 172,
    172f, 173g, 176
  summary and review questions,
    192–93
  transmission-based. *See*
    Isolation procedures
Infection(s), 153–65
  aging process and, 162–63,
    543
  bacterial, 157–59
  body flora and, 156
  burns and, 149
  catheters and, 348, 351
  chain of, 155, 155f, 156f
  clinical focus and objectives,
    153
  diarrhea and, 327
  emphysema and, 545
  fungal, 155f, 162
  immunity to and immunizations
    for, 157
  increase of, 157
  microbes in, 154–55, 154f, 155f

Infection(s)—*cont'd*
  natural defenses against, 156–57, 157*f*
  outbreaks of, 163–64
  prevention measures, 163, 163*f*
  protozoan, 162
  respiratory, 543
  sexually transmitted, 572–73
  skin breakdown and, 257*g*, 258
  summary and review questions, 164–65
  types of, 156
  urinary tract, 347
  viral, 159–62, 160*f*, 161*f*
Inferior body part division, 75, 76*f*
Inferior vena cava, 521, 522*f*, 523, 523*f*
Inflammation, 157, 157*f*
  of GI tract, 313
  signs in elderly, 163
Influenza, 154, 160, 543
  infection control and, 177
  outbreaks of, 164
  vaccine, 157
Informed consent, 117
Inguinal hernia, 312
Injury prevention, 133
  *See also* Safety
In-service education, 680–81, 681*f*
Inspiration, respiratory, 541
Instrumental activities of daily living (IADL), 200, 200*f*, 437
Insulin, 552, 554, 556
  home administration of, 414*f*, 415
  injections, 558, 559
Insulin-dependent diabetes mellitus (IDDM), 556, 558
Insulin shock, 556, 557, 557*f*, 558
Intake and output (I&O) of fluids, 299, 301–2, 302*f*, 352–56
  measurement and recording procedure for, 302, 303*f*
  specimen collection and, 359, 359*f*, 361
  urination and, 352
Integumentary system, 79*f*, 252
  effects of aging on, 225*f*, 253–54, 253*f*, 254*f*
  observation of, 88
  prevention of inactivity effects on, 434*t*
  *See also* Skin
Intelligence quotient (IQ), 636
Intention tremor, from multiple sclerosis, 607

Interdisciplinary health care team, 20–21, 20*f*, 22–23*f*, 24–26, 24*f*
  assessment of new resident by, 404, 404*f*
  discharge planning and, 410, 411–15
  and mental retardation diagnosis and evaluation, 636
  nursing assistant in, 37
  process of, 92, 93*f*, 94
  and psychosocial needs of residents, 106
  restorative care and, 431–32, 437–39, 444–45
Intermittent positive pressure breathing (IPPB), 548
Internal rotation
  hip, 454, 454*f*
  shoulder, 450, 450*f*
Interpersonal skills. *See* Communication
Intervention, in care plan, 93*f*, 94
Interviews
  employment, 678–79, 678*f*, 679*f*
  of residents during facility survey, 671
Intestines, 291, 291*f*, 292–93
Intravenous (IV) therapy, 656–57, 656*f*, 657*f*, 658*g*
Invasion of privacy, 117
Inversion, 447, 455, 455*f*
Involuntary seclusion, 102
Iris, 597, 597*f*
Iron, dietary, 327
Ischemia, 521, 531
Islam, 213*f*
  death and dying beliefs and practices, 649*f*
  dietary practices, 300*f*
Islets of Langerhans, 552, 553*f*, 554
Isolation, 176–79
  preparation of resident room for, 179
  psychological aspects of, 176
Isolation procedures
  gloving, 181, 181*f*
  gowning, 180
  linen care in isolation unit, 185
  mask donning, 179
  meals in isolation unit, 186–87
  patient transport to and from isolation unit, 189–90, 190*f*
  removal of contaminated gloves, mask, and gown, 182–83, 183*f*, 184*f*
  specimen collection, 187–88, 188*f*

transfer of nondisposable equipment, 189
  vital signs measurement, 185–86

**J**
Jacket restraint, 131*f*
Jehovah's Witnesses, death and dying beliefs and practices, 649*f*
Jejunum, 292
Jewelry
  nursing assistants and, 34
  residents' rights to, 116, 116*f*
Job description, 35–36, 36–37*f*
Joints, 579, 581, 581*f*
  movements of, 446–47, 446*f*, 447*f*
Judaism, 213*f*
  death and dying beliefs and practices of, 649*f*
  dietary practices, 300*f*

**K**
Kaposi's sarcoma, 161, 161*f*
Kardex, 14
Ketones, diabetes and, 557
Kidney dialysis, 363, 363*f*, 403
  caring for resident receiving, 661–62, 661*f*
  subacute care unit and, 654
Kidney stones, 363
Kidneys, 78, 344, 345*f*
  edema and, 352
  effect of aging on, 346, 346*f*
  urine production and, 346
Kilogram measurements, 370, 391
Kitchen, 16
Knee exercises, 454
Kyphosis, 582

**L**
Labia majora, 566, 567*f*
Labia minora, 566, 567*f*
Laceration prevention, 133
Language of health care. *See* Terminology
Large intestine. *See* Colon
Laryngectomies, 542
Larynx, 540*f*, 541
  cancer of, 542
Last rites, 647, 647*f*, 649*f*
Lateral division of body, 75, 76*f*, 77*f*
Lateral position, 457
  procedures for, 468–69, 469*f*
Laundry, 16
  *See also* Linens

Leg bag drainage, 356, 356*f*
  catheter connection procedure
    for, 357–58, 358*f*
  emptying procedure for, 357
Legal aspects of health care,
  116–17
Legal guardian, 100
Lens, eye, 597, 597*f*
Letter of resignation, 681
Leukemia, 157, 526
Leukocytes, 526
  HIV and, 161
  and infectious disease, 156
Lhermitte's sign, 607
Libel, 117
Licensed practical nurses (LPNs),
  21, 22*f*
Licensed vocational nurses
  (LVNs), 21, 24*f*
Licensure of facility, 668
Lifting, rules for, 124*f*
Ligaments, 579
Lighting
  maintaining adequacy of, 236,
    237, 238*g*
  prevention of falls and, 134
Linens
  caring for in isolation unit, 185
  handling of, 241–42*g*, 243, 247
  infection control and, 170, 172*f*,
    174*g*
Liver, 291, 291*f*
Liver disease, diet for, 298, 298*f*
Liver spots, 254, 254*f*
Living Will, 108, 109–10*f*
Log rolling procedure, 465–66, 466*f*
Long-term care (LTC) facilities,
  3–19
  assisting new residents to
    adjust to living in, 218
  certification and licensure for,
    668
  clinical focus and objectives, 3
  comparison with other health
    care facilities, 5*f*
  computers and fax machines in,
    14–15, 15*f*
  dining room/day room in, 13
  environment of. *See*
    Environment
  functional areas in, 11–16
  kitchen and laundry, 16
  nurses' station, 13*f*, 14
  rehabilitation areas, 15–16
  resident rooms, 11–13, 12*f*
  residents' right to remain in,
    115–16

residents' right to work in, 115
  standards and regulations for,
    10–11
  subacute care units of. *See*
    Subacute care units
  summary and review questions,
    16–18
  surveys of. *See* Survey of facility
  types of, 8–10
  younger resident in, 203, 203*f*,
    204*g*
Lou Gehrig's disease, 609–10, 610*g*
Low fat diet, 298, 298*f*
Low residue diet, 298*f*, 299
Low sodium diet, 298, 298*f*
LTC. *See* Long-term care facility
Lumen, arterial, 527, 527*f*
Lung disease, 198
  cancer, 542
  COPD, 545–48, 546*f*, 547*f*
Lungs, 523*f*, 540*f*, 541
Lutherans, death and dying beliefs
  and practices, 649*f*
Lymph and lymph nodes, 521, 523,
  526

**M**
Macular degeneration, 599
Magnetic resonance imaging
  (MRI), 607, 638, 639
Maintenance, survey and, 670
Maintenance activities, 113
Maladaptive behaviors, 219–20
Malignancies
  of digestive system, 313
  of reproductive system, 569
  of respiratory system, 542
  *See also* Cancer
Mammography, 569
Manipulative behavior, 219
Mantoux test, 159
Manuals, policy and procedure,
  52, 52*f*
Mask(s)
  donning procedure, 179
  infection control and, 177,
    177*f*
  removal procedure, 182–84
  as standard precaution, 172*f*,
    173*g*
Maslow, Abraham, 208
Masturbation, 214, 214*f*
Material Safety Data Sheets
  (MSDS), 126, 127*f*
Mattresses and pads, 259–61, 259*f*,
  260*f*, 261*f*
Maturity, nursing assistant, 32

Meals
  cleanliness after, 236, 238*g*
  dietitian and, 21
  discharge planning and, 410–11
  infection control and, 170
  serving procedure in isolation
    unit, 186–87
  *See also* Diet; Feeding;
    Nutritional needs
Measles, 154, 157, 177, 177*f*
Measurements
  abbreviations for, 74
  metric units for, 301, 370, 371,
    391
Meatus, urinary, 348, 348*f*, 350,
  351, 361
Mechanical aids, pressure-
  reducing, 259–61, 259*f*, 260*f*,
  261*f*
Mechanical lift, 123*g*, 496
  transfer procedure with,
    496–98, 497*f*, 498*f*
  weight measurement with, 391,
    392*f*
Mechanical soft diet, 297, 297*f*
Medial division of body, 75, 76*f*,
  77*f*
Medicaid/Medicare, 9
  residents' right to benefits from,
    114
Medical asepsis, 168–70, 169*f*, 322
Medical chart, 14, 54, 54*f*
  DNR orders on, 142*f*
  documenting observations on,
    90–92, 90*f*, 91*f*
  fluid intake and output chart of,
    303*f*
Medical record practitioner, 22*f*
Medical terminology. *See*
  Terminology
Medical treatment, residents' right
  to refuse, 108
Medications
  as chemical restraints, 102
  diabetic, 558–59
  diarrhea and, 327
  dispensing of, 14
  and immunosuppression, 157
  observations of effectiveness,
    87
  residents' right to refuse, 108
  as risk factor for accidents, 129
Membranes, 78, 81
Memory loss, as stage of
  Alzheimer's disease, 620
Memos, 52, 52*f*
Meninges, 81, 594

Menopause, 568
Menstrual cycle, 568
Menstruation, 568
Mental abuse, 102
Mental retardation, 635–37
Mental status
    examination for, 92
    observation of, 87, 88
Mentally ill, facilities for, 4*f*, 7
Mercury manometer, 386*f*, 387*g*,
    388*g*
Mercury thermometer
    reading procedure, 372, 372*f*
    safety precautions, 372–73
    temperature measurement
        procedures with, 373–77,
        374*f*, 375*f*, 376*f*, 377*f*
Metabolism
    definition of, 554
    glucose, 555–56
Methicillin-resistant
    *Staphylococcus aureus*
    (MRSA), 158, 158*f*, 164
Metric system units, 301, 370, 371,
    391
Microbes, 154–55, 236
    antibiotic resistance of, 158
    in chain of infection, 155, 156*f*
    linens and, 241*g*
    as normal body flora, 156
Micturition, 347
Milliliter measurements, 301
Minerals, 294
    food groups containing, 294–96
    functions of, 292*f*
Minimum Data Set (MDS) 2.0, 92
    new resident admission and,
        404
    physical functioning and
        structural problems in, 431*f*,
        432
Mitered corner in bedmaking, 244,
    244*f*, 246, 248
Mobility
    and accidents, 129
    observation of, 88
    physical therapists and, 25, 25*f*
    task segmentation for, 438*t*
    typical duties for, 37*f*
Mobility restoration, 484
    ambulation guidelines and
        procedures, 504–6, 504*g*, 506*f*
    assistive devices for, 501–2,
        502*f*, 503*f*, 504*f*
    clinical focus and objectives,
        483
    evaluation for ambulation, 500

gait patterns and training,
    500–1, 501*f*
    summary and review questions,
        514–15
    transfers in. *See* Transfer
        procedures
    wheelchair use and, 506–10,
        507*f*, 508*f*, 509*f*, 510*f*, 511*f*
Mobility skills, 432, 432*f*
Moist cold applications, 418*f*, 425
Moist warm applications, 418*f*,
    419, 421
Moribund period, 644–48
    *See also* Death and dying
Mormons, dietary practices, 300*f*
Moslems, 213*f*
    dietary practices, 300*f*
Motor nerves, 594
Mottling, skin, 648
Mouth, 290, 291–92, 291*f*
    care of, oxygen therapy and,
        548
    *See also* Oral hygiene
Mucous membranes, 81
    infection and, 156, 172, 172*f*
    STD transmission and, 572
Mucus, 81
Multi-infarct dementia, 619*f*
Multiple sclerosis (MS), 198, 203*f*,
    607, 607*f*
    care guidelines for, 608*g*
    and gait, 500
    as reason for admission to LTC,
        402
Mumps, 154, 157
Muscle cells and tissue, 78
Muscles, 578–79, 580*f*
Musculoskeletal disorders, 577–90
    amputation, 587
    arthritis, 585–87, 588*f*
    bursitis, 581
    clinical focus and objectives,
        577
    foot and toenail problems, 587,
        589
    fractures, 582–85, 582*f*, 583*f*,
        584*f*
    osteoporosis, 582
    summary and review questions,
        589–90
Musculoskeletal system, 79*f*,
    578–79, 579*f*, 580*f*, 581, 581*f*
    effects of aging on, 225, 226*f*,
        227, 227*f*, 581
    observation of, 88, 88*f*
    prevention of inactivity effects
        on, 433–34*t*

Myasthenia gravis (MG), 610–11,
    610*g*
*Mycobacterium tuberculosis*, 158
Myocardial infarction (MI),
    527–28, 527*f*, 528*f*, 531, 531*f*
    acute 531–32
Myths. *See* Stereotypes and myths
Myxedema, 554

**N**
N95 respirator, 177*f*
Narcotic, in PCA pump, 659
Nasal catheter, 546, 547
Nasogastric tube feedings, 311–12
Native Americans
    health/illness belief systems of,
        212*f*
    personal space and, 234, 235*f*
Neglect, 102, 117
    residents' right to file
        complaints about, 115
*Neisseria gonorrheae*, 572
Nephron, 344, 345*f*, 346
Nerve cells, 78
Nerve impulses, 593
Nerves, 593–94, 594*f*
Nervous system, 593–94, 593*f*, 594*f*
    autonomic, 596
    central, 593, 594, 595*f*, 596, 596*f*
    effects of aging on, 225*f*, 598
    observation of, 88
    sense organs, 596–98, 597*f*, 598*f*
Nervous system disorders,
    591–613
    amyotrophic lateral sclerosis,
        609–10, 610*g*
    clinical focus and objectives,
        591
    hearing loss, 600–1
    Huntington's disease, 608–9, 609*g*
    multiple sclerosis, 607, 607*f*,
        608*g*
    Parkinson's disease, 603, 603*f*,
        604*g*
    signs and symptoms of, 602–3
    stroke, 604–7, 605*f*, 606*f*, 606*g*
    summary and review questions,
        611–13
    vision impairment, 598–600, 600*g*
Nervous tissue, 78
Networking, employment and, 677
Neurons, 593, 593*f*, 619
    seizures and, 637–38
Neurotransmitters, 593–94, 594*f*
    Alzheimer's disease and, 619
    Parkinson's disease and, 603
Nitroglycerin, 532

No-code orders, 108, 142, 142*f*
Nocturia, 346
Noise control, 237, 237*f*, 238*g*
Non-insulin-dependent diabetes
    mellitus (NIDDM), 556
Nonverbal communication, 48, 49
Non–weight bearing activity, 484
Nosocomial infections, 154, 158
Nourishments and supplements,
    309–10
Nurse Aide Competency
    Evaluation Program
    (NACEP), 10
Nurse practitioners, 21
Nurse's notes, 90, 90*f*
Nurses' station, 13, 13*f*, 14
Nursing assistant(s), 21, 24*f*,
    31–44
  admissions procedure
     responsibilities, 404–5
  assignments of, 38, 38*f*
  care plan responsibilities, 92, 94
  certification of, 10–11
  in chain of command, 50*f*
  characteristics and attitude of,
    32–33, 32*f*, 33*f*
  clinical focus and objectives, 31
  and communication, 48, 48*f*
  in community health care
    facilities, 4–5, 5–6*f*, 6–8, 8*f*
  diabetic care responsibilities,
    559
  dying process responsibilities,
    648
  hygiene of, 34, 34*f*
  in interdisciplinary health care
    team, 22*f*, 92, 93*f*, 94
  job description of, 35–36, 36–37*f*
  mealtime responsibilities, 304
  and organization of time, 40
  and physical therapy, 25
  restorative program
    responsibilities, 443–44*g*
  self-care and, 40–41, 41*f*
  sexual harassment and, 41–42
  specific duties of, 39–40, 39*f*
  staff development and, 42, 42*f*
  staff relations and, 37
  summary and review questions,
    42–44
  survey responsibilities, 671–72
  uniforms of, 34–35, 35*f*
Nursing diagnosis, 92, 93*f*
Nursing facility (NF), 8, 10
Nursing organizational chart, 49,
    50*f*
Nursing policy manual, 52

Nursing staff
  discharge planning, 414*f*, 415
  members of, 21
Nutrients, 290, 291, 292*f*, 293–94
Nutrition
  artificial, right to refuse, 101
  in cardiac care, 533
  infection prevention and, 163
Nutritional needs, 289–318
  aging and, 293, 293*f*
  assessment of, 21, 297, 303–4
  assistance with meeting, 105,
    105*f*
  basic nutrients and their
    function, 292*f*, 293–94
  clinical focus and objectives,
    289
  dietary practices and
    restrictions, 299, 300*f*, 301*f*
  digestive process and, 291–93,
    291*f*, 292*f*
  feeding assistance. *See* Feeding
  fluid intake/output and, 299,
    301–3, 302*f*, 303*f*
  food groups, 294–97, 295*f*
  food thickeners and, 305, 307
  nourishments and supplements
    for, 309–10
  summary and review questions,
    314–18
  types of diets for, 297–98, 297*f*,
    298*f*
  typical duties for, 37*f*
  water and, 310–11, 310*f*
Nystagmus, 607

# O

Obesity, 297, 604
Objective observations, 86, 86*f*
Observations, 86–90, 86*f*, 87*f*
  clinical focus and objectives, 85
  summary and review questions,
    95–96
Occupational exposure, 172
Occupational Safety and Health
    Administration (OSHA),
    125–26, 133
Occupational therapist, 25, 25*f*, 26
  discharge planning and, 414*f*,
    415
  in interdisciplinary health care
    team, 22*f*
Occupational therapy, 15–16, 484*f*
Odor control, 237, 238*g*
Oil glands, 252*f*, 253
Oil-retention enema, 328, 329
  procedure for, 330–31, 330*f*

Oliguria, 363
Ombudsman, 115, 668
Omnibus Budget Reconciliation
    Act (OBRA), 10, 28, 404
  in-service education
    requirements of, 680–81
  and reporting cases of abuse,
    116
  restorative care and, 431
Oncology
  subacute care unit and, 654
  treatments, 662
Open reduction/internal fixation
    (ORIF), 585
Ophthalmologist, 26, 599
Opposition, 447, 453, 453*f*
Optic nerve, 597, 597*f*
Optometrist, 22*f*, 26
Oral communications, 49–51
  *See also* Communication
Oral hygiene, 278–84
  brushing procedure, 279*f*, 280,
    280*f*
  denture care procedure, 278–80,
    282–83, 282*f*
  flossing procedure, 281–82, 281*f*
  special procedure for, 283–84,
    283*f*
Oral temperature, 371
  contraindications to, 372
  measurement procedures,
    373–75, 374*f*, 375*f*, 377–78,
    378*f*
  normal ranges of, 371*f*
Oral thermometer, 371, 372*f*, 374*f*
Orders and charting
    abbreviations, 72–73
Organ donation, religious beliefs
    and practices regarding, 649*f*
Organic mental syndrome, 618
Organizational chart
  administrative, 27*f*
  nursing, 49, 50*f*
Organs of body, 77, 78, 79*f*, 80*f*
Orthopedic bedpan, 322, 322*f*
Orthopedic injuries
  dislocations, 461
  fractures, 582–84, 582*f*, 583*f*,
    584*f*
  treatment for, 149–50
Orthopnea, 532
Orthopneic position
  for congestive heart failure,
    532
  for COPD, 546, 546*f*
Orthoses (orthotic devices), 25,
    25*f*, 460–61, 460*f*, 461*f*

Orthotist, 22*f*
OSHA, 125–26, 133
Osteoarthritis, 585–86, 586*f*
Osteoporosis, 582, 586*f*
  prevention of, 434*t*
Ostomies, 37*f*, 39, 338–42, 339*f*,
  340*f*, 341*f*
Ovaries, 78, 552, 553*f*, 554, 566,
  566*f*, 567*f*
Oviducts, 566*f*, 567*f*, 568
Ovulation, 568
Ovum, 566, 568
Oxygen, 540, 541, 541*f*
Oxygen mask, 546, 547, 547*f*
Oxygen safety, 128, 128*f*, 547
Oxygen therapy
  in cardiac care, 533
  for COPD, 546–48, 546*f*, 547*f*
  pulse oximetry and, 655, 655*f*
Oxygenated blood, 523

**P**
Pacemaker, 534–35, 535*f*
  as transfer belt
    contraindication, 487
Pacing and wandering,
    Alzheimer's disease and, 621,
    628
Pain, 86
  management of, 654, 657,
    659–60, 660*f*
  observations of, 89–90
Pancreas, 78, 291, 291*f*, 292*f*, 552,
    553*f*
Paralysis, 436
  motor nerves and, 594
  positioning and , 457, 471
Paraplegia, 436
  from multiple sclerosis, 607
  sliding board transfers for,
    499–500
Parathormone, 554
Parathyroid glands, 552, 553*f*,
    554
Parkinson's disease, 198, 198*f*,
    603, 603*f*, 618
  care guidelines for, 604*g*
  features and course of, 619*f*
  and gait, 500
  as reason for admission to LTC,
    402
Partial bath, 268–69
Partial weight bearing ability, 484
Passive range of motion
    exercises, 445
  *See also* Range of motion
    exercises

Pathogens, 154–55, 154*f*
  asepsis and, 168
  immunity and immunization
    and, 157
  transmission of, 155, 156, 156*f*
  urinary tract and, 347
Pathology, 75
Patient-care equipment, infection
    control and, 172*f*, 174*g*
Patient-controlled analgesia
    (PCA), 657, 659
Patient orders and charting
    abbreviations, 72–73
Patient transport, infection
    control and, 177, 177*f*, 178*f*,
    179
Patients
  definition of, 6
  health care services for, 5*f*
  *See also* Resident(s)
Pelvic cavity, 80*f*
Penis, 564, 565*f*
  bathing of, 272, 272*f*
  catheter care and, 349–50, 350*f*
  urinary drainage with condom
    over, 361, 362, 362*f*
Perceptual deficits, 436–37
Pericardium, 81
Perineal care, 269, 323
  for clean catch specimen
    collection, 361
  female, 270–71, 270*f*, 271*f*
  male, 271–73, 272*f*
  urinary incontinence and, 347
Perineum, 66, 566, 567*f*
Peripheral intravenous central
    catheter (PICC), 656, 656*f*
  gown changing procedure with,
    658–59, 659*f*
Peripheral nervous system (PNS),
    593
Peripheral vascular disease, 528,
    528*f*, 529, 529–30*g*, 557
Peritoneal cavity, 80*f*
Peritoneal dialysis, 654, 662
Peritoneum, 66, 81
Perseveration, 621
Personal funds, residents' right to
    manage, 114
Personal hygiene, 251–88
  assisting with, 104–5
  backrubs, 261–62, 262*f*
  bathing, general care and safety,
    261–63, 263*f*
  bed baths, 264–67, 264*f*, 265*f*, 266*f*
  in cardiac care, 533
  clinical focus and objectives, 251

  dressing, 284–86
  foot and toenail care, 277, 278
  guidelines for dementia
    residents, 626*g*
  hair care, 273, 273*f*, 274, 274*f*
  hand and fingernail care, 276–77
  infection control and, 163, 163*f*,
    169
  of nursing assistants, 34, 34*f*
  oral hygiene, 278–84, 279*f*, 280*f*,
    281*f*, 282*f*, 283*f*
  partial baths, 268–69
  perineal care, 269, 270–73, 270*f*,
    271*f*, 272*f*
  shaving, 274–76, 274*f*, 275*f*, 276*f*
  for skin, 253–56, 254*f*, 255*f*,
    256*f*, 257*g*, 258–61, 258*f*, 259*f*
  summary and review questions,
    286–88
  survey and, 670
  tub baths/showers, 267–68
  typical duties for, 37*f*
Personal inventory, 405, 406*f*,
    407
Personal possessions
  as part of personal space,
    234–35
  residents' right to, 116, 116*f*, 117
Personal protective equipment
    (PPE), 179
  and hazardous chemicals, 126
  infection control and, 172*f*,
    173*g*, 176
Personal space, 234–35, 235*f*
Personality, 209
  development of, 210*f*
  stroke and change in, 604,
    605
Perspiration
  effect of renal failure on, 363
  fluid output recording and, 354,
    354*f*, 355
  as sign of acute MI, 532
Pet therapy, 627
Petit mal seizure, 638
Phantom pain, 587
Pharmacist, 22*f*
Pharynx, 290, 291*f*, 540*f*, 541
Phlebitis, 528
Phlegm, 543, 545, 546
Phocomelia, 635*f*
Physical abuse, 57, 102
Physical condition
  assessment of, 94*f*
  observations and, 87
Physical needs, 104–5, 104*f*, 105*f*,
    208–9, 208*f*

Physical restraints, 102–3, 103*f*, 129*f*
  guidelines for use of, 131–33*g*
  resident safety and, 129–30, 130*f*
  right to freedom from, 102–3
  unauthorized use of, 117
Physical therapist, 22*f*, 25, 25*f*
  and ambulation, 500–1, 501*f*, 502*f*
  discharge planning and, 413, 414, 414*f*
  on interdisciplinary health care team, 22*f*
Physical therapy, 15, 640*f*
Physician, 21, 23*f*
Physician's offices, 4*f*, 7
Physician's orders
  for enemas, 330
  for restraints, 131*g*
  over telephone, 50, 51
Physiology, 75
Piggyback, 656, 656*f*
Pigmentation, skin, 254, 254*f*
Pillaging and hoarding, Alzheimer's disease and, 629
Pillows, 260
Pineal body, 552, 553*f*, 553
Pituitary gland, 552, 553*f*, 553
Plan of correction, after survey, 672
Plantar flexion, 454, 455*f*
Plaques, arterial, 527, 527*f*
Plasma, 526
Platelets, 526
Platform crutches, 502, 503*f*
Pleura, 81, 541
Pneumonia, 543
  as complication of HIV, 161
  and COPD, 545
  prevention of, 435*t*
  vaccine for, 157
Podiatrist, 23*f*, 26, 589
Points of attachment, 76, 77*f*
Poisoning
  prevention of, 133
  treatment for, 150
Policy book, 14, 14*f*, 35
Polio, 157
Polydipsia, 556, 556*f*
Polyphagia, 556, 556*f*
Polyuria, 556, 556*f*
Pores, 252*f*, 253
Position sense, loss of, 605
Positioning of resident, 457–61
  bridging, 472
  in chairs, 472–73, 472*f*, 475, 475*f*
  for congestive heart failure, 532

for COPD, 546, 546*f*
Fowler's position procedure, 470–71, 471*f*
guidelines for, 457–58*g*
with hip prosthesis, 587*f*, 588*f*
lateral procedures, 468–69, 469*f*
to prevent pressure ulcers, 257*g*, 258–59
purposes of, 457
semiprone procedure, 470, 470*f*
semisupine procedure, 468, 468*f*
special considerations for, 471, 472*f*
for stroke patients, 606*g*
supine procedure, 467, 467*f*
supportive equipment for, 458–61, 458*f*, 459*f*, 460*f*, 461*f*
survey and, 670, 671*f*
wheelchair procedures, 473–75, 474*f*, 475*f*, 511–13, 511*f*, 512*f*, 513*f*
Posterior body surface, 75, 76*f*, 77*f*
Postmortem care, 644, 650–51
Postmortem period, 644
Postoperative care, 655
Postural supports, 458–61, 458*f*, 459*f*, 460*f*, 461*f*
Posture, observation of, 88
Potentially infectious material, 172
Power of Attorney for Health Care, 108, 111–12*f*
Preadmission activities, 403
Prefixes, 67, 67*f*, 70
Presbycusis, 600–1
Presbyopia, 598
Pressure ulcers, 87*f*, 255–56, 256*f*, 258–59, 434*f*
  common sites for, 258*f*
  as complication of multiple sclerosis, 608*g*
  exercise and, 163
  infection control and, 178
  mechanical aids for protection from, 259–61, 259*f*, 260*f*, 261*f*
  positioning and, 472
  prevention of, 257*g*, 258–59, 434*t*
  restraints and, 130
  risk assessment, 92
Privacy, 215, 215*f*, 239*f*
  invasion of, 117
  personal care procedures for, 239*f*
  residents' right to, 103–4, 103*f*

Procedure book, 14, 35, 52, 52*f*
Procedures
  basic, 35–36
  for personal care of residents, 237–38, 239–40*f*
Progesterone, 554, 566
Progress notes, 90, 90*f*
Progressive diet, 299
Progressive mobilization, 445
  continuing with, 477
  independent bed movement and, 476
Projection, 217
Prolapsed uterus, 571
Pronation, 447, 451, 451*f*
Prone position, 457
Prostate gland, 345–46, 345*f*, 564, 565*f*, 566
  enlargement of, 571
  urinary obstruction and, 347
Prostheses, 15, 105
  hip, 586–87, 586*f*, 587*f*
  lower extremity, 587
Prosthetist, 23*f*
Proteins, 294
  enzymatic breakdown of, 291, 292*f*, 293
  food groups containing, 296
  functions of, 292*f*
Protestantism, 213*f*
Protozoa, 155
Protozoan infections, 155, 162
Protraction, lateral positioning and, 468–69
Proximal anatomic location, 76, 77*f*
Pruritis, 571
*Pseudomonas aeruginosa*, 158
Psychosocial aspects of aging. *See* Aging process
Psychosocial needs, 105–6, 106*f*, 208, 208*f*, 209, 209*f*
  assisting residents in fulfilling, 217–18
  reactive behaviors and, 218–20
Psychosocial reactions, inactivity and, 436*t*
Puberty, 568
Pubic area, bathing of, 266
  *See also* Perineal care
Pulmonary artery and veins, 521, 522*f*
Pulse, 381
  measurement of, 381–84, 382*f*, 383*f*, 384*f*
  observation and, 88
Pulse deficit, 382

Pulse oximetry, 655, 655*f*
Pulse points, 146, 146*f*, 382*f*
Pulse rate, 370
  average, 383, 383*f*
  heart rate and, 382
Pupil, 597, 597*f*
Pureed diet, 298, 298*f*

**Q**
Quadrants, abdominal, 76–77, 77*f*
Quadriplegia, 436
  in cerebral palsy, 637
  multiple sclerosis and, 607
Quality assurance manual, 52
Quality assurance program, 28
Quality of life
  in facility survey, 670
  residents' rights and, 100

**R**
RACE steps, 136, 136*f*
Radial artery, 381
Radial deviation, 447, 451, 452*f*
Radial pulse, 381, 382*f*
  blood pressure measurement
    and, 389, 390*f*
  procedure for counting, 382–83,
    383*f*
Radiation therapy, 157, 662
Rales, 384*f*
Range of motion exercises,
  445–56
  ankle and toes procedure,
    454–56, 455*f*, 456*f*
  elbow and wrist procedure,
    450–51, 450*f*, 451*f*
  fingers and thumb procedure,
    452–53, 452*f*, 453*f*
  guidelines for, 445–46*g*
  hip and knee procedure,
    453–54, 453*f*, 454*f*
  joint movement terminology,
    446–47, 446*f*, 447*f*
  shoulder procedure, 449–50,
    448*f*, 449*f*, 450*f*
  surveyors and, 671*f*
Rapport, in grief and adjustment
  period, 216, 216*f*
Rash, 86*f*
Rationalization, 217
Reaching aids, 135
Reality orientation (RO), 629–30
Receptors, skin, 252, 252*f*
Records, at nurses' station, 14
Recreational activities, for
  dementia residents, 627, 627*f*
Rectal suppositories, 336–37, 337*f*

Rectal temperature, 371
  contraindications to, 372–73
  measurement procedures,
    375–76, 376*f*, 378–79, 378*f*
  normal ranges of, 371*f*
Rectal thermometer, 371, 372*f*,
  376*f*
Rectal tube and flatus bag, 337,
  338, 338*f*
Rectoceles, 363, 571
Rectum, 565*f*
References, employment, 677, 678
Reflexes
  gag, 292, 293, 293*f*
  mechanics of, 594
Registered nurse (RN), 21, 94*f*
  discharge planning and, 410
  on interdisciplinary health care
    team, 23*f*
Regularity, fiber and, 294
Regurgitation, for esophageal
  speech, 542
Rehabilitation
  areas for, 15–16
  differences from restorative
    care, 432
  facilities for, 4*f*, 7
  in nursing facility, 9–10, 9*f*
  as reason for admission to LTC,
    402
  subacute care unit and, 654
  typical duties for, 37*f*
Rehabilitation aides, 23*f*, 25
Rehabilitation nurse, 21, 413, 414,
  414*f*
Rehabilitation staff, 410
Religion, 212–13, 213*f*
  activities related to, 114, 114*f*
  death and dying beliefs and
    practices, 647–48, 647*f*, 649*f*
  dietary practices, 300*f*
Reminiscing, 630, 630*f*
Renal calculi, 363
Renal failure, 363
Reporting
  clinical focus and objectives, 85
  of observations, 89*f*, 90
  of resident care procedures, 240*f*
  summary and review questions,
    95–96
  *See also* Documentation
Reprisal, 108
Reproductive disorders, 563–75
  benign prostatic hypertrophy, 571
  breast self-examination
    procedure, 569–70, 570*f*
  clinical focus and objectives, 563

  malignancies, 569
  prolapsed uterus, 571
  rectoceles and cystoceles, 571
  STDs, 571–73
  summary and review questions,
    574–75
  vaginitis and pruritis, 571
Reproductive system, 78, 79*f*
  effects of aging on, 226*f*, 568–69
  female, 566, 566*f*, 567*f*, 568
  male, 564–66, 565*f*
  observation of, 88–89
Resident care plan, 92, 93*f*, 94
  *See also* Care plan
Resident councils, 113
Resident profile, 14
Resident unit(s), 11–13, 235
  infection control and, 170
  isolation preparation of, 179
  preparation for new admission,
    403–4
  privacy in, 103–4, 103*f*
  spousal sharing rights in, 115
Residential care facilities, 4*f*
Resident(s), 197–206
  clinical focus and objectives,
    197
  definition of, 8
  health care services for, 5*f*
  in interdisciplinary health care
    team, 23*f*
  summary and review questions,
    204–6
  women, 199, 200
  younger, 203, 203*f*, 204*g*
Residents' rights, 99–120
  to accommodation of needs,
    104–6, 104*f*, 105*f*, 106*f*
  clinical focus and objectives, 99
  dementia and, 625, 625*f*
  of environmental needs, 106–7,
    106*f*, 107*f*
  ethics and, 117
  to file complaints about abuse,
    neglect, or misappropriation
    of property, 115
  of free choice, 101–2
  of freedom from abuse and
    restraints, 102–3
  to immediate and unlimited
    access to family/relatives,
    115
  to information about advocacy
    groups, 115
  to information about
    Medicare/Medicaid benefits,
    99

to inspect facility surveys and records, 114

legal aspects of health care and, 116–17

to make advance directives, 107–8

to manage personal funds, 114

to notification of change in condition, 116

to organize and participate in family and resident groups, 113

to participate in social, religious, and community activities, 113–14, 114*f*

to perform or not perform work for the facility, 115

of personal/clinical record confidentiality, 104

of privacy, 103–4, 103*f*

to refuse food and/or medication, 108

to remain in facility, 115–16

of resuscitative orders and/or hospitalization, 108

to share room with spouse, 115

typical duties for protecting, 36*f*

to use personal possessions, 116, 116*f*

to voice grievances, 108, 113, 113*f*

Residents' Rights document, 403

legal foundation of, 116–17

purpose of, 100–1

restorative care and, 431

Residual limb, positioning considerations for, 471, 472*f*

Resignation, letter of, 681

Respiration, 381

checking of in emergency response, 140*g*

factors affecting, 385*f*

measurement of, 384–85

observation of, 88

rate of, 370

Respiratory arrest, 141

Respiratory disorders, 539–51

clinical focus and objectives, 539

COPD, 545–48

Fowler's position for, 471

infections, 543

malignancies, 542

sputum specimen collection for, 543–44, 544*g*

summary and review questions, 549–50

Respiratory system, 79*f*, 540–41, 540*f*, 541*f*

effects of aging on, 226*f*, 542, 542*f*

observation of, 88

prevention of inactivity effects on, 435*t*

Respiratory therapist, 23*f*

Rest home, 8

Restoration. *See* Rehabilitation

Restorative care, 429–82

adaptive devices for, 440–42*f*

ADL and, 436–37

bowel and bladder programs for, 477–78, 478–80*g*

clinical focus and objectives, 429–30

dependent resident positioning in, 467–75, 468*f*, 469*f*, 470*f*, 471*f*, 472*f*, 474*f*, 475*f*

environment of, 444–45, 444*f*

independent bed movement and, 476–77

interdisciplinary health care team and, 431–32, 431*f*

mobility restoration. *See* Mobility restoration

positioning of resident and, 457–61, 457–58*g*, 458*f*, 459*f*, 460*f*, 461*f*

prevention of inactivity complications in, 433, 433–36*t*

program setup for, 437–40, 438*t*, 439*f*

progressive mobilization in, 445, 477

purposes of, 432–33, 432*f*

range of motion exercises, 445–47, 456

range of motion exercises, guidelines for, 445–46*g*

range of motion exercises, procedures for, 448–56

responsibility guidelines, 443–44*g*

turning and moving resident procedures, 461–66, 462*f*, 464*f*, 465*f*, 466*f*

Restraints, 129*f*

guidelines for use of, 131–33*g*

resident safety and, 129–30, 130*f*

right to freedom from, 102–3

unauthorized use of, 117

Résumés, 677–78

Resuscitation, 646

residents' right and, 108

Retention, urinary, 346, 347

Retina, 597, 597*f*

Retraction, 469

Retroperitoneal space, 80*f*

Rheumatoid arthritis, 586*f*, 587, 588*f*

Rhythm, pulse, 381

Rigor mortis, 648, 650, 650*f*

Ringworm, 155

Roman Catholics, 213*f*

death and dying beliefs and practices, 647, 647*f*, 649*f*

dietary practices, 300*f*

Rooms. *See* Resident unit(s)

Rotation, 447, 447*f*

Rubella, 157

Ruptures, 312–13

**S**

Sacrament of the Sick, 647, 647*f*, 649*f*

Safety, 121–38

assessment of resident, 92

bathing and, 263, 263*f*

choking prevention, 134

cleanliness and order of rooms and, 236, 238*g*

clinical focus and objectives, 121

for employees, 122, 123*g*, 124*f*, 125*f*

environmental maintenance and, 238*g*

fire, 135–36, 135*f*, 136*f*

injury and falling prevention, 133–34

lighting and, 236

personal care procedures for, 239*f*, 240*f*

physical restraints for, 129–30, 129*f*, 130*f*, 131–33*g*

poisoning prevention, 133

precautions for thermometer use, 372–73

residents' need for, 208, 208*f*, 209

risk factors and, 129

summary and review questions, 136–38

surveys and, 670

during toileting, 323

typical duties for, 36*f*

for using assistive devices, 501–2

when using oxygen, 128, 128*f*, 547

with warm and cold applications, 418, 419, 419*f*, 421

wheelchair, 134–35, 507

work environment hazards and, 125–26, 128, 128*f*

Safety devices. *See* Restraints
Salivary glands, 291, 291*f*, 292*f*
Salmonella, 158
Salt, in diet, 296
Scabies
    infection control and, 178
    outbreaks of, 164
Scales, 391, 391*f*, 392*f*
    chair, 395
    upright, 392–94, 393*f*, 394*f*
    wheelchair, 394–95, 395*f*
Scarlet fever, 154*f*
Sclera, 597, 597*f*
Scrotum, 554, 565, 565*f*
Second-degree burns, 149
Security devices, for wandering
        residents, 130, 130*f*
Security thermometer, 371, 372*f*
Seizures, 148, 148*f*, 637–39, 639*f*
    causes of, 638*f*
    emergency treatment for, 148–49
Self-appraisal, in job application
        process, 676, 676*f*
Self-care
    with diabetes, 558
    and infection prevention and,
        156, 163
    for nursing assistants, 40–41
Self-care deficits, 199, 436
    evaluation of, 437–39
Self-Determination Act, 107–8
Self-esteem, 213
    defense mechanisms and, 217
    promotion of, 218
Self range of motion exercises,
        445, 456, 456*f*
Self-stimulation, 214, 214*f*
Seminal vesicles, 564, 565, 565*f*
Semiprone positioning procedure,
        470, 470*f*
Semisupine positioning
        procedure, 468, 468*f*
Senescent changes, 224–25,
        225–26*f*, 227–28
Senile lentigines, 254, 254*f*
Senility, 618
    *See also* Alzheimer's disease
Senses
    effects of aging on, 226*f*, 227–28
    observations and, 86, 88
    organs of, 596–598, 597*f*, 598*f*
Sensitivity, 32, 32*f*
Sensors, for wandering residents,
        130, 130*f*
Sensory deprivation, prevention
        of, 436*t*
Sensory nerves, 593

Sensory-perceptual changes
    seizures and, 148
    as stage of Alzheimer's disease,
        621, 621*f*
    from stroke, 605
Sensory stimulation
    positioning and, 457
    for prevention of inactivity
        effects, 436*t*
Sepsis, 347
Septicemia, 347
Seroposivity, HIV and, 161, 162
Serous membranes, 81
Serum, 526
Seventh-Day Adventists, dietary
        practices, 300*f*
Sexual abuse, 215
    definition of, 102
    STDs as indication of, 572
Sexual harassment, 41–42
Sexual intercourse, 57, 214, 564
    aging and, 228
Sexuality, 213–15, 215*f*, 216*f*, 564
    myths regarding elderly, 202
    reproductive disorders and, 569
    residents' rights and, 106
    younger residents and, 204*g*
Sexually transmitted diseases
        (STDs), 571–73
Sharps
    disposal of, 173*g*
    infection control and, 172*f*
    safety and, 126, 128*f*, 133
Shaving, 274, 274*f*, 275–76, 275*f*,
        276*f*
Shearing
    Fowler's position and, 471
    positioning and, 457
    and skin breakdown, 255, 255*f*
Sheath, thermometer, 373, 373*f*,
        378*f*
Sheepskin pads, 259, 259*f*
Shift report, 49–50, 50*f*
Shingles, 154, 159
Shoulder exercises, 448–50, 448*f*,
        449*f*, 450*f*
Side rails
    prevention of falls and, 134
    seizures and, 148*f*
Sign language, 58, 59*f*
Signal cords, 13, 13*f*, 126
Signs and symptoms of disease,
        86–87, 86*f*, 87*f*
Sitz bath, 418*f*
Skeletal muscles, 78, 79*f*, 578–79,
        580*f*
Skeletal traction, 583, 583*f*

Skilled nursing facility (SNF), 8,
        9–10, 9*f*
    subacute care units in. *See*
        Subacute care units
Skin, 79*f*, 81, 252
    burns, 149
    cancer, 254
    cross section of, 252*f*
    depression and, 219
    effects of aging on, 225*f*,
        253–54, 253*f*, 254*f*
    functions of, 253
    infection control and, 168
    injury prevention, 133
    layers of, 252–53, 252*f*
    lesions, 254–56, 254*f*, 256*f*,
        258–61
    mechanical aids for protection
        of, 259–61, 259*f*, 260*f*, 261*f*
    mottling of, 648
    observation of, 88
    pressure ulcers, 255–56, 256*f*,
        258–59
Skin breakdown, 254–55, 254*f*,
        255*f*
    common sites for, 258*f*
    Fowler's position and, 471
    incontinence and, 477, 478
    perineal care and, 269
    prevention guidelines for, 257*g*
    prolonged urine exposure and,
        347
Skin tears, 255
Skin traction, 583, 583*f*
Slander, 117
Sliding board transfers, 499–500,
        499*f*, 499*g*
Slings, 461, 461*f*
Small intestine, 291, 291*f*, 292–93,
        292*f*
Smoking
    of nursing assistants, 34
    supervision of, 133
Smooth muscles, 78, 79*f*, 578
Soapsuds enema, 328, 329, 330
    procedure for, 331–34, 331*f*,
        332*f*, 333*f*
Social activities, 113
    residents' right to participate in,
        113–14
    younger resident and, 204*g*
Social services, 21, 24*f*
    in chain of command, 27*f*
    preadmission activities and, 403
Social worker
    and communication, 49*f*
    discharge planning and, 410, 412

on interdisciplinary health care team, 23*f*
responsibilities of, 21
Sodium-restricted diet, 298, 298*f*
Spastic cerebral palsy, 637
Spasticity, 457
  as complication of multiple sclerosis, 608*g*
  footboards and, 459
Spatial-perceptual deficits, 605
Special procedures, 37, 39, 39*f*
Specimen collection
  from resident in isolation unit, 187–88, 188*f*
  stool, 343–44, 344*f*
  urine, 353, 353*f*, 358–61, 359*f*, 360*f*
Speech-language pathologist, 23*f*, 26
Speech therapy, 16
Sperm, 565
Sphincter muscle
  bladder, 345, 347
  rectal, 336, 337*f*
Sphygmomanometer, 370, 371, 389, 390*f*, 391*f*
  guidelines for using, 387*g*, 388*g*
  types of, 386*f*
Spinal cavity, 80*f*
Spinal cord, 594, 595*f*
Spinal injury, logrolling procedure for, 465–66, 466*f*
Spirituality, 210, 212*f*
  *See also* Religion
Splints, 25, 460–61, 460*f*
Spousal right to share room, 115
Sprain, 149, 150
Sputum, 543
  culture for tuberculosis, 159
  specimen collection, 543–44, 544*f*
Square corner in bedmaking, 244, 245, 245*f*, 246, 248
Staff
  communication among, 49
  nursing, 21, 24*f*, 50*f*
  relations, 37
Staff development, 28, 42, 42*f*
Standard diets, 297–98, 297*f*, 298*f*
Standard precautions, 172, 172*f*, 176
  bathroom equipment and, 322
  guidelines for, 173*g*
  isolation precautions with, 176.
    *See also* Isolation procedures
  personal care procedures for, 239*f*, 240*f*
  with respiratory infections, 543

Standards and regulations, for health care facilities, 10–11
Staphylococci, 158, 158*f*
Status epilepticus, 638
STDs. *See* Sexually transmitted diseases
Stereotypes and myths about elderly, 200–3, 201*f*, 202*f*
Sterile procedures, 191–92, 192*f*
Sterilization, 190–91, 191*f*
Stethoscope, 371, 387*f*, 390*f*
  guidelines for using, 387*g*, 388*g*
Stoma, 338, 339–41, 339*f*, 340*f*, 341*f*
Stomach, 291, 291*f*, 292, 292*f*
Stool, 290, 291, 321, 327
  characteristics, in relation to colostomy site, 339*f*
  constipation and, 312
  enemas and, 329
  specimen collection, 343–44, 344*f*
Strain, muscle, 149, 150
Strengths of resident, and restorative care, 433
Strep throat, 154*f*, 154
Streptococcus A, 158
Stress
  reactions of residents, 218
  reduction, for nursing assistants, 41, 41*f*
Stroke, 527, 528*f*, 604–7
  care guidelines for, 606*g*
  as complication of diabetes, 557
  and gait, 500
  transient ischemic attack and, 529
Subacute care units, 4, 4*f*, 8, 199, 653–64
  clinical focus and objectives, 653
  definition of, 654
  dialysis in, 661–62, 661*f*
  intravenous therapy in, 656–57, 656*f*, 657*f*, 658–59, 658*g*
  oncology treatment in, 662
  pain management in, 657, 659–60, 660*f*
  pulse oximetry in, 655, 655*f*
  special procedures and, 655
  summary and review questions, 663–64
  tracheostomy care, 660–61, 660*f*
  types of care provided in, 654–55
Subcutaneous tissue, 252, 252*f*
  burns and, 149
  skin breakdown and, 256, 256*f*

Subjective observations, 86–87, 87*f*, 90
Subluxation, 461
Suffixes, 67, 67*f*, 70–71
Sugars, dietary, 296
Suicide, indications of possibility of, 219
Sundowning, 621, 628–29, 629*f*
Superior body part division, 75, 76*f*
Superior vena cava, 521, 522*f*, 523, 523*f*
Supervising nurse, 21, 27
  assignments and, 38, 38*f*
  communication with, 49–50
Supination, 447, 451, 451*f*
Supine position, 457
Supplements, nutritional, 309–10
Support services, 26, 26*f*, 39–40, 39*f*
Supportive activities, 113–14
Supportive equipment, for positioning resident, 458–61, 458*f*, 459*f*, 460*f*, 461*f*
Suppositories, 328, 336–37, 337*f*
Suppression defense mechanism, 217
Surgical asepsis, 191
Surrogates, 109–10*f*, 111–12*f*
Survey of facility, 11, 667–73
  clinical focus and objectives, 667
  completion of, 672
  preparation for, 668–69, 669*f*
  process of, 669–70, 669*f*
  purpose of, 668
  residents' right to examine, 114
  responsibilities during, 671–72, 672*f*
  summary and review questions, 672–73
Surveyors, 668
Sweat glands, 252*f*, 253
Symbols, communication and, 48
Symptoms of disease, 86–87
Syncope, 150
  as sign of acute MI, 532
Synovial membranes, 81
Syphilis, 572, 619*f*
Systems, body, 77, 78, 79*f*
  *See also specific body systems*
Systole, 522
Systolic pressure, 387, 390, 391

**T**
T cells, HIV and, 161
Tachycardia, 383

Tachypnea, 384*f*, 543

Talismans, 212

Tap water enema (TWE), 330

Task segmentation, ADL, 438, 438*t*

TED hose, 532, 533–34, 533*f*, 534*f*

Telephone etiquette, 50–51, 51*f*

Temperature, 370
  abbreviations, 74
  axillary measurement
    procedure, 376–77, 377*f*, 379
  as defense against disease, 157
  of facility, 236, 238*g*
  observation of, 88
  oral measurement procedure,
    373–75, 374*f*, 375*f*, 377–78,
    378*f*
  rectal measurement procedure,
    375–76, 376*f*, 378–79, 378*f*
  thermometers for measuring,
    371–73, 372*f*, 373*f*
  tympanic measurement
    procedure, 380–81, 380*f*, 381*f*
  variations in related to method
    of measurement, 371*f*

Tendons, 579

Terminal condition/illness, 199
  grieving process and, 646–47,
    646*f*
  hospice care for, 4, 4*f*, 5, 6*f*
  Living Will and, 108
  reactions to diagnosis of,
    644–45, 645*f*
  religious beliefs and practices
    and, 647–48, 647*f*, 649*f*
  resuscitation and, 646
  and right to refuse food, 108
  in skilled nursing facility, 9
  subacute care units and, 654

Terminology, 65–83
  anatomic, 75–77, 75*f*, 76*f*, 77*f*
  of body structure and function,
    77–78, 78–80*f*, 81
  clinical focus and objectives, 65
  combining word forms in, 67*f*,
    68–70
  common abbreviations in, 71–74
  expansion of vocabulary for,
    67–68, 67*f*
  prefixes and suffixes, 67*f*, 70–71
  word parts, 66–67, 67*f*

Testes (testicles), 552, 553*f*, 554,
  564, 565, 565*f*

Testosterone, 554, 565

Test(s)
  abbreviations, 73–74
  for Alzheimer's disease, 618
  blood sugar, 559

culture and sensitivity, 158
  for level of mental retardation,
    636–37
  for tuberculosis, 159

Tetanus, 157

Theft, 117

Therapeutic bath, 263, 263*f*

Therapeutic diets, 21, 298–99, 298*f*

Therapeutic recreational
  specialist, 23*f*, 26

Thermal blanket, 421, 423–24

Thermal injury prevention, 133

Thermometers, 371–73, 372*f*, 373*f*,
  379

Third-degree burns, 149

Thoracic cavity, 80*f*

Thorax, 541

Thrombocytes, 526

Thrombophlebitis, 528

Thrombus
  prevention of, 435*t*
  stroke from, 604

Thrush, 155, 155*f*

Thumb exercises, 453, 453*f*

Thymus, 553*f*

Thyrocalcitonin, 552, 554

Thyroid gland, 552, 553*f*, 554

Thyroxine, 552, 554

Tilt positioning procedure, 468,
  468*f*

Time
  abbreviations, 74
  on medical chart, 91–92, 91*f*
  organization of, 40

Tissue breakdown
  signs of, 255–56, 256*f*
  *See also* Skin breakdown

Tissues, 77, 78

Toe exercises, 455–56, 455*f*, 456*f*

Toilet equipment, 321–22, 322*f*
  odor control and, 237, 238*g*
  seats, 105, 321, 322*f*

Toileting
  assistance procedures for, 105,
    326–27
  guidelines for dementia
    residents, 626*g*
  task segmentation for, 438*t*
  transfer procedures to and from
    wheelchair, 492–94, 493*f*

Tongue-jaw lift method for airway
  obstruction, 144, 144*f*

Toothbrushing and flossing, 278,
  279*f*, 280–82, 280*f*, 281*f*

Total care, 21

Total parenteral nutrition (TPN),
  311, 312, 656–57

Touch
  communication through, 57–58,
    57*f*
  in restorative care, 444*f*
  sexuality and, 215

TPN. *See* Total parenteral
  nutrition

Trachea, 540*f*, 541, 541*f*

Tracheostomy, 542, 548
  care of, 654, 660–61, 660*f*
  intubation through, 548

Trachoma, 573

Traction, 583, 583*f*

Transcutaneous electrical nerve
  stimulation (TENS), 660,
  660*f*

Transfer belt, 123*g*, 485
  contraindications to, 487
  prevention of falls and, 134
  procedure using, 485–87, 486*f*

Transfer procedures,
  sitting/standing, 484–500
  assisted standing, 489–90, 490*f*,
    491–92, 492*f*
  chair to bed, 490–91, 491*f*
  gait belt, 485–87, 86*f*
  guidelines for, 485*g*
  lying to sitting position, 487–88,
    488*f*
  mechanical lift, 496–98, 497*f*,
    498*f*
  sliding board, 499–500, 499*g*
  types of, 485, 487
  wheelchair to bed, 495–96
  wheelchair to toilet and toilet to
    wheelchair, 492–94, 493*f*
  wheelchair to tub/shower chair,
    494–95, 495*f*

Transfer within/outside facility,
  407–8, 407*f*, 409*f*
  clinical focus and objectives,
    401
  form for, 408–9*f*
  to and from isolation unit,
    189–90, 190*f*
  procedure for, 410
  summary and review questions,
    415–16

Transient ischemic attack (TIA),
  527, 528–29, 604

Transitional care, 654
  *See also* Subacute care units

Transmission of infection, 155,
  156*f*

Transmission precautions, 176–79,
  177*f*, 178*f*, 543
  *See also* Isolation procedures

Transurethral prostatectomy (TURP), 571
Trauma, 198
  as admission reason for younger residents, 203, 203*f*
Tremors, Parkinsonian, 603
*Treponema pallidum*, 572
*Trichomonas vaginalis*, 572
Trichomonas vaginitis, 572
Trochanter roll, 458–59, 459*f*, 467, 467*f*
Tub bath/shower, 267–68
Tube feedings, 311–12, 311*f*, 312*f*
  advance directives and, 108
Tubercle, 159
Tuberculosis, 158–59
  as complication of HIV, 161
  and COPD, 545
  infection control and, 176, 177*f*
  outbreaks of, 164
Tuberculosis disease, 159
Tuberculosis infection, 159
Tumors
  breast, 569
  urinary obstruction and, 347
Turning schedule, 257*g*
Turning sheet, 457, 461
  moving procedures with, 462–63, 462*f*
  turning procedures with, 464–66, 464*f*, 465*f*, 466*f*
  for wheelchair positioning, 474, 511, 511*f*
Tympanic temperature, 371, 380–81, 380*f*, 381*f*
Tympanic thermometer, 373, 373*f*, 379

**U**
Ulnar deviation, 447, 451, 451*f*
Umbilicus, 77, 77*f*
Uniforms, 34–35, 35*f*
Unilateral neglect, 605
Unit secretary, 21, 23*f*
Universal distress sign, 142, 142*f*
Upright scale, 391, 391*f*
  accurate reading of, 392–93, 393*f*
  measurement procedure with, 393–94, 394*f*
Uremia, 363
Uremic frost, 363
Ureters, 344, 345*f*, 567*f*
Urethra, 345–46, 345*f*, 564, 565*f*, 567*f*
Uric acid, 363
Urinals, 325, 325*f*

Urinalysis, 346
Urinary catheter drainage, 347–52, 348*f*
  catheter care procedure, 349–50, 350*f*
  connection procedure, 357–58
  disconnection procedure, 351–52, 352*f*
  emptying procedures, 355–56, 355*f*, 356*f*, 357
  with leg bag, 356, 356*f*, 357–58, 358*f*
  routine checking procedure for, 348–49, 349*f*
Urinary system, 79*f*, 344–46, 345*f*
  effects of aging on, 226*f*, 227, 346, 346*f*
  observation of, 88, 89*f*
  prevention of inactivity effects on, 435*t*
Urinary tract infections, 158, 162, 347, 477, 478
Urination, 347
  conditions affecting, 363, 363*f*
  through condom catheter, 361, 362, 362*f*
  fluid intake/output and, 352
  indwelling catheters for, 347–52, 348*f*, 350*f*, 352*f*
  observation of, 88
  output measurement procedures, 353–56, 353*f*, 354*f*, 355*f*, 356*f*
  retention and incontinence and, 347
Urine specimen collection
  clean-catch procedure, 360–61
  for measuring fluid output, 353, 353*f*
  routine procedure, 359–60, 359*f*, 360*f*
Uterine tubes, 566*f*, 567*f*, 568
Uterus, 566*f*, 567*f*, 568
  prolapsed, 571

**V**
Vaccines, 157, 160
Vagina, 566*f*, 567*f*, 568
Vaginitis, 155, 571, 572
Validation therapy, 630–31
Valley fever, 162
Value system, 203
Valves, heart, 521–22
Vancomycin-resistant enterococci (VRE), 158
Varicose veins, 528, 529*f*
Vas deferens, 564, 565, 565*f*

Vascular disease, peripheral, 528, 528*f*, 529, 529–30*g*, 557
Vasoconstriction, 421
Vasodilation, 419
Vasodilators, 532
Veins, 522, 523, 525*f*, 529*f*
Venereal warts, 573
Ventilation
  in facility, 236, 238*g*
  respiratory, 541
Ventilator weaning, 654
Ventral body surface, 75, 76*f*, 77*f*
Ventral cavity, 80*f*, 81
Ventricles, 521, 522*f*, 523*f*
Venules, 523
Verbal abuse, 102
Verbal communication
  with residents, 48–49
  with staff, 49–51
  *See also* Communication
Vertigo, 607
Viral infections, 159–62, 160*f*, 161*f*, 543
Viruses, 154
Vision
  effects of aging on, 226*f*, 227
  mechanics of, 597
Vision impairment
  and accidents, 129
  assistance guidelines for, 600*g*
  causes of, 598–600
  and communication, 58–60, 59*f*
  diabetes and, 557
  HIV and, 161
Vital signs, measurement and recording of, 369–91, 396–99
  apical pulse, 382–84, 384*f*
  axillary temperature, 376–77, 377*f*, 379
  blood pressure, 385–87, 385*f*, 386*f*, 387*f*, 387–88*g*, 389–91, 389*f*, 390*f*
  in cardiac care, 533
  clinical focus and objectives, 369
  equipment for, 371
  in isolation unit, 185–86
  oral temperature, 373–75, 374*f*, 375*f*, 377–78, 378*f*
  radial pulse, 381, 382–83, 382*f*, 383*f*
  rectal temperature, 375–76, 376*f*, 378–79, 378*f*
  respiration, 384–85, 384*f*, 385*f*
  sample form for, 397*f*
  summary and review questions, 398–99

Vital signs, measurement and
recording of—*cont'd*
thermometers for, 371–73, 371*f*,
372*f*, 373*f*, 379
tympanic temperature, 380–81,
380*f*, 381*f*
Vitamins, 294
food groups containing, 294–96
functions of, 292*f*
Vocal cords, 541
Voice production, 541
after laryngectomies, 542
Voiding, 347
Volume, pulse, 381
Volunteers, 23*f*
Vomiting
aspiration during, 143, 147
fluid output recording and, 354,
354*f*
Vulva, 566
bathing of, 270, 270*f*
Vulvovaginitis, 571

**W**
Walkers, 15, 25
ambulation procedure with,
505, 506
assisting residents with, 105
use of, 502
Walking. *See* Ambulation
Wandering, Alzheimer's disease
and, 621, 628
Warm applications, 418*f*, 419–21
Aquamatic K-pad® application
procedure, 420, 420*f*

clinical focus and objectives,
417
safety when using, 418, 419*f*
summary and review questions,
425–26
Warm soaks, 418*f*, 419
Water, 310–11
functions of, 292*f*
nutrition and, 304
Water temperature, thermal
injuries and, 133
Weight bearing activity, 484
Weight measurement and
recording, 391–96
abbreviations, 74
accuracy in, 392–93, 393*f*
chair scale procedure, 395
electronic wheelchair scale
procedure, 394–95, 395*f*
equipment for, 391, 391*f*, 392*f*
in-bed procedure for, 396
upright scale procedure, 393–94
Wet compresses
cold, 425
warm, 418*f*, 421
Wheelchair pushups, 474–75, 475*f*,
513, 513*f*
Wheelchair scale, 394–95, 395*f*
Wheelchair(s)
activities to relieve pressure in,
474–75, 475*f*, 513, 513*f*
catheter drainage bag and,
351
positioning in, 472, 511–13, 511*f*,
512*f*, 513*f*

repositioning procedure,
473–74, 474*f*
restraints for, 131*f*
special maneuvers with, 507–10,
508*f*, 509*f*, 510*f*, 511*f*
transfer to bed procedure,
495–96
transfer to toilet procedure,
492–93, 493*f*
transfer to tub/shower chair
procedure, 494–95, 495*f*
use and safety of, 134–35,
506–7, 507*f*
Wheezing, 384*f*
Whirlpool bath, 263, 263*f*
White blood cells, 67, 526
HIV and, 161
and infectious disease, 156
Whooping cough, 157
Women residents, 199, 275
Word parts, 66–67, 67*f*
combining forms, 68–70
prefixes and suffixes, 70–71
Word roots, 67, 67*f*
Work, residents' right to, 115
Work environment, hazards in,
125–26, 128, 128*f*
Work practice controls, 176
Wound management, 654–55
Wrist exercises, 451, 451*f*
Written communications, 52, 52*f*,
53*f*, 54, 54*f*

**Y**
Younger residents, 203, 203*f*, 204*g*